# Children With Complex Medical Issues in Schools

**Christine L. Castillo, PhD, LSSP,** is a licensed psychologist in the Neuropsychology Service, in the Department of Psychiatry, at Children's Medical Center Dallas, and is an Assistant Professor in the Department of Psychiatry at the University of Texas Southwestern Medical Center at Dallas. She holds the National Certification in School Psychology and is a Licensed Specialist in School Psychology. Dr. Castillo is coauthor of numerous book chapters and peer-reviewed articles and presents nationally to school districts and state school psychology associations on the topics of emotional disturbance, social maladjustment, and executive functioning. She is actively involved in grant-funded research investigating the neuropsychological sequelae of antiepileptic medication and the efficacy of nonpsychopharmacologic treatment for children with Attention Deficit Hyperactivity Disorder. Dr. Castillo's primary clinical interest includes facilitating successful school experiences for children with a variety of chronic and acute medical disorders, including those with epilepsy, neurofibromatosis, central nervous system cancers, meningitis/encephalitis, brain tumors, and traumatic brain injuries.

# Children With Complex Medical Issues in Schools

*Neuropsychological Descriptions and Interventions*

Christine L. Castillo, PhD, LSSP
*Editor*

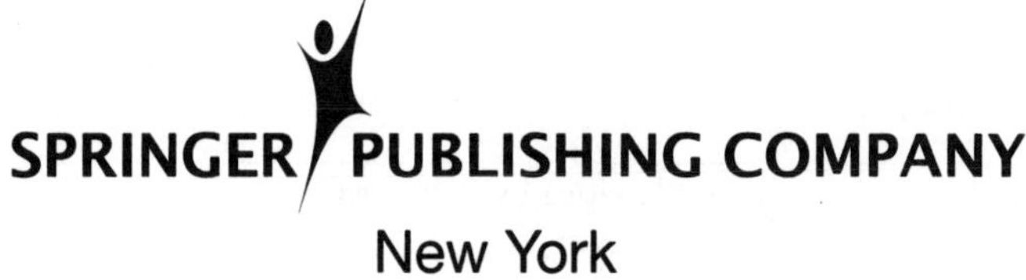


New York

Springer Publishing Company, LLC
11 West 42nd Street
New York, NY 10036
www.springerpub.com

*Acquisitions Editor:* Philip Laughlin
*Production Editor:* Rosanne Lugtu
*Cover design:* Joanne E. Honigman
*Composition:* Apex CoVantage, LLC

08 09 10 11/ 5 4 3 2 1

**Library of Congress Cataloging-in-Publication Data**

Children with complex medical issues in schools : neuropsychological descriptions and interventions / [edited by] Christine L. Castillo.
p. ; cm.
Includes bibliographical references and index.
ISBN 978-0-8261-2472-2 (alk. paper)
1. Pediatric neuropsychology. 2. Learning disabilities—Etiology. 3. Chronically ill children—Education. 4. Children with disabilities—Education. 5. School psychology. I. Castillo, Christine L. [DNLM: 1. Child. 2. Neuropsychology. 3. Disease—psychology. 4. Early Intervention (Education) 5. Needs Assessment. 6. School Health Services. WL 103.5 C536 2008]

RJ486.5.C47 2008
618.92′8—dc22 2007045878

Printed in the United States of America by Bang Printing.

# Contents

# Contributors

**Denise Phalon Cascio, MS**
Mount Washington Pediatric Hospital
Baltimore, Maryland

**Christine L. Castillo, PhD, LSSP**
Children's Medical Center Dallas
Dallas, Texas

**Peter J. Duquette, PhD**
Children's National Medical Center
Washington, D.C.

**Eve N. Fontaine, PhD**
Duke University Medical Center
Durham, North Carolina

**Bonny J. Forrest, JD, PhD**
Loyola College in Maryland
Baltimore, Maryland
and
Private Practice
Bethesda, Maryland, and Washington, D.C.

**Kristy S. Hagar, PhD**
Children's Medical Center Dallas
Dallas, Texas

**Ann C. Halbower, MD**
Johns Hopkins University
Baltimore, Maryland

**Joette James, PhD**
Children's National Medical Center
Washington, D.C.

**Jennifer A. Janusz, PsyD, ABPP-CN**
Private Practice, and University of Colorado at Denver and Health Sciences Center
Denver, Colorado

**Lauren S. Krivitzky, PhD**
Children's National Medical Center
Washington, D.C.

**Emily F. Law, MA**
University of Maryland, Baltimore County
Baltimore, Maryland

**Nirupama S. Madduri, MD**
Baylor College of Medicine and Texas Children's Hospital
Houston, Texas

**Michelle Murray, PhD**
Children's Medical Center Dallas
Dallas, Texas

**Julie A. Panepinto, MD, MSPH**
Medical College of Wisconsin
and

The Children's Research Institute of the Children's Hospital of Wisconsin
Milwaukee, Wisconsin

**Roger Perez, PhD**
Advanced Neurobehavioral Health of Southern California
San Diego, California

**Sarika U. Peters, PhD**
Baylor College of Medicine and Texas Children's Hospital
Houston, Texas

**Krestin J. Radonovich, PhD**
University of Florida, College of Medicine
Gainesville, Florida

**Kimberly M. Rennie, PhD**
NeuroBehavioral Health Clinic
Glendale, Wisconsin

**Julie K. Ries, PsyD**
Mount Washington Pediatric Hospital
Baltimore, Maryland

**Jennifer L. Riff, PhD**
Private Consultation/Practice
Edina, Minnesota

**Shahal Rozenblatt, PhD**
Advanced Psychological Assessment, P.C.
Lake Success, New York

**Susan A. Scarvalone, MSW, LCSW-C**
Prevention and Research Center, Mercy Medical Center
Baltimore, Maryland

**Jillian C. Schneider, PhD**
Children's National Medical Center
Washington, D.C.

**Sarah Schnoebelen, PhD**
Private Practice
Austin, Texas

**Laura Slap-Shelton, PsyD**
Southern Maine Medical Center
Biddeford, Maine
and
The University of New England
Biddeford, Maine

**Anne-Marie Slinger-Constant, MD, FAAP**
University of Florida, College of Medicine
Gainesville, Florida

**Cynthia A. Smith, PhD**
Mount Washington Pediatric Hospital, Johns Hopkins Medical School, and University of Maryland Medical School
Baltimore, Maryland

**Gregory Snyder, PhD**
Children's Hospital
Omaha, Nebraska

**Peter L. Stavinoha, PhD**
Children's Medical Center Dallas
Dallas, Texas

**Karin S. Walsh, PsyD**
Children's National Medical Center
Washington, D.C.

**Crista E. Wetherington, PhD**
Children's Medical Center Dallas
Dallas, Texas

**Dixie J. Woolston, PhD**
University of Texas Southwestern Medical Center
Dallas, Texas

# Foreword

In the course of training in pediatric neuropsychology, clinicians and students need to be familiar with a range of disorders and their phenotypes. All too often, the focus is on the high incidence disorders, such as learning disabilities and attention deficit hyperactivity disorder, rather than on the multitude of other conditions that can affect children's educational and social-emotional functioning. A neuropsychological approach to assessment and case conceptualization incorporates information from various behavioral domains believed to be related to functional neurological systems. The major premise of neuropsychological assessment is that different behaviors involve the interaction of differing neurological structures or functional systems with subsequent inferences drawn about brain integrity based on performance across a variety of specialized assessment tasks. The case studies included in this text provide examples of both the variability and similarities in the ways medical conditions, some of which do not have obvious neurological underpinnings (like endocrine disorders, diabetes) as well as those that more emphatically involve the central nervous systems (e.g., seizure disorder, encephalitis, meningitis) can affect day-to-day functioning in the crucial developmental period of life.

The range of conditions covered is broad, ambitious, and successful. This text provides information on 21 such disorders that clinicians and educators alike may encounter. From asthma to traumatic brain injury, each chapter is written by clinicians with practical expertise with the disorder. In addition to standard descriptions of etiology, course, and comorbid disorders, each chapter includes a case study, with results from neuropsychological evaluations and recommendations for educational modifications and accommodations. With those conditions that include pharmacotherapy as a component of treatment, some of the more frequently included medications, and their side effects, are discussed as well.

The position held by the editor seems to be that all children can learn and that the best way for them to learn is in the general education classroom for as much of the school day as is feasible. At the same time, there is increased awareness of chronic medical conditions and neurogenetic disorders that can affect the educational outcomes of children with these disorders. Given the potential effects of various disorders and conditions on educational prognosis, it is important for neuropsychologists, pediatric psychologists, school psychologists, and other professionals who are working with these children to be aware of the nature and course of these many disorders and avenues for rehabilitation, accommodation, and classroom modification. As such, this compendium is a major contribution to the literature and is formulated in such a way to address questions from a variety of perspectives. Our expectation is that this text will fill a void in discerning best educational practices for children with these lower incidence disorders and stimulate additional research across disciplines.

Cynthia A. Riccio
Cecil R. Reynolds
*College Station, TX*
*September, 2007*

# Preface

*To know that we know what we know, and to know that we do not know what we do not know, that is true knowledge.*

—Nicolas Copernicus

It was six men of Indostan
To learning much inclined,
Who went to see the elephant
(Though all of them were blind),
That each by observation
Might satisfy his mind.

The *First* approached the elephant,
And happening to fall
Against his broad and sturdy side,
At once began to bawl:
'God bless me! but the elephant
Is very like a wall!'

The *Second,* feeling of the tusk,
Cried, 'Ho! what have we here
So very round and smooth and sharp?
To me 'tis mighty clear
This wonder of an elephant
Is very like a spear!'

The *Third* approached the animal,
And happening to take
The squirming trunk within his hands,
Thus boldly up and spake:
'I see,' quoth he, 'the elephant
Is very like a snake.'

The *Fourth* reached out his eager hand,
And felt about the knee.
'What most this wondrous beast is like
Is mighty plain,' quoth he;

'"Tis clear enough the elephant
Is very like a tree!'

The *Fifth* who chanced to touch the ear,
Said: 'E'en the blindest man
Can tell what this resembles most:
Deny the fact who can,
This marvel of an elephant
Is very like a fan!'

The *Sixth* no sooner had begun
About the beast to grope,
Than seizing on the swinging tail
That fell within his scope,
'I see,' quoth he, 'the elephant
Is very like a rope!'

And so these men of Indostan
Disputed loud and long,
Each in his own opinion
Exceeding stiff and strong,
Though each was partly in the right,
And all were in the wrong!

So, oft in theologic wars,
The disputants, I ween,
Rail on in utter ignorance
Of what each other mean,
And prate about an Elephant
Not one of them has seen!

—John Godfrey Saxe (based on an original fable)

For individuals who are true students of life, there is never a finish line. There is not an absolute end point in which one can possibly obtain all the knowledge and expertise available to them. For me, the more time passes, the more I find myself amazed at how much I don't know. Although as a field we may be, as Henry Miller states, pushing back the "horizon of ignorance," we can all benefit from others' experiences. There are (fortunately) some things that I have learned and experienced. I consider myself one of the blind men from John Godfrey Saxe's poem, "The Blind Men and the Elephant." Many of us have heard this story in different forms, and may even use it as an analogy to describe how different medical and mental health practitioners each uncover varied issues in a single child. However, unlike the men of Indostan, we do not have to continue in disagreement about what issues are primary in medically complex children. Communication among professionals, and education in areas that we may fall short, can only benefit the children and families that we serve.

As most readers of this book can attest, children with significant medical issues are increasingly being incorporated into the general school environment in order to maintain the least restrictive environment and provide these students with access to the general education curriculum and age-appropriate social interaction. As a result, teachers, counselors, school administrators, and especially school psychologists find themselves working with these students without the resources needed to delineate the effects on neurocognitive, academic, behavioral, and emotional functioning as impacted by specific medical issues and their respective treatments. Without this information, proposed interventions may not target the specific and unique needs of each group. Likewise, for professionals in the field of pediatric neuropsychology, understanding of appropriate expectations for educational interventions and accommodations may be somewhat limited, especially for those who may not have had an opportunity to spend much time in public schools other than their own early education. With the recent publication of books regarding school neuropsychology (D'Amato, Fletcher-Janzen, & Reynolds, 2005; Hale & Fiorello, 2004; Miller, 2007), it is clear that the field is changing. Because children with complex medical issues are being reintegrated into schools more frequently, school personnel are attempting to supplement their knowledge through these and other means in order to provide the most appropriate educational environment for all students.

In my initial musings about *Children With Complex Medical Issues in Schools,* I felt the need to bridge the gap between research and practice for school psychologists and other related school personnel by detailing specific neuropsychological outcomes for medical disorders more commonly seen in schools, providing ideas for educational interventions, and presenting additional resources for teachers and families. I hope that the reader will find that this goal has been met. The chapters included in this book were chosen with purpose and include commonly seen medical disorders that may affect school functioning. Included in each chapter the reader will find helpful data regarding morbidity and mortality rates, related medical issues, and common medical treatments. Each chapter provides information and assessment data from a neuropsychological evaluation of a child with the respective medical disorder in an attempt to elicit understanding and greater insight into how a student's school functioning may be affected by their medical history. Finally, interventions that may be helpful to a child with the specific medical disorder will be provided, along with educational resources that may be accessed via the internet or through other literature.

My hope is that school psychologists and other school evaluation professionals will appreciate the hands-on, practical applications that *Children With Complex Medical Issues in Schools* provides via presentations of case studies and provision of additional resources for each specific disorder. This book in no way is the final authority and does not provide a comprehensive review of all possible medical disorders in schools, but hopefully readers will find it to be a launching pad in which additional information searches and research can begin. I hope you will join me in increasing our understanding of these special children and pushing back our "horizon of ignorance."

## REFERENCES

D'Amato, R. C., Fletcher-Janzen, E., & Reynolds, C. R. (2005). *Handbook of school neuropsychology.* Hoboken, NJ: John Wiley & Sons, Inc.

Hale, J. B., & Fiorello, C.A (2004). *School neuropsychology: A practitioner's handbook.* New York: The Guilford Press.

Miller, D.C. (2007). *Essentials of school neuropsychological assessment.* Hoboken, NJ: John Wiley & Sons, Inc.

Christine L. Castillo

# Acknowledgments

A book such as this is the culmination of years of clinical practice and research. I first want to acknowledge the contributions of all of the authors. Their clinical expertise, combined with diligent research and thoughtful application of their knowledge, has resulted in a very unique way of helping school personnel and other clinical practitioners better understand how children are affected by complex medical disorders.

Secondly, I would like to thank Philip Laughlin, senior editor at Springer Publishing, for his guidance, encouragement, and support in this large undertaking. He has been a cheerleader from the beginning and has made my experience all that much better.

This book would not have been a consideration if not for the gentle prodding and tremendous support I have been fortunate enough to experience. I specifically want to thank my previous supervisors and mentors, Robert Leark, Cynthia Riccio, Cecil Reynolds, Antolin Llorente, Glenn Brown, Cynthia Smith, and Julie Ries, and for their leadership and guidance. In many different ways, they have fostered my unrelenting desire to facilitate successful school functioning for children and adolescents with complex medical disorders.

Finally, I want to thank my family and friends for their unwavering support. My husband, in particular, has been a source of strength and optimism throughout this endeavor. I am eternally blessed to have such a support system and cannot imagine undertaking such an enterprise without the support and contribution of all of these individuals.

# Acknowledgments

# Special Note

Readers are reminded that the names and identifying information of all children presented in the case studies have been changed to protect confidentiality. When reviewing evaluation data, the following rules apply unless otherwise noted: Z Scores have an average of 0 and a standard deviation of 1; Scaled Scores have an average of 10 and a standard deviation of 3; T Scores have an average of 50 and a standard deviation of 10; and Standard Scores have an average of 100 and a standard deviation of 15.

## CHAPTER ONE

# Asthma

Christine L. Castillo, PhD, LSSP, and
Jennifer L. Riff, PhD

Asthma is one of the most chronic health problems in children (Akinbami, 2006; American Lung Association [ALA], 2006; Centers for Disease Control and Prevention [CDC]/National Center for Environmental Health [NCEH], n.d.). It is a chronic inflammatory disease of the airways that is caused by an increased reaction of the airways to various stimuli (i.e., triggers) and reversible airway obstruction (ALA; McQuaid & Walders, 2003). Asthma is exacerbated by any number of acute triggers and is complicated by numerous issues, including substandard living conditions, low socioeconomic status, and limited resources.

## DESCRIPTION OF THE DISORDER

### Description and Etiology

Asthma does not have a singular etiology; rather, it results from several variables that interact. These variables include genetic predisposition to allergy, environmental influences, and exposure to triggers, in addition to psychological influences such as stress (McQuaid & Walders, 2003). Previous research has found that parenting difficulties at 3 weeks of age are an independent predictor of asthma status between 6 and 8 years of age (Klinnert et al., 2001).

Some of the symptoms of asthma include shortness of breath, wheezing, gasping, chest tightness, and coughing during the night or early morning (CDC/NCEH, n.d.; Fiorello & McLaughlin, 2004). An asthma attack may be preceded by these symptoms, as well as by increased breathing rate and chest retractions (Plaut, 1998). Diagnosis of asthma is made by a health care provider based on questions regarding the aforementioned symptoms, family history, and impact on school attendance and physical activity. Pulmonary specialists may complete pulmonary function tests using a spirometer that measures the amount of air an individual can exhale after taking a very deep breath (CDC/NCEH).

Diagnosing asthma in infants is difficult, especially when there are no genetic markers. It is often mistaken for pneumonia, bronchitis, or bronchiolitis (National Asthma Education and Prevention [NAEP], 1997; Plaut, 1998). To make a firm diagnosis in this young patient group, information regarding parental history of asthma, immunologic tests, eczema, and other biological markers are collected (Fiocchi, Terracciano, Martelli, Guerriero, & Bernardo, 2006).

## Triggers

Asthma is a chronic condition that is exacerbated by acute triggers. Triggers are activities and environmental stimuli that worsen an individual's asthma and can lead to an asthma attack or episode. Some of the most common triggers include allergens (e.g., dust mites, cockroaches, pollen, mold, pet dander, foods), irritants (e.g., tobacco smoke, nitrogen dioxide, pollution, extreme temperature, candles), chemicals (e.g., perfume, household cleaners), and medications (e.g., aspirin, Advil, Motrin) (ALA, 2006; Fiorello & McLaughlin, 2004; McQuaid and Walders, 2003). Exercise and overexertion are the most common triggers (Plaut, 1998). Respiratory infections and influenza in children with asthma may cause a child to become more sensitive to allergens or irritants that do not typically cause an episode. Even strong emotional reactions, such as intense fear, laughing, or crying, may cause an episode.

Some triggers are somewhat avoidable, such as exposure to certain allergens and irritants, and control of these allergens should be a first-line defense against asthma exacerbation (Phipatanakul, 2006). Food allergies are often detected early in life. As a result, exposure to certain foods can be limited if the family is diligent. Reducing exposure to dust mites can be accomplished by using covers for mattresses and pillows (Shedd et al., 2007) and by limiting the use of down-filled bedding and stuffed animals (CDC/NCEH, n.d.). Placing stuffed animals in the freezer for a short time has been known to reduce allergens. Although frequent laundering of bed linens had previously been shown to reduce asthma symptoms, Shedd and colleagues (2007) found that laundering bed linens more than once per week resulted in decreased quality of life for caregivers of pediatric patients as well as increased asthma symptoms. This finding appears counterintuitive, but increased frequency of laundering may lead to increased humidity or increased exposure to detergents with fragrance. Nevertheless, the National Institute of Allergy and Infectious Diseases (NIAID, 2004) continues to urge frequent laundering of bed linens in water that has a minimum temperature of 130 degrees Fahrenheit.

Cockroaches are often difficult to eradicate but can be eliminated by maintaining a clean home environment. Pet dander is another trigger that it may be difficult to limit exposure to, but frequent bathing of pets and keeping them outside as much as possible may reduce the likelihood of dander causing an episode.

As noted by Abramson and colleagues (2006), although exposure to indoor allergens is greatest in the home, schools and day care centers may also harbor significant levels of environmental allergens. Levels of allergens depend on physical, structural, and behavioral factors. In fact, it was found that allergens from dust mites, cats, and cockroaches were at detectable levels in Birmingham, Alabama, and Houston, Texas, schools, with a higher dust mite allergen level in lower grade classrooms and libraries due to the greater numbers of allergen-friendly accoutrements (e.g., upholstered furniture, floor pillows, books; Abramson et al., 2006). In addition, indoor air pollution (e.g., nitrogen dioxide) caused by gas stoves or space heaters may result in poor indoor air quality and can therefore trigger asthma episodes (Kattan et al., 1997).

Limiting exposure to tobacco smoke may be difficult for some children, as caregivers may continue to smoke in the house or car. In one study examining inner-city children with asthma, 59% of families included at least one smoker, and someone was smoking in the home during 10% of the home visits (Kattan et al., 1997). Not only does exposure to tobacco smoke increase the possibility of a child experiencing an asthma episode, but it may also worsen their condition overall (ALA, 2006). Although pollen, air pollution, or high concentrations of ozone cannot necessarily be avoided altogether, limiting outdoor activities on days when levels are higher is advised (Babin et al., 2007). It is important to realize that seasons for high pollen counts differ among geographical regions (Babin et al.). Overall, the number of visits to the emergency room increased for children between 5 and 12 years of age when there were higher levels of pollen, increased ozone concentration, or higher temperatures; these outdoor pollutants did not cause children under 4 years of age to be at as great a risk for emergency room visits as their older peers because they likely spend less time outdoors (Babin et al.).

Mold is a serious trigger and causes illness even in individuals without asthma, but it can be prevented by ensuring that leaks are fixed quickly to thwart mold growth. Also, humidity levels between 35% and 50% in the home are ideal and reduce the likelihood of mold (CDC/NCEH, n.d.). Very cold or hot weather, or high humidity, can be avoided by remaining indoors if conditions are well regulated via climate-control appliances (e.g., heaters, air conditioners, dehumidifiers). Unfortunately, not all families have access to these appliances.

Other triggers may be more difficult to avoid. Strong emotional reactions may also be hard to prevent, as they may occur rather suddenly due to an event. In fact, asthma attacks were once believed to be psychogenic in nature (McQuaid & Walders, 2003). Overall, for children with asthma, it is important that caregivers understand the possible triggers for an asthma episode and then both reduce the exposure to such triggers as much as possible by maintaining an adequate environment and assist the individual with coping techniques to manage the symptoms.

## Biological Mechanisms

An asthma episode begins as a result of exposure to a trigger to which the immune system reacts. In order to fight off the allergens or irritants, a defensive antibody, immunoglobulin E (IgE), is produced and released into the airway, which then causes airway constriction and inflammation. In fact, an episode may include one or all of the following events: swelling of the airway lining, tightening of the muscles surrounding the airway (i.e., bronchoconstriction), and secretion of mucus in the airway causing the characteristic wheezing (ALA, 2006). As a result, less air flows in and out of the lungs, which causes an increased breathing rate and chest retractions (Plaut, 1998). Episodes range from very mild to severe and have characteristics that are reversible, intermittent, and variable (Fiorello & McLaughlin, 2004). *Status asthmaticus* is a severe episode of asthma during which the symptoms do not subside after use of prescribed medications and that threatens an individual's ability to breathe, possibly requiring intubation.

## Prevalence

Of all chronic conditions in childhood and adolescence, asthma is the most common (McQuaid & Walders, 2003). According to a study conducted by the CDC in 2004, approximately 6.5 million children under 18 years of age (8.9% of children) have asthma, with 9 million children being diagnosed with asthma at some point in their lives and over 4 million having experienced an asthma episode during the last 12 months (CDC,

2004b, 2007). Although the diagnosis of asthma can occur at any age, most individuals are diagnosed by 3 years of age (Fiorello & McLaughlin, 2004). Without a currently specified cause, asthma prevalence rates more than doubled between 1980 and the mid-1990s and remain historically high (Akinbami, 2006).

Male children are more likely to have had an asthma diagnosis and an asthma attack in the last year than female children; this pattern is reversed for adolescents (Akinbami, 2006) and adults (Akinbami; CDC/Health Data for All Ages [HDAA], n.d.), although the reason for this pattern is not clear. Overall, asthma prevalence increases with age, but this may result in part from the difficulty of diagnosing asthma in young children, who tend to experience a higher incidence of wheezing due to respiratory infections and other transient episodes (Akinbami; CDC/NCEH, n.d.). The increased prevalence of asthma as children enter adolescence also may result from the reduced roles that caregivers play in managing their child's asthma (Bruzzese et al., 2004). However, prevalence of asthma attacks, which provides a crude estimate of control and outcome, was noted to decrease with age (CDC/HDAA) and be highest in children under 10 years of age (McCoy et al., 2006). However, two-thirds of children suffering from asthma experienced at least one attack during 2005 (Akinbami), indicating that a large number of children have asthma that is not well controlled.

In a large sample of 17-year-old Israeli adolescents, asthma was diagnosed in 8.6% of males and 6.9% of females (Goldberg et al., 2007). It is interesting that in Israeli families with four or more children, asthma prevalence in children was found to be inversely related to family size. Specifically, 7.3% of only children were reported to have asthma; although prevalence increased to 8.95% in families with three children, the prevalence then progressively declined to 0.58% in families with 15 to 20 siblings (Goldberg et al.).

Data collected by the CDC and the National Center for Health Statistics (NCHS) between 2000 and 2005 for children ranging in age from birth to 17 years indicated that children living in poverty were more likely to suffer from asthma than those who were classified as "near poor" or "nonpoor" (CDC/NCHS, n.d.). In fact, whereas 10.4% of poor children under 17 years of age suffered from asthma during that time period, only 8.6% of "near poor" children and 8.1% of "nonpoor" children had asthma (CDC/NCHS). Other studies (Babin et al., 2007) also suggest increased risk of asthma-related complications for children living in poverty, especially for those with additional levels of stress (Chen et al., 2006).

According to the study conducted by the CDC/NCHS (n.d.), there are also morbidity differences based on ethnicity. For children under 17 years of age, Puerto Rican children had higher asthma prevalence rates (19.6%) than other groups of children (Akinbami, 2006; Lara, Akinbami, Flores, & Morgenstern, 2006). Thirteen percent of non-Hispanic black children and 12.2% of American Indian/Alaska Native children suffered from asthma. Non-Hispanic white, Mexican, and Asian children suffered from asthma at much lower rates (7.9%, 5.9%, and 4.8%, respectively; CDC/NCHS). Data also suggest that asthma prevalence rates differ according to region within the United States. According to Akinbami (2006), prevalence rates are higher in the northeast, where higher numbers of Puerto Rican children reside, with recent data indicating that Massachusetts had the highest asthma prevalence rates.

## Health Care Use

During 2004, children and adults with asthma made 13.6 million visits to office-based physicians, 1 million hospital outpatient department visits, and 1.8 million emergency room visits (CDC, 2007). Children and adults with asthma were seen in outpatient settings at approximately the same rate, but females had a 50% higher outpatient visit rate compared to their male counterparts (CDC/HDAA, n.d.). Notably, outpatient monitoring of children with asthma is very important for overall quality of ambulatory care. It is fortunate that although prevalence rates have plateaued and visits to the emergency room have reportedly remained stable, ambulatory care for children with asthma has continued to increase (Akinbami, 2006), suggesting increased access to preventive medications and services.

Based on previous studies, the rate of emergency room visits and subsequent hospitalizations was highest among children under 4 years of age (Akinbami, 2006; Babin et al., 2007; CDC/HDAA, n.d.). Children who have asthma and behavioral or emotional difficulties (e.g., depression) have more frequent and prolonged hospitalizations and greater overall impairment (McQuaid & Walders, 2003). There were significant differences among rates for emergency room visits and hospitalization based on ethnicity. In 2002, the emergency room visit rate was 380% higher for blacks compared to whites (CDC/HDAA); for children with asthma the numbers are comparable (Akinbami). The data demonstrating that black children with asthma had lower rates for ambulatory care yet higher rates of emergency room visits and hospitalizations indicate underutilization of ambulatory (and therefore preventive) care (Akinbami).

Socioeconomic status also affects patterns of health care utilization for acute asthma episodes. Previous research (Babin et al., 2007) indicates that children living in high-poverty zip codes in the District of Columbia have an increased likelihood of needing care in an emergency room. Also, because these children visit the emergency room with more severe symptoms, they have an increased number of subsequent hospital admissions (Babin et al.). Along with these severe symptoms, a history of previous intubation and previous hospitalization places children at even greater risk for additional admissions (Pollack et al., 2002). Other risk factors for subsequent hospital admissions include age at first admission (i.e., less than 12 months) and severity of asthma symptoms (Lasmar, Camargos, Goulart, & Sakurai, 2006). Reasons for the increased severity of symptoms for this select group of children include deferment of medical care until symptoms become more severe, lack of air conditioning, poor indoor air quality, and restricted access to and availability of health care (Babin et al.).

Based on a study investigating emergency room visits for children under 18 years of age during 2002, asthma ranked as the third most frequent diagnosis, with fever and acute upper respiratory infections ranking first and second, respectively (Alpern et al., 2006). In 2004, children with asthma made 750,000 emergency room visits (Akinbami, 2006). "Unspecified asthma" was the most common emergency room diagnosis for children between 5 and 14 years of age, and it ranked among the top five most common diagnoses for children between ages 1 and 4 years and ages 15 and 18 years (Alpern et al.). Furthermore, of all the patients who were transported to the emergency room via emergency medical services, asthma was the second most common diagnosis; convulsions were the most common diagnosis (Alpern et al.). For children, hospitalization for asthma represented about 3% of all hospitalizations (Akinbami).

## Impact on Education, Work, and Daily Life

Asthma and asthma-related illnesses cause children to miss nearly 15 million days of school each year (CDC/HDAA, n.d.). This indicates that children with asthma miss two additional days of school per year compared to their nonaffected peers (Silverstein et al., 2001). Data from a study completed in the mid-1990s indicated that children missed approximately 4 to 6.5 days of school during a 3-month period (Kattan et al., 1997). The 4 million children who have experienced at least one asthma attack miss nearly 13 million days of school (Akinbami, 2006). Only 3.5% of adolescents with controlled asthma missed one or more day of school, compared to 34% of adolescents with poorly controlled asthma (Schmier et al., 2007). Overall, asthma is the leading cause of school absences due to a chronic condition (Fiorello & McLaughlin, 2004; McQuaid & Walders, 2003; Rhee, Wenzel, & Steeves, 2007; Smart, 2004).

Although asthma-related issues clearly impact a child's ability to attend school, other activities also are impacted. According to a study that asked parents about the effect of asthma on their child's play activity and sleep, approximately 2 out of 14 days were reportedly characterized by reduced play activity and sleep disruption for the children (Kattan et al., 1997). Children with asthma report a "perception of loss" and occasionally have to give up preferred physical activities such as sports (Rhee et al., 2007).

Not only do asthma-related issues affect the diagnosed children, but caregivers also experienced approximately 2 days of disrupted sleep during a 2-week period and had to change their plans on nearly 3 days out of a 3-month period (Kattan et al., 1997). Caregivers missed just as many days of work as their children missed of school due to caring for children with asthma (Smart, 2004). Overall, inadequately controlled asthma had a significant impact on quality of life and school/work productivity and attendance (Schmier et al., 2007).

## Mortality

Mortality rates for asthma reached 1.3 deaths per 100,000 individuals during 2004, for a total of 3,780 deaths (CDC, 2007). Fortunately, mortality rates have declined after an increase in asthma-related deaths from 1980 through the mid-1990s (Akinbami, 2006) and even into 2001, when mortality rates reached 1.5 deaths per 100,000 individuals for a total of 4,269 (CDC, 2004a). Throughout childhood, boys are more likely to die from asthma than girls (Akinbami). Although the prevalence of asthma is greater in children under 17 years of age, mortality rates do not follow this statistic (CDC/HDAA, n.d.). In 2002, 4,261 individuals died from asthma, which included 1.9 adult deaths and 0.3 child deaths per 100,000 (CDC/HDAA). Notably, there is a higher rate of asthma-related deaths in adolescents compared to younger children (Akinbami).

Mortality due to asthma-related complications was much more common in non-Hispanic black children and adults, with the death rate more than 200% higher in this group of individuals compared to non-Hispanic whites (CDC/HDAA, n.d.); black children have a death rate that is 500% higher than white children have (Akinbami, 2006). Hispanic individuals had a mortality rate of 1.4 deaths per 100,000 (CDC/HDAA), although some of the mortality differences among Mexican and Puerto Rican subgroups may be masked by grouping them together (Akinbami). According to Akinbami (2006), "the disparity in asthma mortality between black and white children has increased in recent years" (p. 2) and may be due to numerous factors, not limited to lack of asthma education or difficulty in adopting asthma control methods.

Overall, the data suggest that repeated visits to the emergency room for acute asthma management are a risk factor for mortality

(McFadden & Warren, 1997). Issues affecting mortality rates include lack of proper diagnosis of asthma severity, difficulty managing medication use, limited ability to avoid triggers, and restricted or lacking access to appropriate medical treatment due to limited financial or transportation resources (Akinbami, 2006). Other risk factors for asthma-related deaths include poor control of symptoms, recurrent hospitalizations, previous intubation, or a history of a near-fatal asthma attack (McFadden & Warren), as well as poor adherence to medication regimens and difficulty perceiving symptom severity (McQuaid & Walders, 2003).

## Prevention and Intervention of Asthma Episodes

Asthma episodes are best prevented by identifying and avoiding all known triggers. Airway functioning should be monitored using a peak flow meter and diary (Plaut, 1998), and early warning signs of an impending attack should be identified (Fiorello & McLaughlin, 2004). Early identification of episode symptoms will assist children in managing the severity of their asthma.

When the first signs of an asthma attack appear, several things can be done to prevent exacerbation of the episode. Cessation of all physical activity for a period of time until the symptoms subside is of utmost importance (Fiorello & McLaughlin, 2004). It may be helpful to use prescribed medication and slowly drink warm liquids to encourage relaxation of the airways. The child also may find reduction in symptoms by engaging in previously learned relaxation techniques (e.g., diaphragmatic breathing, guided imagery) as well as cognitive-behavioral techniques to reduce anxiety.

Chronic asthma is treated with long-term medication that is designed to prevent acute episodes. Acute episodes are treated with quick-relief medications designed to control the symptoms and prevent escalation of an attack (CDC/NCEH, n.d.). Asthma medications serve to reduce inflammation of the airways and to relieve or prevent narrowing of the airways (ALA, 2006). The two classes of asthma medications are known as anti-inflammatory agents and bronchodilators and can be administered in several forms, including tablet, liquid, inhaled, and nebulized. A nebulizer is a machine that changes liquid medicine into a mist that can be inhaled through a mouthpiece or mask. In the case of status asthmaticus, use of an EpiPen and intubation may be warranted. A new medication for patients with severe asthma is Xolair, which blocks the antibodies that increase sensitivity to allergies that may trigger asthma symptoms (ALA). Notably, children with similar asthma severity will not necessarily respond the same to similar treatments (Stoloff & Boushey, 2006), which makes it necessary for them to be seen by an asthma specialist, especially if they have moderate to severe asthma.

According to the ALA (2006), anti-inflammatory medications are used for long-term control and prevention of episodes, as well as termination of ongoing airway inflammation. These medications include inhaled corticosteroids (e.g., Flovent, Pulmicort), cromolyn and nedocromil (e.g., Intal, Tilade), and leukotriene modifiers (e.g., Singulair, Zyflo), among others. Inhaled corticosteroids are the preferred medication for long-term asthma control (NAEP, 1997; Szefler, 2007). Leukotriene modifiers are administered in tablet form, whereas cromolyn sodium medications are given via inhalers or nebulizers. Advair, which is administered via an inhaler, is a medication that combines inhaled corticosteroid with a long-acting beta-2 agonist to reduce inflammation and open the airways (McQuaid & Walders, 2003). Some of the associated side effects of these medications may include headache, tremor, hyperactivity, upset stomach/nausea, dizziness, and fatigue (Plaut, 1998).

Bronchodilators include short-acting beta-adrenergic agonists, methylxanthines, oral/systemic corticosteroids, and anticholinergics, which serve to rapidly open the airways by relaxing the bronchial muscles. These are sometimes called "rescue medicines" and are intended to be used on an as-needed basis. Some children may be managed only on these medications. However, if a child experiences frequent episodes requiring repeated use of these quick-relief medications, his or her asthma is probably not well controlled (McQuaid & Walders, 2003). Oral corticosteroids are administered in tablet or liquid form and include medications such as prednisone (e.g., Prednisone Intensol, Sterapred), prednisolone (e.g., Prelone), and methylprednisolone (e.g., Medrol). Anticholinergics, such as ipratropium bromide (e.g., Atrovent), may be administered via an inhaler or nebulizer but are not intended to reduce symptoms brought on by exercise. Other medications classified as "quick relief" include albuterol (e.g., Ventolin, Proventil, and Airet), levalbuterol (e.g., Xopenex), and pirbuterol (e.g., Maxair). Some bronchodilators have side effects that can impact a child's functioning in school. These side effects include attention and memory difficulties, drowsiness, anxiety, depression, and tremors (Fiorello & McLaughlin, 2004). Other possible physiological side effects include tremor, increased heart rate, increased appetite (with oral corticosteroid use), and sleeping difficulties (Henry & DuPaul, 2004; Plaut, 1998).

Multidisciplinary management and treatment are becoming more common for children and adolescents with asthma. Medical professionals, such as primary care physicians, pulmonologists, and allergists, are the main feature of the multidisciplinary team and are involved in creating an asthma action plan that includes instruction on how to prevent and reduce symptoms and on when to access a particular level of health care depending on symptom severity (McQuaid & Walders, 2003).

Other individuals on this multidisciplinary team include pediatric psychologists and health educators. Pediatric psychologists are well suited for intervention with this population based on their training with medically complex children and their understanding of psychological concepts and behavioral management. According to McQuaid and Walders (2003), roles that pediatric psychologists can assume in working with children with asthma include providing asthma education, intervening with barriers to effective management of asthma, and employing techniques to promote appropriate asthma management.

## RELATED ISSUES

### Medical Comorbidities

There are several medical comorbidities of pediatric asthma, including otitis media (i.e., middle ear infection), sinusitis, and allergic rhinitis (Abramson et al., 2006). Other medical issues frequently seen in pediatric asthma include obesity and sleep disturbances.

Sinusitis, or rhinosinusitis, is a condition that is characterized by inflammation of the paranasal sinuses and nasal passages and that can be considered acute (i.e., lasting up to 4 weeks), subacute (i.e., lasting between 4 and 12 weeks), or chronic (i.e., lasting longer than 12 weeks) (Lai, Hopp, & Lusk, 2006). It has been estimated that 20% to 30% of children with asthma also suffer from sinusitis (Rachelefsky et al., 1978). Especially for children whose asthma symptoms are difficult to control, research indicates that aggressive treatment for sinusitis also can improve asthma symptoms (Virant, 2000).

Another common comorbidity of asthma is childhood obesity, although the relationship between the two remains unclear. In one study, over 20% of children with asthma were rated as obese whereas only 6.6% of children without asthma were obese (Glazebrook et al., 2006). Hypotheses regarding the underlying mechanisms include shared genetic risk factors (Hallstrand et al., 2005), changes in lung volumes related to smooth muscle function (Shore & Fredberg, 2005), and decreased activity level for those with asthma (Glazebrook et al.; van Gent et al., 2007).

Although some studies have previously shown no associations between asthma and sleep disturbances (Ronchetti et al., 2002), sleep disturbances are actually quite common among children with asthma. Nocturnal awakenings among children with asthma often result from coughing, wheezing, or breathlessness (Stores, Ellis, Wiggs, Crawford, & Thomson, 1998). Chronic cough and rhinosinusitis alone have been noted to be strongly associated with impaired sleep quality (Desager, Nelen, Weyler, & De Backer,

2005). Nocturnal wheezing has been associated with decreased quality of sleep, including poor sleep onset and restless sleep, resulting in increased somnolence (i.e., sleepiness) during the day (Desager et al., 2005). In fact, children with asthma are reported to fall asleep more frequently than children without asthma (Stores et al., 1998). This pattern of increased daytime somnolence has been coined *allergic—tension—fatigue syndrome* (Naudé & Pretorius, 2003). Not only will daytime somnolence impact multiple domains of functioning and inhibit learning, but sleeping during school may also be followed by office referrals and additional periods of missed learning opportunities. Research has shown that sleep disturbances in children with asthma are associated with impaired functioning in multiple psychological and neuropsychological domains; the reader is directed to the appropriate chapter in this volume for a thorough review of sleep-related effects on cognition.

## Neurocognitive, Emotional, and Behavioral Comorbidities

Children with any chronic medical condition are more likely to experience difficulties in cognitive, psychological, and social functioning (McQuaid & Walders, 2003; Richards, 1994). A study completed in 1980 revealed impaired neuropsychological functioning in a group of children with asthma (Dunleavy & Baade, 1980). Academic underachievement was correlated to frequent school absences due to asthma-related illnesses (Naudé & Pretorius, 2003). In fact, problems with attention, mood changes, and daydreaming greatly influenced poor academic achievement in approximately 60% of children between 6 and 13 years of age (Naudé & Pretorius). In severe cases of respiratory arrest and resulting hypoxia (i.e., reduced oxygen supply to the brain), children may experience specific neurocognitive effects due to lack of oxygen in select centers of the brain that tend to be sensitive to reduced oxygen levels (Bender, 1995; de Mesquita & Fiorello, 1998; Fletcher-Janzen, 2005). For instance, the hippocampus, which is partly responsible in consolidating new information, can be damaged after periods of reduced oxygen supply.

In contrast, two other studies examining neuropsychological performance in children with asthma did not demonstrate significantly different performance on measures of intelligence, memory, concentration, or school performance compared to matched controls (Annett, Aylward, Lapidus, Bender, & DuHamel, 2000; Rietveld & Colland, 1999). In an examination of the cognitive ability of children with asthma living in urban environments, their performance was comparable to that of other urban samples (Wade et al., 1997). It is suspected, however, that the impact on development, and therefore select neuropsychological domains, is likely moderated by asthma severity and adherence to medical interventions (Fritz & McQuaid, 2000).

In addition to the association between asthma and neuropsychological and psychological functioning, many studies have demonstrated an association between corticosteroid and bronchodilator use and declarative and verbal memory deficits, depression, drowsiness, fatigue, inattention, hyperactivity, mania or hypomania, psychotic symptoms, and other cognitive changes (for a review of these studies, see Creer & Bender, 1995; Fiorello & McLaughlin, 2004; Naudé & Pretorius, 2003; Plaut, 1998). For children with asthma who have received corticosteroids since they were very young, often due to the long-term consequences of bronchopulmonary dysplasia (i.e., a disease characterized by need for supplemental oxygen and/or mechanical ventilation beyond 28 days of age and by persistently abnormal chest X-rays and respiratory examinations), adverse effects on brain development have been cited (Papile et al., 1998). The side effects of asthma medications, especially corticosteroids, are concerning and confirm the importance of adherence to prescribed medication regimens and frequent communication with medical professionals to ensure the best control of asthma symptoms with the fewest possible side effects.

Research suggests that children with more severe asthma have more emotional symptoms (Glazebrook et al., 2006); increased feelings of loneliness, sadness, despair, frustration, and anger (Rhee et al., 2007); limited self-efficacy (van der Meer et al., 2007); and more internalizing difficulties than their peers (McQuaid, Kopel, & Nassau, 2001). Although some studies found that those with less severe asthma did not demonstrate significant differences in emotional or behavioral functioning compared to healthy peers (McQuaid et al., 2001), others have found that approximately one in four pediatric asthma patients being treated in an inner-city asthma clinic had increased symptoms of anxiety or depression (Goodwin, Messineo, Bregante, Hoven, & Kairam, 2005). Children seen in a pediatric emergency department due to asthma symptoms were also more likely to demonstrate increased levels of anxiety and depression on select measures than the normative samples (Wood et al., 2006). Similarly, teachers have reported greater prevalence of anxiety and anxiety-related habits (e.g., nail biting, fidgeting, etc.), depression, and problems with psychosocial functioning in children with asthma than in their nonasthmatic peers (Naudé & Pretorius, 2003). It is important to note that children who experience greater levels of psychological distress have more difficulty managing their asthma, have more adherence issues, and require higher doses of steroids (McQuaid & Walders, 2003). Other factors contributing to increased levels of anxiety and depression in children with asthma include negative family emotional climate, children's perception of poor relational security with their parents, and increased disease severity (Wood et al.). Also, independent of adherence to prescribed treatments, depression was significantly correlated to disease severity (Wood et al.). Quality of life is also impacted for children with asthma and even more greatly for children with asthma who are also obese (van Gent et al., 2007).

With regard to behavioral factors, children with mild to moderate asthma have been found to exhibit greater difficulty with impulse control and behavioral inhibition (Annett et al., 2000; Butz et al., 2001). They also show greater numbers of behavior problems as rated by their parents on the Child Behavior Checklist (CBCL; Achenbach & Edelbrock, 1983), with 35% of children in one sample demonstrating clinically significant levels of behavior problems (Wade et al., 1997). Many children, due to lethargy and difficulty with sustained attention following restless nights, are misdiagnosed with attention-deficit disorder (Celano & Geller, 1993).

## Case Study

The following case study details the background and medical history leading to repeat neuropsychological evaluations of an African American adolescent female, Sarah Smith.

### Initial Neuropsychological Evaluation

At the time of the initial neuropsychological evaluation, Sarah was 14 years old. She had an uncomplicated gestational period and achieved developmental milestones within normal limits. Her medical history was significant for seasonal and food allergies and chronic asthma. She was receiving albuterol, Flonase, Singulair, Advair, and Claritin on a daily basis.

With regard to her educational history, Sarah and her mother reported passing grades of B's and C's without any concerns of premorbid learning, behavioral, or emotional difficulties. However, she had failed to pass the eighth-grade state-mandated assessments and therefore was not promoted to ninth grade. Although school had started approximately three weeks before the initial evaluation, Sarah was not attending school at that time.

Prior to hospitalization and evaluation, Sarah was living in substandard inner-city housing with her mother, sisters, and five other extended family members. Several family members smoked cigarettes, and there were reports of high levels of mildew, dust, pet dander, and cockroaches in the home.

Sarah had developed symptoms of a cold. On the third morning following the onset of these symptoms, she woke with shortness of breath and self-administered albuterol via an inhaler, followed by administration of medication with the nebulizer. These medications reportedly were not helpful, and her mother found her to be anxious with severe shortness of breath as Sarah was administering her second dose of albuterol. Emergency medical services were called to the home, and Sarah had lost consciousness by the time they arrived. They transferred her to the local hospital's pediatric intensive care unit (PICU) where she was intubated for 1 day. She remained in the PICU for one week and was then transferred to a rehabilitation hospital. PICU discharge documents indicated that Sarah had suffered from a hypoxic brain injury secondary to status asthmaticus. She was referred for a neuropsychological evaluation due to concerns with select areas of neurocognitive functioning, including slow processing speed, poor sustained attention, emotional lability, expressive language difficulties, and fine motor weaknesses. During her hospitalization, she received speech, occupational, and physical therapies. Sarah also received therapy and support from pediatric psychology and child life services.

### *Behavioral Observations*

Sarah presented as a quiet but cooperative young girl who developed a good rapport with the examiner. Subjective complaints included concentration and memory difficulties and fatigue. She expressed symptoms of depression and had a sullen and somber affect. She did not appear to have difficulty in comprehending instructions, but she evidenced dysnomia (i.e., word-finding difficulties) and dysfluent speech due to retrieval difficulties. Sarah was slow in initiation and completion of tasks and was very concerned about errors. Her level of attention waned at times, and she often asked for repetition or explanation of directions. It became obvious that she was becoming cognitively fatigued after working for more than an hour. A very mild tremor was noticed in her left hand, and her gait was slow and deliberate, characterized by a wide stance and limited arm swing.

### *Evaluation Results*

Sarah was administered a battery of measures in order to estimate premorbid functioning and determine her profile of strengths and weaknesses. Specific test scores from select measures administered during the initial neuropsychological evaluation are presented in Table 1.1.

Sarah performed in the low average range on a brief measure of verbal intelligence and in the borderline range on measures of nonverbal cognition. Her cognitive processing speed fell in the mildly impaired range. Based on a brief assessment of her academic skills, Sarah performed in the average range on measures of word reading, reading comprehension, and applied mathematics. She performed in the borderline range on measures of numerical operations. However, it should be noted that on nearly all of the math problems that she answered incorrectly, she did so as a result of misreading the signs and adding instead of subtracting. Sarah obtained scores in the mildly impaired to borderline range on measures of nonverbal processing speed and verbal fluency. Although she made few mistakes on these tasks, her speed of processing impaired her ability to achieve higher scores.

Her attempt to copy a complex figure was executed very poorly; she began with smaller figures and details before drawing the larger figures. The qualitative observations of her copying the figure revealed that Sarah had few organizational and planning strategies that she could use before attempting similar tasks for the first time. However, on subsequent drawings performed from memory, Sarah was more adept at drawing the figure, leading with larger figures and filling in the details in a more organized manner, suggesting that, once attempted, her completion of a complex task becomes more organized and efficient. On another task that measures a person's ability to recognize patterns and demonstrate cognitive flexibility, Sarah performed well within the average range with regard to her response to feedback; however, upon starting this task, it took 32 trials for Sarah to complete the first category, which is in the low average range.

Sarah completed the Test of Variables of Attention (TOVA; Leark, Dupuy, Greenberg, Kindschi, & Corman, 1996) on two separate occasions. The initial completion of the TOVA was administered without stimulant medication. During the first administration, Sarah had a significant amount of omission errors (i.e., not responding when a visual target appeared), indicating that Sarah had significant difficulty sustaining attention during boring activities. However, on the second administration of the TOVA, after Sarah had begun a trial of Ritalin, her omission and commission errors were drastically reduced, and she performed well within the average range with regard to accuracy of her responses. Consequently, however, a significantly increased response time was noted. Comparing her performance during the two administrations of the TOVA, it was apparent that the stimulant medication was a positive addition to Sarah's treatment regimen. The scores from the two administrations of the TOVA can be viewed in Table 1.2.

On measures of language, Sarah's overall abilities were within the average range. However, she demonstrated significant difficulty primarily due to the extended amount of time it took for her to provide responses to questions. On these verbal and visual memory tasks, Sarah in general

**TABLE 1.1 Select Neuropsychological Testing Data from the Initial Evaluation**

| | Scaled Score | T Score | Standard Score |
|---|---|---|---|
| **Intellectual Functioning** | | | |
| WASI Full Scale IQ | | | 71 |
| Verbal IQ | | | 89 |
| Performance IQ | | | 77 |
| WISC-IV Processing Speed Index | | | 67 |
| **Academic Achievement** | | | |
| WJ-III Letter-Word Identification | | | 92 |
| Passage Comprehension | | | 90 |
| Calculation | | | 72 |
| Applied Problems | | | 91 |
| **Executive Functioning** | | | |
| D-KEFS Trail Making Test | | | |
| Visual Scanning | 5 | | |
| Number Sequencing | 1 | | |
| Letter Sequencing | 5 | | |
| Number-Letter Sequencing | 1 | | |
| Motor Speed | 7 | | |
| D-KEFS Verbal Fluency Test | | | |
| Letter Fluency | 4 | | |
| Category Fluency | 5 | | |
| Category Switching | 6 | | |
| **Learning/Memory** | | | |
| CVLT-C Trials 1-5 | | 43 | |
| List B Free Recall | | 35 | |
| List A Short Delay Free Recall | | 50 | |
| List A Short Delay Cued Recall | | 50 | |
| List A Long Delay Free Recall | | 45 | |

*Continued*

**TABLE 1.1** *(Continued)*

| | Scaled Score | T Score | Standard Score |
|---|---|---|---|
| List A Long Delay Cued Recall | | 55 | |
| Recognition | | 50 | |
| Visuospatial Functioning | | | |
| JLO | | | 103 |
| Fine Motor Skills | | | |
| Finger Tapping Test (Preferred Right) | | | 80 |
| Finger Tapping Test (Nonpreferred) | | | 64 |
| Grooved Pegboard (Preferred Right) | | | 108 |
| Grooved Pegboard (Nonpreferred) | | | <50 |

*Note.* CVLT-C, California Verbal Learning Test—Children's Version (Delis, Kramer, Kaplan, & Ober, 1994); D-KEFS, Delis-Kaplan Executive Function System (Delis, Kaplan, & Kramer, 2001); Finger Tapping Test (Reitan, 1969); Grooved Pegboard Test (Trites, n.d.); JLO, Judgment of Line Orientation (Benton, Hamsher, Varney, & Spreen, 1983); WASI, Wechsler Abbreviated Scale of Intelligence (Wechsler, 1999); WISC-IV, Wechsler Intelligence Scale for Children—Fourth Edition (Wechsler, 2003); and WJ-III, Woodcock-Johnson Tests of Achievement—Third Edition (Woodcock, McGrew, & Mather, 2001).

performed in the average range. However, she demonstrated difficulty learning multiple chunks of information.

On tasks that measure Sarah's fine motor skills, she evidenced significant weaknesses in her nondominant (left) hand. Although she demonstrated average fine motor dexterity with her dominant (right) hand, she had substantial difficulty completing these tasks with her nondominant hand. Sarah performed well within the average range on a measure of visual perception. However, she performed in the severely impaired range when asked to draw a complex geometric figure, indicating significant visual-motor weaknesses.

With regard to emotional and behavioral functioning, Sarah was shy and extremely reticent to engage in conversation with individuals when she first entered the rehabilitation hospital setting. She reported feelings of sadness because she wanted to return home and exhibited symptoms of depression, including somber affect, lethargy, and emotional lability. Sarah also reported numerous symptoms of anxiety,

**TABLE 1.2 Results from the Test of Variables of Attention**

| | Standard Score | |
|---|---|---|
| | Before Ritalin | After Ritalin |
| Omission Errors | 68 | 102 |
| Commission Errors | 102 | 114 |
| Response Time | 92 | 65 |

including fear of another asthma attack, intubation, and loss of consciousness. During the 2 weeks that Sarah spent at the hospital, she was able to develop relationships with the staff and other patients. She participated in group activities and looked forward to seeing her family when they visited.

## Neuropsychological Reevaluation

Approximately 1 year after her initial evaluation, Sarah returned for a reevaluation of her neuropsychological functioning. During the previous year, she and her immediate family had relocated to the home of an extended family member within the area. The new home did not have excessive levels of dust, mildew, pet dander, or insects; however, family members continued to smoke in the home. She had one visit to the emergency room because of breathing difficulties; she was treated and released. At the time of the reevaluation, Sarah was receiving Flonase, Advair, and Claritin on a daily basis; her Ritalin prescription had not been refilled since she left the hospital the previous year.

Sarah had not attended school for the entire school year since her release from the hospital. Due to concerns about extreme environmental triggers in the school setting, attempts were reportedly made to access homebound instruction but without success. Some of the more prominent concerns at school included poor ventilation in a cosmetology class in which fumes were emitted from acrylic nails and other procedures; several instances of fires set by students; overcrowding; and poor heating or air conditioning during extreme temperatures.

Concerns shared by Sarah included poor sleep hygiene. In fact, her sleep pattern consisted of going to bed very early in the morning (i.e., 2:00 or 3:00 a.m.), waking up multiple times after falling asleep, and waking up at 2:00 p.m. on most days. This pattern was reinforced through family members, and there was no in-home support for changing this behavior. Sarah also shared that she had a very poor appetite and typically ate only once per day. Because of her sleep schedule and lack of schooling, all of her social contacts had been eradicated.

### *Behavioral Observations*

Sarah presented as a quiet but cooperative young woman who developed good rapport with the examiner. She was thin, well groomed, and dressed appropriately. Sarah's mood and range of affect were appropriate for the situation. However, she appeared tearful when explaining that she often felt sad and did not have friends. During the testing, she did not appear to have difficulty comprehending instructions but was slow in completing tasks and concerned about making errors. When she was sure of an answer, she responded quickly and confidently. However, she was more hesitant when she was unsure of an answer and often needed encouragement to respond. She remained persistent when completing tasks even when frustrated. She was not impulsive when completing tasks and took time to think about an answer thoroughly before responding. She became fidgety at times, shaking her leg or bouncing in her chair, although she maintained good attention and persistence throughout the testing. She claimed that her hands were weak despite her average performance on tests of hand strength.

### *Evaluation Results*

Specific test scores from select measures administered during the neuropsychological reevaluation are presented in Table 1.3. Sarah's overall cognitive ability, as measured by the Wechsler Intelligence Scale for Children—Fourth Edition (WISC-IV; Wechsler, 2003), fell in the average range. Her abilities on verbal, perceptual reasoning, and working memory tasks fell in the average range, with scores in the low average range on processing speed tasks.

With regard to academic achievement, Sarah's ability to read sight words, comprehend sentences or short paragraphs, complete applied math problems, spell words, and write sentences fell in the average range. It is impressive that she was able to perform to this level considering that she had not attended school for over a year. Her reading fluency skills fell in the low average range, and she performed in the borderline range on math fluency tasks. Her ability to complete numerical operations fell in the borderline range.

Sarah performed in the average range on measures of nonverbal processing speed. On tests of verbal fluency and rapid word-finding ability, Sarah achieved scores in the low average range. She performed in the average range when she was asked to name colors and read words

**TABLE 1.3 Select Neuropsychological Testing Data From the Re-evaluation**

| | Scaled Score | Standard Score |
|---|---|---|
| **Intellectual Functioning** | | |
| WISC-IV Full Scale IQ | | 90 |
| Verbal Comprehension | | 93 |
| Perceptual Reasoning | | 98 |
| Working Memory | | 94 |
| Processing Speed | | 85 |
| **Academic Achievement** | | |
| WJ-III | | |
| Letter-Word Identification | | 94 |
| Passage Comprehension | | 91 |
| Reading Fluency | | 88 |
| Calculation | | 78 |
| Applied Problems | | 90 |
| Math Fluency | | 77 |
| Spelling | | 95 |
| Writing Samples | | 100 |
| **Executive Functioning** | | |
| D-KEFS Trail Making Test | | |
| Visual Scanning | 7 | |
| Number Sequencing | 8 | |
| Letter Sequencing | 9 | |
| Number-Letter Sequencing | 7 | |
| Motor Speed | 9 | |
| D-KEFS Verbal Fluency Test | | |
| Letter Fluency | 7 | |
| Category Fluency | 7 | |
| Category Switching | 9 | |

*Continued*

**TABLE 1.3** *(Continued)*

| | Scaled Score | Standard Score |
|---|---|---|
| D-KEFS Color-Word Interference | | |
| Color Naming | 8 | |
| Word Reading | 10 | |
| Inhibition | 3 | |
| Inhibition/Switching | 7 | |
| **Learning/Memory** | | |
| CMS Dot Locations | | |
| Learning | 14 | |
| Total Score | 13 | |
| Long Delay | 12 | |
| CMS Stories | | |
| Immediate | 10 | |
| Delayed | 10 | |
| Delayed Recognition | 10 | |
| **Visuospatial and Visual-Motor Functioning** | | |
| JLO | | 88 |
| VMI-V | | 82 |
| **Fine Motor Skills** | | |
| Hand Dynamometer (Preferred Right) | | 104 |
| Hand Dynamometer (Nonpreferred) | | 108 |
| Grooved Pegboard (Preferred Right) | | 73 |
| Grooved Pegboard (Nonpreferred) | | 64 |

*Note*. CMS, Children's Memory Scale (Cohen, 1997); D-KEFS, Delis-Kaplan Executive Function System (Delis, Kaplan, & Kramer, 2001); Grooved Pegboard Test (Trites, n.d.); Hand Dynamometer (Smedley, n.d.); JLO, Judgment of Line Orientation (Benton, Hamsher, Varney, & Spreen, 1983); VMI-V, Beery-Buktenica Developmental Test of Visual-Motor Integration—Fifth Edition (Beery, Buktenica, & Beery, 2005); Wechsler Intelligence Scale for Children—Fourth Edition (Wechsler, 2003); and WJ-III, Woodcock-Johnson Tests of Achievement—Third Edition (Woodcock, McGrew, & Mather, 2001).

quickly, but on inhibition tasks, she achieved scores in the mildly impaired range. On verbal and nonverbal cognitive flexibility tasks, she performed in the low average to average range. Her pattern of performance on these tasks suggests difficulty with cognitive inhibition.

Sarah obtained a score in the average range on a test of receptive vocabulary. Her ability to recall and formulate sentences fell in the average to high average range. On most verbal and visual memory tasks, Sarah performed in the average range or better. However, when asked to recognize photographs of faces, she demonstrated difficulty during the immediate recognition tasks, which may allude to difficulties with encoding strategies during initial presentation.

On tasks that measured Sarah's fine motor, visual-motor, and visual-perceptual skills, her performance was variable. On a test measuring hand strength, she performed in the average range bilaterally, although she reported subjective weakness in both hands. On a fine motor dexterity task, she performed in the borderline range with her right hand and in the mildly impaired range with her left hand. She performed in the low average range when given a measure that assessed her ability to copy geometric figures and also on a task that measured visual-perceptual skills.

Sarah completed a questionnaire that assessed her emotional and behavioral functioning. She had general concerns with her emotional functioning. She also noted feelings of inadequacy and poor interpersonal relations. In addition, she mentioned feelings of sadness and worries about having no friends. She denied suicidal ideation or psychotic symptoms. Her mother indicated that Sarah cried easily over what would otherwise be considered insignificant issues (i.e., a preferred television show being interrupted by the news).

## Comparison of Evaluation Results

Based on a review of the results of the initial and repeat evaluations, Sarah made progress in many areas, with significant gains in perceptual reasoning skills, visual sequencing, verbal fluency, and left-hand dexterity. She also demonstrated gains in processing speed, although she clearly had not returned to an average level, which continued to hamper her overall level of performance on cognitive tasks. Her academic achievement levels remained stable as expected, as did her verbal comprehension. This is not surprising as these skills (academic achievement, general cognition) are typically robust to hypoxic events. Although it may appear that declines in fine motor dexterity and visual-perceptual skills occurred, it is likely that inattention to detail and slow overall processing speed significantly affected Sarah's performance on tasks measuring these skills.

## Case Summary

Overall, Sarah's neuropsychological profile indicated diffuse, dampened, and relatively impaired executive functioning skills. This pattern of performance is not surprising given a hypoxic episode, which typically results in slower processing speed, poor inhibition and attention, and difficulty with emotional regulation. Although lack of oxygen to the brain for sustained periods of time, such as that experienced by Sarah during status asthmaticus, typically results in damage to hippocampal and temporal structures, leading to impairments in memory functioning, Sarah appears to be doing quite well in these areas.

With regard to differential diagnosis, Sarah was demonstrating characteristics of dysthymic disorder. Although her responses on a self-report questionnaire did not lead to elevations on the Depression subscale, she acknowledged experiencing a mild sense of inadequacy and poor interpersonal relationships. Reports from Sarah and her mother further supported this hypothesis and included concerns with emotional lability, poor sleep patterns, poor appetite, and a relatively lethargic presentation. In addition to a mood disorder, Sarah's pattern of performance on tasks measuring cognitive ability and academic achievement revealed a significant discrepancy between her cognitive skills and mathematics achievement. As a result, Sarah also met criteria as a student with a specific learning disability in math calculation.

# INTERVENTIONS

## Case-Specific Interventions

Due to Sarah's significant risk of incurring further impairment in neuropsychological functioning if she were to suffer another hypoxic episode, an environment that is free from asthma triggers is extremely important for her. Sarah and her family, the school nurse, and all of her teachers and other school personnel must be aware of Sarah's vulnerability to another life-threatening asthma attack. They should be aware of any triggers, including activity, dust, pollen, insects, smoke, and other things that may prompt an attack. Her classrooms and general school environment should be carefully considered. She should not be placed in situations where there is construction, mildew, mold, or poor ventilation. There must be adequate air conditioning or heat to regulate the air temperature.

In addition, if Sarah is required to complete any physical education courses, her health status should be closely monitored and she should not overexert herself. On days during which any notable levels of air pollution occur, Sarah should be exempt from participating in strenuous physical activities. Furthermore, a school health nurse or other medical staff should be on campus at all times in order to intervene if Sarah is in medical crisis. It is suggested that the school have a full supply of Sarah's medication, including an inhaler, a nebulizer, and an EpiPen in case of severe allergic reactions. Any concerns about limited airway should be addressed immediately by contacting emergency medical services and Sarah's caregivers.

With regard to special education services, the school team should meet to discuss the results of this evaluation. Based on the evaluation, Sarah may be eligible to receive special education services under the categories of Other Health Impairment and Specific Learning Disability. Consideration regarding eligibility under the category of Emotional Disturbance may also be considered due to her diagnosis of dysthymic disorder. Even if the school team does not agree that special education services are warranted, educational accommodations and modifications can be implemented under Section 504. Pull-out special education services may be necessary to assist Sarah in developing her mathematics skills. In order to strengthen her math skills and increase her success in this area, Sarah should be presented with math problems that apply to everyday situations or that are paired with pictures. Manipulatives should be provided so as to reduce frustration.

It is recommended that Sarah be reintegrated into the school environment as soon as possible. Although homebound services may be useful during times of medical instability and recuperation, extended periods of absence from school may increase her social isolation and school refusal behaviors and make reintegration even more difficult. Reintegration may occur slowly, with Sarah attending half a day of school for a select period of time before attending for an entire school day. In order to assist in this process, a guidance counselor or special education counselor may facilitate Sarah's successful transition into high school, considering her delayed entrance and significant life events.

Because Sarah is at significant risk for dropping out of school, her caregivers, teachers, and guidance counselor should help in her decision making. They should encourage her to complete her education, even if this means taking the General Educational Development (GED) examination. Furthermore, a guidance counselor or vocational teacher may be an excellent resource for Sarah. These individuals can provide her with information to facilitate her interdependent search for a career path and help her navigate the process to apply for the Job Corp, trade school, or other work preparation programs.

In order to address her emotional functioning, Sarah should undergo a psychiatric consultation to address the possible benefits of both cognitive-behavioral therapy and antidepressant medication. If medication is provided to address these concerns, there should be close monitoring of its benefits and side effects, including sleep disturbances, mood swings, or a change in energy/activity level or appetite. As Sarah matures, her medication regimen may need to be altered in order to ensure the least amount of harmful effects. In combination with psychopharmacologic treatment, Sarah would benefit from psychotherapy in order to obtain active coping skills to address her depressive symptoms, her social skill needs, and her anxiety regarding further asthma exacerbations. A combination of therapy and medication is one of the most effective treatment combinations for depression. Because she has average cognitive skills and insight into her difficulties, therapy using cognitive-behavioral methods would likely be helpful in allowing her to gain positive momentum and initiate problem solving. Therapy should focus on changing sleeping and eating patterns, as well as on assisting her in setting specific personal and educational goals for herself.

With regard to attention, it appears that Sarah benefited greatly from the trial of stimulant medication (i.e., Ritalin). With this in mind, if antidepressant medication does not significantly alter her ability to maintain attention, it is suggested that she also receive stimulant medication in order to address difficulties with sustained attention. Caregivers should gain her full and undivided attention before assigning tasks, chores, or assignments and keep her highly involved in activities during which her attention may wane. Use hands-on or interactive activities when possible to engage her in the task. Work periods can be assigned giving Sarah preestablished time limits to prevent her from feeling overwhelmed by the task; occasional breaks and changes of task should be provided for her in the classroom and at home. Also, isolating distractions in the classroom via barriers or preferential seating arrangements may alleviate some of the distractions that inhibit her full attention to a task.

In order to address social skills and interpersonal relationships, it is very important that Sarah return to school, at least on a part-time basis, so that she may meet the developmentally appropriate goal of having relationships with same-age peers. She is clearly feeling isolated from others her age, which is one of the causes of her mild depression. In addition, Sarah's caregivers should look into getting her involved in other activities outside of the home. She may enjoy organized sports through her city's Parks and Recreation department or life enrichment classes offered by local community colleges at a reduced rate. This would serve to increase her self-esteem and decrease her social isolation.

Because of her slower processing speed, Sarah may be pressured to rush through tasks and therefore complete tasks incorrectly; therefore, she must not be pressured by strict time limits. She should be allowed extra time to complete tests, homework assignments, or other classroom tasks. Accuracy should be encouraged over speed. Assignments may need to be shortened so that Sarah can complete them within a given time period. Also, due to Sarah's diminished processing speed, it will be very difficult for her to take notes in class and ensure that she has gathered all the information. With this in mind, provide Sarah with annotated notes, allowing her to fill in the blanks with key concepts so that she is an active participant in the lecture but is not negatively impacted by slow processing speed. Otherwise, a copy of a peer's notes or teacher notes may need to be provided to her.

A related issue is the rate of presentation for new material, which may need to be altered for Sarah. She may need additional processing time or time to rehearse the information. When learning large amounts of information, Sarah will need to take a break between sections. Otherwise, her new learning will be impaired by interference from material already learned.

With regard to organization and planning, Sarah needs to be encouraged to take time to prepare for a task, especially a multistep task, prior to attempting it. It might be helpful to write out the steps before attempting the task or to review an already-made list. This will give her time to think through the process of completing such tasks. It will also be important for Sarah to find the right studying place and keep it consistent. At home, gather the necessary materials and keep them in a common location near her work area. At school, create an organizational system using a notebook with dividers for each individual class. Maintain an agenda book to keep track of assignments and due dates.

## General Interventions

Every child with asthma will have different needs. If children have severe asthma and have been hospitalized on numerous occasions due to respiratory difficulty or failure, they may demonstrate greater neurocognitive weaknesses, especially with regard to attention, processing speed, memory, and other select skills.

Primary interventions should be targeted at preventing the onset of an asthma attack by reducing or eliminating the exposure to triggers and ensuring that the child has easy access to their necessary medications (Fletcher-Janzen, 2005). In order to provide children with asthma a safe environment and access to medications when needed, families and schools must be given education and training.

With regard to family education, pulmonologists and other specialized health care workers should ensure that caregivers are provided with detailed information about their child's health needs. Research has shown that poor parental literacy is associated with greater incidence of emergency room visits, hospitalizations, and school absences (DeWalt, Dilling, Rosenthal, & Pignone, 2007). Even more, poor parental health literacy (i.e., the ability to comprehend the complexities of medical treatments) is linked to generally poor health outcomes (Rudd et al., 2004; Wittich, Mangan, Grad, Wang, & Gerald, 2007).

In addition to the importance of parental literacy and comprehension of complex medical terminology and routines, general family processes have also been found to impact health outcomes for children with asthma. Caregiver stress (especially after experiencing their child's life-threatening asthma episode), maternal depression, and caregiver anxiety were found to be related to adherence to long-term medications and general asthma severity (Bartlett et al., 2004; Kean, Kelsay, Wamboldt, & Wamboldt, 2006; Silver, Warman, & Stein, 2005). Interestingly, although high levels of parental criticism led to poorer adherence to medication, criticism was also associated with better outcomes following inpatient treatment for adolescents with severe asthma (Wamboldt, Wamboldt, Gavin, Roesler, & Brugman, 1995). In addition, research has documented that children whose families are characterized by high levels of conflict experience a greater number of lifetime hospitalizations (Chen, Bloomberg, Fisher, & Strunk, 2003). Taking a family-systems perspective, it is clear that family variables (psychosocial functioning, level of conflict, communication) are related to management of asthma and its neurocognitive and psychological effects (Celano, 2006). Family-focused intervention through education regarding important medical issues; psychoeducation, including training in problem solving and novel coping strategies; and therapy to address dysfunctional patterns within the family have been supported in the literature as increasing positive outcomes for children with asthma and other chronic medical disorders (Campbell, 2003). It is recommended that a pediatric psychologist collaborate with children, their families, and the medical team in order to positively impact health outcomes by addressing family processes that influence asthma morbidity (Celano).

School personnel also must be provided with education and support in order to positively impact the health and general educational performance of children with asthma. The CDC (2002) offers six strategies to consider when addressing asthma in the schools through maintaining a systems perspective that includes school health services, psychological/social services, health education, nutrition services, family involvement, physical education, and environmental considerations. These strategies include management of support systems for asthma-friendly schools; arrangement of health and mental health services; provision of asthma education and awareness to all students and staff; creation of a healthy school environment; preparation of safe physical activity opportunities; and coordination of all involved individuals (i.e., family, school, community) to manage asthma symptoms and reduce absences.

It is apparent that everyone within the school community plays a vital role in the prevention and treatment of asthma and its effects. Although school nurses may be the members of a school's faculty who most frequently intervene directly with children with asthma, school nurses are not always available. Research has determined that classroom teachers can learn to effectively recognize the visual signs and symptoms of increasing respiratory difficulty for their students with asthma and can increase their comfort level of identifying symptoms through a very brief (i.e.,1-hour) education session (Sapien, Fullerton-Gleason, & Allen, 2004). Increased proficiency in symptom identification, and therefore increased comfort with symptom identification, could lead to better outcomes for the affected children by means of a shorter response time for acute medication use and faster initiation of emergency medical services, if the situation warrants (Sapien et al., 2004). As a result, children with asthma may have better outcomes if their respiratory difficulties do not escalate into very severe episodes that lead to intubation or hypoxic episodes. However, even prior to the onset of asthma symptoms, teachers may be able to learn about antecedents and other triggers for a child's asthma episodes, including high ambient temperature or high levels of air pollution that may be reported by the media or accessed through other local resources. Teachers may also better serve their students with asthma by recognizing that difficulties in academic performance may be partially due to the side effects of medication (de Mesquita & Fiorello, 1998).

Finally, school psychologists are greatly underutilized in terms of managing asthma symptoms and preventing increased respiratory difficulties. In fact, school psychologists have special training to assist in stress reduction and instruct in relaxation methods (Fletcher-Janzen, 2005). Because children may experience increased anxiety upon the initiation of respiratory difficulties, training in relaxation methods may delay the progression of symptoms so that they do not become life threatening.

Education and support of families and school personnel is clearly important for children with asthma. However, education of and direct intervention with the children themselves is essential. The NAEP (1997) recommended that patient-focused asthma education include information on asthma medication, including medications' mechanisms of action and appropriate use; avoidance of triggers; and response plans for increased symptom severity. One study instituted a multimedia, Web-based asthma management program in several inner-city schools, which focused on increasing controller medication adherence, increasing availability of rescue medications, and reducing smoking (Joseph et al., 2007). At 12 months following completion of the intervention, adolescents in the treatment group reported fewer symptom days/nights, days of restricted activity, and school absences compared to the control group. They also reported better quality of life compared to the control group, which was only exposed to generic asthma Web sites.

Another study utilized daily Web-based monitoring of asthma symptoms and found that adolescents with poorly controlled asthma reported positive experiences and a greater likelihood to incorporate such an intervention into the regular treatment regimen (van der Meer et al., 2007). Other technology-based asthma management tools are currently in development or being investigated and have shown promise as a successful component of multisystemic asthma monitoring (for descriptions of some of these tools, see Bensley et al., 2004; Bruzzese et al., 2004; Guendelman, Meade, Benson, Chen, & Samuels, 2002; Krishna et al., 2003).

Besides the aforementioned media-based instruction and monitoring for children and adolescents with asthma, a private online computer network was made available to children and adolescents who were hospitalized due to their increase in asthma symptoms (Hazzard, Celano, Collins, & Markov, 2002). The computer network provided health education via access to specific programs and selected Web sites, participation in online recreational activities (e.g., games, crafts), and communication (e.g., video conference, email, chatrooms) with hospitalized peers. Although significant changes were not found for children in the treatment group, adolescents demonstrated a trend toward increased knowledge about asthma.

In addition to education and monitoring, interventions should also focus on reduction of asthma-related psychological symptoms (i.e., anxiety, depression, stress, anger; Abrams, 1990). Research has shown that even preschool children with asthma can demonstrate increased cooperation with necessary asthma-related management and interventions after participating in a family asthma education program that utilized storytelling, imagery, and relaxation (Kohen & Wynne, 1997). This has implications for techniques used in asthma clinics by social workers and pediatric psychologists.

For adolescents, perceptions of breathlessness, which is not related to actual lung function, were decreased slightly by positive imagery (Rietveld, Everaerd, & van Beest, 2000). Similarly, children reported less shortness of breath when viewing movie clips that elicited a positive emotional state (Von Leupoldt, Riedel, & Dahme, 2006). These results lead to two counterintuitive hypotheses. First, probably the most prominent message is the potential benefit of inducing positive emotional states when children with asthma are feeling short of breath. However, a second, more threatening issue is the tendency to underreport the seriousness of breathlessness when in a positive emotional state, which could then perhaps lead to delayed treatment and increased risk of serious complications. Both of these issues must be seriously considered prior to eliciting positive emotional states during episodes of breathlessness for children with asthma.

In addition to elicitation of positive imagery, several other methods have also been investigated in the literature as possible psychological interventions for children with asthma in order to prevent the onset or reduce the intensity of their episodes (for a review of the following methods, see McQuaid & Nassau, 1999). Relaxation training, especially for children with emotionally triggered asthma attacks, has been shown to be correlated with small positive pulmonary function changes. Several different types of biofeedback have been shown to possibly decrease respiratory resistance and reduce muscle tension in the face and neck that lead to increased airway constriction. Family therapy is the third method of intervention for children with asthma. Specifically, family therapy may reduce maladaptive interactions that affect the course of asthma.

## CONCLUSION

Children and adolescents with asthma have the opportunity to control their symptoms through a variety of methods including management of the environment and limited exposure to triggers and intervention by means of medication. While these children are still young, family members and school personnel have the responsibility to monitor the environment and their symptoms and intervene when necessary. As children with asthma enter adolescence, issues regarding self-efficacy and independence may conflict with good asthma management practice. However, although asthma is one of the most chronic health problems in children, it does not have to lead to negative outcomes regarding cognitive functioning, academic achievement, or psychological functioning if the appropriate prevention and intervention methods are applied.

## RESOURCES

### Books and Pamphlets

Allen, J. L., Bryant-Stephens, T., & Pawlowski, N. A. (Eds.). (2004). *Guide to asthma: How to help your child live a happier life.* Hoboken, NJ: John Wiley & Sons.

Centers for Disease Control and Prevention (CDC). (2002). *Strategies for addressing asthma within a coordinated school health program.* Atlanta, GA: CDC National Center for Chronic Disease Prevention and Health Promotion. Available at http://www.cdc.gov/HealthyYouth/asthma/strategies.htm

Farber, H., & Boyette, M. (2001). *Control your child's asthma: A breakthrough program for the treatment and management of childhood asthma.* New York: Henry Holt and Company.

Gosselin, K. (1996). *ZooAllergy: A fun story about allergy and asthma triggers.* Plainview, NY: Jayjo Books.

Gosselin, K. (1997). *SPORTSercise!* Plainview, NY: Jayjo Books.

Gosselin, K. (1998). *The ABCs of asthma: An asthma alphabet book for kids of all ages.* Plainview, NY: Jayjo Books.

Gosselin, K. (1998). *Taking asthma to school* (2nd ed.). Plainview, NY: Jayjo Books.

Kroll, V. L. (2005). *Brianna breathes easy: A story about asthma.* Morton Grove, IL: Albert Whitman and Company.

London, J. (1992). *The lion who had asthma.* Morton Grove, IL: Albert Whitman and Company.

Plaut, T. F. (1998). *Children with asthma: A manual for parents.* Amherst, MA: Pedipress.

Weiss, J. H. (2003). *Breathe easy: Young people's guide to asthma.* New York: Magination.

## Organizations and Web Sites

American Academy of Allergy, Asthma, and Immunology (AAAAI)

The AAAAI supplies information for patients and professionals through provision of current pollen counts, medication guides, and tip sheets.

Mailing Address: 555 East Wells Street, Suite 1100
Milwaukee, Wisconsin 53202
Web Site: www.aaaai.org

American Lung Association (ALA)

The ALA provides information for patients, families, educators, and others regarding asthma management, treatment, and research.

Mailing Address: 61 Broadway, 6th Floor
New York, New York 10006
Phone Number: (800) LUNG-USA
Web Site: www.lungusa.org

Asthma and Allergy Foundation of America (AAFA)

The AAFA provides practical information, community-based services, and support through a national network of chapters and support groups.

Mailing Address: 1233 20th Street Northwest, Suite 402
Washington, D.C. 20036
Phone Number: (800) 7-ASTHMA
Web Site: www.aafa.org/index_noflash.cfm

Asthma Publications

This Web site, sponsored by the Pedipress, Inc., provides access to relatively inexpensive resources to track and manage asthma symptoms through diaries and action plans. They are available in English and Spanish.

Mailing Address: 125 Red Gate Lane
Amherst, Massachusetts 01002
Phone Number: (800) 611-6081
Web Site: www.pedipress.com/dap_main.html

National Asthma Education and Prevention Program (NAEPP)

The NAEPP works with major medical associations, voluntary health organizations, and community programs to educate patients, health professionals, and the public in order to enhance the quality of life for patients with asthma and decrease asthma-related morbidity and mortality. The Web site provides information for patients and their families, health care professionals, and school personnel.

Web Site: www.nhlbi.nih.gov/about/naepp/index.htm

## REFERENCES

Abrams, R. B. (1990). Adolescent health problems: A model for their solution. *Henry Ford Hospital Medical Journal, 38,* 160–161.

Abramson, S. L., Turner-Henderson, A., Anderson, L., Hemstreet, M. P., Tang, S., Bartholomew, L. K., et al. (2006). Allergens in school settings: Results of environmental assessments in three city school systems. *Journal of School Health, 76,* 246–249.

Achenbach, T. M., & Edelbrock, C. (1983). *Manual for the Child Behavior Checklist and Revised Behavior Profile.* Burlington: Department of Psychiatry, University of Vermont.

Akinbami, L. J. (2006). The state of childhood asthma, United States, 1980–2005. *Advance Data From Vital and Health Statistics, 281.* Hyattsville, MD: National Center for Health Statistics. Retrieved May 24, 2007, from http://www.cdc.gov/nchs/data/ad/ad381.pdf

Alpern, E. R., Stanley, R. M., Gorelick, M. H., Donaldson, A., Knight, S., Teach, S. J., et al. (2006). Epidemiology of a pediatric emergency medicine research network: The PECARN core data project. *Pediatric Emergency Care, 22,* 689–699.

American Lung Association (ALA). (2006). *Asthma and children fact sheet.* Retrieved May 29, 2007, from http://www.lungusa.org/site/pp.asp?c=dvLUK9O0E&b=44352

Annett, R. D., Aylward, E. H., Lapidus, J., Bender, B. G., & DuHamel, T. (2000). Neurocognitive functioning in children with mild and moderate asthma in the Childhood Asthma Management Program. *Journal of Allergy and Clinical Immunology, 105,* 717–724.

Babin, S. M., Burkom, H. S., Holtry, R. S., Tabernero, N. R., Stokes, L. D., Davies-Col, J. O., et al. (2007). Pediatric patient asthma-related emergency department visits and admissions in Washington, DC, from 2001–2004, and associations with air quality, socio-economic status and age group. *Environmental Health, 6,* 1–11. Retrieved May 10, 2007, from the PubMed database.

Bartlett, S. J., Krishnan, J. A., Riekert, K. A., Butz, A. M., Malveaux, F. J., & Rand, C. S. (2004). Maternal depressive symptoms and adherence to therapy in inner-city children with asthma. *Pediatrics, 113,* 229–237.

Beery, K. E., Buktenica, N. A., & Beery, N. A. (2005). *Beery-Buktenica Developmental Test of Visual-Motor Integration* (5th ed.). Lutz, FL: Psychological Assessment Resources, Inc.

Bender, B. G. (1995). Are asthmatic children educationally handicapped? *School Psychology Quarterly, 10,* 274–291.

Bensley, R. J., Mercer, N., Brusk, J. J., Underhile, R., Rivas, J., Anderson, J., et al. (2004). The eHealth Behavior Management Model: A stage-based approach to behavior change and management. *Preventing Chronic Disease, 1*(4), 1–13.

Benton, A. L., Hamsher, K. deS., Varney, N. R., & Spreen, O. (1983). *Judgment of Line Orientation.* New York: Oxford University Press.

Bruzzese, J., Bonner, S., Vincent, E. J., Sheares, B. J., Mellins, R. B., Levison, M. J., et al. (2004). Asthma education: The adolescent experience. *Patient Education and Counseling, 55,* 396–406.

Butz, A. M., Eggleston, P., Huss, K., Kolodner, K., Vargas, P., & Rand, C. (2001). Children with asthma and nebulizer use: Parental asthma self-care practices and beliefs. *Journal of Asthma, 38,* 565–573.

Campbell, T. L. (2003). The effectiveness of family interventions for physical disorders. *Journal of Marital and Family Therapy, 29,* 263–281.

Celano, M. P. (2006). Family processes in pediatric asthma. *Current Opinion in Pediatrics, 18,* 539–544.

Celano, M. P., & Geller, R. J. (1993). Learning, school performance, and children with asthma: How much at risk? *Journal of Learning Disabilities, 26,* 23–32.

Centers for Disease Control and Prevention (CDC). (2002). *Strategies for addressing asthma within a coordinated school health program.* Atlanta, GA: CDC National Center for Chronic Disease Prevention and Health Promotion. Retrieved May 6, 2007, from http://www.cdc.gov/HealthyYouth/asthma/strategies.htm

Centers for Disease Control and Prevention (CDC). (2004a). *National Center for Health Statistics fast stats: Asthma.* Retrieved February 25, 2005, from http://www.cdc.gov/nchs/fastats/asthma.htm

Centers for Disease Control and Prevention (CDC). (2004b). *Nine million U.S. children diagnosed with asthma, new report finds.* Retrieved February 25, 2005, from http://www.cdc.gov/nchs/pressroom/04news/childasthma.htm

Centers for Disease Control and Prevention (CDC). (2007). *National Center for Health Statistics fast stats: Asthma.* Retrieved May 24, 2007, from http://www.cdc.gov/nchs/fastats/asthma.htm

Centers for Disease Control and Prevention (CDC) and Health Data for All Ages (HDAA). (n.d.). *Asthma prevalence, health care use and mortality, 2002.* Retrieved May 24, 2007, from http://209.217.72.34/HDAA/tTableviewer/document.aspx?FileID=54

Centers for Disease Control and Prevention (CDC) and National Center for Environmental Health (NCEH). (n.d.). *You can control your asthma.* Retrieved May 24, 2007, from http://www.cdc.gov/asthma/pdfs/faqs.pdf

Centers for Disease Control and Prevention (CDC) and the National Center for Health Statistics (NCHS). (n.d.). *Asthma, all ages: US, 2000–2005.* Retrieved May 24, 2007, from http://209.217.72.34/HDAA/TableViewer/tableView.aspx

Chen, E., Bloomberg, G. R., Fisher, E. B., & Strunk, R. C. (2003). Predictors of repeat hospitalizations in children with asthma: The role of psychosocial and socioenvironmental factors. *Health Psychology, 22,* 12–18.

Chen, E., Hanson, M. D., Paterson, L. Q., Griffin, M. J., Walker, H. A., & Miller, G. E. (2006). Socioeconomic status and inflammatory processes in childhood asthma: The role of psychological stress. *Journal of Allergy and Clinical Immunology, 177,* 1014–1020.

Cohen, M. J. (1997). *Children's Memory Scale.* New York: The Psychological Corporation.

Creer, T. L., & Bender, B. G. (1995). Pediatric asthma. In M. C. Roberts (Ed.), *Handbook of pediatric psychology* (pp. 219–239). New York: Guilford Press.

de Mesquita, P. B., & Fiorello, C. A. (1998). Asthma (childhood). In L. Phelps (Ed.), *Health-related disorders in children and adolescents: A guidebook for understanding and educating* (pp. 74–81). Washington, DC: American Psychological Association.

Delis, D., Kaplan, E., & Kramer, J. (2001). *The Delis-Kaplan Executive Function System: Examiner's manual.* San Antonio, TX: The Psychological Corporation.

Delis, D. C., Kramer, J. H., Kaplan, E., & Ober, B. A. (1994). *California Verbal Learning Test—Children's Version.* San Antonio, TX: The Psychological Corporation.

Desager, K. N., Nelen, V., Weyler, J. J. J., & De Backer, W. A. (2005). Sleep disturbance and daytime symptoms in wheezing school-aged children. *Journal of Sleep Research, 14,* 77–82.

DeWalt, D. A., Dilling, M. H., Rosenthal, M. S., & Pignone, M. P. (2007). Low parental literacy is associated with worse asthma care measures in children. *Ambulatory Pediatrics, 7,* 25–31.

Dunleavy, R. A., & Baade, L. E. (1980). Neuropsychological correlates of severe asthma in children 9–14 years old. *Journal of Consulting and Clinical Psychology, 48,* 214–219.

Fiocchi, A., Terracciano, L., Martelli, A., Guerriero, F., & Bernardo, L. (2006). The natural history of childhood-onset asthma. *Allergy and Asthma Proceedings, 27,* 178–185.

Fiorello, C. A., & McLaughlin, E. M. (2004). Asthma: Information for parents and educators. *Communiqué, 33*(2), insert 1–3.

Fletcher-Janzen, E. (2005). The school neuropsychological examination. In R. C. D'Amato, E. Fletcher-Janzen, & C. R. Reynolds (Eds.), *Handbook of school neuropsychology* (pp. 172–212). Hoboken, NJ: John Wiley & Sons.

Fritz, G. K., & McQuaid, E. L. (2000). Chronic medical conditions: Impact on development. In A. J. Sameroff, M. Lewis, & S. M. Miller (Eds.), *Handbook of developmental psychopathology* (2nd ed., pp. 277–289). New York: Kluwer Academic/Plenum Press.

Glazebrook, C., McPherson, A. C., Macdonald, I. A., Swift, J. A., Ramsay, C., Newbould, R., et al. (2006). Asthma as a barrier to children's physical activity: Implications for body mass index and mental health. *Pediatrics, 118,* 2443–2449.

Goldberg, S., Israeli, E., Schwartz, S., Schochat, T., Izbicki, G., Toker-Maimon, O., et al. (2007). Asthma prevalence, family size and birth order. *Chest, 131,* 1747–1752. Retrieved May 8, 2007, from the PubMed database.

Goodwin, R. D., Messineo, K., Bregante, A., Hoven, C. W., & Kairam, R. (2005). Prevalence of probably mental disorders among pediatric asthma patients in an inner-city clinic. *Journal of Asthma, 42,* 643–647.

Guendelman, S., Meade, K., Benson, M., Chen, Y., & Samuels, S. (2002). Improving asthma outcomes and self-management behaviors of inner-city children: A randomized trial of the Health Buddy interactive device and an asthma diary. *Archives of Pediatrics and Adolescent Medicine, 156,* 114–120.

Hallstrand, T. S., Fischer, M. E., Wurfel, M. M., Afari, N., Buchwald, D., & Goldberg, J. (2005). Genetic pleiotropy between asthma and obesity in a community-based sample of twins. *Journal of Allergy and Clinical Immunology, 116,* 1235–1241.

Hazzard, A., Celano, M., Collins, M., & Markov, Y. (2002). Effects of STARBRIGHT World on knowledge, social support, and coping in hospitalized children with sickle cell disease and asthma. *Children's Health Care, 31,* 69–86.

Henry, C. N., & DuPaul, G. J. (2004). Pediatric asthma among African American children: The emerging role of the school psychologist. *Communiqué, 33*(2), 30–33.

Joseph, C. L. M., Peterson, E., Havstad, S., Johnson, C. C., Hoerauf, S., Stringer, S., et al. (2007). A web-based, tailored asthma management program for urban African-American high school students. *American Journal of Respiratory and Critical Care Medicine, 175,* 888–895.

Kattan, M., Mitchell, H., Eggleston, P., Gergen, P., Crain, E., Redline, S., et al. (1997). Characteristics of inner-city children with asthma: The national cooperative inner-city asthma study. *Pediatric Pulmonology, 24,* 253–262.

Kean, E. M., Kelsay, K., Wamboldt, F., & Wamboldt, M. Z. (2006). Posttraumatic stress in adolescents with asthma and their parents. *Journal of the American Academy of Child and Adolescent Psychiatry, 45,* 78–86.

Klinnert, M. D., Nelson, H. S., Price, M. R., Adinoff, A. D., Leung, D.Y.M., & Marzek, D. A. (2001). Onset and persistence of childhood asthma: Predictors from infancy. *Pediatrics, 108,* e69–77.

Kohen, D. P., & Wynne, E. (1997). Applying hypnosis in a preschool family asthma education program: Uses of storytelling, imagery, and relaxation. *American Journal of Clinical Hypnosis, 39,* 169–181.

Krishna, S., Francisco, B., Balas, A., Konig, P., Graff, G., & Madsen, R. (2003). Internet-enabled interactive multimedia asthma education program: A randomized trial. *Pediatrics, 111,* 503–510.

Lai, L., Hopp, R. J., & Lusk, R. P. (2006). Pediatric chronic sinusitis and asthma: A review. *Journal of Asthma, 43,* 719–725.

Lara, M., Akinbami, L., Flores, G., & Morgenstern, H. (2006). Heterogeneity of childhood asthma among Hispanic children: Puerto Rican children bear a disproportionate burden. *Pediatrics, 117,* 43–53.

Lasmar, L. M., Camargos, P. A., Goulart, E. M., & Sakurai, E. (2006). Risk factors for multiple hospital admissions among children and adolescents with asthma. *Jornal Brasileiro de Pneumologia, 32,* 391–399.

Leark, R. A., Dupuy, T., Greenberg, L., Kindschi, C., & Corman, C. (1996). *Test of Variables of Attention: Professional manual.* Los Alamitos, CA: Universal Attention Disorders.

McCoy, K., Shade, D., Irvin, C. G., Mastronarde, J. G., Hanania, N. A., Castro, M., et al. (2006). Predicting episodes of poor asthma control in treated asthmatics. *Journal of Allergy and Clinical Immunology, 117,* 557–562.

McFadden, E. R., Jr., & Warren, E. L. (1997). Observations on asthma mortality. *Annals of Internal Medicine, 127,* 142–147.

McQuaid, E. L., Kopel, S. J., & Nassau, J. H. (2001). Behavioral adjustment in children with asthma: A meta-analysis. *Journal of Developmental and Behavioral Pediatrics, 22,* 430–439.

McQuaid, E. L., & Nassau, J. H. (1999). Empirically supported treatments of disease-related symptoms in pediatric psychology: Asthma, diabetes, and cancer. *Journal of Pediatric Psychology, 24,* 305–328.

McQuaid, E. L., & Walders, N. (2003). Pediatric asthma. In M. C. Roberts (Ed.), *Handbook of pediatric psychology* (3rd ed., pp. 269–285). New York: Guilford Press.

National Asthma Education and Prevention (NAEP). (1997). *Practical guide for the diagnosis and management of asthma expert panel report 2: Guidelines for the diagnosis and management of asthma* (NIH Publication No. 97-4053). Hyattsville, MD: U.S. Department of Health and Human Services. Retrieved June 7, 2007, from http://www.nhlbi.nih.gov/health/prof/lung/asthma/practgde/practgde.pdf

National Institute of Allergy and Infectious Diseases (NIAID). (2004). *How to create a dust-free bedroom.* Retrieved May 29, 2007, from http://www.niaid.nih.gov/factsheets/dustfree.htm

Naudé, H., & Pretorius, E. (2003). Investigating the effects of asthma medication on the cognitive and psychosocial functioning of primary school children with asthma. *Early Child Development and Care, 173,* 699–709.

Papile, L. A., Tyson, J. E., Stoll, B. J., Wright, L. L., Donovan, E. F., Bauer, C. R., et al. (1998). A multicenter trial of two dexamethasone regimens in ventilator-dependent premature infants. *New England Journal of Medicine, 338,* 1112–1118.

Phipatanakul, W. (2006). Environmental factors and childhood asthma. *Pediatric Annals, 35,* 646–656.

Plaut, T. F. (1998). *One minute asthma: What you need to know.* Amherst, MA: Pedipress.

Pollack, C. V., Jr., Pollack, E. S., Baren, J. M., Smith, S. R., Woodruff, P. G., Clark, S., et al. (2002). A prospective multicenter study of patient factors associated with hospital admission from the emergency department among children with acute asthma. *Archives of Pediatrics and Adolescent Medicine, 156,* 934–940.

Rachelefsky, G. S., Goldberg, M., Katz, R. M., Boris, G., Gyepes, M. T., Shapiro, M. J., et al. (1978). Sinus disease in children with respiratory allergy. *Journal of Allergy and Clinical Immunology, 61,* 310–314.

Reitan, R. (1969). *Finger Tapping Test.* Tucson: Reitan Neuropsychological Laboratories, University of Arizona.

Rhee, H., Wenzel, J., & Steeves, R. H. (2007). Adolescents' psychosocial experiences living with asthma: A focus group study. *Journal of Pediatric Health Care, 21,* 99–107.

Richards, W. (1994). Preventing behavior problems and allergies. *Clinical Pediatrics, 33,* 617–624.

Rietveld, S., & Colland, V. T. (1999). The impact of severe asthma on schoolchildren. *Journal of Asthma, 36,* 409–417.

Rietveld, S., Everaerd, W., & van Beest, I. (2000). Excessive breathlessness through emotional imagery in asthma. *Behaviour Research and Therapy, 38,* 1005–1014.

Ronchetti, R., Villa, M. P., Matricardi, P. M., La Grutta, S., Barreto, M., Pagani, J., et al. (2002). Association of asthma with extra-respiratory symptoms in school-children: Two cross-sectional studies 6 years apart. *Pediatric Allergy and Immunology, 13,* 113–118.

Rudd, R. E., Zobel, E. K., Fanta, C. H., Surkan, P., Rodriguez-Louis, J., Valderrama, Y., et al. (2004). Asthma: In plain language. *Health Promotion Practice, 5,* 334–340.

Sapien, R. E., Fullerton-Gleason, L., & Allen, N. (2004). Teaching school teachers to recognize respiratory distress in asthmatic children. *Journal of Asthma, 41,* 739–743.

Schmier, J. K., Manjunath, R., Halpern, M. T., Jones, M. L., Thompson, K., & Diette, G. B. (2007). The impact of inadequately controlled asthma in urban children on quality of life and productivity. *Annals of Allergy, Asthma, and Immunology, 98,* 245–251.

Shedd, A. D., Peters, J. I., Wood, P., Inscore, S., Forkner, E., Smith, B., et al. (2007). Impact of home environment characteristics on asthma quality of life and symptom scores. *Journal of Asthma, 44,* 183–187.

Shore, S. A., & Fredberg, J. J. (2005). Obesity, smooth muscle, and airway hyperresponsiveness. *Journal of Allergy and Clinical Immunology, 115,* 925–927.

Silver, E. J., Warman, K. L., & Stein, R. E. (2005). The relationship of caretaker anxiety to children's asthma morbidity and acute care utilization. *Journal of Asthma, 42,* 379–383.

Silverstein, M. D., Mair, J. E., Katusic, S. K., Wollan, P. E., O'Connell, E. J., & Yunginger, J. W. (2001). School attendance and school performance: A population-based study of children with asthma. *Journal of Pediatrics, 139,* 278–283.

Smart, B. A. (2004, Fall). The costs of asthma and allergy. *Allergy and Asthma Advocate.* Retrieved May 29, 2007, from http://www.aaaai.org/patients/advocate/2004/fall/costs.stm

Smedley, F. (n.d.). *Smedley Hand Dynamometer.* Wood Dale, IL: Stoelting.

Stoloff, S. W., & Boushey, H. A. (2006). Severity, control, and responsiveness in asthma. *Journal of Allergy and Clinical Immunology, 117,* 544–548.

Stores, G., Ellis, A. J., Wiggs, L., Crawford, C., & Thomson, A. (1998). Sleep and psychological disturbance in nocturnal asthma. *Archives of Disease in Childhood, 78,* 413–419.

Szefler, S. J. (2007). Advances in pediatric asthma 2006. *Journal of Allergy and Clinical Immunology, 119,* 558–562.

Trites, R. (n.d.). *Grooved Pegboard Test.* Lafayette, IN: Lafayette Instruments.

van der Meer, V., van Stel, H. F., Detmar, S. B., Otten, W., Sterk, P. J., Sont, J. K., et al. (2007). Internet based self-management offers and opportunity to achieve better asthma control in adolescents. *Chest, 132,* 112-119. Retrieved June 29, 2007, from the PubMed database.

van Gent, R., van der Ent, C. K., Rovers, M. M., Kimpen, J. L. L., van Essen-Zandvliet, L. E. M., & de Meer, G. (2007). Excessive body weight is associated with additional loss of quality of life in children with asthma. *Journal of Allergy and Clinical Immunology, 119,* 591–596.

Virant, F. S. (2000). Sinusitis and pediatric asthma. *Pediatric Annals, 29,* 434–437.

Von Leupoldt, A., Riedel, F., & Dahme, B. (2006). The impact of emotions on the perception of dyspnea in pediatric asthma. *Psychophysiology, 43,* 641–644.

Wade, S., Weil, C., Holden, G., Mitchell, H., Evans, R., III, Kruszon-Moran, D., et al. (1997). Psychosocial characteristics of inner-city children with asthma: Description of the NCICAS psychosocial protocol. *Pediatric Pulmonology, 24,* 263–276.

Wamboldt, F. S., Wamboldt, M. Z., Gavin, L. A., Roesler, T. A., & Brugman, S. M. (1995). Parental criticism and treatment outcome in adolescents hospitalized for severe chronic asthma. *Journal of Psychosomatic Research, 39,* 995–1005.

Wechsler, D. (1999). *Wechsler Abbreviated Scale of Intelligence.* San Antonio, TX: The Psychological Corporation.

Wechsler, D. (2003). *Wechsler Intelligence Scale for Children* (4th ed.). San Antonio, TX: The Psychological Corporation.

Wittich, A. R., Mangan, J., Grad, R., Wang, W., & Gerald, L. B. (2007). Pediatric asthma: Caregiver health literacy and the clinician's perception. *Journal of Asthma, 44,* 51–55.

Wood, B. L., Miller, B. D., Lim, J., Lillis, K., Ballow, M., Stern, T., et al. (2006). Family relational factors in pediatric depression and asthma: Pathways of effect. *Journal of the American Academy of Child and Adolescent Psychiatry, 45,* 1494–1502.

Woodcock, R. W., McGrew, K. S., & Mather, N. (2001). *Woodcock-Johnson Tests of Achievement* (3rd ed.). Rolling Meadows, IL: Riverside.

# CHAPTER TWO

# Brain Tumors

Sarah Schnoebelen, PhD, Roger Perez, PhD, and
Peter L. Stavinoha, PhD

## DESCRIPTION OF THE DISORDER

### Incidence and Prevalence

Recent statistics indicate that 16.6% of all childhood cancer cases are brain or other central nervous system (CNS) tumors (Gurney, Smith, & Bunin, 1999). Nonetheless, pediatric brain tumor is relatively uncommon in the general population, with the Central Brain Tumor Registry of the United States (CBTRUS) estimating 3,410 new cases of pediatric primary brain and CNS tumor in 2005. It should be noted that incidence rates vary among sources depending on whether nonmalignant tumors are also included in the statistic. For example, data collected by the National Cancer Institute includes only malignant tumors and estimates that approximately 2,200 individuals under the age of 20 years are diagnosed with malignant CNS tumors annually (Gurney et al.). When both malignant and nonmalignant tumors are considered, there is an overall pediatric incidence of 4.3 per 100,000, with the rate slightly higher for males (4.5 per 100,000) than females (4.1 per 100,000) (CBTRUS, 2005). Significant medical advances have resulted in improved survival rates, such that approximately 73% of children who have been diagnosed with a brain or other CNS tumor are expected to survive for at least five years (Jemal et al., 2005). However, survival rates vary widely by tumor type and location. It is estimated that there are over 21,000 children living in the United States who have been diagnosed with brain tumor (CBTRUS). When considered from this perspective, it is not at all unlikely that any given school district may serve a child who is a survivor of brain tumor.

## Etiology and Underlying Causes

In the vast majority of cases, the underlying etiology for brain tumors is unknown. However, it is believed that two processes are related to the pathogenesis of brain tumors: the increased expression of growth-promoting factors (i.e., proto-oncogenes) that cause cells to grow in an out-of-control manner and the inactivation of those genes that in general function to suppress cell growth (i.e., tumor suppressor genes; Menkes & Till, 1995). Therefore, the disruption of normal restraints allows for unusual cellular proliferation.

Several genetic conditions increase the risk of CNS tumors as well as tumors of other systems, including neurofibromatosis (types 1 and 2), tuberous sclerosis, and von Hippel-Lindau, Li-Fraumeni, Turcot, and Gorlin syndromes (Melean, Sestini, Ammannati, & Papi, 2004). Some tumor types are congenital, including craniopharyngiomas and some medulloblastomas, and result from an area of neural mal-development (Menkes & Till, 1995). Research suggests that certain viruses may be involved in the development of tumor, although the specific role such viruses play in human brain tumors remains unclear and is likely moderated by a number of other factors, including environmental and patient variables (White et al., 2005). Other known risk factors include gender, with males demonstrating a higher incidence for specific tumor types (e.g., medulloblastoma and ependymoma), and therapeutic doses of ionizing radiation delivered to the head, for example, to treat previous brain tumor or leukemia (for a review, see Gurney et al., 1999). Possible risk factors include the inclusion of cured meat in the maternal diet during pregnancy, a parent or sibling diagnosed with brain tumor, and a family history of bone cancer, leukemia, or lymphoma (Gurney et al.). However, as the authors point out, these data are not conclusive as confounding factors exist, including other aspects of diet and the possibility that the genetic syndromes described above explain the increased risk in children with a family history of cancer. A recent literature review indicated that research suggests no causal link between brain tumor and exposure to cell phones and to high residential electromagnetic fields, but some literature implicates exposures to carcinogenic industrial, residential, and personal chemicals as a cause of brain tumors, although the data are far from conclusive or consistent (Wrensch, Minn, Chew, Bondy, & Berger, 2002).

## Factors Affecting Neuropsychological Outcome

Several factors are critical to consider when predicting the effect a primary brain tumor may have on ultimate medical and neuropsychological outcome. These include the location of the tumor, type of tissue involved, growth rate and invasiveness of the tumor, and the treatments the child has undergone. Although new treatment methods are continually being explored, the three primary treatment options at the current time are neurosurgery, radiation therapy (including craniospinal and focal radiation, as well as radiosurgery), and chemotherapy.

### *Neurosurgery*

Neurosurgery is typically the first intervention in the treatment of pediatric brain tumor. The goal of surgery is complete removal of tumor tissue while limiting injury to the surrounding healthy tissue (Sills, 2005). Surgical resection of a tumor also is used to determine a diagnosis, to alleviate symptoms caused by the tumor, or to potentially cure the illness (Schold et al., 1997). Complications following neurosurgery to treat brain tumors occur in approximately 5% to 8% of cases and include seizures, accumulation of blood (i.e., hematoma) or fluid (i.e., edema) surrounding the surgical site, and temporary or permanent neurological deficits (Sills). Despite advanced surgical techniques, death during the course of surgery occurs in approximately 5% of brain tumor cases (Grant, 2004). However, as indicated previously, the rate of brain tumor survivorship has increased over the past several decades, and this has led to an increased focus on the negative effects of cancer treatment on cognitive functioning. Surgery on the developing brains of children can result in a variety of short- and long-term cognitive deficits.

Such deficits can vary in type and severity. A study conducted by Carpentieri and colleagues (2003) on children surgically treated for brain tumors (e.g., craniopharyngioma, optic glioma, low-grade/pilocytic astrocytoma, and ependymoma) found deficits in nonverbal intellectual ability, perceptual organization, and visual memory. Verbal deficits were observed in the areas of word retrieval, memory, and recognition, in addition to impairments in fine motor speed and dexterity. In terms of specific tumor types, children surgically treated for craniopharyngiomas have been shown to demonstrate deficits in verbal and visual-spatial memory (Carpentieri et al., 2001). Similarly, studies have shown that surgical resection of pituitary tumors in adults can result in impaired anterograde memory (Guinan, Lowly, Stanhope, Lewis, & Kopelman, 1998). Deficits in verbal and visual memory, executive functions, and manual speed and dexterity also have been noted in children and adults who underwent surgery for third-ventricle tumors (Friedman, Meyers, & Sawaya, 2003).

In the past, children treated for posterior fossa tumors were thought to have minimal cognitive impairment if they did not undergo cranial radiation or chemotherapy; however, recent research suggests a number of cognitive deficits in children following surgery for posterior fossa tumors. Deficits in memory, language abilities, attention, processing speed, and executive functions have been noted in children who have undergone surgical resection of posterior fossa tumors (Aarsen, Van Dongen, Paquier, Van Mourik, & Cateman-Berrevoets, 2004; Ater et al., 1996; Levisohn, Cronin-Golomb, & Schmahmann, 2000; Riva & Giorgi, 2000; Steinlin et al., 2003). Mixed results have been found for other cognitive functions. Some studies have noted declines in verbal, nonverbal, and overall intellectual functioning following surgery for posterior fossa tumors (Beebe et al., 2005; Steinlin et al.), whereas other studies have found no deficits in these intellectual domains (Karatekin, Lazareff, & Asarnow, 2000). Several studies have also demonstrated that surgical resection of posterior fossa tumors results in visual-spatial and visual-motor deficits (Aarsen et al., 2004; Levisohn et al., 2000; Steinlin et al.); however, others have found these skills to be intact (Ater et al.).

Neurosurgery to treat posterior fossa tumors can result in specific patterns of cognitive and behavioral changes in some children. One such condition is the cerebellar cognitive affective syndrome, which has been observed in patients following lesions to the cerebellum. This syndrome is characterized by deficits in executive function, including abstract reasoning, set shifting, planning, verbal fluency, and working memory. Impaired visual-spatial abilities, expressive language problems, changes in personality, and poor affect regulation and behavioral control also are observed. Overall, the cognitive impairments observed in cerebellar cognitive affective syndrome result in reduced intellectual ability (Schmahmann, 2004; Schmahmann & Sherman, 1998). The posterior fossa syndrome has also been documented in approximately 15% to 30% of children who underwent resection of a cerebellar tumor. These children initially may demonstrate mutism following surgery, which usually remits over a period of several months. Speech problems such as dysarthria (i.e., articulation difficulties) and oral apraxia (i.e., difficulty performing learned movements on command with the face, lips, tongue, cheeks, larynx, and pharynx) often develop during the recovery from mutism. The children exhibit personality changes that include emotional lability, regressed behavior, and reduction in voluntary movements (Schmahmann, 2004; Turkel et al., 2004). Studies have shown expressive language difficulties and irritability to be among the most common symptoms of posterior fossa syndrome (Kirk, Howard, & Scott, 1995). In general, the most common findings following neurosurgery for brain tumor relate to cognitive, behavioral, emotional, and verbal functioning.

### *Radiation*

Radiation therapy is frequently utilized in the treatment of malignant brain tumor and is often cited as having the greatest rate of neurocognitive morbidity of the various cancer treatments, especially when administered to the entire brain in high doses. Several different delivery approaches may be utilized. For more aggressive tumors or when there is risk of spread of disease, craniospinal radiation may be utilized, in which the entire neuroaxis (i.e., brain and spinal cord) is irradiated. Some tumor types can be treated with conformal (i.e., focal) radiation therapy, which targets the highest doses of radiation to the tumor and the surrounding site and thereby limits the overall amount of radiation delivered to the surrounding brain tissue. A recent advent has been stereotactic radiosurgery, which allows for focused, high doses of radiation to be delivered to delineated small targets within the brain. Common trade names for radiosurgical devices include Gamma Knife (manufactured by Elekta) and Cyberknife (manufactured by Accuray).

Whole-brain radiation can result in long-term declines in overall intellectual functioning (Palmer et al., 2001, 2003; Ris, Packer, Goldwein, Jones-Wallace, & Boyett, 2001; Spiegler, Bouffet, Greenberg, Rutka, & Mabbott, 2004), with a steeper decline observed for those with higher baseline performance (Palmer et al., 2003; Ris et al., 2001). It is important to note that the onset of these intellectual declines is generally delayed, occurring 1 to 2 years after the completion of radiation therapy and continuing for time periods of at least 5 to 7 years and possibly longer (e.g., Jankovic et al., 1994; Palmer et al., 2003); however, younger patients generally show a more immediate decline (Palmer et al., 2003).

Declines in intellectual functioning associated with radiation can be significant. In one study, 58% of patients demonstrated IQs above 80 at 5 years after treatment, but only 15% scored above this cutoff at 10 years posttreatment, with the children youngest at treatment faring the worst (Hoppe-Hirsch et al., 1990). It has been hypothesized that the observed declines in intelligence subsequent to cranial radiation therapy reflect problems in the development of some basic cognitive skills such as processing speed and working memory (Schatz, Kramer, Ablin, & Matthay, 2000), which are thought to be impacted by the effect of radiation on developing white matter (Mulhern et al., 1999; Reddick et al., 2003). Furthermore, these declines are likely representative of a reduced rate of learning new material as opposed to an actual loss of previously acquired skills, with one study finding that children treated for brain tumor demonstrated a learning rate that was 49% to 62% of that expected for same-age peers (Palmer et al., 2001). It is important to note that reduced doses of craniospinal radiation appear to offer some preservation of cognitive functioning; however, intellectual declines may be present even with reduced dosages, especially for younger patients (e.g., Kieffer-Renaux et al., 2000; Mulhern et al., 2005; Ris et al., 2001; Silber et al., 1992). Those children treated with focal radiation tend to demonstrate IQs comparable to those who have not received radiation (Merchant et al., 2004).

The most frequently cited specific neuropsychological impairments secondary to radiation therapy are problems with memory and attention (for a review, see Mulhern, Merchant, Gajjar, Reddick, & Kun, 2004). Deficits in processing speed also have been noted in children who have received cranial radiation therapy (Anderson, Godber, Smibert, Weiskop, & Ekert, 2004; Schatz et al., 2000). Problems in fine motor speed and coordination, visual-motor integration skills, visual-spatial functioning, verbal fluency, memory, and mathematics have been described in the pediatric brain tumor population as well (Johnson et al., 1994; Packer et al., 1987, 1989).

Clearly, the deficits described above have direct implications for educational performance, and research suggests academic impairments in children who have received radiation for brain tumor. As articulated by Butler and Mulhern (2005), academic failure is a "secondary deficit" resulting from the "core deficits" in executive functioning, attention, information processing, and fluid abilities that occur subsequent to the white matter damage sustained during radiation (Mulhern et al., 1999; Reddick et al., 2003). Deficits in academic performance have been noted whether the metric is standardized achievement testing or utilization of special education services. In a study conducted in France, Hoppe-Hirsch and colleagues (1990) noted that 34% of patients who had been diagnosed with a malignant posterior fossa tumor (i.e., medulloblastoma) showed academic delays of 2 or more years at 5 years posttreatment and that an additional 26% of the sample had been enrolled in a specialized school because of their inability to complete a normal curriculum. A recent study that analyzed the contributors to poor academic functioning revealed that children who had received radiation therapy demonstrated extremely poor academic fluency even though their basic academic skills remained within the average range (Stavinoha & Burrows, 2004), which is consistent with the research cited above regarding the effects of radiation on processing speed. In general, performance on measures of math achievement in the irradiated population is more impaired than reading (Buono et al., 1998; Packer et al., 1987), especially in those children who require a shunt to treat hydrocephalus (Mabbott et al., 2005). However, reading development appears particularly vulnerable in young children who receive radiation therapy (Mabbott et al.; Mulhern et al., 2005).

### *Chemotherapy*

Chemotherapy is another frequently used treatment for brain tumor and is administered orally, intravenously, or intrathecally (i.e., use of lumbar puncture to deliver medication to the fluid surrounding the spinal cord). Most chemotherapy agents function by impairing cell division (i.e., mitosis), thereby targeting those cells that are dividing in a rapid manner. The fact that chemotherapy affects cells undergoing mitosis explains many of the side effects. For example, cells in the hair, skin, and lining of the digestive system are constantly dividing and renewing, explaining hair loss (i.e., alopecia), sensitive or dry skin, and stomach problems for those patients on active chemotherapy. Because at any given point some cancer cells will be dividing and some will be resting, chemotherapy is generally given in cycles in order to increase the chances of attacking as many cancer cells as possible. Furthermore, children are generally on a combination of chemotherapy drugs as individual agents target cells at different stages of division.

Relatively few studies investigate the effects of chemotherapy without radiation in patients with brain tumors. An important exception would be in the treatment of optic pathway tumors. Within this population, a recent study suggested that treatment with chemotherapy in the absence of radiation may result in preserved neurocognitive functioning (Lacaze et al., 2003). In general, chemotherapy is thought to be a less toxic form of treatment (Ris & Noll, 1994) and, in some studies, has not been associated with significant declines in intellectual functioning (Copeland, Moore, Francis, Jaffe, & Culbert, 1996; Ellenberg, McComb, Siegel, & Stowe, 1987; Palmer et al., 2003). With the exception of visual-spatial skills, children who do not receive radiation, instead being treated with surgery only or surgery and chemotherapy, demonstrate better performance on a variety of neuropsychological tasks compared to patients receiving radiation (Moore, Ater, & Copeland, 1992). Nonetheless, the results of one study indicated that perhaps the number of different treatments a child receives may be a more accurate predictor of deficits than whether or not the child received radiation therapy (Carlson-Green, Morris, & Krawiecki, 1995). As with radiation, children treated with chemotherapy at a younger age appear to be affected more than older children, especially on nonverbal and perceptual-motor tasks and when chemotherapy is administered intrathecally as opposed to other delivery methods (Copeland et al., 1996). Possible neurocognitive effects associated with intrathecal chemotherapy include problems with attention, nonverbal memory, fine motor speed and coordination, and academic achievement, especially mathematics (Moleski, 2000). There is evidence that intrathecal methotrexate, a chemotherapy agent that blocks the metabolism of cells and is frequently used in the treatment of cancer, may compound the negative cognitive effects of radiation and intravenous chemotherapy in children with malignant brain tumors, especially in those patients younger than 10 years of age (Riva et al., 2002).

### *Other Variables Affecting Outcome*

In addition to the specific treatment modalities utilized to treat brain tumor, a variety of other factors impact ultimate neuropsychological outcome. For example, a number of studies suggest that females appear to be at higher risk for IQ declines associated with some treatments used to address malignancy (Bleyer et al., 1990; Ris et al., 2001; Waber, Tarbell, Kahn, Gelber, & Sallan, 1992). Age at diagnosis is an important consideration, as younger ages are associated with poorer neurocognitive outcome regardless of treatment type (Chapman et al., 1995). For children under 3 years of age, who represent approximately 20% of the pediatric brain tumor population, significant declines in intellectual functioning have been noted in those who have received craniospinal radiation (Copeland, deMoor, Moore, & Ater, 1999; Fouladi et al., 2005). Because of the neurocognitive vulnerability of children under 3 years of age, an attempt is often made to use chemotherapy to delay radiation.

Time since treatment is an essential variable as the neuropsychological deficits associated with brain tumor and its treatment are considered late effects, or consequences that become observable only over long-term follow-up. As was described above, particularly in the case of craniospinal radiation therapy, these effects may not appear for up to a year or more after treatment, and decrements in performance may become more obvious as time goes on.

Furthermore, tumor type and location are important considerations, especially in terms of how these variables guide treatment decisions. In broad terms, tumors are classified as infratentorial (i.e., below the tentorium and including the cerebellum and brain stem) and supratentorial (i.e., including the cerebral hemispheres and midline structures). In children, one-half to two-thirds of brain tumors occur infratentorially, many of them referred to as posterior fossa (meaning "back vault") tumors. Supratentorial tumors have been shown to result in greater neuropsychological deficits than infratentorial tumors (Ris & Noll, 1994). Finally, it is important to note that poor academic performance may be associated with other factors beyond simply a decline in cognitive functioning, including fatigue and absenteeism (Mabbott et al., 2005), as well as psychosocial variables such as coping resources and family functioning.

Although an exhaustive discussion of the various types of primary tumors is beyond the scope of this chapter, the most commonly observed primary brain tumors and their characteristics will be described briefly. The two most common pediatric tumor types, which account for the large majority of all pediatric brain tumors (Gurney et al., 1999), are gliomas and primitive neuroectodermal tumors (PNETs). Gliomas are tumors that arise from the glial cells, which are nonneuronal cells in the brain that provide support and nutrition and form myelin. The most common type is the astrocytoma, which develops from the astrocytes (i.e., star-shaped glial cells) and ranges from the more common low-grade pilocytic astrocytoma, which accounts for approximately 20% of all childhood tumors, to the highly aggressive glioblastoma multiforme, which accounts for approximately 3% of pediatric tumors (CBTRUS, 2005). Whereas pilocytic astrocytomas in general are treated with surgery alone, children with more aggressive astrocytomas may also receive radiation and chemotherapy. Other gliomas include ependymoma, ganglioglioma, and oligodendroglioma.

The single most common malignant childhood tumor is the medulloblastoma, a type of PNET. Other types of primitive neuroectodermal tumors, labeled as such because they are believed to arise from primitive, or undeveloped, neuroepithelial cells in the brain, include retinoblastoma, pineal blastoma, neuroblastoma, esthesioneuroblastoma, ganglioblastoma, and ependymoblastoma. Medulloblastomas occur in the posterior fossa and are treated with neurosurgery, radiation therapy, and chemotherapy.

Another tumor type that it is important to mention is the craniopharyngioma, which accounts for approximately 3% of all pediatric brain tumors (CBTRUS, 2005). Although these are generally considered to be histologically benign tumors, the fact that they are in general located in the hypothalamic-pituitary region results in a number of unique behavioral and emotional sequelae. These children often present with significant social and behavioral difficulties, school problems, visual complications, endocrine deficiency, and obesity (Poretti, Grotzer, Ribi, Schönle, & Boltshauser, 2004).

## RELATED MEDICAL ISSUES

Children presenting with brain tumor often exhibit a number of other medical conditions that must be considered when designing educational plans. During active stages of treatment, especially chemotherapy, patients may experience a number of side effects, although these are likely to vary depending on the specific agents utilized. Common side effects include fatigue, nausea, vomiting, and changes in appetite. Various problems are associated with low blood cell counts, including neutropenia (i.e., low white blood cell count), anemia (i.e., low red blood cell count), and thrombocytopenia (i.e., low blood platelet count). Therefore, there may be periods of time when it is not safe for students to attend school due to a depressed immune system, and homebound services may be necessary. Clinical experience suggests that it is imperative for good communication to exist between the school and the medical team as a percentage of children who have been on extended homebound services may demonstrate some degree of school refusal behavior when cleared to return to school, and it is important that this issue be addressed proactively. Short-term fatigue is also associated with radiation therapy, and a permanent loss or thinning of hair may occur around the area to which the radiation was administered.

A multitude of body systems are affected by treatment for a brain tumor, and the interested reader is referred to the National Cancer Institute's document *Late Effects of Treatment for Childhood Cancer* (2006) for a comprehensive review. Common late effects include problems with hearing, especially in those children who have received high doses of radiation therapy and platinum-containing chemotherapy agents (Landier, 1998). Visual impairments are also observed frequently in survivors of pediatric brain tumor (Macedoni-Luksic, Jereb, & Todorovski, 2003). In addition, endocrine abnormalities, including growth hormone deficiency, precocious puberty, and hypothyroidism, may be observed after radiation therapy (Duffner, 2004; Gurney et al., 2003). It is important to note that survivors of pediatric brain tumor have higher rates of epilepsy than the general population. Epilepsy could be related to either the tumor or the treatment, and one study indicated an overall epilepsy rate of 14.6% in brain tumor survivors, increasing to 38% in children treated for cortical tumors (Shuper et al., 2003). The presence of epilepsy in brain tumor survivors is associated with a higher risk of disability (Macedoni-Luksic et al., 2003). Furthermore, many children exhibit obstructive hydrocephalus associated with the tumor. If the hydrocephalus is acute, there may not be significant long-term effects (Ris & Noll, 1994). However, should a tumor be slow-growing and the child experience an extended period of hydrocephalus, those deficits generally associated with this condition in other clinical groups, specifically problems with attention, memory, and nonverbal abilities, may become apparent. For further information about hydrocephalus, please refer to the relevant chapter in this volume.

# RESULTS FROM NEUROPSYCHOLOGICAL EVALUATION

As discussed above, a number of factors affect the ultimate neuropsychological outcome of children who have been diagnosed with and treated for brain tumor. Because medulloblastomas are the most common malignant tumor type seen in the pediatric population and generally receive multiple forms of treatment, including neurosurgery, radiation therapy, and chemotherapy, a case with this tumor type has been selected for presentation. However, because brain tumor survivors are so variable in their presentation, comprehensive evaluation and long-term follow-up is necessary to document their profile of strengths and weaknesses and to note changes in status, both necessary functions for educational planning.

## Background and Demographic Information

At 8 years of age, Sophia, a right-handed Latina girl, presented for a magnetic resonance imaging (MRI) scan of her brain after an ophthalmologist noted diplopia (i.e., double vision), papilledema (i.e., optic disc swelling secondary to increased intracranial pressure), and a right VI cranial nerve palsy (i.e., paralysis of the lateral rectus muscle, affecting lateral eye movement from midline and often resulting in an inward turning of the eyes). The MRI revealed a large mass lesion within the posterior fossa with associated obstructive hydrocephalus. She underwent brain surgery, and the biopsy revealed tissue consistent with medulloblastoma. Shortly after the surgery, a 6-week course of craniospinal radiation was initiated. Chemotherapy was subsequently administered, lasting approximately 18 months. Sophia's cognitive function had not been assessed previously.

At the time of the evaluation, Sophia was 11 years old and in the fifth grade. The primary language spoken in the home was Spanish, although English was also spoken, and her mother was fluent in English. According to her mother, Sophia had been placed in a bilingual classroom from kindergarten through third grade. Since that time, all of her instruction was provided in English, and Sophia reported that she was more fluent in English than in Spanish. She received homebound services for much of fourth grade and the beginning of fifth grade secondary to her medical condition. At the time of the assessment, Sophia was placed in mainstream classes and had access to the Content Mastery classroom (i.e., supplemental instruction or assistance provided outside of the regular education classroom in an individual or small-group format, generally after receiving instruction in the regular education environment). She was receiving special education services under the disabling condition of Other Health Impairment (OHI).

Further information about Sophia's functioning in the school environment was obtained via a telephone interview with her teacher, who indicated that Sophia was a very hard worker and got along well with others. However, she reportedly fatigued very easily. Although the teacher indicated that she believed Sophia's comprehension of the English language to be adequate, it was also noted that she occasionally appeared to have difficulty grasping the concepts presented in class. Because of her visual difficulties, all of her work was presented in larger font, and she sat at the front of the classroom.

In the 4 to 5 months preceding the evaluation, Sophia became angry more easily than usual. Her mother reported that, when angry, Sophia would scream and throw things, although she had not broken anything nor been physically aggressive toward anyone. Her mother said that little things appeared to provoke such a reaction. Sophia was also reported to seem sad at times and often went into her room and cried. Sometimes, she would sit down and not do anything, complaining to her mother that she was bored. Although Sophia often did not verbalize why she was upset, she occasionally indicated that she felt lonely and was concerned that her peers no longer wanted to be her friends. Furthermore, Sophia became very frustrated when she had difficulty completing her homework. No significant problems with sleep were noted. On rare occasions, she complained of headaches and stomachaches. Her mother reported no significant behavioral difficulties other than those previously mentioned. Furthermore, she indicated that Sophia's teachers had reported no major problems with sustaining attention. However, Sophia's mother described her as displaying some forgetfulness and a tendency to lose items necessary for daily activities, such as her school folders. Additionally, Sophia's mother noted that her daughter appeared to be easily distracted from her homework by noises and other stimuli.

## Behavioral Observations

Sophia was evaluated over the course of a single testing session. She presented to the evaluation as a casually dressed and adequately groomed girl. Her mother accompanied her to the evaluation, and Sophia separated easily from her when it was time to begin the evaluation. Sophia demonstrated slower-than-average gross and fine motor movements. Although she initially was somewhat reserved, she was polite and socially appropriate. During the interview portion of the evaluation, however, she was very forthcoming with the examiner about her wish for more friends at school and her frustration regarding her difficulties with homework completion. Throughout the evaluation, Sophia was highly cooperative and extended her best effort. Within the one-on-one testing environment, she demonstrated no inattentiveness or hyperactivity. Although Sophia stated that she felt more comfortable communicating in English than Spanish, the results of the verbal tasks were interpreted with some caution, considering that English was her second language. However, given her good effort and cooperation, the test results were generally thought to be a valid and reliable estimate of her current level of functioning.

## Test Results

Data from the administered tests are listed in Tables 2.1 and 2.2. The results of the current evaluation revealed a pattern of neurocognitive deficits along with areas of preserved functioning, which is generally consistent with that of many children who have received craniospinal radiation and chemotherapy to treat malignant brain tumor. Results of intellectual testing indicated verbal reasoning abilities in the low average range, which may be a slight underestimate of her level of functioning given that English was her second language. However, she demonstrated significant difficulty on tasks of nonverbal reasoning and visual-spatial perception. Consistent with the research regarding the late effects of adjuvant treatments for brain tumor, Sophia also demonstrated significantly impaired working memory and processing speed. In addition, deficits were noted in her fine motor speed and dexterity. She also demonstrated some difficulty in the area of executive functions, a group of skills and processes that allow an individual to set an appropriate goal, develop organized plans to achieve it, implement plans and evaluate their effectiveness, and switch strategy as necessary.

Although Sophia's academic skills generally fell at the low end of the average range, her ability to perform academic tasks quickly and efficiently was significantly below average, as would be expected given her slow processing speed. Although she had worked very hard to maintain her academic skills, results of the testing were suggestive of some difficulty in her ability to learn and remember new information. The results indicated that she may be better able to recall information if she is allowed additional time to consolidate that material. Furthermore, her learning suffered when she was required to learn several pieces of information in rapid succession, as the previously learned information interfered with her ability to master new material.

Although Sophia was not described as exhibiting any acting-out behavior at school, both she and her mother reported that she easily became frustrated by her homework. Several months prior to the evaluation, she had exhibited an elevated level of sadness and anger. In part, this may have been due to her difficulties adapting to the demands of the school environment after an extended period of homebound service. Her severe neurocognitive deficits compromised her ability to perform in the academic setting, which is understandably frustrating to Sophia.

**TABLE 2.1 Neuropsychological Testing Data**

| Scale | Z Score | Scaled Score | Standard Score |
|---|---|---|---|
| Wechsler Intelligence Scale for Children—Fourth Edition | | | |
| Full Scale IQ | | | 71 |
| General Ability Index | | | 81 |
| Verbal Comprehension Index | | | 89 |
| Perceptual Reasoning Index | | | 73 |
| Working Memory Index | | | 77 |
| Processing Speed Index | | | 62 |
| Woodcock-Johnson Tests of Achievement—Third Edition | | | |
| Academic Skills | | | 90 |
| Academic Fluency | | | 77 |
| Letter-Word Identification | | | 92 |
| Reading Fluency | | | 78 |
| Passage Comprehension | | | 86 |
| Calculations | | | 83 |
| Math Fluency | | | 69 |
| Spelling | | | 91 |
| Writing Fluency | | | 82 |
| California Verbal Learning Test—Children's Version | | | |
| List A Total Trials 1-5 | | 5 | |
| List A Trial 1 Free Recall | −1.0 | | |
| List A Trial 5 Free Recall | −2.0 | | |
| List B Free Recall | −1.5 | | |
| List A Short-Delay Free Recall | −1.5 | | |
| List A Short-Delay Cued Recall | −1.5 | | |
| List A Long-Delay Free Recall | −1.0 | | |

**TABLE 2.1** *(Continued)*

| Scale | Z Score | Scaled Score | Standard Score |
|---|---|---|---|
| List A Long-Delay Cued Recall | −1.0 | | |
| Recognition | −0.5 | | |
| Wide Range Assessment of Memory and Learning—Second Edition | | | |
| Story Memory | | 6 | |
| Story Memory Recall | | 7 | |
| Story Recognition | | 7 | |
| Design Memory | | 8 | |
| Design Recognition | | 9 | |
| Picture Memory | | 3 | |
| Picture Memory Recognition | | 8 | |
| Wisconsin Card Sorting Test | | | |
| Total Errors | | | 71 |
| Perseverative Responses | | | 79 |
| Perseverative Errors | | | 78 |
| Nonperseverative Errors | | | 73 |
| Grooved Pegboard Test | | | |
| Preferred Hand (right) | −5.88 | | |
| Non-preferred Hand (left) | −8.29 | | |
| Beery-Buktenica Developmental Test of Visual-Motor Integration—Fifth Edition | | | |
| VMI | | | 85 |

*Note.* Beery-Buktenica Developmental Test of Visual-Motor Integration—Fifth Edition (VMI-5; Beery, Buktenica, & Beery, 2004); California Verbal Learning Test—Children's Version (CVLT-C; Delis, Kramer, Kaplan, & Ober, 1994); Grooved Pegboard Test (Lafayette Instrument Company, n.d.); Wechsler Intelligence Scale for Children—Fourth Edition (WISC-IV; Wechsler, 2003); Wide Range Assessment of Memory and Learning—Second Edition (WRAML-2; Adams & Sheslow, 2003); Wisconsin Card Sorting Test (WCST; Grant & Berg, 1993); Woodcock-Johnson Tests of Achievement—Third Edition (WJ-III; Woodcock, McGrew, & Mather, 2001).

**TABLE 2.2 Behavioral and Emotional Testing Data**

| Scale | T Score |
|---|---|
| Behavior Assessment System for Children—Second Edition, Parent Rating Scale | |
| Hyperactivity | 41 |
| Aggression | 55 |
| Conduct Problems | 40 |
| Anxiety | 84 |
| Depression | 85 |
| Somatization | 78 |
| Atypicality | 54 |
| Withdrawal | 53 |
| Attention Problems | 48 |
| Adaptability | 44 |
| Social Skills | 48 |
| Leadership | 59 |
| Activities of Daily Living | 57 |
| Functional Communication | 57 |
| Behavior Assessment System for Children—Second Edition, Self-Report | |
| Attitude to School | 43 |
| Attitude to Teachers | 46 |
| Anxiety | 55 |
| Depression | 50 |
| Sense of Inadequacy | 56 |
| Attention Problems | 49 |
| Hyperactivity | 46 |
| Atypicality | 45 |
| Locus of Control | 42 |
| Social Stress | 50 |
| Relations with Parents | 52 |
| Interpersonal Relations | 56 |
| Self-Esteem | 47 |
| Self-Reliance | 50 |

*Note.* Behavior Assessment Scale for Children—Second Edition (BASC-2; Reynolds & Kamphaus, 2004).

## Interventions

*Case-Specific Interventions*

Specifically for this case, the following recommendations were made:

1. To address Sophia's emotional symptoms associated with the challenges of adjusting to the consequences of her illness, we strongly recommended a course of individual therapy. During the interview, Sophia appeared rather insightful as to the underlying causes of her distress, and she was able to articulate her concerns. She also appeared to be able to identify and employ some basic coping strategies. Therefore, we believed that Sophia was likely to benefit from psychotherapy. A treatment plan that included cognitive-behavioral techniques as well as supportive counseling was suggested as being the most beneficial for Sophia.
2. As engagement in pleasant events is known to have a positive effect on mood, we strongly encouraged Sophia's parents to ensure that time is set aside each day for play and socialization. We noted that it would be beneficial to create opportunities for Sophia to spend time with friends, uninterrupted by siblings. Furthermore, facilitating Sophia's participation in extracurricular activities or going over to friends' houses also was described as important.
3. We highlighted the fact that it was necessary for Sophia's neurocognitive limitations to be considered in the development of her educational programming. For example, given her slowed processing speed, consideration of reduced assignments was encouraged. In addition, it was noted that Sophia may benefit from a brief break between the presentation of different concepts or ideas or between studying different subjects. Given her extremely impaired fine motor functioning, the amount of information to be copied from the board or projection screen should be limited, and Sophia should be allowed to obtain notes from peers or her teachers. During the feedback session, it was further suggested that as Sophia enters middle school and adjusts to the requirements for independent organization and planning, a specific time at the end of the day should be established for Sophia to meet with a teacher or a peer to ensure that assignments are recorded correctly and that she has all of the necessary materials to bring home. Such accommodations and interventions should be documented in her Individualized Education Program (IEP). It was noted that although Sophia's basic academic skills generally fell in the low average range during the current evaluation, we were concerned that she would increasingly struggle to develop her skills at the same pace

as her peers and that at some point a more restrictive educational environment might become necessary in order to provide Sophia with the type of individualized instruction she might require.

4. It was also important to note that Sophia's difficulties in the area of executive functioning may impact her ability to flexibly adapt to new situations or changes in plans. For example, Sophia may struggle to adjust her expectations when she is not allowed to do something for which she had already made plans. To accommodate for this weakness, her parents and teachers should be aware of her difficulties in switching set and provide advanced and clear warning about upcoming transitions.
5. High-frequency hearing loss is one of the common effects of the type of treatment that Sophia received. Therefore, we strongly recommended that the district's audiology specialist be consulted to determine whether additional interventions, such as a classroom amplification system, were necessary.
6. Finally, given that neurocognitive changes secondary to treatment for brain tumor continue to be observed for several years after the completion of therapy, we recommended that Sophia return for reevaluation in approximately 12 to 18 months. At that time, the effectiveness of the proposed interventions will be reviewed, and modifications can be made as necessary.

### *General Recommendations*

The recommendations listed above were generated based on an analysis of Sophia's specific needs. As indicated previously, a significant degree of heterogeneity exists within the pediatric brain tumor population depending on a multitude of factors, including age at diagnosis, type of treatment, and tumor type and location. It is important to note that many children with a history of pediatric brain tumor will not necessarily demonstrate testing results that are suggestive of a diagnosis of a specific learning disability. Nonetheless, their neurocognitive difficulties significantly impact their educational performance, and intervention often is required. Like Sophia, these children are likely to be eligible for special education services under the disabling condition of OHI.

Other accommodations and modifications that are commonly recommended to address the neurocognitive effects of brain tumor and its associated treatments involve modification of the school environment. For example, in Sophia's case, enlarged print text was required to accommodate her visual difficulties, and a classroom amplification system may be necessary to ensure that she can hear the teacher adequately above other classroom noise. Other environmental modifications include early release from class in order to facilitate navigation of the hallways without large crowds, as many children demonstrate residual gross motor impairment. Furthermore, especially during the active course of therapy, these children may be extremely fatigued. Therefore, they may need to rest in the nurse's office at various points in the day. Some children may require a shortened class day or the scheduling of core classes at a time when they feel the most alert. It may be necessary to reduce distractions and external stimuli in the classroom because problems with attention and concentration are commonly noted after brain tumor. In addition, the role of stimulant medication in an overall treatment package should be acknowledged. A few studies have examined the safety and efficacy of methylphenidate in survivors of pediatric cancer, finding improvement on direct measures of attentional functioning (Thompson et al., 2001), as well as on parent and teacher reports of attention and teacher reports of social skills and academic functioning (Mulhern, Khan, et al., 2004).

One of the keys to successful school reentry is close collaboration between the medical team at the hospital and the school education team (Upton & Eiser, 2006). In many hospitals, child life specialists, professionals trained to assist patients and their families in coping with stressful medical experiences, may be available to visit the school to share information about the child's condition and treatment with teachers and classroom peers. Furthermore, contact with the treatment team regarding the medical limitations of the child is essential. Certainly, some children, especially those who experience immunosuppression as a result of their treatment, may require a period of homebound instruction. However, as noted previously, clinical experience suggests that physicians generally attempt to encourage children to return to a normal school experience as early as it is safely possible to do so. Nonetheless, it has been the case that, due to poor communication, the school has not been aware that a child has been cleared to return to school, resulting in an unnecessarily protracted period of homebound services, which can increase the anxiety associated with returning to school and result in school-refusal behaviors. Therefore, the essential nature of proactive communication between the hospital and school cannot be stressed enough.

Finally, in addition to recognizing the traumatic nature of the experience of brain tumor and associated treatment for the child, it is also important to note the effect such an event has on the parents. Certainly, the parental response to a child's diagnosis and prognosis will vary, but some parents display significant difficulty coping with the condition and may benefit from efforts to increase their support network, including referrals to community-based support groups and possibly even psychotherapy. In addition to the emotional stress of caring for an ill child, practical and financial challenges also may be present, with some parents reducing the amount of time they work in order to care for their child or attempting to fit additional responsibilities, including bringing the child to numerous doctor's appointments, into an already-busy schedule. Therefore, referrals to community agencies that offer respite care could be helpful. Clinical experience suggests that some parents may be hesitant to employ the consistent discipline strategies that were used prior to the diagnosis for a variety of reasons, including fears about the fragility of the child and a sense that routine daily issues pale in comparison to the life-threatening nature of the child's disease. In these cases, parents may need support and encouragement to resume their normal parenting and discipline practices.

## RESOURCES

### Books

Deasy-Spinetta, P., & Irvin, E. (Eds.). (1993). *Educating the child with cancer.* Kensington, MD: The Candlelighters Childhood Cancer Foundation.

Henry, C. S., & Gosselin, K. (2001). *Taking cancer to school.* Plainview, NY: Jayjo Books.

Keene, N., Hobbie, W., & Ruccione, K. (2006). *Childhood cancer survivors* (2nd ed.). Sebastopol, CA: Patient Centered Guides.

Keene, N., & Romain, T. (2002). *Chemo, craziness and comfort: My book about childhood cancer.* Kensington, MD: The Candlelighters Childhood Cancer Foundation.

Klett, A., & Klett, D. (2001). *The amazing Hannah: Look at everything I can do!* Kensington, MD: The Candlelighters Childhood Cancer Foundation.

Maze, A. (2004). *Cutting up: Laughing and crafting ideas that helped one teenager through cancer treatment.* Oxon, England: Amazing Publications.

Woznick, L. A., & Goodheart, C. D. (2001). *Living with childhood cancer: A practical guide to help families cope.* Washington, DC: American Psychological Association.

### Organizations and Web Sites

American Brain Tumor Association

The American Brain Tumor Association provides funding for brain tumor research and offers educational and support services for patients and families.

Mailing Address: 2720 River Road, Suite 146
Des Plaines, Illinois 60018-4110
Phone Number: (800) 886-2282
Web Site: www.abta.org

American Cancer Society

The American Cancer Society is dedicated to eliminating cancer through research, education, advocacy, and service.

Phone Number: (800) ACS-2345
Web Site: www.cancer.org

The Brain Tumor Society

The Brain Tumor Society provides information, resources, and support for people affected by brain tumors.

Mailing Address: 124 Watertown Street, Suite 3H
Watertown, Massachusetts 02472
Phone Number: (800) 770-TBTS
Web Site: www.tbts.org

Candlelighters Childhood Cancer Foundation (CCCF)

CCCF was founded by parents and provides information and awareness for children and adolescents with cancer and their families.

Mailing Address: P.O. Box 498
Kensington, Maryland 20895
Phone Number: (800) 366-2223
Web Site: www.candlelighters.org

The Children's Brain Tumor Foundation

The Children's Brain Tumor Foundation is committed to improving treatments, quality of life, and long-term outcomes for children with brain and spinal cord tumors through research, support, education, and advocacy.

Mailing Address: 274 Madison Avenue, Suite 1004
New York, New York 10016
Phone Number: (914) 238-7658
Web Site: www.cbtf.org

National Brain Tumor Foundation

The National Brain Tumor Foundation provides information about brain tumors and their treatment. Information on clinical trials and medical centers specializing in brain tumors is also available.

Mailing Address: 22 Battery Street, Suite 612
San Francisco, California 94111-5520
Phone Number: (800) 934-CURE
Web Site: www.braintumor.org

National Cancer Institute

The National Cancer Institute supports and conducts research, provides education and training, and disseminates information regarding cancer.

Mailing Address: 6116 Executive Boulevard, Room 3036A
Bethesda, Maryland 20892-8322

Phone Number: (800) 4-CANCER
Web Site: www.cancer.gov

OncoLink

Oncolink provides comprehensive and accurate information about cancer, treatments, and research advances.

Web Site: www.oncolink.upenn.edu/

## REFERENCES


Aarsen, F. K., Van Dongen, H. R., Paquier, P. F., Van Mourik, M., & Catsman-Berrevoets, C. E. (2004). Long-term sequelae in children after cerebellar astrocytoma surgery. *Neurology, 62,* 1311–1316.

Adams, W., & Sheslow, D. (2003). *Wide Range Assessment of Memory and Learning* (2nd ed.). San Antonio, TX: The Psychological Corporation.

Anderson, V. A., Godber, T., Smibert, E., Weiskop, S., & Ekert, H. (2004). Impairments of attention following treatment with cranial irradiation and chemotherapy in children. *Journal of Clinical and Experimental Neuropsychology, 26,* 684–697.

Ater, J. L., Moore, B. D., Francis, D. J., Castillo, R., Slopis, J., & Copeland, D. R. (1996). Correlation of medical and neurosurgical events with neuropsychological status in children at diagnosis of astrocytoma: Utilization of neurological severity score. *Journal of Clinical Neurology, 11,* 462–469.

Beebe, D. W., Ris, M. D., Armstrong, F. D., Fontanesi, J., Mulhern, R., Holmes, E., et al. (2005). Cognitive and adaptive outcome in low-grade pediatric cerebellar astrocytomas: Evidence of diminished cognitive and adaptive functioning in national collaborative research studies (CCG 9891/POG 9130). *Journal of Clinical Oncology, 23,* 5198–5204.

Beery, K. E., Buktenica, N. A., & Beery, N. A. (2004). *Beery-Buktenica Developmental Test of Visual-Motor Integration* (5th ed.). Bloomington, MN: Pearson Assessments.

Bleyer, W. A., Fallavollita, J., Robison, L., Balsom, W., Meadows, A., Heyn, R., et al. (1990). Influence of age, sex, and concurrent intrathecal methotrexate therapy on intellectual function after cranial irradiation during childhood: A report from the Children's Cancer Study Group. *Pediatric Hematology and Oncology, 7,* 329–338.

Buono, L. A., Morris, M. K., Morris, R. D., Krawiecki, N., Norris, F. H., Foster, M. F., et al. (1998). Evidence for the syndrome of nonverbal learning disabilities in children with brain tumors. *Child Neuropsychology, 4,* 1–14.

Butler, R. W., & Mulhern, R. K. (2005). Neurocognitive interventions for children and adolescents surviving cancer. *Journal of Pediatric Psychology, 30,* 65–78.

Carlson-Green, B., Morris, R. D., & Krawiecki, N. (1995). Family and illness predictors of outcome in pediatric brain tumor. *Journal of Pediatric Psychology, 20,* 769–784.

Carpentieri, S. C., Waber, D. P., Pomeroy, S. L., Scott, R. M., Goumnerova, L. C., Kieran, M. W., et al. (2003). Neuropsychological functioning after surgery in children treated for brain tumors. *Neurosurgery, 52,* 1348–1357.

Carpentieri, S. C., Waber, D. P., Scott, R. M., Goumnerova, L. C., Kieran, M. W., Cohen, L. E., et al. (2001). Memory deficits among children with craniopharyngiomas. *Neurosurgery, 49,* 1053–1058.

Central Brain Tumor Registry of the United States (CBTRUS). (2005). *Statistical report: Primary brain tumors in the United States, 1998–2002.* Hinsdale, IL: Central Brain Tumor Registry of the United States.

Chapman, C. A., Weber, D. P., Bernstein, J. H., Pomeroy, S. L., LaVally, B., Sallan, S. E., et al. (1995). Neurobehavioral and neurologic outcome in long-term survivors of posterior fossa brain tumors: Role of age and perioperative factors. *Journal of Child Neurology, 10,* 209–212.

Copeland, D. R., deMoor, C., Moore, B. D., III, & Ater, J. L. (1999). Neurocognitive development of children after a cerebellar tumor in infancy: A longitudinal study. *Journal of Clinical Oncology, 17,* 3476–3486.

Copeland, D. R., Moore, B. D., III, Francis, D. J., Jaffe, N., & Culbert, S. J. (1996). Neuropsychologic effects of chemotherapy on children with cancer: A longitudinal study. *Journal of Clinical Oncology, 14,* 2826–2835.

Delis, D. C., Kramer, J. H., Kaplan, E., & Ober, B. A. (1994). *California Verbal Learning Test—Children's Version.* San Antonio, TX: The Psychological Corporation.

Duffner, P. K. (2004). Long-term effects of radiation therapy on cognitive and endocrine function in children with leukemia and brain tumors. *The Neurologist, 10,* 293–310.

Ellenberg, L., McComb, G., Siegel, S. E., & Stowe, S. (1987). Factors affecting intellectual outcome in pediatric brain tumor patients. *Neurosurgery, 21,* 638–644.

Fouladi, M., Gilger, E., Kocak, M., Wallace, D., Buchanan, G., Reeves, C., et al. (2005). Intellectual and functional outcome of children 3 years old or younger who have CNS malignancies. *Journal of Clinical Oncology, 23,* 7152–7160.

Friedman, M. A., Meyers, C. A., & Sawaya, R. (2003). Neuropsychological effects of third ventricle tumor surgery. *Neurosurgery, 52,* 791–793.

Grant, D. A., & Berg, E. A. (1993). *Wisconsin Card Sorting Test.* San Antonio, TX: The Psychological Corporation.

Grant, R. (2004). Overview: Brain tumour diagnosis and management/Royal College of Physicians guidelines. *Journal of Neurology, Neurosurgery, and Psychiatry, 75*(Suppl. 2), ii18–ii23.

Guinan, E. M., Lowly, C., Stanhope, N., Lewis, P. D. R., & Kopelman, M. D. (1998). Cognitive effects of pituitary tumours and their treatments: Two case studies and an investigation of 90 patients. *Journal of Neurology, Neurosurgery, and Psychiatry, 65,* 870–876.

Gurney, J. G., Kadan-Lottick, N. S., Packer, R. J., Neglia, J. P., Sklar, C. A., Punyko, J. A., et al. (2003). Endocrine and cardiovascular late effects among adult survivors of childhood brain tumors: Childhood cancer survivor study. *Cancer, 97,* 663–673.

Gurney, J. G., Smith, M. A., & Bunin, G. R. (1999). CNS and miscellaneous intracranial and intraspinal neoplasms. In L. A. G. Ries, M. A. Smith, J. G. Gurney, M. Linet, T. Tamra, J. L. Young, et al. (Eds.), *Cancer incidence and survival among children and adolescents: United States SEER program 1975–1995* (NIH Publication No. 99-4649). Bethesda, MD: National Cancer Institute, SEER Program.

Hoppe-Hirsch, E., Renier, D., Lellouch-Tubiana, A., Sainte-Rose, C., Pierre-Kahn, A., & Hirsch, J. F. (1990). Medulloblastoma in childhood: Progressive intellectual deterioration. *Child's Nervous System, 6,* 60–65.

Jankovic, M., Brouwers, P., Valsecchi, M. G., Veldhuizen, A. W., Huisman, J., & Kamphuis, R. (1994). Association of 1800 cGy cranial irradiation with intellectual function in children with acute lymphoblastic leukemia. *Lancet, 344,* 224–227.

Jemal, A., Murray, T., Ward, E., Samuels, A., Tiwari, R. C., Ghafoor, A., et al. (2005). Cancer statistics, 2005. *CA: A Cancer Journal for Clinicians, 55,* 10–30.

Johnson, D. L., McCabe, M. A., Nicholson, H. S., Joseph, A. L., Getson, P. R., Byrne, J., et al. (1994). Quality of long-term survival in young children with medulloblastoma. *Journal of Neurosurgery, 80,* 1004–1010.

Karatekin, C., Lazareff, J. A., & Asarnow, R. F. (2000). Relevance of the cerebellar hemispheres for executive functions. *Pediatric Neurology, 22,* 106–112.

Kieffer-Renaux, V., Bulteau, C., Grill, J., Kalifa, C., Viguier, D., & Jambaque, I. (2000). Patterns of neuropsychological deficits in children with medulloblastoma according to craniospatial irradiation doses. *Developmental Medicine and Child Neurology, 42,* 741–745.

Kirk, E. A., Howard, V. C., & Scott, C. A. (1995). Description of posterior fossa syndrome in children after posterior fossa brain tumor surgery. *Journal of Pediatric Oncology Nursing, 4,* 181–187.

Lacaze, E., Kieffer, V., Streri, A., Lorenzi, C., Gentaz, E., Habrand, J. L., et al. (2003). Neuropsychological outcome in children with optic pathway tumours when first-line treatment is chemotherapy. *British Journal of Cancer, 89,* 2038–2044.

Lafayette Instrument Company. (n.d.). *Grooved Pegboard Test.* Retrieved February 15, 2007, from http://www.lafayetteinstrument.com

Landier, W. (1998). Hearing loss related to ototoxicity in children with cancer. *Journal of Pediatric Oncology Nursing, 15,* 195–206.

Levisohn, L., Cronin-Golomb, A., & Schmahmann, J. D. (2000). Neuropsychological consequences of cerebellar tumour resection in children: Cerebellar cognitive affective syndrome in a pediatric population. *Brain, 123,* 1041–1050.

Mabbott, D. J., Spiegler, B. J., Greenberg, M. L., Rutka, J. T., Hyder, D. J., & Bouffet, E. (2005). Serial evaluation of academic and behavioral outcome after treatment with cranial radiation in childhood. *Journal of Clinical Oncology, 23,* 2256–2263.

Macedoni-Luksic, M., Jereb, B., & Todorovski, L. (2003). Long-term sequelae in children treated for brain tumors: Impairments, disability, and handicap. *Pediatric Hematology and Oncology, 20,* 89–101.

Melean, G., Sestini, R., Ammannati, F., & Papi, L. (2004). Genetic insights into familial tumors of the nervous system. *American Journal of Medical Genetics Part C (Seminar in Medical Genetics), 129C,* 74–84.

Merchant, T. E., Mulhern, R. K., Krasin, M. J., Kun, L. E., Williams, T., Li, C., et al. (2004). Preliminary results from a Phase II trial of conformal radiation therapy and evaluation of radiation-related CNS effects for pediatric patients with localized ependymoma. *Journal of Clinical Oncology, 22,* 3156–3162.

Menkes, J. H., & Till, K. (1995). Tumors of the nervous system. In J. H. Menkes (Ed.), *Textbook of child neurology* (pp. 635–694). Baltimore: Williams & Wilkins.

Moleski, M. (2000). Neuropsychological, neuroanatomical, and neurophysiological consequences of CNS chemotherapy for Acute Lymphoblastic Leukemia. *Archives of Clinical Neuropsychology, 15,* 603–630.

Moore, B. D., III, Ater, J. L., & Copeland, D. R. (1992). Improved neuropsychological outcome in children with brain tumors diagnosed during infancy and treated without cranial irradiation. *Journal of Child Neurology, 7,* 281–290.

Mulhern, R. K., Khan, R. B., Kaplan, S., Helton, S., Christensen, R., Bonner, M., et al. (2004). Short-term efficacy of methylphenidate: A randomized, double-blind, placebo-controlled trial among survivors of childhood cancer. *Journal of Clinical Oncology, 22,* 4795–4803.

Mulhern, R. K., Merchant, T. E., Gajjar, A., Reddick, W. E., & Kun, L. E. (2004). Late neurocognitive sequelae in survivors of brain tumours in children. *The Lancet Oncology, 5,* 399–408.

Mulhern, R. K., Palmer, S. L., Merchant, T. E., Wallace, D., Kocak, M., Brouwers, P., et al. (2005). Neurocognitive consequences of risk-adapted therapy for childhood medulloblastoma. *Journal of Clinical Oncology, 23,* 5511–5519.

Mulhern, R. K., Reddick, W., Palmer, S. L., Glass, J. O., Elkin, T. D., & Kun, L. E. (1999). Neurocognitive deficits in medulloblastoma survivors and white matter loss. *Annals of Neurology, 46,* 834–841.

National Cancer Institute. (2006, February 17). *Late effects of treatment for childhood cancer* (PDQ®). Retrieved October 16, 2006, from http://www.cancer.gov/cancertopics/pdq/treatment/lateeffects/HealthProfessional/page2

Packer, R. J., Sposto, R., Atkins, T. E., Sutton, L. N., Bruce, D. A., Siegel, K. R., et al. (1987). Quality of life in children with primitive neuroectodermal tumors (medulloblastoma) of the posterior fossa. *Pediatric Neuroscience, 13,* 169–175.

Packer, R. J., Sutton, L. N., Atkins, T. E., Radcliffe, J., Bunin, G. R., D'Angio, G., et al. (1989). A prospective study of cognitive function in children receiving whole-brain radiotherapy and chemotherapy: Two-year results. *Journal of Neurosurgery, 70,* 707–713.

Palmer, S. L., Gajjar, A., Reddick, W. E., Glass, J. O., Kun, L. E., & Wu, S., et al. (2003). Predicting intellectual outcomes among children treated with 35–40 Gy craniospinal irradiation for medulloblastoma. *Neuropsychology, 17,* 548–555.

Palmer, S. L., Goloubeva, O., Reddick, W. E., Glass, J. O., Gajjar, A., Kun, L., et al. (2001). Patterns of intellectual development among survivors of pediatric medulloblastoma: A longitudinal analysis. *Journal of Clinical Oncology, 19,* 2302–2308.

Poretti, A., Grotzer, M. A., Ribi, K., Schönle, E., & Boltshauser, E. (2004). Outcome of craniopharyngioma in children: Long-term complications and quality of life. *Developmental Medicine and Child Neurology, 46,* 220–229.

Reddick, W. E., White, H. A., Glass, J. O., Wheeler, G. C., Thompson, S. J., Gajjar, A., et al. (2003). Developmental model relating white matter volume to neurocognitive deficits in pediatric brain tumor survivors. *Cancer, 97,* 2512–2519.

Reynolds, C. R., & Kamphaus, R. W. (2004). *Behavior Assessment Scale for Children* (2nd ed.). Circle Pines, MN: AGS Publishing.

Ris, M. D., & Noll, R. B. (1994). Long-term neurobehavioral outcome in pediatric brain-tumor patients: Review and methodological critique. *Journal of Clinical and Experimental Neuropsychology, 16,* 21–42.

Ris, M. D., Packer, R., Goldwein, J., Jones-Wallace, D., & Boyett, J. M. (2001). Intellectual outcome after reduced-dose radiation therapy plus adjuvant chemotherapy for medulloblastoma: A Children's Cancer Group Study. *Journal of Clinical Oncology, 19,* 3470–3476.

Riva, D., & Giorgi, C. (2000). The cerebellum contributes to higher functions during development: Evidence from a series of children surgically treated for posterior fossa tumours. *Brain, 123,* 1051–1061.

Riva, D., Giorgi, C., Nichelli, F., Bulgheroni, S., Massimino, M., Cefalo, G., et al. (2002). Intrathecal methotrexate affects cognitive function in children with medulloblastoma. *Neurology, 59,* 48–53.

Schatz, J., Kramer, J. H., Ablin, A., & Matthay, K. K. (2000). Processing speed, working memory, and IQ: A developmental model of cognitive deficits following cranial radiation therapy. *Neuropsychology, 14,* 189–200.

Schmahmann, J. D. (2004). Disorders of the cerebellum: Ataxia, dysmetria of thought, and the cerebellar cognitive affective syndrome. *Journal of Neuropsychiatry and Clinical Neurosciences, 16,* 367–378.

Schmahmann, J. D., & Sherman, J. C. (1998). The cerebellar cognitive affective syndrome. *Brain, 121,* 561–579.

Schold, S. C., Jr., Burger, P. C., Mendelsohn, D. B., Glatstein, E. J., Mickey, B. E., & Minna, J. D. (1997). *Primary tumors of the brain and spinal cord.* Boston: Butterworth-Heinemann.

Shuper, A., Yaniv, I., Michowitz, S., Kornreich, L., Schwartz, M., Goldberg-Stern, H., et al. (2003). Epilepsy associated with pediatric brain tumors: The neuro-oncologic perspective. *Pediatric Neurology, 29,* 232–235.

Silber, J. H., Radcliffe, J., Peckham, V., Periolongo, G., Kishnani, P., Fridman, M., et al. (1992). Whole-brain irradiation and decline in intelligence: The influence of dose and age on IQ score. *Journal of Clinical Oncology, 10,* 1390–1396.

Sills, A. K. (2005). Current treatment approaches to surgery for brain metastases. *Neurosurgery, 57*(Suppl. 5), S24–32.

Spiegler, B. J., Bouffet, E., Greenberg, M. L., Rutka, J. T., & Mabbott, D. J. (2004). Change in neurocognitive functioning after treatment with cranial radiation in childhood. *Journal of Clinical Oncology, 22,* 706–713.

Stavinoha, P. L., & Burrows, F. (2004). Academic speed in childhood brain tumor survivors treated with cranial radiation. *Brain Impairment, 5,* 99.

Steinlin, M., Imfeld, S., Zulauf, P., Boltshauser, E., Lövblad, K. O., Lüthy, A. R., et al. (2003). Neuropsychological long-term sequelae after posterior fossa tumour resection during childhood. *Brain, 126,* 1998–2008.

Thompson, S. J., Leigh, L., Christensen, R., Xiong, X., Kun, L. E., Heideman, R. L., et al. (2001). Immediate neurocognitive effects of methylphenidate on learning-impaired survivors of childhood cancer. *Journal of Clinical Oncology, 19,* 1802–1808.

Turkel, S. B., Chen, L. S., Nelson, M. D., Hyder, D., Gilles, F. H., Woodall, L., et al. (2004). Case series: Acute mood symptoms associated with posterior fossa lesions in children. *Journal of Neuropsychiatry and Clinical Neuroscience, 16,* 443–445.

Upton, P., & Eiser, C. (2006). School experiences after treatment for a brain tumour. *Child: Care, Health, and Development, 32,* 9–17.

Waber, D. P., Tarbell, N. J., Kahn, C. J., Gelber, R. D., & Sallan, S. E. (1992). The relationship of sex and treatment modality to neuropsychologic outcome in childhood acute lymphoblastic leukemia. *Journal of Clinical Oncology, 10,* 810–817.

Wechsler, D. (2003). *Wechsler Intelligence Scale for Children* (4th ed.). San Antonio, TX: The Psychological Corporation.

White, M. K., Gordon, J., Reiss, K., Del Valle, L., Croul, S., Giordano, A., et al. (2005). Human polyomaviruses and brain tumors. *Brain Research Reviews, 50,* 69–85.

Woodcock, R. W., McGrew, K. S., & Mather, N. (2001). *Woodcock-Johnson Tests of Achievement* (3rd ed.). Rolling Meadows, IL: Riverside.

Wrensch, M., Minn, Y., Chew, T., Bondy, M., & Berger, M. S. (2002). Epidemiology of primary brain tumors: Current concepts and review of the literature. *Neuro-Oncology, 4,* 278–299.

CHAPTER THREE

# Cerebral Palsy

Krestin J. Radonovich, PhD, and Anne-Marie Slinger-Constant, MD, FAAP

## DESCRIPTION OF THE DISORDER

Cerebral palsy (CP) is a neurodevelopmental disorder with hallmark impairments in motor control, movement, and posture. CP is a descriptive term that refers to a wide variety of motor impairments or motor control problems that are usually apparent in the first few years of life. These motor impairments range from mild to severe. Cerebral palsies are the most common cause of physical disability in childhood, with a prevalence of approximately 2.5 per 1,000 live births (Koman, Smith, & Shilt, 2004). About 500,000 children and adults in the United States have CP (March of Dimes, n.d.). Prematurity entails a markedly elevated risk for CP, but the majority (over 60%) of children who are diagnosed with CP were born at term (Thorngren-Jerneck & Herbst, 2006). Advances in medical care have led to a marked decrease in infant mortality and improved survival of very-low-birth-weight, premature infants. This led to a slight increase in the prevalence of CP in the 1980s; however, more recently, indicators suggest this may be leveling off with further advancements in perinatal care (Paneth, Hong, & Koreniewski, 2006). CP may be diagnosed in early infancy, particularly if an infant has severe symptoms and is known to be at high risk, but a definitive diagnosis usually is not made until the second or third year of life.

CP results from abnormal development of or injury to the motor areas of the developing brain occurring before, during, or following birth or in the first few years of life. The anomalies of the central nervous system (CNS) that result in the motor impairments characteristic of CP can lead to impairments in cognitive functioning, including mental retardation (52% of persons with CP), vision and ocular motility (28%), hearing (12%), as well as speech, language, and other domains (Ashwal et al., 2004). The constellation of impairments varies with the extent and location of the underlying lesion, and symptoms differ from individual to individual. Development within cognitive, motor, and behavioral domains is often further compromised by limitations in mobility, resulting in secondary complications that may develop later (Menkes & Sarnat, 2000). By definition, CP is a nonprogressive disorder, which distinguishes this condition from neurodegenerative disorders; however, the motor and associated functional impairments typically change over the course of the child's growth and development. The goal of treatment for children with developmental disabilities is to promote function, prevent secondary impairments, increase developmental capabilities, and thereby facilitate maximum participation and function in society.

## Types of Cerebral Palsy

There is no one condition called CP; rather, CP is an umbrella term used to refer to a group of disorders with primary impairments in motor functioning. CP is usually classified by the body region affected (*hemi-*, *di-*, and *quadriplegia*) and by the type of movement impairment (*spastic, dyskinetic [dystonic* or *athetoid]*, and *ataxic*). *Hemi-* refers to involvement of the arm and leg on one side (left or right) of the body. *Di-* refers to involvement of two limbs but is also used when referring to bilateral involvement with all four limbs affected, the legs more so than the arms. *Quadri-* means that all four limbs are affected, as well as the trunk of the body. These body region prefixes are then combined with descriptors that indicate muscle weakness (*paresis*) or muscle paralysis (*plegia*). For example, *hemiparesis* indicates muscle weakness on one side of the body, whereas *quadriplegia* indicates that all four limbs are affected with muscle paralysis. Other descriptors are also used. *Spasticity* refers to abnormal muscle stiffness, while *dyskinesia* refers to impairment in the control of muscles, leading to abnormal movements. The term *ataxia* refers to the inability to coordinate movements of voluntary muscles.

It is common for children to have symptoms that do not correspond to any single type of CP and are thus referred to as mixed types of CP. For example, a child with mixed CP may have some muscles that are too tight and others that are too relaxed, creating a mix of stiffness and floppiness. Below are descriptions of some of the more common clinical forms of CP.

*Spastic Hemiplegia/Hemiparesis*

The name indicates that there is impairment on one side of the body, typically affecting the arm more than the leg, and that it involves spastic muscle tone. These children often are identified by delays in developmental milestones, such as delayed walking. Depending on the location and extent of neural involvement, a child with spastic hemiplegia may also have seizures. Half of children with this type of CP have intelligence within normal limits, although speech may be delayed (Nelson & Ellenberg, 1982).

*Spastic Diplegia/Diparesis*

The hallmark of this type of CP is muscle spasticity, predominantly in the legs. Clinical features vary with the degree of severity. A "scissored" gait is characteristic. This type of gait occurs when the legs develop spasticity, and the child walks by crossing one leg in front of the other. Some children require a walker or leg braces. The muscles of the arms and face also may be affected, and hand movements may be clumsy. In cases of spastic diplegia, there tends to be a general correlation between the severity of the motor deficit and the level of intellectual impairment (Menkes & Sarnat, 2000).

*Spastic Quadriplegia/Quadriparesis*

This is the most severe form of CP. It is associated with widespread damage to the brain or significant brain malformations. Children are, in most cases, severely intellectually impaired (Nelson & Ellenberg, 1982). Children will often have severe stiffness in their limbs but a floppy neck. They are rarely able to walk. Nearly all have seizures that occur frequently and do not respond well to medications. Expressive speech and language, including articulation, are often impaired.

*Dyskinetic Cerebral Palsy*

This type of CP is characterized by slow and uncontrollable writhing movements of the hands, feet, arms, or legs. Other terms used to describe the observed movements are athetoid (i.e., slow, writhing), choreoathetoid (i.e., continual rapid, jerky, complex), and dystonic (i.e., sustained muscle contractures). Children with these unwanted movements find it difficult to sit comfortably or walk, and they may also have problems coordinating the muscle movements required for speaking. Intelligence is rarely affected in these forms of CP.

## How Is Cerebral Palsy Diagnosed?

Signs of CP usually appear early in life. Most children with CP are diagnosed during the first few years of life. If the impairments are mild, it can be difficult to make a reliable diagnosis before the age of 4 or 5 years. Infants with CP are frequently slow to reach developmental milestones such as learning to roll over, sit, crawl, smile, or walk. Many infants first present with hypotonia or flaccid (i.e., floppy) muscle tone; this typically progresses to hypertonia or muscle spasticity. Some young children appear stiff from the beginning. Others have variability in their muscle tone, sometimes being floppy and sometimes being stiff. A child with CP also might develop an unusual limb posture (e.g., arm contracture) or favor one side of the body.

Doctors diagnose CP by clinical evaluation including a detailed medical history and neurological examination. The medical evaluation involves development of a differential diagnosis and consideration of other conditions that may have similar symptoms to CP or may occur concurrently. A history of progressive deterioration in motor functioning or psychomotor regression would prompt further investigation to exclude, for example, a neurodegenerative condition, metabolic disorder, or CNS lesion or mass. In addition to neuroimaging studies, laboratory studies including cytogenetic analyses may be performed. Electromyography (EMG) and nerve conduction velocity (NCV) studies are done when a nerve or muscle disorder is suspected. An electroencephalogram (EEG) traces electrical activity in the brain and is used to determine the presence of seizures in symptomatic children.

Neuroimaging techniques, such as cranial ultrasound, computed tomography (CT) scan, or magnetic resonance imaging (MRI) can help identify whether there is a brain lesion. Ultrasound uses high-frequency sound waves that cannot be heard by humans that enter the body and bounce back; the sound-wave echoes produce a picture called a *sonogram*. This procedure is typically used in the early neonatal period when the fontanels (e.g., soft spots) are still open to detect gross abnormalities in brain structures and signs of hemorrhage (i.e., bleeding) or injury related to lack of oxygen and blood flow. MRI and CT scans both involve placing the child in a large imaging machine, requiring that the child lie very still, which can be difficult. CT scans, formerly called CAT scans (computed axial tomography), use low-dose X-ray radiation imaging to create images of the brain and/or body. Head CT scans can identify intracranial hemorrhage, malformations, and CNS lesions associated with tissue damage. MRI uses a powerful magnetic field that passes through the body to create pictures of the internal structures of the brain. MRI is used to detect bleeding and structural damage, similar to CT scans, but MRI can also create images that are better for detecting abnormalities of white matter pathways and smaller brain structures. Neuroimaging is recommended in all cases of CP to establish cause and likely clinical course (Ashwal et al., 2004).

A common finding on CT or MRI in children with CP is periventricular leukomalacia (PVL). PVL is caused by a lack of blood supply and insufficient oxygenation of tissue surrounding the cerebral ventricles, which results in tissue death and subsequent "softening." PVL may be accompanied by a hemorrhage or bleeding in the area around and inside the ventricles. In some children, neuroimaging studies show no abnormalities. This does not necessarily mean that the brain is unaffected; sometimes, microscopically small areas of brain damage are present. In general, the prognosis is worse with larger areas of brain damage, although this is not always a direct correlation. Some children with no imaging findings are severely impaired, and some children with observable brain damage function relatively well. A recent large-scale study examined MRI findings in children with CP (Bax, Tydeman, & Flodmark, 2006). The study determined that the most common MRI findings involved white matter damage, such as PVL, in 42.5% of cases. Other findings included basal ganglia lesions (12.8%), cortical/subcortical lesions (9.4%), structural malformations (9.1%), focal infarcts (i.e., bleeds, 7.4%), and a variety of other miscellaneous lesions (7.1%). Normal MRI brain scans were observed in 11.7% of cases.

## Causes of Cerebral Palsy

Though many risk factors have been identified, the many causal pathways that lead to the various cerebral pathologies resulting in the spectrum of clinical entities seen in CP are still not fully understood. The specific cause of most cases of CP is often unknown, and in most cases the etiology is likely multifactorial. For many years, CP was thought to result from problems during birth; however, we now know that CP can result from a variety of prenatal, perinatal, and postnatal causes. Evidence suggests that prenatal factors, such as congenital malformations, play a significant role in the etiology of CP, accounting for over 70% of cases (Jacobsson & Hagberg, 2004). Though infants born prematurely with very low birth weights have a high incidence of CP, more than half of all cases of CP occur in term or near-term infants (Nelson, 1996, 2002).

Reduction in, or loss of, oxygen during delivery accounts for approximately 10% to 14% of CP cases; known congenital factors have been identified that account for about 50% of cases (Tomlin, 1995; Torfs, Van den Berg, Oeschsli, & Cummins, 1990). Several other causes of CP have been identified: migrational neural defects, hemorrhagic brain lesions, cerebrovascular malformations, intrauterine infections, CNS infections, maternal hemodynamic disturbances, placental emboli, Rh incompatibility, anomalous fetal circulation, and rubella (German measles; Lou, 1998). Some causes of CP after birth include head injury, jaundice, bacterial meningitis, viral meningoencephalitis, and vascular accidents (e.g., stroke; Lou, 1998; Menkes & Sarnat, 2000). It should be noted that some of these causes, such as infections or head injury, are preventable or treatable.

## RELATED MEDICAL ISSUES

Many children with CP are also affected by other problems that can impact functioning. The most common related medical condition in CP is seizures, co-occurring in as many as 28% to 50% of children with CP (Bax et al., 2006; Vargha-Khadem, Isaacs, van der Werf, Robb, & Wilson, 1992). The presence of seizures often results in greater cognitive impairment, beyond that expected based on the size or timing of brain lesions (Vargha-Khadem et al., 1992).

Children with CP often have impaired vision, hearing, or speech. Common vision problems include strabismus, in which the eyes deviate due to weakness and poor control of ocular muscles. Strabismus can result in double vision because the images coming in from the two eyes are different. In many children, the brain adapts to the condition by ignoring signals from one of the misaligned eyes. Untreated, this can lead to poor vision in one eye and can interfere with the ability to judge distance. In some cases, doctors will recommend surgery to realign the muscles. Children with CP, particularly those who were born prematurely, also can have retinopathy of prematurity (ROP). ROP involves disordered growth and development of the blood vessels of the retina. Typically, the retina develops in utero, and therefore full-term infants are born with a mature retina. However, when an infant is born prematurely, the experiences outside the uterus affect the development of the retina. Also, the use of high levels of supplemental oxygen can result in damage to these fragile blood vessels. Mild ROP often resolves as the child gets older but can result in permanent blindness.

A syndrome called *failure to thrive* is common in children with moderate to severe CP, especially those with spastic quadriparesis/plegia. Failure to thrive is used to describe children who lag behind in growth and development. The term does not imply a cause. Infants can have poor weight gain, and children are often shorter than their peers. During adolescence many children show a lack of sexual development. The muscles and limbs affected by CP tend to be smaller than normal. This is especially noticeable in children with spastic hemiplegia because limbs on the affected side of the body may not grow as quickly or as long as those on the unaffected side. CP also is associated with deformities of the spine, such as curvature (i.e., scoliosis), humpback (i.e., kyphosis), and saddle back (i.e., lordosis). These spinal deformities can make sitting, standing, and walking even more difficult and can cause chronic back pain.

Some children with CP have abnormal sensations and perceptions. They may have difficulty feeling simple sensations, such as touch. They may have stereognosia, which makes it difficult to perceive and identify objects using only the sense of touch. Children with stereognosia, for example, would have trouble sensing the difference between a hard ball and a sponge ball placed in their hands when their eyes are closed.

A common complication of CP is incontinence due to poor control of the muscles that keep the bladder closed. Incontinence can take the form of bed-wetting, uncontrolled urination during physical activities, or slow leaking of urine throughout the day. Many children with CP use diapers or have catheters that collect urine and stool in special bags ("leg bags"), which can be difficult to change. These continence issues can result in additional social problems due to odor and social stigmatization.

Another common associated problem seen in CP is drooling because of poor control of the muscles of the throat, mouth, and tongue. Drooling may initially seem like an inconsequential problem; however, because it is socially unacceptable, drooling can impact interactions with other children. Drooling can also cause severe skin irritation.

Children with CP often experience a great deal of pain and fatigue. Children, teachers, and parents report that complaints of pain interfere with the child's functioning at school, and research has supported this claim (Varni et al., 2006), as well as increased school absenteeism due to pain (Houlihan, O'Donnell, Conaway, & Stevenson, 2004). Recent findings have shown that pain and fatigue, independently and in combination, affect school functioning deleteriously, particularly for children with different spastic CP subtypes (Berrin et al., 2007). Coping with these related issues may be even more of a challenge than coping with the motor impairments of CP itself.

The presence of CP indicates some degree of alteration in brain functioning. As might be expected, impairments in motor functioning may be associated with impaired intellectual development. It is estimated that 50% to 70% of children with CP have mental retardation (Fennell & Dikel, 2001). Yet cognitive functioning may or may not be affected in children with CP, and the amount of motor impairment does not necessarily indicate the level of cognitive functioning. For example, a child who has severe spasticity of the lower limbs, is wheelchair bound, and has difficulty speaking may have no impairment in cognitive function.

Poor cognitive abilities are more common in cases of spastic quadriplegia and those who have epilepsy and observable brain abnormalities. Few studies, however, have examined specific neuropsychological functioning in the specific subtypes of CP. In general, the laterality of the brain lesion site relates to observed cognitive impairments, with left-hemisphere lesions typically affecting language functions and right-hemisphere lesions usually impacting nonverbal reasoning, spatial abilities, and/or math skills. Studies examining neuropsychological abilities in CP have reported lateralized findings on syntactic awareness, sentence repetition, and math skills (Kiessling, Denckla, & Carlton, 1983). Others have reported language impairments related to prematurity and PVL in CP (Feldman, Evans, Brown, & Wareham, 1992). Impairments in constructional dyspraxia (i.e., difficulty in performing tasks involved with construction, for example, drawing a figure) have been reported in children with spastic diplegia, regardless of level of visual impairments (Koeda, Inoue, & Takeshita, 1997). An important caution in reviewing these studies is that studies are lacking that examine neuropsychological functioning in CP with regards to specific brain lesion sites (Fennell & Dikel, 2001). In a sample of adolescents and adults with CP, those with dyskinetic CP demonstrated better auditory comprehension, visuospatial abilities, immediate visual memory, and verbal working memory when compared with individuals with spastic CP, despite comparable abilities in nonverbal reasoning (as assessed with the Raven's Colored Progressive Matrices) (Pueyo, Junqué, & Vendrell, 2003).

Intelligence tests are often administered to determine the level of cognitive functioning; however, results on traditional IQ tests can be misleading for individuals with CP. Because cognitive testing typically requires a motor output to indicate a response, there is a risk of underestimating the true level of intelligence. Responses often require a verbal or written response, which can be nearly impossible for some children with CP. Administration procedures may need to be modified to require decreased levels of motor output. For example, responses can be presented in a multiple-choice format that allows for a pointing response. Yet it can still be difficult for a child with CP to point accurately. A further modification that is used is to allow an eye-gaze response or a squeeze response (e.g., squeeze my right hand for "yes," left hand for "no"). These types of modifications are very laborious, and the child should be tested in brief sessions to minimize problems with fatigue. The goal of modifications should be to require the least amount of energy expenditure by the child. Testing procedures should ensure that the child's responses are clearly understood and leave no room for misinterpretation. Responses also should not be influenced by the examiner. Of course, any modification from the standard procedure renders the test results suspect, and comparison with normative scores provided in the test manuals should be done with caution. It is important to report any accommodations during testing or modifications to standardized testing procedures and to provide a statement of the validity of results reported.

It is important to conduct a comprehensive evaluation of the neuropsychological abilities of a child with CP. Without a detailed examination of these abilities, one can over- or underestimate the child's true functioning level. A comprehensive evaluation should cover common domains of functioning seen in most neuropsychological exams: intelligence, achievement, language, memory, motor skills, visuoperception, executive functioning, adaptive functioning, and emotional functioning. Examination in each of these domains should ideally include multimodal-multimethod assessments using a variety of tests and respondent questionnaires, particularly because the child may evidence inconsistent performance based on the demands of the task or situation.

Communication impairments that are commonly seen in CP can impact results in testing of general cognitive abilities, as well as other areas of functioning, such as social skills. The examiner may consider using a measure that places lower demands on language or communication. Such measures include the Universal Nonverbal Intelligence Test (UNIT; Bracken & McCallum, 1998), the Wechsler Nonverbal Scale of Ability (WNV; Wechsler & Naglieri, 2006), and the Leiter Performance Scales—Revised (Leiter-R; Roid & Miller, 1997). For children with severe motor impairments, a measure involving limited motor output demands should be considered, such as the Reynolds Intellectual Assessment Scales (RIAS; Reynolds & Kamphaus, 2003) and the Comprehensive Test of Nonverbal Intelligence (C-TONI; Hammill, Pearson, & Wiederholt, 1997). One approach to assessing the child with CP is to administer tests first in the standardized format and then with modifications, such as in an untimed setting, to determine the relative impact of motor slowing on scores. Some clinicians prefer to begin testing with language and memory tasks before deciding what IQ measure to use, as some assessments rely more heavily on language and memory in determining general cognitive ability.

## CEREBRAL PALSY IN THE SCHOOL ENVIRONMENT

Several of the primary and secondary medical issues associated with CP can affect the child's ability to function in the school setting. Physical limitations can make it challenging for the child to ambulate through a busy school hallway and navigate a classroom. Children can become fatigued easily by the physical demands. For instance, the amount of energy expended on simply sitting upright often results in fewer cognitive resources available to maintain attention to the teacher's instruction and to actually learn, retain, and reproduce material.

Medical issues, such as recurrent seizures, certainly affect school attendance and functioning. After experiencing a seizure, the child often becomes lethargic and may need to sleep for a period of time. Medication side effects can affect energy levels, sleep, and cognitive functioning. Difficulty with breathing compounds other issues that lead to fatigue. Vision and sensory problems can make it challenging to encode new material. Social issues, such as embarrassment and avoidance by classmates due to toileting concerns, drooling, and poor communication, compound the situation. Families of children with CP are often stressed, and children can become depressed and overwhelmed.

CP is considered an orthopedic impairment according to the Individuals With Disabilities Education Act (IDEA), which is defined in the *Code of Federal Regulations* Section 300.8 (c) (8) (United States Department of Education, 2004) as:

> a severe orthopedic impairment that adversely affects a child's educational performance. The term includes impairments caused by a congenital anomaly, impairments caused by disease (e.g., poliomyelitis, bone tuberculosis), and impairments from other causes (e.g., cerebral palsy, amputations, and fractures or burns that cause contractures).

## CASE PRESENTATION

We recently evaluated a 9-year-old boy with spastic diplegic CP in order to help with educational planning. Peter Jones is in the fourth grade in a public school where he receives special education services. His parents reported concerns about his academic progress, particularly in mathematics, and his socioemotional functioning at school. They stated that Peter works very hard when given appropriate help and encouragement, but without this individualized instruction and support, he becomes overwhelmed and discouraged, and his performance declines.

Peter was born prematurely for unknown reasons at 31-weeks gestation, weighing 2 pounds 14 ounces. Labor was complicated by fetal distress, prompting delivery via emergency cesarean section. He required resuscitation for several minutes after delivery. During the neonatal period, he experienced typical complications of prematurity, including respiratory problems (i.e., transient tachypnea of the newborn), clinical sepsis (i.e., a severe infection in the blood), and hyperbilirubinemia (i.e., jaundice). He did not require mechanical ventilation. There was no history of neonatal seizures, and results of cranial ultrasounds were normal.

He was discharged home at 6½ weeks. By parental report, he was an irritable infant who fussed when handled and was difficult to feed. Delayed emergence of early motor skills along with persistent concerns about his feeding problems and overall development led to neurological evaluation and diagnosis of CP at 6 months of age. Magnetic resonance imaging (MRI) of the brain revealed bilateral PVL.

Peter received speech and language therapies until approximately 4 years of age. In contrast to his motor skills, his parents reported that Peter's language development progressed age-appropriately. He has received occupational and physical therapies (OT, PT) since infancy and underwent surgery to decrease spasticity of his legs and improve his ability to stand and walk. He is able to ambulate for short distances with the aid of a walker and ankle-foot orthoses but otherwise uses a wheelchair. Contractures of his left arm and wrist limit the use of his left hand. He uses his right hand for writing. He passed recent vision and hearing screening tests. Peter had a full-time aide to assist him with completion of his homework in the afterschool program until recently. At the time of evaluation, his parents reported that he had difficulty getting through all of his assignments after school and indicated that he tends to become frustrated.

## Behavioral Observations

Peter was a very friendly and outgoing boy. He worked diligently throughout the assessment, although he had to be guided back to tasks repeatedly because he had a tendency to engage in extraneous conversation during test administration. Rapport was easily established and maintained throughout the course of the evaluation. Peter's performance on tasks varied throughout the testing. He persisted well on tasks at some times, whereas at other times he was highly distractible. As tasks became more difficult, he often asked to play a game or go to the bathroom. Peter benefited from verbal praise and tangible reinforcers and reminders of progress toward completion. Furthermore, he responded well to earning a reward (e.g., playing a game) after the completion of a set number of tasks. Peter's speech and language engagement was largely commensurate with his same-age peers, although his articulation became somewhat less intelligible when he spoke quickly and became animated.

## Overall Cognitive Abilities

Peter's overall cognitive abilities were within the average range with commensurate functioning in overall verbal and nonverbal abilities. Peter displayed a relative strength in visual/auditory learning of novel information, in which he was required to recall words that stood for symbols. He had more difficulty with visual discrimination of abstract shapes; his performance on this task was in the below-average range and significantly different than other areas assessed (see Table 3.1).

## Academic Achievement

Peter's overall reading score was within the average range, and he demonstrated stable performance on each reading subcomponent. Peter read aloud and verbalized much of his thought processing. As Peter encountered more difficult reading items, his persistence declined and his answers were inconsistent, appearing haphazard.

Peter's overall mathematics score was within the average range. He also scored in the average range for math fluency and applied problems, while he scored in the low average range on the calculation subtest. Peter used his fingers as a strategy to help him solve math problems. In addition, he often drew objects to assist in solving problems. He frequently encountered difficulties when mentally manipulating the objects. Peter experienced difficulty during the math portions of the examination, and he frequently skipped problems without attempting them.

Peter scored in the average range for spelling and writing samples. Despite concerns regarding fine motor development, Peter's handwriting was legible, and he seemed to write with minimal difficulty.

## Language

Based on the results of formal testing, Peter's receptive (listening) and expressive (speaking) language skills were within normal limits for his age. His phonological processing skills also were within normal limits. Although Peter's scores were in the average range for his age, he made errors during testing, consisting mainly of semantic errors. This indicates that he has more difficulty using meaningful language than forming grammatically correct sentences. This difficulty was evident when he was asked to complete the sentence "I am as sick as a ____." He responded with "doornail."

According to the results of the Test of Word Finding-2 (German, 2000), Peter's ability to retrieve words was below average. The difficulty was evident throughout the test because Peter labeled many pictures as "the thingy" and acted out how you would use the object rather than supplying the correct word.

## Visuospatial Organization and Memory

Peter's performance on the Rey-Osterrieth Complex Figure tasks (Bernstein & Waber, 1996) demonstrated a below-average to average ability to integrate nonverbal, visually complex information. He demonstrated significant deficits in copying, encoding, and reconstructing the general structure and the inner and outer details of the figure. His approach to the drawing was part-oriented and did not reflect the overall configuration. Given structural support, Peter was able to copy the figure with greater accuracy; however, his scores for the immediate-recall trial remained below average, consisting only of fragmented elements of the design. His scores reflected poor graphomotor skills and visual construction skills in addition to impaired ability to plan and organize the reproduction of the figure. His motor deficits likely impacted his performance on this task.

## Memory

Peter's general memory abilities were in the average range. He demonstrated a significant strength in short-term verbal memory. While he scored above average in all of the free-recall trials, he did not appear to benefit from semantic cuing on the cued-recall trials. This is not uncommon for children his age. Peter received a significantly high scaled score for perseveration errors; research suggests that elevated perseveration rates could indicate a possible verbal learning disability (Wiig & Roach, 1975). On longer term recall, Peter demonstrated a relative strength for recognition memory as opposed to free recall without a verbal cue.

Peter's performance across visual tasks was inconsistent. When he was required to remember meaningful visual information, such as faces, he performed within the average range. However, his performance was in the below-average range when he was asked to remember visuospatial locations.

## Attention/Executive Functioning

Peter's attention was assessed both through formal assessments, as well as through classroom observations and parent ratings. During formal testing, he was observed to be easily distracted, and it was difficult to keep him on task. Peter was also observed in his classroom where he exhibited on-task behaviors throughout the lesson. His teacher and mother indicated no concerns with attention problems. Scores on formalized testing also did not indicate problems with working memory or problem solving.

## Emotional and Adaptive Functioning

Peter was at ease with the examiners, and rapport was established quickly. He was comfortable talking about most things but needed to be asked direct specific questions to elicit responses regarding his emotions. He seemed concerned with what the examiner was writing throughout testing and expressed concerns regarding what he should or should not say to the examiner.

Peter was asked to tell a story about a series of pictures portraying children and adults in social scenarios. His responses indicated that he was able to identify simple emotions, whereas he had difficulty dealing with strong negative emotions. For example, in response to a picture of a boy hiding while his parents appear to be arguing, Peter described the situation as the family playing hide-and-seek and said that everyone was happy. Furthermore, throughout the evaluation, Peter had a tendency to retreat to fantasy when asked personal or emotionally loaded questions. For example, when asked to draw his family, he wanted to draw superheroes (e.g., the Fantastic Four). Also, when asked to describe what he wished for, he said he wished to be the Invisible Woman.

Parent and teacher reports did not indicate any concerns regarding symptoms of anxiety, depression, or other emotional problems. Overall, Peter's adaptive functioning was within the average range. He functions well in the community and home environments. He has some relative weaknesses in functioning independently in self-care activities due to his motor impairments.

## IMPRESSIONS AND RECOMMENDATIONS

Peter is a friendly, engaging 9-year-old boy with spastic diplegic CP. Current evaluation results suggest that he is progressing well from an academic standpoint, with basic reading and math skills commensurate with his average overall cognitive abilities. Given his profile, Peter will continue to benefit from a supportive learning environment including services that minimize the impact of his motor impairments on his educational progress and socioemotional development. Furthermore, occupational and physical therapies, which are currently in place, should continue along with regular communication with school personnel and other providers to facilitate close monitoring of his socioemotional well-being. Below are some specific recommendations targeted at the needs identified through the evaluation process:

1. Peter would benefit from learning about his cognitive strengths, including his verbal reasoning skills. It will be important to emphasize these strengths to him so that he is willing to take a risk when tasks are perceived as difficult. Increased independence, personal thought, and responsibility should be fostered, as Peter was noted to frequently seek approval from the evaluator. This could

**TABLE 3.1 Selected Neuropsychological Testing Data**

| | Scaled Score | T Score | Standard Score | Percentile |
|---|---|---|---|---|
| **Intellectual Functioning** | | | | |
| WJ-III Cognitive | | | | |
| General Intellectual Ability | | | 92 | |
| Verbal Ability | | | 103 | |
| Thinking Ability | | | 97 | |
| Cognitive Efficiency | | | 84 | |
| Fluid Reasoning | | | 92 | |
| Spatial Relations | | | 78 | |
| **Adaptive Functioning** | | | | |
| ABAS-II Global | | | 105 | |
| Communication | 9 | | | |
| Community Use | 11 | | | |
| Functional Academics | 11 | | | |
| Home Living | 14 | | | |
| Health and Safety | 12 | | | |
| Leisure | 12 | | | |
| Self-Care | 7 | | | |
| Self-Direction | 9 | | | |
| Social | 10 | | | |
| **Academic Skills** | | | | |
| WJ-III Achievement | | | | |
| Broad Reading | | | 101 | |
| Broad Math | | | 90 | |
| Broad Written Language | | | 115 | |
| **Attention/Executive Functioning** | | | | |
| WCST-64 | | | | |
| Total Errors | | | 82 | |

*Continued*

**TABLE 3.1** *(Continued)*

| | Scaled Score | T Score | Standard Score | Percentile |
|---|---|---|---|---|
| Perseverative Responses | | | 97 | |
| Perseverative Errors | | | 95 | |
| Nonperseverative Errors | | | 77 | |
| Conceptual-Level Responses | | | 79 | |
| Visuospatial Organization and Memory | | | | |
| RCFT Standard Admininstration: Organization | | | | |
| Copy | | | | 10 |
| Immediate Recall | | | | 10 |
| Long-Delay Recall | | | | 10 |
| RCFT Structural Elemental Accuracy | | | | 10 |
| Copy | | | | 10 |
| Immediate Recall | | | | 10 |
| Long-Delay Recall | | | | |
| RCFT Incidental Elemental Accuracy | | | | |
| Copy | | | | 10 |
| Immediate Recall | | | | 10 |
| Long-Delay Recall | | | | 10 |
| Socioemotional Functioning | | | | |
| BASC-2 (Parent) | | | | |
| Hyperactivity | | 61 | | |
| Aggression | | 46 | | |
| Conduct Problems | | 43 | | |
| Anxiety | | 59 | | |
| Depression | | 43 | | |
| Somatization | | 36 | | |
| Atypicality | | 41 | | |

**TABLE 3.1** *(Continued)*

| | Scaled Score | T Score | Standard Score | Percentile |
|---|---|---|---|---|
| Withdrawal | | 49 | | |
| Attention Problems | | 45 | | |
| Adaptability | | 73 | | |
| Social Skills | | 63 | | |
| Leadership | | 46 | | |
| BASC-2 (Teacher) | | | | |
| Hyperactivity | | 41 | | |
| Aggression | | 46 | | |
| Conduct Problems | | 42 | | |
| Anxiety | | 39 | | |
| Depression | | 42 | | |
| Somatization | | 47 | | |
| Atypicality | | 43 | | |
| Withdrawal | | 44 | | |
| Attention Problems | | 43 | | |
| Learning Problems | | 48 | | |
| Adaptability | | 66 | | |
| Social Skills | | 49 | | |
| Leadership | | 59 | | |
| Study Skills | | 58 | | |
| Functional Communication | | 44 | | |

*Note.* ABAS-II, Adaptive Behavior Assessment System—Second Edition (Harrison & Oakland, 2003); BASC-2, Behavior Assessment System for Children—Second Edition (Reynolds & Kamphaus, 2004); RCFT, Rey-Osterreith Complex Figure Test (Bernstein & Waber, 1996); WCST-64, Wisconsin Card Sorting Test—64: Computer Version for Windows (Heaton & PAR Staff, 2000 ); WJ-III Achievement, Woodcock-Johnson Tests of Achievement—Third Edition (Woodcock, McGrew, & Mather, 2001); and WJ-III Cognitive, Woodcock-Johnson Tests of Cognitive Abilities (Woodcock, McGrew, & Mather, 2001).

be achieved through the use of a self-monitoring system for behavior and schoolwork completion.

2. Peter will require additional time to complete assignments, assessments, and/or tasks. Peter also may benefit from being provided a copy of the overhead slides or class notes prior to the lesson.
3. Considering Peter's difficulty with visual tasks, it will be important to present information both visually and verbally whenever possible.
4. During the evaluation, Peter experienced difficulty remembering the rules for a particular problem. He may benefit from having visible rules for the different math concepts during instruction, particularly when learning new concepts. Highlighting the signs or target words in math problems will benefit Peter by drawing his attention to which operation the class is working on and allowing him to focus attention on the rules for that particular operation.
5. Conversations with Peter should be very structured. Closed-ended questions such as those with the answers embedded in the questions (e.g., "Is the grass green or red?") or those requiring a yes/no response are recommended so as to give him structure.
6. Consider providing alternative technologies that would promote Peter's independence, such as a scribe, note-taking assistance, or dictation when completing lengthy written work. A voice-activated digital recorder might provide such support for both school and classroom assignments. He would be able to perform classroom work directly on the computer, whereas at home he could use the digital recorder and then transfer his responses to his computer in school the next morning. He should receive instruction in how to edit his work on the computer.
7. Peter would benefit from continued school OT and PT. The educational planning team at his school might consider revising some of the accommodations currently in place based on his specific needs. Ergonomic/adapted seating to accommodate for physical impairments and poor endurance should be considered.
8. Encourage discussion between school PT/OT and physical education teachers to help introduce or modify activities so Peter can actively participate with his peers during physical education class. The therapists should have continued consultation with the adaptive PE teacher so that he can participate as much as possible in the least restricted environment(LRE).

The responsibility and challenges associated with caring for children with CP are extraordinary and often place substantial burdens on families who must rely on professionals in the medical, allied-health, and educational communities to assist their children through their collective efforts. The goal of treatment for children with developmental disabilities is to promote function, prevent secondary impairments, and increase developmental capabilities, thus maximizing participation and function in society. Unfortunately, there is still limited empirical evidence to guide decisions about therapeutic interventions, including what types of treatment approaches are most effective, how intensively they should be delivered, and for how long (Mayston, 2005). Outcomes of children with CP are influenced by the quality of their motor control and the efficiency of movements, along with environmental, emotional, and cognitive factors. Therefore, treatment using a multidisciplinary approach will be most beneficial for a child with CP. Further, the targets and goals for treatment should change with the child's age (Iannaccone, 1994).

Medications can be used to control seizures and muscle spasms. Surgery and mechanical aids, such as special limb braces, can help overcome motor impairments and muscle imbalance. Counseling for emotional and psychological needs as well as speech and behavioral therapy may be employed. Physical therapy and occupational therapy are the hallmark treatments of choice for children with CP. Some evidence suggests that early intervention, when the child is very young, has beneficial outcomes (Blauw-Hospers & Hadders-Algra, 2005).

A nice review of treatments used for children with CP is provided by Tupper (2007). A common treatment target in CP involves the management of muscle spasticity. There are three main goals in treating spasticity: (a) to improve limb range of motion, (b) to make it easier for the child to move, and (c) to make the child more comfortable (Brunstrom, 2001). The use of braces, splints, or serial casting can help prevent contractures by stretching out the muscles (Tupper, 2007). Some medications can inactivate or relax muscles, such as baclofen, dantrolene, and diazepam (Valium). More patients are being fitted with an intrathecal baclofen pump that is surgically implanted around the spinal cord and delivers the medication continuously (Brunstrom, 2001; Goldstein, 2004). A specific surgical intervention called dorsal root rhizotomy involves cutting dorsal root fibers that overstimulate the muscles (Mittal et al., 2002). Another somewhat invasive procedure involves injecting botulinum toxin A into the muscle; this procedure has been shown to be effective, but its results are temporary and it must be repeated approximately every 6 months (Russman, Tilton, & Gormley, 1997; Speth, Leffers, Janssen-Potte, & Vies, 2005). Children with CP may have resultant orthopedic deformities that can be corrected, at least to some extent, with limb-lengthening procedures. In these procedures, a surgeon uses various devices to slowly lengthen the bones in the leg. These procedures, and the subsequent therapy involved, can be extremely painful.

Constraint-induced movement therapy (CIMT) is another treatment that has shown promise, particularly in individuals with hemiplegia (Taub, Uswatte, & Pidikiti, 1999). CIMT involves restraining the more functional limb, thus forcing the individual to use the impaired limb exclusively.

Many children with CP will also use a variety of accommodations to navigate through society and the school environment. These may include special wheelchairs, saddle seats, and splints. In order to assist with communication they are provided with different types of augmentive communication systems, such as electronic communication boards or picture exchange systems (PECS).

Whatever combination of treatments or accommodations is used, it is most important that the child be encouraged to function independently as much as possible. Despite the obvious motor impairments, the child should get as much physical activity as possible (Brunstrom, 2001; Tupper, 2007). Regular aerobic activity can improve muscular strength, physical endurance, and emotional energy levels.

It is important to remember that a diagnosis of CP does not provide information regarding the functional capabilities of a child. There are important neurodevelopmental interactions of cognitive, communicative, executive, behavioral, and motor abilities within the child and environmental issues that all come to bear on a child's daily functioning (Shapiro, 2004). These interactions are complex and can change over time. It is important not to focus exclusively on the motor impairments but to consider the child in the whole context.

## RESOURCES

### Books

Anderson, M. E. (2000). *Taking cerebral palsy to school.* Plainview, NY: Jayjo Books.

Miller, F., & Bachrach, S. J. (2006). *Cerebral palsy: A complete guide for caregiving.* Baltimore: Johns Hopkins University Press.

Parker, J. N., & Parker, P.M. (Eds.). (2002). *The official parent's sourcebook on cerebral palsy: A revised and updated directory for the internet age.* San Diego, CA: ICON Health Publications.

Shriver, M. (2001). *What's wrong with Timmy?* New York: Little, Brown and Company Books for Young Readers.

Wright, P.W.D., & Wright, P. D. (2006). *Wrightslaw: From emotions to advocacy—The special education survival guide* (2nd ed.). Hartfield, VA: Harbor House Law Press.

## Organizations and Web Sites

American Academy for Cerebral Palsy and Developmental Medicine (AACPDM)

The AACPDM is a multidisciplinary scientific society devoted to studying cerebral palsy and other childhood-onset disabilities, to promoting professional education for the treatment and management of these conditions, and to improving the quality of life for people with these disabilities.

Mailing Address: 555 East Wells Street, Suite 1100
Milwaukee, Wisconsin 53202
Phone Number: (414) 918-3014
Web Site: www.aacpdm.org/index?service=page/Home

American Academy of Pediatrics (AAP)

The AAP provides information to professionals and families regarding identification of and care for CP, as well as additional resources.

Web Site: www.medicalhomeinfo.org/health/cer_palsy.html

Centers for Disease Control and Prevention and the National Center on Birth Defects and Developmental Disabilities (NCBDDD)

The NCBDDD Web site offers information to professionals and families, including answers to common questions and additional resources for families.

Web Site: www.cdc.gov/ncbddd/dd/ddcp.htm

Cerebral Palsy Magazine

This is a subscription-based publication that is the only magazine in the country dedicated to CP. A free issue of the magazine can be obtained by contacting the magazine.

Mailing Address: P.O. Box 7005
Bloomfield Hills, Michigan 48302
Phone Number: (877) 843-7278
Web Site: www.cerebralpalsymagazine.com/

Individuals With Disabilities Education Act (IDEA) 2004

The IDEA is a law that ensures services to children with disabilities throughout the nation, governing how states and public agencies provide early intervention, special education, and related services to more than 6.5 million eligible infants, toddlers, children, and youth with disabilities.

Web Site: idea.ed.gov/

National Institute of Neurological Disorders and Stroke (NINDS)

The NINDS CP information Web site offers answers to frequently asked questions, as well as information about current research and related associations.

Web Site: www.ninds.nih.gov/disorders/cerebral_palsy/cerebral_palsy.htm

United Cerebral Palsy (UCP)

UCP is the leading source of information on CP and is a pivotal advocate for the rights of persons with any disability, dedicated to advancing the independence, productivity, and full citizenship of people with disabilities through an affiliate network.

Mailing Address: 1660 L Street NW, Suite 700
Washington, DC 20036
Phone Number: (800) 872-5827
Web Site: www.ucp.org

Wrightslaw

Parents, educators, advocates, and attorneys come to Wrightslaw for accurate, reliable information about special education law, education law, and advocacy for children with disabilities.

Web Site: www.wrightslaw.com

## REFERENCES

Ashwal, S., Russman, B. S., Blasco, P. A., Miller, G., Sandler, A., Shevell, M., et al. (2004). Practice parameter: Diagnostic assessment of the child with cerebral palsy. *Neurology, 62,* 851–863.

Bax, M., Tydeman, C., & Flodmark, O. (2006). Clinical and MRI correlates of cerebral palsy: The European Cerebral Palsy Study. *Journal of the American Medical Association, 296,* 1602–1608.

Bernstein, J. H., & Waber, D. P. (1996). *Developmental scoring system for the Rey-Osterrieth Complex Figure: Professional manual.* Lutz, FL: Psychological Assessment Resources.

Berrin, S. J., Malcarne, V. L., Varni, J. W., Burwinkle, T. M., Sherman, S. A., Artavia, K., et al. (2007). Pain, fatigue, and school functioning in children with cerebral palsy: A path-analytic model. *Journal of Pediatric Psychology, 32,* 330–337.

Blauw-Hospers, C. H., & Hadders-Algra, M. (2005). A systematic review of the effects of early intervention on motor development. *Developmental Medicine and Child Neurology, 47,* 421–432.

Bracken, B. A., & McCallum, R. S. (1998). *Universal Nonverbal Intelligence Test.* Itasca, IL: Riverside.

Brunstrom, J. E. (2001). Clinical considerations in cerebral palsy and spasticity. *Journal of Child Neurology, 16,* 10–15.

Feldman, H. M., Evans, J. L., Brown, R. E., & Wareham, N. L. (1992). Early language and communicative abilities of children with periventricular leukomalacia. *American Journal of Mental Retardation, 97,* 222–234.

Fennell, E. B., & Dikel, T. N. (2001). Cognitive and neuropsychological functioning in children with cerebral palsy. *Journal of Child Neurology, 16,* 58–63.

German, D. J. (2000). *Test of Word Finding* (2nd ed.). Austin, TX: ProEd.

Goldstein, M. (2004). The treatment of cerebral palsy: What we know, what we don't know. *Journal of Pediatrics, 145*(2 Suppl.), S42–S46.

Hammill, D. D., Pearson, N. A., & Wiederholt, J. L. (1997). *Comprehensive Test of Nonverbal Intelligence.* Austin, TX: Pro-Ed.

Harrison, P., & Oakland, T. (2003). *Adaptive Behavior Assessment System* (2nd ed.). San Antonio, TX: The Psychological Corporation.

Heaton, R. K., & PAR Staff. (2000). *Wisconsin Card Sorting Test—64: Computer version for Windows.* Odessa, FL: Psychological Assessment Resources.

Houlihan, C. M., O'Donnell, M., Conaway, M., & Stevenson, R. D. (2004). Bodily pain and health-related quality of life in children with cerebral palsy. *Developmental Medicine and Child Neurology, 46,* 305–310.

Iannaccone, S. T. (1994). Pediatric aspects of spinal cord rehabilitation. *Journal of Neurological Rehabilitation, 8,* 41–46.

Jacobsson, B., & Hagberg, G. (2004). Antenatal risk factors for cerebral palsy. *Best Practice and Research: Clinical Obstetrics and Gynaecology, 18,* 423–436.

Kiessling, L. S., Denckla, M. B., & Carlton, M. (1983). Evidence for differential hemispheric function in children with hemiplegic cerebral palsy. *Developmental Medicine and Child Neurology, 25,* 727–734.

Koeda, T., Inoue, M., & Takeshita, K. (1997). Constructional dyspraxia in preterm diplegia: Isolation from visual and visual perceptual impairments. *Acta Paediatrica, 86,* 1068–1073.

Koman, L. A., Smith, B. P., & Shilt, J. S. (2004). Cerebral palsy. *Lancet, 363,* 1619–1631.

Lou, H. C. (1998). Cerebral palsy and hypoxic-hemodynamic brain lesions in the newborn. In C. E. Coffey & R. A. Brumback (Eds.), *Textbook of pediatric neuropsychiatry* (pp. 1073–1092). Washington, DC: American Psychiatric Association.

March of Dimes. (n.d.). *Cerebral palsy.* Retrieved May 25, 2007, from http://www.marchofdimes.com/pnhec/4439_1208.asp

Mayston, M. (2005). Evidence-based physical therapy for the management of children with cerebral palsy. *Developmental Medicine and Child Neurology, 47,* 795.

Menkes, J. H., & Sarnat, H. B. (2000). Perinatal asphyxia and trauma. In J. H. Menkes & H. B. Sarnat (Eds.), *Child neurology* (pp. 401–466). Philadelphia: Lippincott, Williams & Wilkins.

Mittal, S., Farmer, J. P., Al-Atassi, B., Gibis, J., Kennedy, E., Galli, C., et al. (2002). Long-term functional outcome after selective posterior rhizotomy. *Journal of Neurosurgery, 97,* 315–325.

Nelson, K. B. (1996). Epidemiology and etiology of cerebral palsy. In A. J. Capute & P. J. Accardo (Eds.), *Developmental disabilities in infancy and childhood: Vol. 2. The spectrum of developmental disabilities* (2nd ed., pp. 73–79). Baltimore: Paul H. Brookes.

Nelson, K. B. (2002). The epidemiology of cerebral palsy in term infants. *Mental Retardation and Developmental Disabilities Research Reviews, 8,* 146–150.

Nelson, K. B., & Ellenberg, J. H. (1982). Children who "outgrew" cerebral palsy. *Pediatrics, 69,* 529–536.

Paneth, N., Hong, T. H., & Koreniewski, S. (2006). The descriptive epidemiology of cerebral palsy. *Clinics in Perinatology, 33,* 251–267.

Pueyo, R., Junqué, C., & Vendrell, P. (2003). Neuropsychologic differences between bilateral dyskinetic and spastic cerebral palsy. *Journal of Child Neurology, 18,* 845–850.

Reynolds, C. R., & Kamphaus, R. W. (2003). *Reynolds Intellectual Assessment Scales.* Lutz, FL: Psychological Assessment Resources.

Reynolds, C. R., & Kamphaus, R. W. (2004). *Behavior Assessment System for Children* (2nd ed.). Bloomington, MN: Pearson Assessments.

Roid, G. H., & Miller, L. J. (1997). *The Leiter International Performance Scale* (rev. ed.). Lutz, FL: Psychological Assessment Resources.

Russman, B. S., Tilton, A., & Gormley, M. E., Jr. (1997). Cerebral palsy: A rational approach to a treatment protocol, and the role of botulinum toxin in treatment. *Muscle Nerve Supplement, 6,* S181–S193.

Shapiro, B. K. (2004). Cerebral palsy: A reconceptualization of the spectrum. *Journal of Pediatrics, 145,* S3–S7.

Speth, L. A., Leffers, P., Janssen-Potte, Y. J., & Vies, J. S. (2005). Botulinum toxin A and upper limb functional skills in hemiparetic cerebral palsy: A randomized trial in children receiving intensive therapy. *Developmental Medicine and Child Neurology, 47,* 468–473.

Taub, E., Uswatte, G., & Pidikiti, R. (1999). Constraint-induced movement therapy: A new family of techniques with broad application to physical rehabilitation—a clinical review. *Journal of Rehabilitation Research and Development, 36,* 237–251.

Thorngren-Jerneck, K., & Herbst, A. (2006). Perinatal factors associated with cerebral palsy in children born in Sweden. *Obstetrics and Gynecology, 108,* 1499–1505.

Tomlin, P. I. (1995). The static encephalopathies. In R. W. Newton (Ed.), *Color atlas of pediatric neurology* (pp. 203–216). London: Times-Wolfe International.

Torfs, C.P.P., Van den Berg, B. J., Oechsli, F. W., & Cummins, S. (1990). Prenatal and perinatal factors in the etiology of cerebral palsy. *Journal of Pediatrics, 116,* 615–619.

Tupper, D. (2007). Management of children with disorders of motor control and coordination. In S. Hunter & J. Donders (Eds.), *Pediatric neuropsychological intervention.* Cambridge, England: Cambridge University Press.

United States Department of Education. (2004). *Individuals with Disabilities Education Act (IDEA).* Retrieved May 25, 2007, from http://idea.ed.gov/explore/view/p/,root,regs,300,A,300%252E8

Vargha-Khadem, F., Isaacs, E., van der Werf, S., Robb, S., & Wilson, J. (1992). Development of intelligence and memory in children with hemiplegic cerebral palsy: The deleterious consequences of early seizures. *Brain, 115*(Pt. 1), 315–329.

Varni, J. W., Burwinkle, T. M., Berrin, S. J., Sherman, S. A., Artavia, K., Malcarne, V. L., et al. (2006). The PedsQL in pediatric cerebral palsy: Reliability, validity, and sensitivity of the Generic Core Scales and Cerebral Palsy Module. *Developmental Medicine and Child Neurology, 48,* 442–449.

Wechsler, D., & Naglieri, J. A. (2006). *Wechsler Nonverbal Scale of Ability.* San Antonio, TX: Harcourt Assessment.

Wiig, E. H., & Roach, M. A. (1975). Immediate recall of semantically varied "sentences" by learning-disabled adolescents. *Perceptual and Motor Skills, 40,* 119–125.

Woodcock, R. W., McGrew, K. S., & Mather, N. (2001a). *Woodcock-Johnson Tests of Achievement* (3rd ed.). Rolling Meadows, IL: Riverside.

Woodcock, R. W., McGrew, K. S., & Mather, N. (2001b). *Woodcock-Johnson Tests of Cognitive Abilities* (3rd ed.). Itasca, NY: Riverside.

CHAPTER FOUR

# Cystic Fibrosis

Michelle Murray, PhD

Cystic fibrosis (CF) is a complicated illness that affects multiple organ systems. When a child has CF, the disease impacts not only the child but also the family, friends, school community, and health care providers. With good health care and treatment, most children with CF have the opportunity to attend school, participate in extracurricular activities, and pursue college and vocational goals. A collaborative relationship among a child's caregivers, school personnel, and health care team can make an enormous difference in the quality of life and consistency of care obtained by the child. In order to understand the psychosocial and emotional issues often presented by children and adolescents with CF, some background about the disease is warranted. Natalie, a teen with CF who presented for neuropsychological evaluation, will be discussed, and suggestions for interventions and accommodations at the school level to assist students with CF will be provided in this chapter.

## DESCRIPTION OF THE DISORDER

### Overview of Cystic Fibrosis

CF is a genetically transmitted disease that affects approximately 30,000 individuals in the United States (Cystic Fibrosis Foundation, 2005). It is the most common life-shortening genetic disease among Whites, with an incidence of about 1 in 2,500 White births (Dodge et al., 1993). The disease also appears, in lesser numbers, among Hispanic, African American, and Asian populations. In general terms, CF is caused by an imbalance of salt in the body. This defect causes the buildup of thick, abundant mucus that clogs organs and traps infection. Chronic infections in the lungs cause gradual, progressive deterioration of lung tissue.

Despite its genetic origin, most families who have a child with CF are not aware of CF in their family medical history. CF is an autosomal recessive disease; both parents must supply a copy of the gene mutation in order for the child to present with the illness. As a result, the CF gene can be passed through many generations of symptomless carriers before it is identified in a child. In fact, 1 in 29 Whites is believed to be a symptomless carrier of the CF gene (National Institutes of Health, 1997). CF is caused by a single gene, which was identified in 1989. In all individuals, the gene controls the production of a protein known as cystic fibrosis transmembrane conductance regulator (CFTR). The role of this protein is to regulate the movement of salt, in the form of sodium and chloride, across cell membranes (Orenstein, 2003). As salt moves through the body's cells, water travels with it. People with CF have a defective or absent CFTR protein, so the regulation of salt in their bodies is faulty. Chloride movement out of cells is blocked; sodium absorption through cells is accelerated. Salt and water are removed from areas of the body that need it. The body's lubricating mucus becomes drier and thicker, most notably in the lungs (Bush, 2001).

## Lung Manifestations

CF lung disease is primarily characterized by thick mucus in the airways. The lungs of an individual with CF quickly become colonized with bacterial growth. Once pathogens are established in the lungs, they are difficult if not impossible to eradicate. Over time, the individual experiences recurrent airway infection and inflammation, bronchial wall thickening, and permanent lung damage. Approximately 95% of CF deaths in the United States are attributable to respiratory failure (Scanlin, 1988).

Lung therapy often entails breathing treatments using an aerosol machine that turns liquid medication into a fine mist that can be inhaled, thus delivering the medication directly to the lungs. Types of medications frequently prescribed for use with an aerosol machine may include bronchodilators to open the airways, mucolytics to thin secretions in the airways, and antibiotics to suppress lung infection (Davis, 2001). Individuals with CF often must take additional oral medications, such as steroids, to decrease airway inflammation.

Another important key to maintaining lung function is airway clearance, by which mucus is loosened from the lungs so it can be coughed up and expelled (Orenstein, 2003). Airway clearance can be performed by having someone who has been trained in the proper technique clap on the patient's back and chest in order to shake the mucus loose. Mechanical forms of airway clearance are often recommended because they give the person with CF more independence and are less taxing to the caregiver. Mechanical airway clearance may involve a device such as a percussive vest worn by the patient (Yankaskas, Marshall, Sufian, Simon, & Rodman, 2004). Handheld devices that create vibrations in the airways can also assist with clearance of mucus.

Finally, exercise is recommended for people with CF, in part because it aids in airway clearance (Andreasson, Jonson, Kornfalt, Nordmark, & Sandstrom, 1987; Zach, Purrer, & Oberwaldner, 1981). A more recent study showed that among patients with CF, regular aerobic exercise slowed the reduction in lung function over 3 years compared to randomized controls (Schneiderman-Walker et al., 2000).

Patients with CF sometimes require the use of supplemental oxygen, especially individuals with advanced disease. Most commonly, people with CF first begin to need extra oxygen only when exercising or while they sleep (Bradley et al., 1999). People who are not receiving adequate oxygen may feel fatigued, experience headaches, and have difficulty with cognitive tasks (Mayo Clinic, 2001–2007).

## Gastrointestinal Manifestations

Because pancreatic ducts become blocked by thick mucus, the pancreas of 85% to 90% of people with CF does not properly secrete digestive enzymes into the intestinal tract. These "pancreatic-insufficient" individuals are at high risk of malnutrition and must take supplementary pancreatic enzymes with all meals and snacks in order to absorb fat (Davis, 2001). Patients with pancreatic insufficiency may present clinically with diarrhea, abdominal pain, and frequent greasy, foul-smelling stools. People with CF are prone to low body weight, requiring high caloric intake (Davis). Those with great difficulty maintaining adequate weight and nutritional status may receive extra calories through nighttime formula feeds, delivered directly into the body through a surgically placed tube. Deficiencies in fat-soluble vitamins (vitamins A, D, E, and K) are common due to insufficient pancreatic function, so vitamin supplementation is usually recommended (Davis). Persons with CF are also at risk for bowel obstructions due to abnormal secretion of digestive fluids; undigested food cannot adequately pass through the gut, causing a blockage that requires medical attention and occasionally surgical intervention (Yankaskas et al., 2004).

## Prognosis

The prognosis for children with CF has improved dramatically, and CF is no longer considered a childhood killer (Lester, 2001). When the illness was first described in medical literature in 1938, most children with CF died in infancy (Bush, 2001). By 1970, children with CF were not expected to live past their high school graduation, with a median life expectancy of 16 years (Yankaskas et al., 2004). In 2006, the predicted age of survival rose to almost 37 years (Cystic Fibrosis Foundation, 2006), and the median survival age predicted for children with CF who were born in the 1990s is estimated to be greater than 40 years (Elborn, Shale, & Britton, 1991). A variety of factors may contribute to this dramatic increase in life expectancy. First, CF treatment centers emphasize techniques for airway clearance that loosen mucus in the lungs so it can be expelled (Lester). Second, efforts aimed at improving the nutritional status of people with CF have not only resulted in improved growth but have also been associated with better pulmonary status (Steinkamp & Wiedemann, 2002). In addition, more effective use of antibiotics to suppress and manage pulmonary infections allows many individuals with CF to maintain healthy lung tissue for many years longer than they would previously have been able to do (Lester).

## Lung Transplantation

Lung transplantation is an option for many patients with CF who have very advanced lung disease. Patients are typically evaluated for transplant when their lung function and other clinical indicators signify to their CF doctor that they have a 50% estimated mortality rate within the next 2 years (Kerem, Reisman, Corey, Canny, & Levison, 1992). The most common procedure in a CF lung transplant involves transplantation of both lungs (Cystic Fibrosis Foundation, 2005). People with CF who pursue lung transplantation are placed on a waiting list. The demand for donated lungs is greater than the supply, and many would-be lung recipients have died while awaiting donor organs. However, new guidelines for allocation of donor organs to patients ages 12 and older were implemented in 2005 by the Organ Procurement Transplant Network and the United Network for Organ Sharing (United Network for Organ Sharing, 2006). Under the new guidelines, patients who are in the most acute need and who are anticipated to obtain the most survival benefit from the transplant move to the top of the list; this is a change from the previous "first-come, first-served" model of lung allocation (United Network for Organ Sharing). Although lung transplantation can extend people's lives for many years, a successful outcome is not guaranteed. Data indicate a survival rate of approximately 50% at 5 years posttransplant (Yankaskas et al., 2004). For more information about lung transplant, refer to the chapter on solid organ transplant in this volume.

## RELATED MEDICAL ISSUES

Although maintaining lung health and nutritional status are most prominent in CF care, other possible manifestations of CF must be considered. For instance, sinus problems are common among individuals with CF (Davis, 2001). Recurrent upper respiratory infections can cause inflammation in the sinuses, facial pain, difficulty breathing through the nose, and headaches.

Yankaskas and colleagues (2004) state that up to 17% of children with CF have clinically significant liver disease, citing separate studies by Colombo and Gaskin and their colleagues. Thick mucus clogs bile ducts in the liver, just as it clogs airways in the lungs. The blocked bile ducts contribute to progressive scarring of the liver tissue, which, in the most severe cases, can cause the development of cirrhosis and eventual liver failure (Davis, 2001). A few patients with CF liver disease will require liver transplants.

As patients with CF grow older, many are diagnosed with CF-related diabetes (CFRD) due to continued deterioration of the pancreas (Davis, 2001). CFRD may be first diagnosed in adolescence, and patients with CF often have difficulty adjusting to the diagnosis. Just as in non-CF diabetes, CFRD may require monitoring of blood sugar levels and insulin injections. For adolescents who may already feel constrained by the demands of their CF treatment regimen, the additional burdens of managing CFRD can feel overwhelming. Poorly controlled CFRD can result in a range of symptoms including blurred vision, drowsiness, and behavior changes (Hardin, Brunzell, Schissel, Schindler, & Moran, 1999).

Like CFRD, bone and joint problems increase in prevalence as patients with CF become older, though they also may be present in children. Osteoporosis, or the loss of bone density, has been associated with poor nutritional status and lung function (Yankaskas et al., 2004). Estimates range widely, but osteoporosis has been found in children and adolescents with CF (Bhudhikanok et al., 1996; Henderson & Madsen, 1996). Cohen and colleagues (cited in Bresnihan, 1988) reported that joint disease occurs in up to 15% of people with CF and may consist of joint inflammation, sensitivity, and pain.

Despite its effect on multiple systems, CF does not directly affect the brain and central nervous system. The intellectual and academic functioning of 52 children and 24 teens with CF was found to range widely and conform to a normal distribution (Thompson et al., 1992). Other studies also have found that children with CF are not significantly different from non-CF controls or normative samples on measures of intelligence, academic achievement, and neuropsychological function (Koscik et al., 2004; Stewart et al., 1995). However, other studies have questioned the effect of poor nutritional status, especially vitamin E deficiency, on cognitive development. A 2005 study indicated that prolonged vitamin E deficiency in infancy was associated with lower cognitive functioning in later childhood compared to controls (Koscik et al., 2005). Additional studies have examined the role of decreased oxygenation in cognitive functioning. In a study of 18 adolescents and adults with advanced CF, neuropsychological evaluation indicated verbal memory problems (Ruchinskas et al., 2000). A 2000 study of 28 children and adolescents with CF found a relationship between reduced oxygenation and impaired neuropsychological performance (Bacon, 2000). Conclusions are difficult to draw, because few studies have been conducted, control groups are not always available, and sample sizes tend to be small. Future research may better elucidate any cognitive deficits common among individuals with CF.

## RESULTS FROM THE NEUROPSYCHOLOGICAL EVALUATION

### Background Information

Natalie is a 15-year-old high school sophomore who was referred by her CF treatment center for a neuropsychological evaluation because of her self-reports of increasing difficulties with memory and organization. She was diagnosed with CF when she was 2 days old due to meconium ileus, an intestinal obstruction that occurs nearly exclusively in newborns with CF. She takes multiple medications for her CF. Natalie has stable lung function but has been hospitalized twice for bowel obstructions in the past 18 months and experiences frequent abdominal pain. Her parents believe her memory and organizational difficulties became more pronounced following her recent hospital admissions. Natalie has no significant psychiatric history. She is involved in school extracurricular activities, including dance squad.

Natalie's diagnosis of CF qualified her for educational accommodations, and she has a written plan under Section 504 on file at her school permitting her to carry her own enzymes to class, take frequent bathroom breaks as needed, and have extra time to complete assignments if she must miss school for a reason related to her illness. However, Natalie reports that recently she has had a great deal of difficulty memorizing facts for history and science tests and cannot remember how to perform multistep math problems. She feels she is more forgetful about keeping track of her schoolwork and less organized, with greater difficulty managing school materials and turning in assignments on time. Natalie also believes that she is slower to learn dance routines than she used to be.

During the evaluation, Natalie presented as a friendly young woman who appeared slightly younger than her stated age. She was cooperative and attentive to tasks, requiring little prompting to stay on task. Natalie responded appropriately to encouragement from the examiner when needed and seemed to gain confidence as the testing proceeded.

## Test Results

Natalie completed a questionnaire that was used to gain information about her emotional functioning. Her scores were suggestive of someone who manifests psychological distress through physical symptoms, although such a score pattern is common for children with chronic medical conditions. Relationships with parents and peers were associated with positive feelings for Natalie, but self-esteem and self-reliance were rated as below average. When Natalie's mother rated her child's behavior, physical expression of psychological needs was also noted. Natalie's mother also completed a scale assessing her executive functioning skills in the home environment; *executive functioning* refers to higher order thinking skills including problem solving, working memory, and planning and organization. The rating of Natalie's behavior suggests that she displays age-appropriate executive functioning skills.

Natalie's intellectual abilities were assessed, and her performance indicated that overall cognitive ability was in the average range, with verbal and nonverbal reasoning skills slightly higher than short-term working memory skills and processing speed. Natalie's knowledge of conventional standards of behavior was in the high average range for children in her age group. She obtained scores in the average range on tasks measuring her word knowledge, verbal reasoning, and sequencing and mental manipulation. She also performed in the average range on nonverbal tasks requiring abstract, categorical reasoning; fluid reasoning and pattern recognition; analysis and synthesis of abstract visual stimuli; and visual scanning ability. Consistent with her self-report, Natalie had greater difficulty with tasks involving auditory short-term memory and short-term visual memory.

When memory tests were administered to assess verbal and visual memory skills, Natalie demonstrated variable performance. While she showed no difficulty immediately remembering the location of dots on a grid or a set of pictures portraying people in familiar, everyday scenes, Natalie's ability to immediately recall faces was below average. After a delay, Natalie's performance was in the average range on all visual memory tasks. Her verbal memory skills were also inconsistent. She performed in the average range on tasks of verbal memory when information was presented in the context of a short story to assist in her encoding. She had greater difficulty when presented with rote, nonmeaningful information. For example, Natalie had trouble remembering a series of word pairs, despite hearing the information over three trials. A similar pattern was apparent on another verbal memory task, on which Natalie had difficulty with list memorization and showed little improvement over a series of trials. Selected test scores from Natalie's evaluation can be reviewed in Table 4.1.

## INTERVENTIONS

### Academic

Recommendations were formulated to assist Natalie specifically with memory and organizational tasks, including breaking schoolwork into smaller increments, taking frequent breaks, making careful notes and lists, utilizing memory tactics such as mnemonics, and creating a folder for completed homework. For a student with CF such as Natalie, a more specific Individualized Education Plan (IEP) may need to be devised in order to anticipate possible medical needs that may arise. The IEP should have specific plans for managing the completion of schoolwork in case of absenteeism due to illness.

Students with CF may have high rates of absenteeism due to doctors' appointments and hospital admissions. Quarterly CF treatment center visits are recommended by the Cystic Fibrosis Foundation's *Clinical Practice Guidelines for Cystic Fibrosis* (1997), and patients may visit their doctors more often if they are ill or experiencing problematic symptoms. Also, the child with CF sees doctors in other fields of specialization. For example, children may visit a pediatrician for immunizations and general care; an endocrinologist regarding CF-related diabetes; and an ear, nose, and throat specialist about management of sinus disease. Some children with CF may require lengthy hospitalizations from time to time. A hospital admission for a child with CF during a respiratory exacerbation is frequently 10 to 13 days and can be longer (Al-Yaman, Bryant, & Sargeant, 2002; Zanni, Shutack, Schuler, Christie, & Holsclaw, 1985). While these children are in the hospital, they often have time to complete schoolwork, and some hospitals have teachers or tutors who can assist with work completion.

**TABLE 4.1 Neuropsychological Evaluation of Natalie: Selected Scores**

| Scale | Scaled Score | Standard Score |
|---|---|---|
| | WISC-IV | |
| Verbal Comprehension Index | | 104 |
| Perceptual Reasoning Index | | 100 |
| Working Memory Index | | 86 |
| Processing Speed Index | | 88 |
| Full Scale IQ | | 95 |
| | CMS | |
| Dot Locations | | |
| Learning | 8 | |
| Total Score | 8 | |
| Long Delay | 9 | |
| Stories | | |
| Immediate | 8 | |
| Delayed | 9 | |
| Delayed Recognition | 9 | |
| Faces | | |
| Immediate | 7 | |
| Delayed | 10 | |
| Word Pairs | | |
| Learning | 7 | |
| Total Score | 5 | |
| Long Delay | 5 | |
| Delayed Recognition | 3 | |
| Family Pictures | | |
| Immediate | 10 | |
| Delayed | 9 | |

*Note*. CMS, Children's Memory Scale (Cohen, 1997); and WISC-IV, Wechsler Intelligence Scale for Children—Fourth Edition (Wechsler, 2003).

Returning to school after a long hospital stay can feel overwhelming if a child has prolific amounts of make-up work to complete. Schools can assist by coordinating with the parents or caregivers to send work to the hospital when possible, allowing extra time to complete work, and modifying the amount of work. Students with advanced illness who are unable to manage a standard school schedule or who require very frequent hospital admissions may be considered for homebound provisions or altered school schedules (e.g., attending for only a few hours each day). In addition, short time periods to travel between classes can be challenging for patients with advanced lung disease, and schools should allow severely affected students extra time to navigate the halls and stairways. Collaboration among school, family, and medical care providers can help determine what level of accommodation is most appropriate for an individual student.

## Lung Health

Because so much of a child's time is spent at school, it can be helpful for a child with CF to feel that the school supports his or her efforts to maintain respiratory health. Some students even take respiratory treatments in the school nurse's office. Physical education classes, playground activities, and school athletic teams can be highly beneficial to the pulmonary health and psychosocial well-being of students with CF. School schedules can be designed to accommodate physical education classes unless the student's doctor recommends otherwise. Physical education teachers should be made aware of the student's illness and asked to allow the student to pace himself or herself appropriately. Children with CF may have reduced exercise tolerance and increased coughing during exercise (Orenstein & Nixon, 1991). These students can also become dehydrated more easily than other children. Accommodations should be made to allow students access to water and more frequent breaks, if needed.

Schools also can assist in minimizing the spread of infectious bacteria at school by encouraging good hand hygiene and asking other parents to keep children home from school when they are ill. CF is not contagious, nor do children with CF spread infectious germs when they cough. However, they are highly susceptible to bacteria in the environment (Bals, Weiner, & Wilson, 1999). Classroom teachers of students with CF should encourage all students to use sanitizing hand gels and wipe down surfaces with disposable antibacterial wipes.

## Nutritional/Gastrointestinal Health

When trying to meet their high caloric needs, some students with CF may be unable to consume all necessary food during a standard school lunch period. Schools can help by allowing students to bring extra snacks to school and permitting students to go to lunch early in order to be first in the cafeteria line. Most children with CF will need to take pancreatic enzymes with meals and snacks. For young children, these enzymes should be administered by the school nurse, but older students (high school and some middle school students) often prefer to carry their own enzymes in order to avoid daily trips to the nurse and gain a greater sense of control. Finally, students with CF may have frequent bowel movements. They should be permitted to use the restroom as needed. Some children feel embarrassed about having numerous, foul-smelling stools and may prefer to have privacy in the bathroom at school whenever possible.

## College and Career Planning

For adolescents with CF who are preparing to complete high school, college and vocational choices are relatively unlimited. A few considerations might be helpful for school counselors to keep in mind when planning for the future with these students. A variety of college scholarships are available specifically for students with CF; a few resources for scholarships are listed at the end of this chapter. For students who plan to move away from home to attend college, it is advisable for them to locate the nearest CF treatment center. Most colleges and universities have a resource center or Office of Disability Services, and it will be helpful if the student establishes a relationship with this center early in case accommodations are needed due to illness.

Students who choose to seek employment might be advised about the importance of job benefits such as health and disability insurance. Workplaces with exposure to environmental lung irritants are not an ideal choice; these might include businesses that use paint and chemical sprayers or restaurants where cigarette smoking is permitted. Patients with CF also should consider the appropriateness of pursuing careers requiring them to complete rigorous physical training (e.g., military service, law enforcement). Other vocations may place people with CF at higher risk of potential exposure to illness, such as work in the health care field.

## Psychosocial Issues

The relationship with a supportive figure at school can have an immeasurable impact on a child with CF. A school counselor, school psychologist, school nurse, or favorite teacher can assist in supporting students and helping them learn how to discuss CF with classmates. A student with CF may seek out reassurance when he or she does not feel well or has been teased by another child about his or her physical limitations. If the child has been prescribed steroids, he or she may feel irritable and require additional patience and encouragement on the part of parents and teachers. States of health can influence children's moods; CF-related diabetes impacts patients' moods and performance when blood sugar levels are too high or too low.

Peer relationships may suffer if a child is absent frequently or if peers develop misunderstandings about CF (e.g., believing it is contagious or that the child is in imminent risk of death). Some children with CF are secretive about their illness because they fear rejection. Body image concerns are numerous, especially as young people with CF become adolescents. They may feel they are too thin or short, feel self-conscious about their chronic coughs, and be frustrated about the late onset of puberty. Adolescence can be particularly difficult for many patients with CF, as they desire greater independence while experiencing fears about an uncertain future.

## CONCLUSION

When children have CF, special challenges may arise in meeting their educational and emotional needs. As in Natalie's case, many young people with CF are actively involved in school and social activities. Through collaboration with parents and medical providers, schools can create individual plans for students with CF, thus providing them the opportunity to obtain academic skills and socialization opportunities that will benefit them throughout their adult lives.

## RESOURCES

### Books

Apel, M. A. (2006). *Cystic fibrosis: The ultimate teen guide (It happened to me)*. Lanham, MD: Scarecrow Press.

Brascia, T., & Flynn, K. (2003). *Cystic fibrosis in the classroom: The problems, the needs, the solutions* [Brochure]. Mountain View, CA: Cystic Fibrosis Research.

Cunningham, J. C., & Taussig, L. M. (2003). *An introduction to cystic fibrosis for patients and families*. Bethesda, MD: Cystic Fibrosis Foundation.

Detrich, T., & Detrich, D. (2000). *The spirit of Lo: An ordinary family's extraordinary journey*. Tulsa, OK: Mind Matters.

Henry, C. S. (2007). *Taking cystic fibrosis to school*. Plainview, NY: Jayjo Books.

Lipman, A. (2002). *Alive at 25: How I'm beating cystic fibrosis*. Atlanta, GA: Longstreet Press.

Lux, C. (2006). *Little brave ones: For children who battle cystic fibrosis*. Charleston, SC: BookSurge.

Novartis Pharmaceuticals. (2007). *CF from the inside out* [Brochure]. East Hanover, NJ: Author.

Orenstein, D. M. (2003). *Cystic fibrosis: A guide for the patient and family* (3rd ed.). Philadelphia: Lippincott-Raven.

Rothenberg, L. (2004). *Breathing for a living: A memoir*. New York: Hyperion.

Smith, D. S. (1997). *Mallory's 65 roses*. Birmingham, AL: Axcan-Scandipharm.

Starbright Foundation. (2000). *Back to school: Teens prepare for school re-entry* [Film]. Available from http://www.starbright.org

## Organizations and Web Sites

Boomer Esiason Foundation

This is an organization dedicated to providing financial support in order to find a cure for CF; heightening education and awareness of CF; and improving quality of life for people with CF, including scholarships for college-bound students.

Web Site: www.esiason.org

cForward.net

This is a Web site designed to provide education, information, and support to children and teens with CF and their parents.

Web Site: www.cForward.net

CysticFibrosis.com

This is an interactive support and education forum for families of children with CF and teens/adults with CF.

Web Site: www.cysticfibrosis.com

Cystic Fibrosis Foundation

This is an organization involved in research, specialized care, education, and advocacy for people with CF, families, friends, and care providers.

Phone Number: (800) FIGHT-CF
Web Site: www.cff.org

Cystic Fibrosis Research, Inc.

This is an organization created to fund research, provide educational and personal support, and spread awareness of CF for families, friends, and care providers.

Web Site: www.cfri.org

Cystic-L

This organization maintains a listserv to provide information and support for adults with CF, families, and care providers.

Web Site: www.cystic-l.org

I.E.P.'s vs. 504 Plans

This is a very helpful Web site that differentiates the types of written plans available to assist students with disabilities; it is useful for parents and educators.

Web Site: www.slc.sevier.org/iepv504.htm

KidsHealth

This is a Web site providing health information about children, designed for parents, children, and teens.

Web Site: www.kidshealth.com

Starlight Starbright Children's Foundation

This is an organization that creates programs for the education, entertainment, and inspiration of seriously ill children.

Web Site: www.starlight.org

### *Organ Transplantation*

Children's Organ Transplant Association

This is an organization providing fundraising assistance and family support to people under age 21 in need of life-saving transplants.

Web Site: www.cota.org

Health Resources Administration/Department of Health and Human Services

This Web site provides access to U.S. government data on organ and tissue donation and transplantation.

Web Site: www.OrganDonor.gov

United Network for Organ Sharing (UNOS)

UNOS is an organization that facilitates all organ transplants in the United States by helping to make sure organs are obtained and distributed in a fair and timely manner.

Web Site: www.unos.org

### *Scholarships*

Cystic Fibrosis Scholarship Foundation

This foundation provides scholarships for students with CF.

Web Site: www.cfscholarship.org

Elizabeth Nash Foundation

This foundation also provides scholarships for students with CF.

Web Site: www.elizabethnashfoundation.org

## REFERENCES

Al-Yaman, F., Bryant, M., & Sargeant, H. (2002). Australia's children 2002: Their health and wellbeing. *Australian Institute of Health and Welfare Report Online*. Retrieved July 6, 2007, from http://www.aihw.gov.au/publications/index.cfm/title/7516

Andreasson, B., Jonson, B., Kornfalt, R., Nordmark, E., & Sandstrom, S. (1987). Long-term effects of physical exercise on working capacity and pulmonary function in cystic fibrosis. *Acta Paediatrica Scandinavica, 76*, 70–75.

Bacon, D. L. (2000). Attention, memory and executive functioning in children with cystic fibrosis (Doctoral dissertation, University of Texas Southwestern Medical Center at Dallas, 2000). *Dissertation Abstracts International, 61*, 1619.

Bals, R., Weiner, D. J., & Wilson, J. M. (1999). The innate immune system in cystic fibrosis lung disease. *The Journal of Clinical Investigation, 103*, 441–445.

Bhudhikanok, G. S., Lim, J., Markus, R., Harkins, A., Moss, R. B., & Bachrach, L. K. (1996). Correlates of osteopenia in patients with cystic fibrosis. *Pediatrics, 97*, 103–111.

Bradley, S., Solin, P., Wilson, J., Johns, D., Walters, E. H., & Naughton, M. T. (1999). Hypoxemia and hypercapnia during exercise and sleep in patients with cystic fibrosis. *Chest, 116*, 647–654.

Bresnihan, B. (1988). Cystic fibrosis, chronic bacterial infection and rheumatic disease. *British Journal of Rheumatology, 27*, 339–341.

Bush, A. (2001). Cystic fibrosis: Cause, course, and treatment. In M. Bluebond-Langner, B. Lask, & D. Angst (Eds.), *Psychosocial aspects of cystic fibrosis* (pp. 1–25). London: Arnold.

Cohen, M. J. (1997). *Children's Memory Scale*. San Antonio, TX: The Psychological Corporation.

Cystic Fibrosis Foundation. (1997). *Clinical practice guidelines for cystic fibrosis*. Bethesda, MD: Author.

Cystic Fibrosis Foundation. (2005). *Patient registry 2005 annual report*. Bethesda, MD: Author.

Cystic Fibrosis Foundation. (2006). New statistics show CF patients living longer. *2006 News Archive*. Retrieved July 4, 2007, from http://www.cff.org/aboutCFFoundation/NewsEvents/2006NewsArchive/index.cfm?ID=2711&TYPE=1132

Davis, P. B. (2001). Cystic fibrosis. *Pediatrics in Review, 22*, 257–264.

Dodge, J. A., Morison, S., Lewis, P. A., Colest, E. C., Geddes, D., Russell, G., et al. (1993). Cystic fibrosis in the United Kingdom, 1968–1988: Incidence, population and survival. *Paediatric and Perinatal Epidemiology, 7*, 157–166.

Elborn, J. S., Shale, D. J., & Britton, J. R. (1991). Cystic fibrosis: Current survival and population estimates to the year 2000. *Thorax, 46*, 881–885.

Hardin, D. S., Brunzell, C., Schissel, K., Schindler, T., & Moran, A. (1999). *Managing cystic fibrosis related diabetes (CFRD)*. Bethesda, MD: Cystic Fibrosis Foundation.

Henderson, R. C., & Madsen, C. D. (1996). Bone density in children and adolescents with cystic fibrosis. *Journal of Pediatrics, 128*, 28–34.

Kerem, E., Reisman, J., Corey, M., Canny, G. J., & Levison, H. (1992). Prediction of mortality in patients with cystic fibrosis. *New England Journal of Medicine, 326*, 1187–1191.

Koscik, R. L., Farrell, P. M., Kosorok, M. R., Zaremba, K. M., Laxova, A., Lai, H. C., et al. (2004). Cognitive function of children with cystic fibrosis: Deleterious effect of early malnutrition. *Pediatrics, 113*, 1549–1558.

Koscik, R. L., Lai, H. C., Laxova, A., Zaremba, K. M., Kosorok, M. R., Douglas, J. A., et al. (2005). Preventing early, prolonged vitamin E deficiency: An opportunity for better cognitive outcomes via early diagnosis through neonatal screening. *Journal of Pediatrics, 147*(3 Suppl), S51–S56.

Lester, L. A. (2001). New therapies and new challenges. In M. Bluebond-Langner, B. Lask, & D. Angst (Eds.), *Psychosocial aspects of cystic fibrosis* (pp. 411–425). London: Arnold.

Mayo Clinic. (2001–2007). *Chronic obstructive pulmonary disease: Overview*. Retrieved July 8, 2007, from http://www.mayoclinic.org/copd/symptoms.html

National Institutes of Health. (1997). Genetic testing for cystic fibrosis. *NIH Consensus Statement Online, 15*, 1–37. Retrieved July 10, 2007, from http://consensus.nih.gov/1997/1997GeneticTestCysticFibrosis106html.htm

Orenstein, D. M. (2003). *Cystic fibrosis: A guide for the patient and family* (3rd ed.). Philadelphia: Lippincott-Raven.

Orenstein, D. M., & Nixon, P. A. (1991). Exercise performance and breathing patterns in cystic fibrosis: Male-female differences and influence of resting pulmonary function. *Pediatric Pulmonology, 10*, 101–105.

Ruchinskas, R. A., Broshek, D. K., Crews, W. D., Jr., Barth, J. T., Francis, J. P., & Robbins, M. K. (2000). A neuropsychological normative database for lung transplant candidates. *Journal of Clinical Psychology in Medical Settings, 7*, 107–112.

Scanlin, T. F. (1988). Cystic fibrosis. In A. P. Fishman (Ed.), *Pulmonary diseases and disorders* (2nd ed., pp. 1273–1294). New York: McGraw-Hill.

Schneiderman-Walker, J., Pollock, S. L., Corey, M., Wilkes, D. D., Canny, G. J., Pedder, L., et al. (2000). A randomized controlled trial of a 3-year home exercise program in cystic fibrosis. *Journal of Pediatrics, 136*, 304–310.

Steinkamp, G., & Wiedemann, B. (2002). Relationship between nutritional status and lung function in cystic fibrosis: Cross sectional and longitudinal analyses from the German CF quality assurance (CFQA) project. *Thorax, 57*, 596–601.

Stewart, S., Campbell, R. A., Kennard, B., Nici, J., Silver, C. H., Waller, D. A., et al. (1995). Neuropsychological correlates of cystic fibrosis in patients 5 to 8 years old. *Children's Health Care, 24*, 159–173.

Thompson, R. J., Gustafson, K. E., Meghdadpour, S., Harrell, E. S., Johndrow, D. A., & Spock, A. (1992). The role of biomedical and psychosocial processes in the intellectual and academic functioning of children and adolescents with cystic fibrosis. *Journal of Clinical Psychology, 48*, 3–10.

United Network for Organ Sharing. (2006). *Information for transplant professionals about the lung allocation score system* [Brochure]. Richmond, VA: Author.

Wechsler, D. (2003). *Wechsler Intelligence Scale for Children* (4th ed.). San Antonio, TX: The Psychological Corporation.

Yankaskas, J. R., Marshall, B. C., Sufian, B., Simon, R. H., & Rodman, D. (2004). Cystic fibrosis adult care: Consensus conference report. *Chest, 125*, S1–S39.

Zach, M. S., Purrer, B., & Oberwaldner, B. (1981). Effect of swimming on forced expiration and sputum clearance in cystic fibrosis. *Lancet, 2*, 1201–1203.

Zanni, R. L., Shutack, J. G., Schuler, P. M., Christie, D., & Holsclaw, D. S. (1985). Peripherally inserted central venous catheters for treatment of cystic fibrosis. *Pediatric Pulmonology, 1*, 328–332.

CHAPTER FIVE

# Diabetes

Eve N. Fontaine, PhD, and
Gregory Snyder, PhD

## DESCRIPTION OF THE DISORDER

Type 1 diabetes, also known as insulin-dependent diabetes mellitus (IDDM), is a chronic metabolic disorder characterized by insulin deficiency. It is the most frequently occurring pediatric endocrine disorder and one of the most common chronic diseases in school-age children. Its onset may occur at any age but most frequently occurs during childhood and adolescence. An estimated 1 in every 400 to 600 children is affected (National Institute of Diabetes and Digestive Diseases, 2005). The incidence of Type 1 diabetes varies by age, with approximately 7 per 100,000 per year in children ages 4 years and under, 15 per 100,000 per year in children 5 to 9 years, and about 22 per 100,000 per year in children and adolescents 10 to 14 years of age (Karvonen et al., 2000). White and Puerto Rican populations have the highest incidence, followed by African Americans and Mexican Americans (LaPorte, Matsushima, & Chang, 1995). In Latino and African American populations, there is a slightly higher incidence rate for females than males, whereas the opposite is seen in Whites (LaPorte et al.).

While the etiology of IDDM is currently believed to include both environmental and genetic factors, the primary disease course and symptoms result from the destruction of the insulin-producing beta cells in the pancreas. Auto-antibodies produced by the autoimmune system attack and destroy these cells. This process results in the absence of insulin production. Insulin is the hormone required for proper glucose (i.e., sugar) metabolism by the body's major organs. This lack of insulin production leads to an accumulation of glucose in the bloodstream and urine and the body's inability to effectively absorb glucose as fuel to produce energy.

Although there is no cure for Type 1 diabetes, it can be treated and controlled through adherence to a complex treatment regimen. The goals of treatment are to maintain appropriate blood glucose levels and to prevent the occurrence of both short- and long-term complications. Short-term assessment of blood glucose occurs multiple (i.e., at least four) times daily. Illness management also involves multiple daily insulin injections (or the continuous infusion of insulin through a pump), dietary regulation, and regular exercise.

In order to achieve optimal management of blood glucose levels, adherence to this treatment plan is required. However, treatment compliance does not guarantee good glycemic control. Other factors may adversely impact blood glucose levels, such as stress, fatigue, physical activity, illness/infection, medications, hormonal changes, and periods of growth. Because triggers for metabolic distress include both environmental and biological factors, Type 1 diabetes should be addressed within a multidisciplinary context, including pediatric endocrinologists, pediatricians, dieticians, nurse educators, psychologists or social workers, ophthalmologists, podiatrists, and child life specialists.

Treatment of diabetes involves multiple daily injections of insulin or the continuous infusion of insulin through a pump. The amount of insulin administered should be individualized, taking into account age, body weight, and pubertal status (Silverstein et al., 2005), and should be balanced with food intake and daily activities. The absorption rates of insulin and the time and duration of maximal action will vary based on the type of insulin, mixture of insulin in the same syringe, site of injection, and individual differences in patient responses.

Due to recent medical advances, many children and adolescents are now using insulin pumps to regulate their blood glucose levels. An insulin pump is a device filled with insulin that is usually attached to the abdomen. It is programmed to deliver insulin continuously, with the dosage based on the unique needs of the individual. The pump allows for flexibility in lifestyle due to its ability to account for variations in timing, amounts of nutritional intake, and physical activity (Plotnick, Clark, Brancati, & Erlinger, 2003). Although this is often a desirable step, individuals are usually required to demonstrate adequate control of their disease with traditional methods of insulin administration and consistent blood glucose monitoring prior to acquiring an insulin pump.

Insulin by injection lacks the accurate feedback control of the normal pancreas, resulting in unstable blood glucose levels. Thus, careful monitoring of glucose levels is an essential component of treatment. Monitoring occurs through the frequent use of a portable blood glucose meter. The goals for optimal blood glucose levels should be individualized and vary based on factors such as the child's age and the time of day (i.e., before meals, before bedtime, overnight), with ideal blood sugars (i.e., euglycemia) ranging between 70 and 130 mg/dL. As treatment progresses, glycosylated hemoglobin derivations (HbA1c), which are the result of nonenzymatic reactions between glucose and hemoglobin, are considered the most effective measure for monitoring medium- to long-term diabetic control. The Diabetes Control and Complications Trial (DCCT) has demonstrated that patients with HbA1c levels around 7% had the best outcomes relative to long-term complications, with values less than 7% marking an increased risk of severe hypoglycemia and values greater than 9% indicating an increased risk for hyperglycemic complications (DCCT Research Group, 1993).

Dietary regulation is an essential component of the treatment regimen. The purpose of appropriate nutrition recommendations is to achieve blood glucose goals without excessive hypoglycemia (Silverstein et al., 2005). Children and adolescents should comply with a diet that is tailored to their specific needs. As this diet is individualized on the basis of each child's specific nutritional needs and metabolism, children and their parents require extensive education that is most often provided by a registered dietician. Adherence to a regulated diet will include the task of monitoring the number of carbohydrates consumed, as this will often coincide with the child's dosage of insulin to regulate blood glucose levels. Typically, dietary regimens include recommendations that carbohydrates be limited to 50% to 60% of the whole caloric intake, with the remaining 40% dispersed among fats (30%) and protein (10%).

Regular exercise is also an important component of successful metabolic regulation. According to the Centers for Disease Control and Prevention (CDC) and the American Academy of Sports Medicine, a minimum of 30 to 60 minutes of moderate physical activity each day is recommended for children and adolescents with Type 1 diabetes (cited in Silverstein et al., 2005). Potential benefits of exercise include improved weight management, improved physical fitness and cardiovascular health, improved lipid profile, and lower pulse and blood pressure (Austin, Warty, Janosky, & Arslanian, 1993; Wasserman & Zinman, 1994). However, exercise also puts individuals at risk for developing a complication of diabetes, acute hypoglycemia. In the pediatric population, 10% to 20% of hypoglycemic episodes are associated with exercise that is generally of greater frequency, intensity, or duration (Silverstein et al.). Thus, the American Diabetes Association (ADA) recommends that blood glucose levels be checked both prior to and following exercise, as well as at hourly intervals during prolonged periods of exercise (cited in Silverstein et al.).

## RELATED MEDICAL ISSUES

Type 1 diabetes may be associated with many short- and long-term complications. Short-term complications include conditions such as hypoglycemia, hyperglycemia, and ketoacidosis. Over time, long-term micro- and macrovascular complications may develop. These may include neuropathy, retinopathy, nephropathy, and cardiovascular disease. Additional complications may include an increased occurrence of infections, poor circulation (especially in the feet and legs), hypertension (i.e., high blood pressure), and coronary heart disease. Children and adolescents with Type 1 diabetes also are at increased risk for thyroid disease, celiac disease, academic difficulties, psychiatric disorders, and neuropsychological impairments. Information related to some of these medical issues and neuropsychological correlates is described below.

### Short-Term Complications

#### *Hypoglycemia*

Hypoglycemia, a condition that occurs when blood glucose levels fall too low, is the most feared short-term complication of Type 1 diabetes. It may be caused by taking too much insulin, missing a meal or snack, or exercising too much. The severity of hypoglycemia varies from mild to severe. In mild hypoglycemic episodes, symptoms may include tremors, palpitations, sweating, pallor (i.e., pale skin), headache, and irritability. Symptoms of moderate hypoglycemia may include drowsiness, confusion, aggression, and autonomic symptoms (e.g., sweating, trembling, nausea). Assistance from others will be required for treatment. In cases of severe hypoglycemia, an altered state of consciousness, seizures, or coma may occur, necessitating hospitalization. The DCCT Research Group (1996) found that intensive insulin treatment was associated with a threefold increase in the incidence of severe hypoglycemia. Thus, frequent blood glucose monitoring is used to maximize the early detection of hypoglycemia.

#### *Hyperglycemia*

Hyperglycemia is a condition that occurs when blood glucose levels rise too high. It may be caused by taking too little insulin, forgetting to take medications on time, eating too much, getting too little exercise, and having an illness or stress. Symptoms may include high levels of glucose in the blood and urine, increased hunger or thirst, and frequent urination. This condition must be treated as soon as detected. Failure to treat hyperglycemia may result in diabetic ketoacidosis (DKA), which is a potentially life-threatening condition.

### *Diabetic Ketoacidosis*

When the body lacks sufficient insulin to utilize blood glucose for cell metabolism, it begins a process of secondary metabolization of fats for energy. This process results in the creation of a toxic substance that is removed from the body by the kidneys. DKA results from the buildup of these ketones in the blood stream. Symptoms of DKA may include high blood glucose levels, high levels of ketones in the urine, abdominal pain, nausea or vomiting, shortness of breath, fatigue, dry mouth, a fruity odor on the breath, and dry or flushed skin. Recurrent extreme episodes of hyperglycemia resulting in DKA are associated with long-term complications, including damage to the kidneys, nerves, blood vessels, eyes, gums, and teeth. Immediate treatment of DKA is required or death may occur. Infections or illnesses, such as a cold or flu, may increase the risk of DKA; therefore, it is recommended that ketones be checked regularly when ill.

## Long-Term Complications

### *Neuropathy*

Neuropathy is a peripheral nerve disorder characterized by the loss of sensation and nerve control of body functions. It is a common complication of diabetes that results from hyperglycemia. Damage to the nerves generally progresses over a period of years and most often occurs in the legs and feet. There are many types of neuropathy, and its clinical presentation varies by type and specific nerve affected. Symptoms may include numbness, pain, tingling, weakness in the muscles, gastrointestinal and bladder problems, and low blood pressure. Symptoms develop gradually, with their onset typically occurring 10 to 20 years after diagnosis.

An estimated 54% of individuals with Type 1 diabetes will develop polyneuropathy, the most common type of neuropathy (Dyck et al., 1993). Neuropathy is uncommon in children, with a reported prevalence of 2% or less (Thomas & Tomlinson, 1993). It is important to identify and begin treatment for neuropathy as early as possible. The purpose of treatment is to reduce symptoms and prevent further nerve damage. Treatment includes optimizing blood glucose levels and improving weight management through diet and exercise. The use of certain medications may assist with pain management. The ADA recommends that all individuals with Type 1 diabetes receive annual screenings for polyneuropathy (ADA, 2007). Regular examinations of the feet are also recommended to identify lesions or injuries that may result from the loss of sensation. Annual foot exams should begin at puberty (Silverstein et al., 2005).

### *Retinopathy*

Retinopathy is a vascular complication that involves damage to the retina of the eye. It is currently the leading cause of blindness in young adults with Type 1 diabetes (Lueder & Silverstein, 2005). There are two types of retinopathy, nonproliferative and proliferative. The nonproliferative form of retinopathy is more common and may lead to ischemia (i.e., restricted blood flow), retinal hemorrhages (i.e., bleeding onto the surface of the retina), leakage of exudative fluid within the retina (Lueder & Silverstein), and macular edema (i.e., swelling of the retina). Over the course of several years, nonproliferative retinopathy may progress to proliferative retinopathy, which may ultimately lead to a complete loss of vision (Lueder & Silverstein).

Retinopathy is most often described as occurring following the onset of puberty. It may also occur in prepubertal children (Murphy et al., 1990), though its incidence is low. The risk for developing retinopathy increases significantly 8 to 10 years after diagnosis (Lueder & Silverstein, 2005), with the majority of individuals developing retinopathy 20 years postdiagnosis (ADA, 2002b). The development of retinopathy is influenced by the duration of diabetes, blood glucose control, blood pressure, and genetics.

Results from the DCCT indicated that the rate of retinopathy can be greatly reduced by improving glycemic control and decreasing hemoglobin A1c concentrations (DCCT Research Group, 1993). In addition, children and adolescents with Type 1 diabetes should receive ophthalmological screenings and regular eye examinations. According to the ADA, the initial evaluation should occur within 3 to 5 years of diagnosis and when the child is at least 10 years of age (cited in Silverstein et al., 2005).

### *Nephropathy*

Nephropathy, or kidney disease, is a life-threatening complication of diabetes in which the kidneys lose their ability to function properly. In the United States and Europe, diabetes is the most common cause of end-stage renal disease, accounting for approximately 40% of new cases (ADA, 2002a). An estimated 20% to 40% of diabetics will be affected (ADA, 2007). Risk factors for developing nephropathy include high blood pressure, high cholesterol, and smoking. The earliest sign of nephropathy is microalbuminuria, which is the presence of low, but abnormal, levels of albumin (i.e., protein found in the blood) in the urine. As damage to the kidneys progresses, greater amounts of this protein are excreted into the urine, resulting in macroalbuminuria. Blood pressure, cholesterol, and triglyceride levels will also rise. Nephropathy may eventually lead to chronic kidney failure and end-stage renal disease.

Early identification of microalbuminuria is important so that further damage to the kidneys can be minimized. Microalbuminuria screenings should be performed annually, beginning 5 years after disease onset (ADA, 2007). Once diagnosed, treatment focuses on managing symptoms and slowing the progression of nephropathy by maintaining optimal blood pressure and glucose control (ADA, 2007).

## Neuropsychological Correlates

### *Metabolic Control*

Poor metabolic control, frequent hypoglycemic episodes, and associated seizures have been implicated as the primary culprits in the long-term neurocognitive sequelae associated with Type 1 diabetes. Acute hypoglycemia alters cerebral blood flow, particularly in the frontal and parietal regions of the brain (Tallroth, Ryding, & Agardh, 1992). This state is also associated with altered neural metabolization and necrosis (i.e., cell death), to which the temporal lobe, basal ganglia, hypothalamus, and brain stem appear the most vulnerable (Auer, Hugh, Cosgrove, & Curry, 1989; Rankins, Wellard, Cameron, McDonnell, & Northam, 2005).

The neuropsychological sequelae associated with hypoglycemia are compounded by recurrent episodes. Ferguson and colleagues (2005) observed an increased incidence of ventricular enlargement and white matter lesions in the hippocampus in patients with a history of recurrent (i.e., more than five) episodes of hypoglycemia. Perros, Deary, Sellar, Best, and Frier (1997) reported an increased likelihood that patients with recurrent episodes of hypoglycemia would exhibit abnormal magnetic resonance imaging (MRI) brain scans, specific to periventricular white matter lesions and generalized cortical atrophy (i.e., wasting away or decrease in size of the cerebral cortex).

Similar results were observed by Northam, Anderson, Werther, Warne, and Andrewes (1999) in their comparison of 123 children between the ages of 3 and 14 years. Comparisons were made based on metabolic control and early onset of disease (EOD) (before 5 years of age). All children were assessed soon after diagnosis and at 2-year follow-up on measures of general reasoning/intelligence, rote verbal learning and memory, visual-perceptual memory and learning, verbal fluency, and complex visuomotor organization. Children with EOD scored more poorly on measures of perceptual reasoning, immediate verbal memory, visual and verbal total learning, and complex visual organization.

Episodes of hyperglycemia also have been implicated in structural central nervous system (CNS) changes and associated neurocognitive performance decrements. Cameron and colleagues (2005) examined hyperglycemic children presenting with and without DKA. They observed CNS edema (i.e., swelling) and abnormal cerebral metabolic changes, primarily in the frontal region of the brain. Similar results were observed in a sample of adults, in which subjects with a history of Type 1 diabetes evidenced significantly greater cerebral spinal fluid, suggesting mild atrophy (Lobnig, Kromeke, Optenhostert-Porst, & Wolf, 2006). The frequency of hyperglycemic episodes also has been associated with declines on measures of motor speed and visuomotor processing speed over time (Jacobson et al., 1990).

### *Age of Onset*

Extant literature has identified EOD as a significant contributor to more pronounced neuropsychological deficits during later childhood, adolescence, and adulthood (Ryan, 1988; Ryan, Vega, & Drash, 1985). This early-onset hypothesis posits that children diagnosed earlier (i.e., before 4 to 7 years of age) are significantly more vulnerable to disrupted neural development (Rovet, Ehrlich, & Czuchta, 1990; Rovet, Ehrlich, & Hoppe, 1988; Ryan et al.). Indeed, there is an increased risk for episodes of severe hypoglycemia in children diagnosed prior to 6 years of age (Davis, Keating, Byrne, Russell, & Jones, 1997).

While children with EOD are at greater risk for developing specific neurocognitive deficits later in childhood and adolescence, such deficits are not readily observable and appear to have a cumulative effect over time (Fox, Chen, & Holmes, 2003; Kovacs, Ryan, & Obrosky, 1994; Rovet et al., 1990; Ryan, 1988). For instance, Ferguson and colleagues (2005) compared 71 adults (early- versus late-onset diagnosis) using both neuropsychological measures and brain imaging (MRI). They observed that adults with EOD had more profound deficits in visual-perceptual skills, processing speed, choice reaction time, and sustained attention than other adults.

# RESULTS FROM NEUROPSYCHOLOGICAL EVALUATION

## Background and Demographic Information

Jonathan Doe is a 7-year-old, right-handed European American male who was referred for a neuropsychological evaluation due to inattention, distractibility, and impulsivity in the classroom. Background information was obtained by a review of available medical and school records, telephone interviews with Jonathan's classroom teachers, and an interview with his mother, Ms. Doe.

Jonathan was the product of an uncomplicated pregnancy and delivery. He was born full-term, weighing 7 pounds 6 ounces. Before 2 years of age, he was hospitalized three times for respiratory syncytial virus (RSV), pneumonia, and fevers. At 4 years of age, Jonathan was hospitalized due to severe nausea and vomiting. He was subsequently diagnosed with Type 1 diabetes and placed on intensive, exogenous insulin replacement therapy.

Since his diagnosis, Ms. Doe reported difficulties maintaining Jonathan's blood sugar levels within acceptable limits. She attributed these difficulties primarily to his frequent refusal to comply with his treatment regimen. Specifically, though Jonathan was required to test his blood glucose levels at least four times per day, he often demonstrated oppositional behavior when required to test his blood glucose or receive insulin. He was also dishonest about his blood glucose results.

Due to his poor treatment adherence and subsequent fluctuations in blood glucose levels, Jonathan was hospitalized four times within 2 years for DKA. His most recent episode of DKA resulted in a seizure. No prior history of seizures was reported. Jonathan was not prescribed any non–diabetes-related medications. His family history was significant for anxiety, depression, and attention problems.

Regarding Jonathan's behavioral and emotional functioning, Ms. Doe indicated that he was dishonest and exhibited defiant and disruptive behavior at home and school. At home, Jonathan frequently lost his temper and became verbally and physically aggressive when given instructions, denied requests, or redirected from enjoyable activities. Those outbursts usually occurred when he was required to test his blood glucose and receive insulin.

Jonathan was in the second grade at a public elementary school. He received some school accommodations for his diabetes under the auspices of a 504 plan. Ms. Doe was unsure of the specific interventions used by the school and believed they were geared mainly toward monitoring his blood sugar. Jonathan's academic achievement was below average, with particular difficulties in computational math. His teacher described him as markedly less mature than his fellow classmates, often inattentive, and easily distracted during class. She contacted Ms. Doe on numerous occasions, and Jonathan received multiple referrals to the principal due to poor conduct and out-of-control behavior. These emotional, behavioral, and academic difficulties led to concerns about Jonathan's learning capacity.

Jonathan lived with his biological mother and 5-year-old sister in a Midwestern city in the United States. He had had little contact with his biological father in the previous 5 years. Ms. Doe characterized Jonathan's relationship with his sister as warm. Regarding peer relationships, Jonathan preferred to play with younger children and maintained few reciprocal friendships with same-age peers. Ms. Doe stated he had recently been picked on and bullied by children at school. Jonathan reported feeling "different" because of his diabetes and targeted by other children because of his illness.

## Behavioral Observations

Jonathan was appropriately dressed and groomed for the evaluation. Gross visual and auditory functioning appeared adequate, and his expressive and receptive language functioning was grossly intact. Throughout testing, Jonathan required repetition of instructions and frequent prompts due to inattention and motoric restlessness. These behaviors resulted in his need for frequent breaks. Toward the end of testing, Jonathan appeared fatigued and became uncooperative or displayed poor effort. Taken together, although this evaluation may have underestimated his true ability, the results likely reflected Jonathan's level of functioning at home and in the classroom.

## Test Results

In neuropsychological assessments, children with Type 1 diabetes generally score within the normal range on tests of intelligence and academic performance but display deficits in information processing (Hagen et al., 1990; Northam et al., 1998), conceptual reasoning abilities, and acquisition of new knowledge when compared to controls (Northam et al., 1998). In contrast to these results, Jonathan's overall cognitive functioning was in the below-average range; however, he exhibited primary weaknesses in information processing and abstract reasoning, consistent with this research. Jonathan's performance across different neuropsychological domains and current research in these areas are described below. For a list of assessment measures administered and scores obtained, see Table 5.1.

**TABLE 5.1 Quantitative Assessment Data for Jonathan Doe**

| Scale | Scaled Score | Standard Score |
|---|---|---|
| WISC-IV | | |
| Full Scale IQ | | 81 |
| Verbal Comprehension index | | 87 |
| Perceptual Reasoning index | | 92 |
| Working Memory index | | 71 |
| Processing Speed index | | 88 |
| GORT-IV | | |
| Rate | 6 | |
| Accuracy | 8 | |
| Fluency | 7 | |
| Oral Reading Quotient | | 82 |
| CTOPP | | |
| Elision | 9 | |
| Blending Words | 10 | |
| Phoneme Reversal | 6 | |
| Blending Nonwords | 7 | |
| Rapid Naming (Numbers) | 8 | |
| Rapid Naming (Letters) | 7 | |
| Rapid Naming (Colors) | 7 | |
| Rapid Naming (Objects) | 5 | |
| WJ-III | | |
| Broad Reading | | 92 |
| Broad Math | | 82 |
| Math Calculation Skills | | 96 |
| GPT | | |
| Dominant (right) Hand | | 86 |
| Nondominant (left) Hand | | 94 |
| VMI | | 92 |
| RCFT | | |
| Copy | | 74 |
| Immediate Recall | | 92 |

*Continued*

**TABLE 5.1** *(Continued)*

| Scale | Scaled Score | Standard Score |
|---|---|---|
| Delayed Recall | | 82 |
| Recognition | | 108 |
| TEA-Ch | | |
| Sky Search | | |
| Targets Found | 6 | |
| Timing | 4 | |
| Score | 2 | |
| Sky Search DT | 2 | |
| Score DT | 1 | |
| Walk, Don't Walk | 4 | |
| CMS | | |
| Dot Locations | | |
| Learning | 7 | |
| Short Delay | 8 | |
| Total Score | 7 | |
| Faces | | |
| Immediate | 11 | |
| Delayed | 9 | |
| Stories | | |
| Immediate Recall | 10 | |
| Delayed Recall | 9 | |
| Delayed Recognition | 11 | |
| Word Lists | | |
| Learning | 6 | |
| Immediate Recall | 4 | |
| Recognition | 5 | |

*Note*. CMS, Children's Memory Scale (Cohen, 1997); CTOPP, Comprehensive Test of Phonological Processing (Wagner, Torgesen, & Rashotte, 1999); GORT-IV, Gray Oral Reading Test—Fourth Edition (Wiederholt & Bryant, 2001); GPT, Grooved Pegboard Test (Trites, 1989); RCFT, Rey Complex Figure Test (Meyers & Meyers, 1995); TEA-Ch, Test of Everyday Attention for Children (Manly, Robertson, Anderson, & Nimmo-Smith, 1999); VMI-V, Beery-Buktenica Developmental Test of Visual-Motor Integration—Fifth Edition (Beery & Beery, 2004); WISC-IV, Wechsler Intelligence Scale for Children—Fourth Edition (Wechsler, 2003); and WJ-III, Woodcock-Johnson Tests of Achievement—Third Edition (Woodcock, McGrew, & Mather, 2001).

### *Verbal Reasoning and Language Skills*

Jonathan's language and verbal reasoning skills were unevenly developed. With respect to his language progression, Jonathan demonstrated average to low average performance on simple phonetic segmentation and blending tasks; however, as task complexity increased, requiring greater phonemic proficiency, he had greater difficulty (e.g., see Elision and Blending Words versus Phoneme Reversal and Blending Nonwords). Challenges with stimulus complexity also were observed. Jonathan's speeded retrieval of numbers and letters remained relatively intact, whereas his recall of objects (involving increased phonetic complexity) was impaired.

Jonathan's verbal reasoning skills were in the low average to borderline range. He had particular difficulty on the Comprehension portion of the Wechsler Intelligence Scale for Children (WISC-IV; Wechsler, 2003), which requires children to verbally describe reasons or solutions for everyday difficulties. On this subtest, Jonathan lacked complexity in his verbal descriptions and rationales, which rarely improved following queries from the examiner. Jonathan's verbal concept formation and crystallized vocabulary skills were low average, and his responses were often limited to three to four words.

Jonathan's language and verbal reasoning deficits were consistent with research that suggests these impairments are associated with EOD. In comparing the verbal and language deficits between children diagnosed with EOD or late-onset diabetes (LOD), Ryan, Vega, and Drash (1985) noted that EOD is associated with a number of traditionally "left-hemisphere" activities, specifically impacting language-mediated concept formation, reading fluency, phonetic skills, and sequencing; however, such observations also revealed intact vocabulary performance. Rovet and Ehrlich (1999) observed significant declines in verbal IQ in children with disease onset at 7 years of age or later. Declines in verbal IQ were also more pronounced in children who had experienced a history of hypoglycemic seizures. In contrast, Holmes and Richman (1985) identified no differences in verbal intelligence regardless of the age of disease onset or disease duration. In a larger, more comprehensive neuropsychological examination of 62 children diagnosed with diabetes prior to 10 years of age, stable blood glucose levels were positively associated with verbal comprehension and academic issues, such that poorer management (i.e., lower blood sugar levels) was related to poorer performance in these children (Kaufman, Epport, Engilman, & Halvorson, 1999).

### *Visual and Spatial Reasoning Abilities*

Jonathan's motor speed and dexterity, visuomotor skills, and visuospatial reasoning also were unevenly developed. In the absence of time demands and speeded motor skills, Jonathan's nonverbal reasoning abilities remained largely intact. Jonathan's fine motor speed and dexterity were low average for his dominant (left) hand and average for his nondominant hand. Whereas his visuomotor integration skills on an untimed task were average, his performance deteriorated when he was required to manipulate objects quickly (i.e., Block Design) or reproduce simple symbols accurately (Digit Symbol Coding). Similar to observations of Jonathan's performance on verbal and language-based assessments, he struggled significantly when presented with increased task and stimulus complexity (i.e., Rey Complex Figure Test [RCFT]; Meyers & Meyers, 1995).

Regarding research in this area, Rovet and Ehrlich (1999) conducted a small ($n$ = 16) prospective study of children whose verbal, visuospatial, visuomotor, memory, attention, and executive functioning were evaluated at 1, 3, and 7 years. The authors observed that motor skills, attention, and executive functioning were impaired for children presenting with a history of hypoglycemic seizures; visuospatial reasoning skills remained intact during the first 7 years following disease onset. Longitudinal data from the DCCT reported similar intact functioning on multiple measures of visuospatial reasoning (cited in Jacobson et al., 1990).

### *Memory and Learning*

In the current case, a number of consistent patterns emerged from the assessments of Jonathan's memory. His rote memory for visual or verbal information represented a significant weakness. On brief measures of verbally mediated short-term and working memory, Jonathan's performance was in the borderline to impaired range. His performance declined on tasks that required mental manipulation (i.e., Letter-Number Sequencing) in addition to simple, brief storage and retrieval. Jonathan's capability for rote memorization of either verbal or visuospatial information was limited, especially for stimuli that were unrelated or became increasingly abstract and complex. Despite these weaknesses, when required to recall or identify more meaningful information, Jonathan performed adequately regardless of complexity.

Jonathan's difficulties in the area of memory and learning were consistent with research in this domain. Children with diabetes have evidenced greater learning difficulties (24%) than controls (13%), with boys demonstrating a higher rate of learning problems (33%) than girls (15%) (Holmes, Dunlap, Chen, & Cornwell, 1992). Deficits across a variety of learning and memory tasks have been reported. For instance, relative to controls, children with diabetes displayed deficits in long-term spatial memory (Hershey et al., 2005) and rote verbal memory (Rovet & Ehrlich,

1999). Despite gaps in rote verbal memory, contextualized verbal memory appears to remain somewhat intact. In a longitudinal investigation of children 8 to 13 years of age, Kovacs and colleagues (1990) observed that performance on logical memory tasks that naturally included increased contextual cues was average despite the children's deficits in rote verbal associative learning and working memory.

Recurrent episodes of hyperglycemia and hypoglycemia have been associated with deficits in visual and verbal learning (Northam et al., 2001). Children with a history of chronic hyperglycemia also performed poorer on the RCFT, which requires complex visuomotor skills, visual organization, and planning skills. Kaufman and colleagues (1999) reported that children diagnosed with diabetes prior to 10 years of age and with a history of hypoglycemic seizures performed worse than those without a history of seizures on tests of memory, including short-term memory and rote verbal learning tasks.

Gender and disease duration have also been associated with the risk for memory deficits in children with diabetes. Fox and colleagues (2003) reported greater risk for memory impairment in their sample of males, relative to females and control subjects. Specifically, boys were at an increased risk for failing to meet age-appropriate gains in verbal learning. The authors also noted that disease duration emerged as the most substantial predictor of overall memory performance for both boys and girls in the sample, with longer disease duration associated with poorer performance, regardless of gender. Given the potential for memory deficits, it is important to consider how these impairments may impact the performance of routine diabetes management tasks.

### *Attention and Executive Functioning*

On standardized assessments of attention, deficits were noted on tests of visual selective attention, divided attention, inhibition, and sustained auditory attention. Jonathan's focused visual attention deteriorated under additional cognitive loading and increased task demands. For instance, when competing demands were of the same modality (i.e., auditory), Jonathan struggled significantly. In the area of executive functioning, results of testing were suggestive of deficits in the inhibition of prepotent responses, mental set shifting, self-initiation, working memory, planning and organization, and self-monitoring.

These deficits are consistent with some research findings. Subtle, inconsistent effects of Type 1 diabetes on children's attention and executive functioning skills have been reported. Attention is a multidimensional construct and includes multiple skills such as the selection of relevant stimuli, inhibition of irrelevant information and responses, and shifting among competing responses and/or stimulus domains. To date, only one study has attempted to ascertain the specific attentional abilities that are affected by Type 1 diabetes. Rovet and Alvarez (1997) reported that children with EOD displayed noticeable deficits on measures of selective attention, whereas other domains of attentional control/shifting (i.e., sustained attention and inhibition) remained intact. Children with a history of hypoglycemic seizures performed worse than their counterparts on selective attention, focused attention, and inhibition.

Executive functions provide a foundation for children to successfully manage school demands. Such skills, traditionally attributed to the prefrontal cortex, include motivation, self-awareness/self-monitoring, planning, and purposive action (Lezak, Howieson, & Loring, 2004). Executive functions allow an individual to regulate attention and behavior to match environmental demands; organize thinking to make tasks easier to complete; demonstrate judgment and foresight; shift flexibly between competing activities/thoughts; generalize learning to new situations; work automatically and efficiently; and inhibit inappropriate responses. Children and adolescents with deficits in these domains can exhibit poor judgment, diminished social tact, inappropriate behaviors, difficulties with abstract reasoning, rigid and perseverative thinking, poor organization, problem-solving and planning difficulties, impaired academic and memory skills, problems with multitasking, and difficulty breaking complex tasks down into logical and manageable steps.

As suggested by the structural CNS changes associated with Type 1 diabetes, Northam and colleagues (2001) reported substantial deficits in multiple facets of executive functioning, including inferential reasoning and problem-solving skills, self-monitoring, and complex visual organization. Similar to findings with learning, memory, and verbal reasoning, these deficits appear more profound in those children with onset of diabetes prior to 4 years of age and/or a history of seizures. Similarly, Rovet and Ehrlich (1999) observed poorer self-monitoring skills, measured by perseverative errors on the Wisconsin Card Sorting Test (WCST; Grant & Berg, 1993) in children with Type 1 diabetes and a seizure history.

### *Academic Achievement*

Although gross measures of reading and mathematics were generally consistent with Jonathan's intellectual abilities, subtle deficits were observed with speeded information processing and phonemic proficiency. For instance, Jonathan's untimed, single-word reading and word-attack skills were average. In contrast, he had difficulty when required to read structured passages aloud to the examiner quickly and accurately. Specifically of concern was the rate at which he completed passages and the frequent phoneme substitution and guessing errors. During this test, Jonathan often guessed prototypical words based on the initial one or two phonemes, especially on more challenging oral vocabulary. Fluency and speed problems were also noted on timed, math-based tasks, where his calculation skills remained intact when not under time constraints.

Despite the number of studies demonstrating subtle fluid reasoning, memory, attention, and executive functioning deficits, two large-scale, multisite studies have indicated little effect on later school achievement. McCarthy, Lindgren, Mengeling, Tsalikian, and Engvall (2002) compared school achievement, as measured by the Iowa Test of Basic Skills (ITBS; Hoover, Hieronymous, Frisbie, & Dunbar, 1993), among children with diabetes and their matched sibling counterparts. In fact, diabetic children with relatively well-controlled blood glucose tended to outperform their sibling controls on many of the academic domains. However, as metabolic control decreased, so too did academic performance and overall grade point average (GPA). McCarthy, Lindgren, Mengeling, Tsalikian, and Engvall (2003) observed that children who had experienced hospitalizations for hyperglycemia or children with poor metabolic control scored lower on overall school achievement, reading scores, and GPA.

### *Behavioral and Emotional Functioning*

On a parent-reported behavior rating scale, Ms. Doe expressed a number of concerns related to the presence of inattention and a mood disturbance. Clinically significant elevations were noted on scales assessing inattention, depression, anxiety, and somatic complaints. However, Jonathan denied the presence of any significant depressive or anxious symptoms. Overall, responses were not indicative of severe emotional or behavioral distress, and Jonathan did not meet criteria for a mood or anxiety disorder. However, his chronic illness, history of academic problems, and inattention place him at risk for the development of emotional and behavioral difficulties in the future.

Due to concerns about the increased risk for adjustment and psychological difficulties in children with diabetes, considerable research has been devoted to this area. Many cross-sectional investigations have revealed that, in comparison with healthy controls, children and adolescents with Type 1 diabetes are similar to controls with respect to their level of psychosocial adjustment (Hanson et al., 1990; Wertlieb, Hauser, & Jacobson, 1986; Wysocki, Hough, Ward, & Green, 1992). Despite these positive results, other research suggests that children and adolescents with diabetes are at greater risk for experiencing psychological distress. For instance, in their meta-analysis, Lavigne and Faier-Routman (1992) reported that children with chronic illnesses, in particular diabetes, are at increased risk for the development of internalizing (e.g., anxiety, depression, somatic disorders) and externalizing symptoms (e.g., aggression, hyperactivity).

Although children present with increased rates of depression and anxiety after diagnosis, these symptoms often remit within 6 months (Kovacs, Brent, Steinberg, Paulauskas, & Reid, 1986); however, children's initial responses to their diagnosis, as reflected by levels of depression, anxiety, and self-esteem, have been predictive of their adjustment 6 years later (Kovacs et al., 1990). Evidence also suggests that age is an important variable; school-age children and their parents reported higher rates of psychological distress than their preschool and adolescent counterparts (Northam, Anderson, Adler, Werther, & Warne, 1996). Glycemic control has also been linked to psychological difficulties. Children who demonstrate poor long-term control of their blood glucose levels are reportedly more likely to exhibit emotional and behavior problems (English & Sills, 1997).

## INTERVENTIONS

Results from Jonathan's evaluation suggest the need for interventions at home and school. The following recommendations are designed to improve his treatment adherence and to address his psychosocial and academic needs. Other interventions that may assist Jonathan and other children and adolescents with diabetes are included as well.

### Increased Parental Involvement in Diabetes Management

Based on Jonathan's reported difficulties complying with the demands of his diabetes regimen, it was recommended that efforts be made to improve his adherence. Treatment adherence is central to successful metabolic control, and noncompliance with insulin regimens has been associated with short- and long-term neurological and systemic problems. Jonathan presented with comorbid behavioral difficulties, which put him at greater risk for treatment noncompliance (Cohen, Lumley, Naar-King, Partridge, & Cakan, 2004; Naar-King, Podolski, Ellis, Frey, & Templin, 2006). To improve Jonathan's adherence, increased parental involvement in diabetes management was strongly recommended.

Parental involvement and monitoring often are critical to the creation of habitual and accurate self-care behaviors. For example, Anderson, Ho, Brackett, Finkelstein, and Laffel (1997) observed that the frequency of blood sugar monitoring and overall glycemic control was greater for children whose parents were more involved with treatment, though adherence declined with increasing age. Indeed, decreased compliance and increased complications over time have been reported (Jacobson et al., 1990). Parents appear to be less involved with the management and oversight of their children treatment as they mature, creating multiple challenges as these children reach adolescence (Ingersoll, Hauser, Herrold, & Golden, 1986; Johnson, 1995).

## Behavior Management Programs

Based on parent and teacher reports, Jonathan exhibited significant inattention and other behavioral difficulties across multiple settings. Parent training was recommended in order to decrease the frequency of generalized defiance, noncompliance, and disruptive behavior. A number of evidence-based, behavior management programs exist (e.g., Helping the Noncompliant Child [Forehand & McMahon, 1981], Parent-Child Interaction Therapy [Hembree-Kigin & McNeil, 1995], Defiant Child [Barkley, 1997]). Behavioral management/parent-training therapies appear to have substantial effects on misbehavior up to 5 years after treatment completion (Forehand & Long, 1988).

Although parent training would likely be helpful with reducing problematic behaviors at home and in community settings, diabetes management behaviors should be concurrently targeted. Contingency management, differential reinforcement, and daily charting would be especially helpful adjunctive interventions. These strategies may be employed by a treating psychologist with the goals of improving compliance and increasing parental involvement with diabetes-related tasks.

### *Family- and Group-Based Approaches*

Other behavioral interventions that may be helpful for Jonathan and his mother include family- or group-based programs. A number of studies have investigated the beneficial effects of family-based behavioral interventions on treatment compliance. For example, using a sample of older school-age children and early adolescents, Anderson and colleagues (1997) observed that families who participated in interventions targeting parent-adolescent teamwork and parent-child conflict resolution demonstrated improved adherence to insulin administration and greater parental involvement in blood glucose monitoring than families who received standard care.

A number of group-based interventions have also been developed to improve coping skills, treatment adherence, diabetes knowledge, and diabetes management. Overall, group-based interventions, either specific or "anchored instruction" (i.e., videotape presentation with subsequent skill training or instruction), appear to have a beneficial effect on adolescent disease-related stress, dietary planning, problem solving, and adherence; however, none of the existing intervention studies have specifically addressed younger populations of children (Boardway, Delemeter, Tomakowsky, & Gutai, 1993; Gross, 1982; Gross, Heimann, Shapiro, & Schultz, 1983; Gross, Johnson, Wildman, & Mullett, 1981; Marrero et al., 1982). Group-based or multifamily interventions focused on conflict resolution and family communication also seem to improve adherence and metabolic control (Satin, LaGreca, Zigo, & Skyler, 1989). Overall, both family- and group-based interventions appear beneficial for children with diabetes and their families.

### *Other Psychosocial Treatments*

Results of this evaluation suggested that Jonathan sometimes exhibited social difficulties. These problems were consistent with his inattention and deficits in verbal reasoning. Consequently, participation in a social skills training program was recommended. Due to Jonathan's relative strengths in visual reasoning, programs incorporating visual aids to support appropriate social interactions could be helpful. In addition, Jonathan was encouraged to increase his participation in organized social activities with peers.

Though Jonathan did not present with significant mood or anxiety symptoms, other children and adolescents with diabetes may exhibit these psychological difficulties. In addition, youth with Type 1 diabetes are at greater risk for the development of eating disorders, which are associated with increased morbidity and mortality (Kelly, Howe, Hendler, & Lipman, 2005). The ADA recommends routine evaluations of psychosocial functioning in children and youth with Type 1 diabetes (cited in Silverstein et al., 2005). Psychiatric screenings are also indicated for adolescents with recurrent DKA or with difficulties achieving their treatment goals (Silverstein et al.). Should psychological difficulties be evident, immediate psychological and/or psychiatric treatment is warranted. Research suggests that cognitive behavioral approaches to treatment are beneficial. Psychological treatments have also been found to improve glycemic control (Winkley, Landau, Eisler, & Ismail, 2006).

## School Interventions

*Recommendations for Learning*

For Jonathan, academic interventions should take into consideration his relative strengths and weaknesses. For instance, providing visual aids and pairing verbal information with visual material may be beneficial. The use of frequent visual aids during instruction, "templates" for more complex assignments, and visually mediated reinforcement also were recommended. These strategies would likely assist with making the classroom environment less taxing.

Although many children benefit from extended rationales and reasoning when new concepts are introduced, it is likely that such explanations would impair Jonathan's ability to parse out meaningful information. It was recommended that instructions, commands, and explanations be kept short and simple. With routine tasks and assignments, he may benefit from the use of lists with pictures and symbols to supplement verbal instructions.

Jonathan's test results also suggested the need for further evaluation. Specifically, he displayed deficits in the areas of language/verbal reasoning and fine motor/visual construction. Both speech/language and occupational therapy evaluations were recommended to better understand the degree of these difficulties. These assessments may be completed as part of a school's full individual evaluation (FIE).

*Recommendations for Diabetes Management*

Diabetes is considered a disability under federal law. These laws, including Section 504 of the Rehabilitation Act of 1973, the Individuals With Disabilities Education Act (IDEA) of 1991, and the Americans With Disabilities Act (ADA) of 1992 protect children and adolescents with diabetes. Not only do these laws make discrimination against children with diabetes by schools or day cares illegal, but they also require any child with diabetes to receive an individual assessment.

To facilitate the appropriate care of children and adolescents with diabetes, school and day care personnel must have an understanding of diabetes. Further, they should be trained in the management of diabetes at school and be equipped to handle diabetic emergencies. According to the ADA (2003), children and adolescents should have an individualized diabetes health care plan at school. The parent/guardian should develop this plan with the assistance of the child's diabetes care team and in coordination with their school. This plan should be tailored to the specific needs of the child and include specific instructions for the management of his or her diabetes at school.

Taken together, interventions for children and adolescents with Type 1 diabetes should focus on improving treatment adherence and addressing their unique psychosocial and academic needs. Strategies for improving treatment compliance include the use of behavior management plans (e.g., parent training, contingency management, differential reinforcement, daily charting) and increased parental involvement in diabetes management. Group- and family-based behavioral interventions also may be beneficial. To address the psychosocial needs of these children and youth, routine evaluations of psychosocial functioning should be performed, and immediate psychological and/or psychiatric treatment should be provided as needed. Academic interventions should be tailored to the individual's relative strengths and weaknesses. In addition, children and adolescents with Type 1 diabetes should have an individualized diabetes health care plan at school.

## RESOURCES

### Books

The following books are recommended to children and adolescents with Type 1 diabetes and their parents, family members, and educators. Some of these books may also be useful to other professionals working with this population.

American Diabetes Association (ADA). (2006). *ADA complete guide to diabetes* (4th ed.). Alexandria, VA: Author.

American Diabetes Association, & Holzmeister, L. A. (2006). *Diabetes carbohydrate and fat gram guide* (3rd ed.). Alexandria, VA: American Diabetes Association.

Chase, H. P. (2004). *A first book for understanding diabetes.* Denver, CO: Children's Diabetes Foundation.

Gosselin, K. (1998). *Taking diabetes to school: Special kids in schools series* (No. 1). Plainview, NY: Jayjo Books.

Hanas, R. (2005). *Type 1 diabetes: A guide for children, adolescents and young adults and their caregivers.* New York: Marlowe & Company.

Hargrave-Nykaza, K. (2006). *My child has diabetes: A parent's guide to a normal life after diagnosis.* Lincoln, NE: iUniverse.

Hendel, E. (2005). *A child in your care has diabetes* (3rd ed.). Paramus, NJ: Hen House Press.

Hieronymus, L., & Geil, P. (2006). *101 tips for raising healthy kids with diabetes.* Alexandria, VA: American Diabetes Association.

Loy, V. N. (2001). *Real life parenting of kids with diabetes.* Alexandria, VA: American Diabetes Association.

McAuliffe, A. (1998). *Growing up with diabetes: What children want their parents to know.* New York: John Wiley & Sons.

McCarthy, M., & Kushner, J. (2007). *The everything parent's guide to children with juvenile diabetes.* Cincinnati, OH: Adams Media.

Peurrung, V. (2001). *Living with juvenile diabetes: A practical guide for parents and caregivers*. Long Island City, NY: Hatherleigh Press.

Warshaw, H. S. (2006). *Diabetes meal planning made easy* (3rd ed.). Alexandria, VA: American Diabetes Association.

## Organizations and Web Sites

The following list includes national foundations and Web sites that provide information to children and adolescents with Type 1 diabetes, their parents, family members, educators, and other professionals. Many of these Web sites include links to additional resources, such as support groups, summer camp listings by state, and recommended school accommodations.

American Association of Diabetes Educators (AADE)

The AADE is a multidisciplinary professional membership organization of health care professionals. It promotes evidence-based diabetes self-management education and practice. Its Web site includes a link to locate diabetes educators by state.

Mailing Address: 100 West Monroe, Suite 400
Chicago, Illinois 60603
Phone Number: (800) 832-6874
Web Site: www.aadenet.org

American Diabetes Association (ADA)

The ADA is a nonprofit health organization that provides diabetes research, information, and advocacy. Its Web site includes links to general information about diabetes, research, nutrition, exercise, and resources available to parents, children, and professionals.

Mailing Address: ATTN: National Call Center
1701 North Beauregard Street
Alexandria, Virginia 22311
Phone Number: (800) 342-2383
Web Site: www.diabetes.org

Barbara Davis Center for Childhood Diabetes

The Barbara Davis Center for Childhood Diabetes is a diabetes and endocrine care program located in Colorado. Its Web site includes links to information about diabetes, its management, and its associated health complications.

Mailing Address: 1775 N. Ursula Street
Aurora, Colorado 80045
Phone Number: (303) 724-2323
Web Site: www.barbaradaviscenter.org

Centers for Disease Control and Prevention (CDC)

The CDC Web site includes general information about diabetes and its management, research, and resources available to parents and professionals.

Phone Number: (800) 311-3435
Web Site: www.cdc.gov/diabetes

Children With Diabetes/Diabetes 123

Children With Diabetes/Diabetes 123 is an online community for children, families, and adults with diabetes. Its Web site includes information about diabetes, products and services, links to family support resources (e.g., chat rooms, conferences, scholarships, books, videos, diabetes camps), and information about managing diabetes in the school setting.

Mailing Address: 5689 Chancery Place
Hamilton, Ohio 45011
Email Address: info@childrenwithdiabetes.com
Web Sites: www.childrenwithdiabetes.com
www.diabetes123.com

Children With Diabetes Foundation

The Children With Diabetes Foundation assists children and adults with diabetes and is committed to seeking a cure for diabetes through scientific research. Its Web site provides a link to recent research in diabetes.

Mailing Address: 685 East Wiggins Street
Superior, Colorado 80027
Phone Number: (303) 475-4312
Web Site: www.cwdfoundation.org

Defeat Diabetes Foundation

The purpose of the Defeat Diabetes Foundation is to provide information and education about diabetes, its prevention, and the consequences of undiagnosed diabetes or poor diabetes management. It provides a free monthly online newsletter, and the Web site includes information about diabetes management, research, resources, and the various programs the foundation conducts each year.

Web Site: www.defeatdiabetes.org

International Diabetes Federation (IDF)

The IDF is an alliance of over 200 diabetes associations in more than 160 countries. The federation seeks to raise awareness of diabetes and promote the prevention of diabetes, appropriate diabetes care, and finding a cure for diabetes.

Mailing Address: Avenue Emile De Mot 19
B-1000 Brussels, Belgium
Phone Number: (+32) 2-5385511
Web Site: www.idf.org

Juvenile Diabetes Research Foundation International

This Web site contains information about diabetes, research, diabetes management in school settings and while traveling, and additional resources.

Mailing Address: 120 Wall Street
New York, New York 10005-4001
Phone Number: (800) 223-1138
Web Site: www.jdf.org

My Child Has Diabetes

This is an e-book and online resource for parents of children with Type 1 diabetes. It contains information about diabetes, school issues, and resources.

Mailing Address: 151 Keeney Street
Manchester, Connecticut 06040
Phone Number: (860) 712-2537
Web Site: www.mychildhasdiabetes.com

National Diabetes Education Program (NDEP)

The NDEP is a partnership of the National Institutes of Health, the CDC, and many public and private organizations. Its Web site includes information about diabetes and prediabetes as well as resources for health, education, and business professionals.

Phone Number: (800) 438-5383
Web Site: www.ndep.nih.gov

National Diabetes Information Clearinghouse

The National Diabetes Information Clearinghouse is a service of the National Institute of Diabetes & Digestive & Kidney Diseases (NIDDK). This Web site provides information about diabetes, its treatment and associated health complications, research, and resources.

Phone Number: (800) 860-8747
Web Site: diabetes.niddk.nih.gov/

National Institute of Diabetes & Digestive & Kidney Diseases (NIDDK)
The NIDDK conducts and supports research on many diseases, including diabetes. Its Web site contains information about diabetes and research.

Phone Number: (800) 891-5390
Web Site: www.niddk.nih.gov

## REFERENCES

American Diabetes Association (ADA). (2002a). Diabetic nephropathy. *Diabetes Care, 25,* S85–S89.

American Diabetes Association (ADA). (2002b). Diabetic retinopathy. *Diabetes Care, 25,* S90–S93.

American Diabetes Association (ADA). (2003). Care of children with diabetes in the school and day care setting. *Diabetes Care, 26*(Suppl. 1), S122–S126.

American Diabetes Association (ADA). (2007). Diabetic retinopathy. *Diabetes Care, 30*(Suppl. 1), S90–S93.

Anderson, B., Ho, J., Brackett, J., Finkelstein, D., & Laffel, L. (1997). Parental involvement in diabetes management tasks: Relationships to blood glucose monitoring adherence and metabolic control in young adolescents with insulin dependent diabetes mellitus. *Pediatrics, 130,* 257–265.

Auer, R. N., Hugh, J., Cosgrove, E., & Curry, B. (1989). Neuropathologic findings in three cases of profound hypoglycemia. *Clinicial Neuropathology, 8,* 63–68.

Austin, A., Warty, V., Janosky, J., & Arslanian, S. (1993).The relationship of physical fitness to lipid and lipoprotein(a) levels in adolescents with IDDM. *Diabetes Care, 16,* 421–425.

Barkley, R. A. (1997). *Defiant child: A clinician's manual for assessment and parent training* (2nd ed.). New York: Guilford Press.

Beery, K. E., & Beery, N. A. (2004). *The Beery-Buktenica Developmental Test of Visual-Motor Integration: Administration, scoring, and teaching manual* (5th ed.). Minneapolis, MN: Pearson.

Boardway, R. H., Delameter, A. M., Tomakowsky, J., & Gutai, J. P. (1993). Stress management training for adolescents with diabetes. *Journal of Pediatric Psychology, 18,* 29–45.

Cameron, F. J., Kean, M. J., Wellard, R. M., Werther, G. A., Neil, J. J., & Inder, T. E. (2005). Insight into the acute cerebral metabolic changes associated with childhood diabetes. *Diabetes Medicine, 22,* 648–653.

Cohen, D. M., Lumley, M. A., Naar-King, S., Partridge, T., & Cakan, N. (2004). Child behavior problems and family functioning as predictors of adherence and glycemic control in economically disadvantaged children with type 1 diabetes: A prospective study. *Journal of Pediatric Psychology, 29,* 171–184.

Cohen, M. J. (1997). *Children's Memory Scale.* San Antonio, TX: The Psychological Corporation.

Davis, E. A., Keating, B., Byrne, G. C., Russell, M., & Jones, T. W. (1997). Hypoglycemia: Incidence and clinical predictors in a large population-based sample of children and adolescents with IDDM. *Diabetes Care, 20,* 22–25.

The Diabetes Control and Complications Trial (DCCT) Research Group. (1993). The effect of intensive treatment of diabetes on the development and progression of long-term complications in insulin-dependent diabetes mellitus. *New England Journal of Medicine, 329,* 977–986.

The Diabetes Control and Complications Trial (DCCT) Research Group. (1996). Effects of intensive diabetes therapy on neuropsychological function in adults in the diabetes control and complications trial. *Annals of Internal Medicine, 124,* 379–388.

Dyck, P. J., Kratz, K. M., Karnes, J. L., Litchy, W. J., Klein, R., Pach, J. M., et al. (1993). The prevalence by staged severity of various types of diabetic neuropathy, retinopathy, and nephropathy in a population-based cohort: The Rochester diabetic neuropathy study. *Neurology, 43,* 817–824.

English, A., & Sills, M. (1997). Psychological factors, stigma and family consequences. In S. Court & B. Lamb (Eds.), *Childhood and adolescent diabetes* (pp. 315–328). New York: John Wiley & Sons.

Ferguson, S. C., Blane, A., Wardlaw, J., Frier, B. M., Perros, P., McCrimmon, R. J., et al. (2005). Influence of an early-onset age of Type 1 diabetes on cerebral structure and cognitive function. *Diabetes Care, 28,* 1431–1437.

Forehand, R. L., & Long, N. (1988). Outpatient treatment for the acting out child: Procedures, long-term follow up data, and clinical problems. *Advances in Behavior Research and Therapy, 10,* 129–177.

Forehand, R. L., & McMahon, R. J. (1981). *Helping the noncompliant child: A clinician's guide to parent training.* New York: Guilford Press.

Fox, M. A., Chen, R. S., & Holmes, C. S. (2003). Gender differences in memory and learning in children with insulin-dependent diabetes mellitus (IDDM) over a 4-year follow-up interval. *Journal of Pediatric Psychology, 28,* 569–578.

Grant, D. A., & Berg, E. A. (1993). *Wisconsin Card Sorting Test.* Lutz, FL: Psychological Assessment Resources.

Gross, A. M. (1982). Self-management training and medication compliance in children with diabetes. *Child and Family Behavior Therapy, 4,* 47–55.

Gross, A. M., Heimann, L., Shapiro, R., & Schultz, R. M. (1983). Children with diabetes: Social skills training and hemoglobin A1c levels. *Behavior Modification, 7,* 151–164.

Gross, A. M., Johnson, W. G., Wildman, H., & Mullett, N. (1981). Coping skills training with insulin-dependent pre-adolescent diabetics. *Child Behavior Therapy, 3,* 141–153.

Hagen, J. W., Barclay, C. R., Anderson, B. J., Feeman, D. J., Segal, S. S., Bacon, G., et al. (1990). Intellective functioning and strategy use in children with insulin-dependent diabetes mellitus. *Child Development, 61,* 1714–1727.

Hanson, C., Rodrigue, J., Henggeler, S., Harris, M., Klesges, R., & Carle, D. (1990). The perceived self-competence of adolescents with insulin-dependent diabetes mellitus: Deficit or strength. *Journal of Pediatric Psychology, 15,* 605–618.

Hembree-Kigin, T. L., & McNeil, C. B. (1995). *Parent-child interaction therapy.* New York: Plenum Press.

Hershey, T., Perantie, D. C., Warren, S. L., Zimmerman, E. C., Sadler, M., & White, N. H. (2005). Frequency and timing of severe hypoglycemia affects spatial memory in children with Type 1 diabetes. *Diabetes Care, 28,* 2372–2377.

Holmes, C. S., Dunlap, W. P., Chen, R. S., & Cornwell, J. M. (1992). Gender differences in the learning status of diabetic children. *Journal of Consulting and Clinical Psychology, 60,* 698–704.

Holmes, C. S., & Richman, L. C. (1985). Cognitive profiles of children with insulin dependent diabetes. *Journal of Developmental and Behavioral Pediatrics, 6,* 323–326.

Hoover, H. D., Hieronymous, D. A., Frisbie, D. A., & Dunbar, S. B. (1993). *Iowa Tests of Basic Skills Complete Battery, Form K.* Chicago: Riverside.

Ingersoll, G. M., Hauser, S. T., Herrold, A. J., & Golden, M. P. (1986). Cognitive maturity and self-management among adolescents with insulin dependent diabetes mellitus. *Pediatrics, 108,* 620–623.

Jacobson, A. M., Hauser, S. T., Lavori, P., Wolfsdorf, J. I., Herskowitz, R. D., Milley, J. E., et al. (1990). Adherence among children and adolescents with insulin-dependent diabetes mellitus over a four-year longitudinal follow-up: I. The influence of patient coping and adjustment. *Journal of Pediatric Psychology, 15,* 511–526.

Johnson, S. B. (1995). Managing insulin dependent diabetes mellitus: A developmental perspective. In J. Wallander & L. Siegel (Eds.), *Adolescent health problems: Behavioral perspectives* (pp. 265–288). New York: Guilford Press.

Karvonen, M., Viik-Kajander, M., Moltchanova, E., Libman, I., LaPorte, R., & Tuomilehto, J. (2000). Incidence of childhood type 1 diabetes worldwide. Diabetes Mondiale (DiaMond) Project Group. *Diabetes Care, 23,* 1516–1526.

Kaufman, F. R., Epport, K., Engilman, K., & Halvorson, M. (1999). Neurocognitive functioning in children diagnosed with diabetes before age 10 years. *Journal of Diabetes Complications, 13,* 31–38.

Kelly, S. D., Howe, C. J., Hendler, J. P., & Lipman, T. H. (2005). Disordered eating behaviors in youth with Type 1 diabetes. *The Diabetes Educator, 31,* 572–583.

Kovacs, M., Brent, D., Steinberg, T. F., Paulauskas, S., & Reid, J. (1986). Children's self-reports of psychologic adjustment and coping strategies during first year of insulin-dependent diabetes mellitus. *Diabetes Care, 9,* 472–479.

Kovacs, M., Iyengar, S., Goldston, D., Stewart, J., Obrosky, D. S., & Marsh, J. (1990). Psychological functioning of children with insulin-dependent diabetes mellitus: A longitudinal study. *Journal of Pediatric Psychology, 15,* 619–632.

Kovacs, M., Ryan, C., & Obrosky, D. S. (1994). Verbal intellectual and verbal memory performance of youths with childhood-onset insulin dependent diabetes mellitus. *Journal of Pediatric Psychology, 19,* 475–483.

LaPorte, R. E., Matsushima, M., & Chang, Y. F. (1995). Prevalence and incidence of insulin-dependent diabetes. In M. Harris (Ed.), *Diabetes in America* (2nd ed., NIH Publication No. 95-1468, pp. 37–46). Bethesda, MD: U.S. Department of Health and Human Services National Institutes of Health.

Lavigne, J. V., & Faier-Routman, J. (1992). Psychological adjustment to pediatric physical disorders: A meta-analytic review. *Journal of Pediatric Psychology, 17,* 133–157.

Lezak, M. D., Howieson, D. B., & Loring, D. W. (2004). *Neuropsychological assessment* (4th ed.). New York: Oxford University Press.

Lobnig, B. M., Kromeke, O., Optenhostert-Porst, C., & Wolf, O. T. (2006). Hippocampal volume and cognitive performance in long standing type 1 diabetic patients without macrovascular complications. *Diabetes Medicine, 23,* 32–39.

Lueder, G. T., & Silverstein, J. (2005). Screening for retinopathy in the pediatric patient with type 1 diabetes mellitus. *Pediatrics, 116,* 270–273.

Manly, T., Robertson, T., Anderson, V., & Nimmo-Smith, I. (1999). *Test of Everyday Attention for Children.* Suffolk, England: Thames Valley Test Company.

Marrero, D. G., Myers, G. L., Golden, M. P., West, D., Kershnar, A., & Lau, N. (1982). Adjustment to misfortune: The use of a social support group for adolescent diabetes. *Pediatric and Adolescent Endocrinology, 10,* 213–218.

McCarthy, A. M., Lindgren, S., Mengeling, M. A., Tsalikian, E., & Engvall, J. C. (2002). Effects of diabetes on learning in children. *Journal of Pediatrics, 109,* E9.

McCarthy, A. M., Lindgren, S., Mengeling, M. A., Tsalikian, E., & Engvall, J. (2003). Factors associated with academic achievement in children with type 1 diabetes. *Diabetes Care, 26,* 112–117.

Meyers, J. E., & Meyers, K. R. (1995). *Rey Complex Figure Test and Recognition Trial professional manual.* Lutz, FL: Psychological Assessment Resources.

Murphy, R. P., Nanda, M., Plotnick, L., Enger, C., Vitale, S., & Patz, A. (1990). The relationship of puberty to diabetic retinopathy. *Archives of Ophthalmology, 108,* 215–218.

Naar-King, S., Podolski, C. L., Ellis, D. A., Frey, M. A., & Templin, T. (2006). Social ecological model of illness management in high risk youths with type 1 diabetes. *Journal of Consulting and Clinical Psychology, 74,* 785–789.

National Institute of Diabetes and Digestive Diseases. (2005). *National diabetes statistics fact sheet: General information and national estimates on diabetes in the United States, 2005.* Bethesda, MD: U.S. Department of Health and Human Services, National Institutes of Health.

Northam, E. A., Anderson, P. J., Adler, R., Werther, G., & Warne, G. (1996). Psychosocial and family functioning in children with insulin-dependent diabetes at diagnosis and one year later. *Journal of Pediatric Psychology, 21,* 699–717.

Northam, E. A., Anderson, P. J., Jacobs, R., Hughes, M., Warne, G. L., & Werther, G. A. (2001). Neuropsychological profiles of children with type 1 diabetes 6 years after disease onset. *Diabetes Care, 24,* 1541–1546.

Northam, E. A., Anderson, P. J., Werther, G. A., Warne, G. L., Adler, R. G., & Andrewes, D. (1998). Neuropsychological complications of IDDM in children 2 years after disease onset. *Diabetes Care, 21,* 379–384.

Northam, E. A., Anderson, P. J., Werther, G. A., Warne, G. L., & Andrewes, D. (1999). Predictors of change in the neuropsychological profiles of children with type 1 diabetes 2 years after disease onset. *Diabetes Care, 22,* 1438–1444.

Perros, P., Deary, I. J., Sellar, R. J., Best, J. J., & Frier, B. M. (1997). Brain abnormalities demonstrated by magnetic resonance imaging in adult IDDM patients with and without a history of severe hypoglycemia. *Diabetes Care, 20,* 1013–1018.

Plotnick, L. P., Clark, L. M., Brancati, F. L., & Erlinger, T. (2003). Safety and effectiveness of insulin pump therapy in children and adolescents with type 1 diabetes. *Diabetes Care, 26,* 1142–1146.

Rankins, D., Wellard, R. M., Cameron, F., McDonnell, C., & Northam, E. (2005). The impact of acute hypoglycemia on neuropsychological and neurometabolite profiles in children with Type 1 diabetes. *Diabetes Care, 28,* 2771–2773.

Rovet, J., & Alvarez, M. (1997). Attentional functioning in children and adolescents with IDDM. *Diabetes Care, 20,* 803–810.

Rovet, J. F., & Ehrlich, R. M. (1999). The effect of hypoglycemic seizures on cognitive function in children with diabetes: A 7-year prospective study. *Journal of Pediatrics, 134,* 503–506.

Rovet, J. F., Ehrlich, R. M., & Czuchta, D. (1990). Intellectual characteristics of diabetes children at diagnosis and one year later. *Journal of Pediatric Psychology, 15,* 775–788.

Rovet, J. F., Ehrlich, R. M., & Hoppe, M. (1988). Specific intellectual deficits in children with early onset diabetes mellitus. *Child Development, 59,* 226–234.

Ryan, C. M. (1988). Neurobehavioral complications of type I diabetes: Examination of possible risk factors. *Diabetes Care, 11,* 86–93.

Ryan, C., Vega, A., & Drash, A. (1985). Cognitive deficits in adolescents who developed diabetes early in life. *Pediatrics, 75,* 921–927.

Satin, W. Q., LaGreca, A. M., Zigo, M. A., & Skyler, J. S. (1989). Diabetes in adolescence: Effects of multifamily group intervention and parent simulation of diabetes. *Journal of Pediatric Psychology, 14,* 259–275.

Silverstein, J., Klingensmith, G., Copeland, K., Plotnick, L., Kaufman, F., Laffel, L., et al. (2005). Care of children and adolescents with type 1 diabetes: A statement of the American Diabetes Association. *Diabetes Care, 28,* 186–212.

Tallroth, G., Ryding, E., & Agardh, C. (1992). Regional cerebral blood flow in normal man during insulin-induced hypoglycemia and in the recovery period following glucose infusion. *Metabolism, 41,* 717–721.

Thomas, P. K., & Tomlinson, D. R. (1993). Diabetic and hypoglycemic neuropathy. In P. Dyck, P. Thomas, J. Griffin, P. Low, & J. Poduslo (Eds.), *Peripheral neuropathy* (3rd ed., pp. 1219–1250). Philadelphia: W. B. Saunders.

Trites, R. (1989). *Grooved Pegboard Test.* Lafayette, IN: Lafayette Instrument.

Wagner, R. K., Torgesen, J. K., & Rashotte, C. A. (1999). *Examiner's manual: The Comprehensive Test of Phonological Processing.* Austin, TX: PRO-ED.

Wasserman, D. H., & Zinman, B. (1994). Exercise in individuals with IDDM. *Diabetes Care, 17,* 924–937.

Wechsler, D. (2003). *Wechsler Intelligence Scale for Children* (4th ed.). San Antonio, TX: The Psychological Corporation.

Wertlieb, D., Hauser, S. T., & Jacobson, A. J. (1986). Adaptation to diabetes: Behavior symptoms and family context. *Journal of Pediatric Psychology, 11,* 463–479.

Wiederholt, J. L., & Bryant, B. K. (2001). *Gray Oral Reading Tests: Examiner's manual* (4th ed.). Austin, TX: PRO-ED.

Winkley, K., Landau, S., Eisler, I., & Ismail, K. (2006). Psychological interventions to improve glycaemic control in patients with type 1 diabetes: Systematic review and meta-analysis of randomised controlled trials [Electronic version]. *British Medical Journal, 333,* 1–5.

Woodcock, R. W., McGrew, K. S., & Mather, N. (2001). *Woodcock-Johnson Tests of Achievement* (3rd ed.). Itaska, IL: Riverside.

Wysocki, T., Hough, B. S., Ward, K. M., & Green, L. B. (1992). Diabetes mellitus in the transition to adulthood: Adjustment, self-care, and health status. *Journal of Developmental and Behavioral Pediatrics, 13,* 194–201.

CHAPTER SIX

# Down Syndrome

Sarika U. Peters, PhD, and
Nirupama S. Madduri, MD

John Langdon Down, an English physician, first published an accurate description of a person with Down syndrome (DS) in 1866. Although others had previously recognized the characteristics of the syndrome, it was Down who described the condition as a distinct and separate entity. In 1959, a French physician, Jerome Lejeune, identified DS as a chromosomal anomaly when he observed 47 chromosomes present in each cell of individuals with DS instead of the usual 46. It was later determined that an extra partial or complete 21st chromosome results in the characteristics associated with DS (Roubertoux & Kerdelhue, 2006).

## DESCRIPTION OF THE DISORDER

DS occurs in 1 out of every 733 live births, and more than 350,000 people in the United States have this genetic condition (Centers for Disease Control and Prevention, 2006). One of the most frequently occurring chromosomal abnormalities, DS affects people of all ages, races, and economic levels. The life expectancy among adults with DS is about 55 years, though life span varies depending on the individual and his or her medical condition.

Parents who have already had a baby with DS, mothers or fathers who have a rearrangement involving chromosome 21, and mothers over 35 years of age are at greater risk for having a child with DS. Table 6.1 illustrates the relationship between the frequency of trisomy 21 and increasing maternal age. However, about 80 percent of babies with DS are born to women under age 35, as younger women have far more babies. In addition to advanced maternal age, some researchers are now demonstrating that polymorphisms in genes (i.e., multiple forms of the same genes) may be responsible for folate metabolism and can lead to an increased risk of having a child with DS (Martínez-Frías et al., 2006; Rai et al., 2006; Scala et al., 2006).

DS is usually identified soon after birth by a characteristic pattern of dysmorphic features. These include hypotonia (i.e., decreased muscle tone); upward-facing palpebral fissures; differences in the structure of frontal sinuses; flattening of the occiput (i.e., back of the skull); small earlobes; dental irregularities; protruding tongue; short, broad hands; and a single palmar crease.

The diagnosis of DS is confirmed by karyotype analysis. A trisomy occurs during cell division, when the chromosome does not divide as expected. Although 95% of individuals have the trisomy, 3% to 4% have a Robertsonian translocation, caused by extra material on chromosome 21. Mosaicism, a mixture of normal diploid and trisomy 21 cells, occurs in 2%. Most chromosome-21 translocations are sporadic (Committee on Genetics, 2001). However, some are inherited from a parent who carries the translocation balanced by a chromosome deletion. Most trisomy 21 pregnancies prove to be nonviable. Only one-quarter of fetuses with trisomy 21 survive to term.

**TABLE 6.1 Maternal Age and Frequency of Trisomy 21**

| Maternal Age | Frequency of DS |
|---|---|
| 20 years | 1/1667 |
| 24 years | 1/1250 |
| 30 years | 1/952 |
| 35 years | 1/385 |
| 40 years | 1/106 |
| 45 years | 1/30 |
| 48 years | 1/14 |
| 49 years | 1/11 |

*Note.* Adapted from Reser (2006).

## RELATED MEDICAL ISSUES

In spite of a distinctive chromosomal abnormality, there is variability in clinical presentation. Children with DS may experience medical problems affecting a range of organ systems. Consequently, children who have significant medical needs also suffer the impact on their developmental progress. Common medical findings for individuals with DS are listed below.

### Cardiology

The most prominent findings are congenital heart anomalies. Reports show that 50% to 60% of all children with DS will have a congenital heart defect noted on an echocardiogram. Infants with a cardiac defect will have difficulty with growth and development (Committee on Genetics, 2001). The heart's ability to pump oxygenated blood to peripheral tissues is compromised, with the brain suffering the most dramatic consequence. In addition, the heart muscle becomes weaker, causing the heart to go into congestive failure when fluid builds up in the lungs. Infants become very exhausted with normal activities, such as feeding. Children do not grow as well, as they have increased nutritional demands and inadequate calorie intake. The most notable cardiac anomalies in children with DS are reviewed below (Torfs & Christianson, 1998):

*Atrioventricular canal.* In 40% of children with DS, the division between the four chambers of the heart fails to form appropriately. In these cases, a mixture of blood with and without oxygen is being distributed to the tissues.

*Ventricular septal defect (VSD).* For 28% of children, this condition occurs when the division between the two lower chambers of the heart does not close. A VSD can close spontaneously during infancy or require a surgical procedure.

*Atrial septal defect (ASD).* In 7% of children, this occurs when the division of the upper chambers of the heart fails to close. There can be shunting of blood between chambers.

*Patent ductus arteriosus (PDA).* In 3.6% of children, the ductus, which is vital in the heart function of the developing fetus, does not close as expected at birth. Generally, it closes spontaneously shortly after birth. If not, surgery may be required.

### Endocrine

The endocrine system is an intricate arrangement of glands, which are organs that secrete hormones. The brain sends signals throughout the body so that glands can secrete hormones, which are proteins that control the growth and development of the body. Children with DS have a higher incidence of endocrine disorders compared to the general population. The disorders listed below are the most commonly occurring endocrine issues for individuals with DS (Committee on Genetics, 2001; Prasher, 1999):

*Hypothyroidism.* This occurs in 15% of children with DS. The thyroid hormone affects growth, metabolism, and cognitive function. In the newborn period, a screen for congenital hypothyroidism may not immediately detect hypothyroidism. As a result, the American Academy of Pediatrics recommends that all children with DS undergo a yearly screen of thyroid function. Children may present with symptoms such as tiredness, weight gain, feeling excessively cold, and constipation. Synthetic thyroid hormone can be administered daily to regulate thyroid function (Committee on Genetics, 2001).

*Congenital hypothyroidism.* This occurs in 1% of the population and is detected by routine newborn screening. Research from the Netherlands shows that treatment with thyroid medication for children with DS who had congenital hypothyroidism resulted in significant improvements in motor and developmental function at 2 years of age (van Trotsenburg et al., 2005).

*Hyperthyroidism.* In individuals with DS, hyperthyroidism is very uncommon and occurs more often in females than males. Symptoms include weight loss, agitation, and heat intolerance (Prasher, 1999).

*Diabetes mellitus.* Diabetes mellitus, also known as Type 1 diabetes, may occur in children with DS and may be attributed to early onset of obesity or an autoimmune process. Type 1 diabetes usually presents in 1% to 10% of young children with DS. Symptoms include increased thirst, frequent urination, and weight loss despite eating more food. Type 2 diabetes is being recognized in older children and adults with DS who have difficulties with obesity. For Type 1 diabetes, diet management and insulin treatment are very effective. For Type 2 diabetes, medications are used as well as diet management and weight reduction.

## Gastrointestinal

Children with DS can present with abnormalities of the gastrointestinal tract at birth. The following gastrointestinal issues are the most common in this population.

*Duodenal atresia.* This occurs in 11% to 33% of children with DS. At birth, when an infant has extensive vomiting upon the first feeding, there is suspicion that the intestinal tract ends at some point in a blind pouch. It called an atresia when there is no connection between portions of the intestine. This requires surgical correction to provide a link between the various portions of the intestinal tract (Committee on Genetics, 2001).

*Hirschprung disease.* Anywhere from 4.5% to 16% of children with DS experience this abnormality of the large intestine. Individuals with this finding have no innervation (i.e., distribution of nerves) to the colon. They are unable to pass stool and may have 5 to 6 days between bowel movements. When impaction of the stool occurs, there can be leakage, presenting similarly to diarrhea. This also requires surgical correction and may result in a long recovery process (Committee on Genetics, 2001).

*Gastroesophageal reflux disease (GERD).* Many children with DS have difficulty with GERD, resulting in extensive feeding difficulty. Some children refuse to take any foods by mouth. Medications are effective, and surgery may be warranted in severe cases of oral aversion.

*Celiac disease.* Between 5 and 15 percent of individuals with DS have celiac disease. These children lack necessary components in their intestinal tract to digest the protein gluten, most commonly found in wheat, oats, and barley. People without DS who have this condition experience bloating, diarrhea, and weight loss when they ingest gluten. However, these symptoms do not always occur in children with DS, so a routine screening test is performed. This disorder is managed by eliminating foods with gluten from the diet (Cohen, 2006).

## Head and Neck

A variety of ear, nose, and throat abnormalities occur very frequently in this population. Children with DS have differences in their facial structure that make them more susceptible to upper respiratory tract infections. Examples of these abnormalities are listed below (Committee on Genetics, 2001):

*Otitis media.* Middle ear infections occur commonly in young children. In children with DS, the ear canals are narrow and fluid stays in the middle ear area, resulting in infection. Antibiotics are the usual mainstay of medical treatment. Tympanostomy tubes may also be useful. Children undergo a simple surgical procedure in which a tube is inserted into their eardrums to help decrease the fluid accumulation in the middle ear.

*Sinusitis.* The sinuses in individuals with DS have differences in the tissue structure as well as facial configuration, increasing vulnerability to infections of the sinus tract. Standard treatment for sinusitis includes a trial of antibiotics, decongestants, antihistamines, and nasally inhaled steroid medication.

*Hearing loss.* Seventy-five percent of children with DS have conductive hearing loss. Amplification devices are useful and encourage language development. Children with DS receive yearly audiological evaluations (Committee on Genetics, 2001).

*Vision problems.* Many children with DS will have eye movement disorders, such as deviations of the orbit to the inside or outside. Cataracts also occur, affecting visual acuity. Also, susceptibility to infections of the conjunctiva (i.e., the delicate membrane lining the eyelids and covering the eyeball) is increased. Children will require yearly evaluations by an ophthalmologist (Committee on Genetics, 2001).

*Atlantoaxial instability (AAI).* Four to 14 percent of children with DS are at increased risk of having instability in the vertebra of the neck, which can cause neurological symptoms if severe, such as loss of bladder control. It is recommended that children receive an X-ray of the neck in neutral, flexed, and extended positions to determine if there is atlantoaxial instability, as there is a potential risk of spinal cord injury. Special Olympics competitions require that children with DS have a documented radiograph (X-ray) of the cervical (i.e., neck) vertebrae (Cohen, 2006). In addition, it is recommended that children with AAI not participate in strenuous and high-impact activity, such as gymnastics or football.

In addition to various medical problems, there is also a phenomenon known as dementia of Alzheimer's type (DAT). DAT occurs in young adults with DS. They have behavior changes and loss of skills, similar to older individuals with Alzheimer's disease. Caregivers report a loss of language skills and difficulty with emotional functioning, such as anxiety and depression. Current research is examining the use of medications that help to improve the outcome of Alzheimer's disease. In particular, medications that affect neurological function are being studied. Studies using donepezil have shown some benefit in improving language over time in adults with DS and documented dementia (Lott, Osann, Doran, & Nelson, 2002).

## GENERAL PSYCHOLOGICAL PROFILE

### Cognitive Development

Most individuals with DS have cognitive abilities that fall within the moderate range of mental retardation. In contrast to typically developing children and other children with developmental disabilities, the cognitive abilities of individuals with DS progressively decrease with age (Pennington, Moon, Edgin, Stedron, & Nadel, 2003). In fact, a recent study found that the cognitive deficits of adolescents and adults fall within the severe range of retardation (Vicari, Marotta, & Carlesimo, 2004). Researchers note that this decline in overall cognitive abilities may be impacted by the increased risk of DAT in DS (Vicari, 2006). Because of the risk of cognitive decline, it is recommended that individuals with DS be routinely assessed (for overall intelligence) throughout their life span; it should not be assumed that their abilities are fixed by a certain age and will not change.

## Language Abilities

Language skills, particularly expressive language skills, are typically noted as a relative weakness for children with DS. A typical developmental progression of language in DS is a slow transition from babbling to speech and, once speech emerges, articulation problems. As in children without DS, the degree of articulation difficulties is associated with hearing acuity. Researchers demonstrate that children with DS exhibit more delays in their expressive language skills, whereas their receptive language skills are typically commensurate with their nonverbal cognitive skills (Chapman & Hesketh, 2001). It is important to note that these delays in expressive language skills are not judged to be a consequence of hearing loss (Chapman, Seung, Schwartz, & Bird, 2000). Children with DS may begin using single words and phrases at expected ages for those milestones, but thereafter the further development of vocabulary and grammar usage is often delayed. In fact, researchers have demonstrated that individuals with DS have difficulties with knowledge and use of grammatical features and also with language pragmatics (Chapman et al., 2000). They typically use less sophisticated sentence structure, and the average length of their utterances (i.e., mean length of utterance; the number of words they use in sentences) is shorter than expected, given their cognitive abilities. In spite of these difficulties with grammar, however, it is also important to note that researchers demonstrated that when asked to perform a task in which they had to narrate a picture story, the group with DS expressed more content than would have been predicted given their mean length of utterances (Miles & Chapman, 2002). Other studies have demonstrated that language learning in individuals with DS continues both in terms of comprehension and production through adolescence and young adulthood.

## Motor Skills

Decreased muscle tone from birth (i.e., hypotonia) contributes to developmental delays in motor skills in individuals with DS. Some studies have demonstrated that emergence of early motor milestones is less delayed than the acquisition of more advanced motor milestones. Specifically, children may roll over between 5 and 6.4 months of age and may sit up without support between 8.5 and 11.7 months of age (Melyn & White, 1973). Crawling on hands and knees may occur between 12.2 and 17.3 months of age, and walking can occur between 15 and 74 months of age (Melyn & White). Regarding the development of fine motor skills, a recent study in individuals with DS found that all of the aspects of fine motor skills assessed were more severely impaired than gross motor skills and showed little development with age (Spanò et al., 1999). More specifically, these researchers found that the accuracy and timing of tasks requiring bimanual coordination were most impaired.

## Memory Skills

Many studies of memory skills in individuals with DS document impairments in verbal short-term and working memory, mostly assessed by a digit or word span (e.g., Bird & Chapman, 1994; Jarrold, Baddeley, & Hewes, 2000; Laws & Gunn, 2004). Working memory is defined as the process of temporarily storing and manipulating information (Baddeley, 1992). Deficits in working memory and verbal short-term memory in DS do not appear to be attributable to any difficulty with articulation but rather to difficulties in phonological memory (Laws, 2004; Laws & Gunn).

Long-term memory skills also have been studied in individuals with DS. Long-term memory consists of explicit memory (i.e., recall or recognition of actual experiences or information) and implicit memory (i.e., the ability to perform perceptual, cognitive, and/or motor tasks). Implicit memories involve a lack of conscious awareness; an example of implicit memory is when an individual rides a bike after many of years of not doing so. Studies have revealed that, compared to typically developing children and children with mental retardation of unknown etiology, individuals with DS perform worse on tasks of explicit memory, whereas their performance on implicit memory tasks does not differ from these groups (Carlesimo, Marotta, & Vicari, 1997). Studies examining the memory changes that occur in early-stage DAT in adults with DS reveal that individuals with DAT show severely diminished long-term storage and retrieval abilities compared to their peers without DAT (Krinsky-McHale, Devenny, & Silverman, 2002). These declines in long-term memory preceded other symptoms of dementia by a full year and, in some cases, by as many as 3 years.

### Results From Magnetic Resonance Imaging Studies

In an effort to link findings from psychological profiles to actual neuroanatomical differences, several groups of researchers have conducted magnetic resonance imaging (MRI) studies in individuals with DS. Volumetric MRI studies, during which the volume/size of different brain regions is examined, confirm that individuals with DS typically have lower overall brain volumes, with disproportionately smaller volumes in the frontal, temporal (i.e., amygdala, hippocampus, and parahippocampul gyrus), and cerebellar regions (Pinter, Eliez, Schmitt, Capone, & Reiss, 2001). MRI studies have also demonstrated hippocampal atrophy, which is more severe in patients with DS and dementia (Raz et al., 1995). Brain volumes in posterior cortical gray matter (i.e., parietal and occipital regions), however, tend to be spared. The psychological profiles in individuals with DS may be explained, in part, by these differences. Specifically, reduced volumes and/or dysfunction in the frontal and cerebellar structures can account for relative difficulties in language and motor tasks. Difficulties in long-term memory may be accounted for by hippocampal dysfunction (Pennington et al., 2003).

## COMMON PSYCHOLOGICAL AND BEHAVIORAL CONDITIONS

Rates of problem behaviors and psychopathology are typically low in individuals with DS. Nevertheless, researchers have demonstrated that children with DS are at greater risk for behavioral difficulties as compared to their typically developing siblings or to typically developing children in general (Gath & Gumley, 1986). On the whole, younger children with DS appear to be more at risk for externalizing disorders (i.e., oppositionality, attention-deficit/hyperactivity disorder [ADHD]), whereas adolescents and adults are more at risk for depression, obsessive-compulsive disorder, and psychosis (Capone, Goyal, Ares, & Lannigan, 2006; Dykens, Shah, Sagun, Beck, & King, 2002). Common comorbid conditions, associated behaviors and symptoms, and associated medical factors will be discussed in turn.

### Attention-Deficit/Hyperactivity Disorder

When evaluating the child with DS for possible ADHD, it is very important to consider attention and impulsivity relative to the child's overall cognitive abilities. Specifically, ADHD is characterized by a pattern of inattention, impulsivity, and hyperactivity that is disproportionate to the child's mental age and results in significant social and academic impairment across multiple environments. In general, researchers have found that hyperactivity and impulsivity with or without comorbid inattention can occur in a proportion of young children with DS, and these deficits are not correlated with mental age and social attributes (Green, Dennis, & Bennets, 1989). Researchers also demonstrated that complaints about inattention in DS are more common between the ages of 4 to 13 years of age and decline significantly thereafter (Dykens et al., 2002).

When evaluating the child with DS for possible comorbid ADHD, associated medical features that can increase risk include sleep apnea (Blunden, Lushington, Lorenzen, Martin, & Kennedy, 2005; Fallone, Owens, & Deane, 2002) or sleep disturbances (Levanon, Tarasiuk, & Tal, 1999). Hearing loss and hyperthyroidism, although uncommon in DS, also may be mistaken for ADHD (Pearl, Weiss, & Stein, 2001). It is therefore important to rule out hyperthyroidism and hearing loss as potential contributors to any inattentive, impulsive, and/or hyperactive symptoms.

## Oppositional Defiant Disorder/Disruptive Behavior Disorder

Oppositional Defiant Disorder (ODD) and Disruptive Behavior Disorder, Not Otherwise Specified (DBD-NOS) are characterized by patterns of oppositional, disruptive, and aggressive behaviors. Again, it is important to consider these behaviors in DS within the context of intellectual functioning. Specifically, some young children with DS may exhibit aggressive behaviors when they are overstimulated, and the aggressive behaviors may be a consequence of impulsivity or a strategy for attention seeking as opposed to being malicious and volitional. In fact, although parents of children with DS often characterize their children as stubborn, researchers demonstrated that only 6% of children with DS engaged in fights and 12% engaged in physically aggressive acts (Dykens et al., 2002). The aggressive behaviors were most common between the ages of 10 through 13 years.

Medical features that may be associated with risks of these problem behaviors include sleep apnea and sleep disturbances, physical pain, and hyperthyroidism.

## Autism

Autism is characterized by deficits in communication and reciprocal social interaction accompanied by repetitive/stereotypic behaviors. Many research studies regarding the coexistence of autism and DS have appeared in the medical and the psychological literature. Some studies have suggested that among persons with DS, about 10% to 11% may have autism (Howlin, Wing, & Gould, 1995; Kent, Evans, Paul, & Sharp, 1999).

Despite these reports, physicians and psychologists may be reluctant to recognize or diagnose autism or an autism spectrum disorder (i.e., Asperger's Disorder, Pervasive Developmental Disorder-Not Otherwise Specified) in children with DS, which can result in inappropriate educational placement for the child and unnecessary emotional hardship for their parents (Ghaziuddin, Tsai, & Ghaziuddin, 1992; Howlin et al., 1995). Arriving at this particular dual diagnosis is often hindered by stereotyped notions about what it means to have DS, autism, or severe cognitive impairment. A recent study conducted by researchers at the Kennedy Krieger Institute at Johns Hopkins Hospital revealed that children with DS and comorbid autism had lower levels of cognition as compared to their peers with DS who did not have autism (Capone, Grados, Kaufmann, Bernad-Ripoll, & Jewell, 2005). Severe mental retardation alone, however, does not account for behaviors related to autism in DS. Specifically, as stated by Capone and colleagues (2005), severe cognitive impairment can and does occur in children with DS who are sociable and have functional communication skills (Waterhouse et al., 1996; Wing & Gould, 1979). In fact, Wing and Gould described 27 of 28 subjects with DS in their study as sociable. Their clinical experiences also suggest that children with DS and comorbid autism have more impaired language abilities as compared to their peers with DS alone; in fact, many are nonverbal. Common behavioral features in children with DS and autism also include social disinterest, impairment in nonverbal communication and use of gestures, unusual use of toys or other objects, unusual sensory interests, anxiety, compulsions and rituals, repetitive motor behaviors, and self-injury.

## Depression

Depression is more common among adolescents and young adults with DS and is typically associated with mild to moderate mental retardation (as opposed to those who are more intellectually impaired) (Määttä, Tervo-Määttä, Taanila, Kaski, & Iivanainen, 2006). Symptoms of depression are usually precipitated in DS by increased perspective-taking skills that allow insight into not being like others, sudden change, or loss of personal relationships. Common symptoms include depressed mood, crying, decreased interest, psychomotor retardation, fatigue, appetite and weight changes, and sleep disturbances (Capone et al., 2006). Researchers have found that symptoms of withdrawal increase with age in DS and are more common among adolescent females with DS as opposed to their male counterparts (Dykens et al., 2002). A history of depression is strongly associated with dementia in DS (Coppus et al., 2006), and it is notable that females with DS are at greater risk of developing Alzheimer's disease as compared to males (Lai et al., 1999). Hypothyroidism in DS can also be associated with depression.

### Obsessive-Compulsive Disorder

Obsessive thoughts are typically quite difficult to assess in populations of individuals with mental retardation and can be especially so in DS because of difficulties with expressive language. Compulsions and rituals, however, do occur in some individuals with DS, and the prevalence rate varies between 0.8% and 4.5% (Myers & Pueschel, 1991; Prasher & Day, 1995). Common symptoms of obsessive-compulsive disorder (OCD) in DS include ordering of materials; an insistence on tidiness; rearranging personal belongings; repeatedly opening/closing doors, cabinets, or blinds; and repeatedly turning light switches on and off (Prasher & Day). Some individuals also may engage in hoarding and increased list making. When individuals are prevented from carrying out these rituals, they can exhibit extreme anxiety, aggression, and distress.

## CASE PRESENTATION

John is a 6-year-old boy who was diagnosed with trisomy 21 (DS) after physicians found notable facial features. Chromosome study confirmed the diagnosis at birth. He was delivered vaginally at full term, with no major complications during pregnancy. He received an echocardiogram, which was normal. He did not appear to have difficulties with feeding. At 1 week of age, John developed jaundice and required treatment with phototherapy. He underwent a tonsilladenoidectomy for sleep apnea and subsequently had a normal sleep study. The only pertinent family history is that his parents were divorced, and there is a history of maternal depression that did not require medical treatment.

At the time of evaluation, John's mother expressed concerns about his activity level. She also noted that he unintentionally engages in rough physical play with other children at times. He is extremely difficult to manage at home, is aggressive toward other children, has tantrums frequently, and will not stay in his car seat. These concerns are not, however, noted within John's school environment. During his developmental assessment using the Capute Scales (Accardo & Capute, 2005), his developmental quotients (developmental age/chronological age × 100) were as follows: Visual Problem-Solving Skills Developmental Quotient, 39; Language, 33; and Gross Motor, 30. He did not exhibit behaviors that would be consistent with an autism spectrum disorder, a disruptive behavior disorder, or ADHD.

At the time of evaluation, John was placed in a life skills classroom. He was receiving speech therapy from his school twice per week for 45 minutes. He was not receiving occupational therapy or physical therapy at school. He also was not receiving any private therapy services, although he was on a waiting list to receive services through the local Mental Health and Mental Retardation (MHMR) division. A recent reevaluation of his overall functioning was conducted by the local school district. At 5 years, 8 months of age, John's cognitive abilities were assessed using the Kaufman Assessment Battery for Children—Second Edition (KABC-II; Kaufman & Kaufman, 2006). Because of his significant language delays, the nonverbal index was administered, and his abilities fell within the moderate range of mental retardation. He was also given the Battelle Developmental Inventory (BDI; Newborg, Stock, Wnek, Guidubaldi, & Svinicki, 1984) and the Vineland Adaptive Behavior Scales (Sparrow, Balla, & Cicchetti, 1984) by the school psychologist at that time. His scores can be found in Table 6.2.

The pattern of John's scores revealed that his overall nonverbal cognitive abilities fell within the moderate range of mental retardation. The pattern of his scores reveals that although no relative strengths or weaknesses were present, his lowest score was in a task that involved short-term memory and motor planning, whereas his highest score was on a task that involved visual-spatial/reasoning skills. This pattern of performance is quite consistent in other children with DS. Based on assessment of his language skills, John's expressive and receptive language skills were significantly lower than what would be predicted given his cognitive abilities. In terms of receptive language skills, he was able to understand body parts, respond to his name, look at pictures, give objects by request, comprehend simple one-step commands, and use signs/gestures. Regarding expressive language, he communicated using single words, had poor grammar skills, and demonstrated a limited vocabulary. He also had difficulties with speech articulation. Thus, his difficulties with expressive language in particular were quite consistent with other children who have DS. It is of concern, however, that his receptive skills were so delayed, since research demonstrates that most children with DS have receptive skills that are commensurate with their nonverbal cognitive abilities.

John's level of adaptive behavior, as reported by his teachers, was broadly consistent with his overall cognitive abilities. Behaviorally, he was cooperative on a one-to-one basis but required praise and encouragement

**TABLE 6.2 Selected Evaluation Data**

| Scale | Scaled Score | Standard Score |
|---|---|---|
| | KABC-II | |
| Nonverbal Index | | 47 |
| Conceptual Thinking | 3 | |
| Face Recognition | 3 | |
| Triangles | 4 | |
| Pattern Reasoning | 5 | |
| Hand Movements | 2 | |
| | BDI[a] | |
| Personal-Social | | 65 |
| Adaptive Total | | 65 |
| Motor Total | | 65 |
| Gross Motor | | 65 |
| Fine Motor | | 65 |
| Communication Total | | 65 |
| Receptive Communication | | 65 |
| Expressive Communication | | 65 |
| Cognitive Total | | 65 |
| BDI Total | | 65 |
| | VABS | |
| Communication | | 62 |
| Daily Living Skills | | 63 |
| Socialization | | 64 |
| Motor | | 62 |
| Adaptive Behavior Composite | | 60 |

*Note.* BDI, Battelle Developmental Inventory (Newborg et al., 1984); KABC-II, Kaufman Assessment Battery for Children—Second Edition (Kaufman & Kaufman, 2006); VABS, Vineland Adaptive Behavior Scales (Sparrow, Balla, & Cicchetti, 1984).

[a]A standard score of 65 is the lowest possible score on this test.

to complete most tasks. At times, he grabbed test materials and refused to release them. With the use of rewards within the school setting, however, he was able to complete testing without difficulty, and his teachers and therapists noted no problem behaviors, except for minor issues with inattention. He therefore did not meet formal criteria for any behavioral diagnoses, despite the concerns noted by his mother.

In general, John's case points out the need to assess children with DS using developmentally appropriate instruments, as opposed to those that are appropriate for chronological age. For the most part, the pattern of strengths and weaknesses that John exhibited is not uncommon in other children with DS. In addition, his case highlights the importance of considering behaviors within a developmental framework and differences in behavior across multiple environments. His mother was educated regarding the pattern of his abilities and how to best manage his behaviors at home; because problem behaviors are more common within the context of significant language delays, she was provided with outside resources for private speech/language therapy to supplement what he was receiving at school.

## INTERVENTIONS

Children with DS are automatically eligible for early intervention services for children from birth to 3 years of age, because of their medical diagnosis and related delays in their language, motor, and cognitive skills. Some studies have suggested benefits in cognition, personal-social skills, and adaptive behaviors in children with DS who receive early intervention services as compared to their peers who did not (Connolly, Morgan, Russell, & Fulliton, 1993). Results are mixed regarding improvements in language and motor skills, and the research regarding the efficacy of these early interventions for children with DS is limited. More research has been conducted that examines the efficacy of interventions to target specific areas of need in individuals with DS.

### Speech/Language Therapy

As previously noted, research demonstrates that the onset of meaningful speech in infants with DS is significantly delayed, and the expansion/growth of their vocabulary is slow once they have acquired meaningful speech. For these reasons, researchers recommend that early speech/language therapy should focus on increasing awareness of words and sounds and how these are meaningful components of communication (Stoel-Gammon, 2001). More specifically, a phonetic approach is recommended by which young children are made aware of speech sounds and syllables. As children acquire single-word speech, most intervention programs continue to target promotion of phonological processes, increasing intelligibility (i.e., addressing difficulties with articulation), providing multiple opportunities for practice, increasing waiting time for verbal responses, and providing visual cues (Chapman & Hesketh, 2001; Stoel-Gammon). Researchers also note that because language comprehension is typically more advanced than language production, goals for comprehension can and should be at higher levels.

## Occupational Therapy

Research indicates that children with DS also have significant delays in their motor skills. The purpose of occupational therapy is to provide individuals with the necessary skills to achieve success and independence in activities of daily living. Occupational therapy may consist of interventions to promote postural reactions, which work to maintain body alignment and proper posture during movement; address the vestibular system, which is responsible for early motor behavior; and address sensory integrative dysfunction (i.e., the inability of the brain to correctly process information brought in by the senses) in children who are hypersensitive or hyposensitive to outside stimuli. Interventions to promote postural stability include training in developmentally appropriate movement patterns and promotion of muscle strengthening. Vestibular stimulation consists of activities such as swinging and developing equilibrium reactions through push/pull movements, through activities on a therapy ball, and by prompting balance. Sensory integration therapy consists of activities to promote visual perception, body awareness, tactile perception, and visual-motor coordination. Children with DS demonstrate difficulties in all of these areas. A recent study demonstrated that all methods of therapy are effective in promoting improvements in children with DS, and therefore all treatment methods should be applied in combination (Uyanik, Bumin, & Kayihan, 2003).

## Physical Therapy

As noted previously, children with DS exhibit considerable delays in their gross motor skills and typically exhibit hypotonia. Because of the increased risk of obesity in DS, physical therapy services as well as adaptive physical education services are essential. Unfortunately, there is limited research regarding the effectiveness of gross motor interventions in children with DS. One study found that when infants with DS were trained on a small, motorized treadmill 5 days a week for 8 minutes per day in their homes, they learned to walk with assistance and to walk independently faster than did the control group who did not receive these interventions (Ulrich, Ulrich, Angulo-Kinzler, & Yun, 2001). The long-term benefits of this intervention are, however, still being studied. Another study advocated for newer treatment paradigms to promote motor development because the results indicated no evidence that motor intervention promoted faster development or improved quality of movement compared to what would be predicted given simple maturation (Mahoney, Robinson, & Fewell, 2001).

Some research suggests the benefits of exercise training programs in individuals with DS. Specifically, a recent study demonstrated that adolescents with DS were able to significantly reduce their fat mass percentage when performing a 12-week exercise training program (Ordonez, Rosety, & Rosety-Rodriguez, 2006). Researchers have also demonstrated that exercise programs can increase the cardiovascular fitness of individuals with DS (Dodd & Shields, 2005).

## MEDICAL AND THERAPEUTIC MANAGEMENT OF PSYCHIATRIC CONDITIONS

Medical reports found that 18% to 38% of individuals with DS have a comorbid psychiatric diagnosis. These comorbid conditions can range from ADHD to depression. Typically, in children with developmental disabilities and comorbid psychiatric concerns, practitioners recommend that behavioral and/or educational modifications be attempted for a specific period of time before initiating medications. Generally, behavioral techniques are effective when consistently enforced. These can include a system of reward/consequence, sticker charts to record positive behaviors, and removal of privileges. If negative behaviors continue that are associated with a coexisting psychiatric disorder that impacts function in multiple settings, a trial of medication is the next option.

For children with DS, a diagnosis of ADHD may be a low priority on the initial differential list. Providers prefer to exclude underlying medical and academic problems before trying medication. The most effective medications for attention problems are psychostimulants. The most widely utilized medication is methylphenidate, which is a central nervous system stimulant. It is available in various strengths and has a mechanism of action in which the chemical compound in the medication binds to receptors in the frontal lobe specific for the neurotransmitter dopamine. Recent work has demonstrated that the level of dopamine increases within the brain, producing greater ability to focus and control impulsive behavior (Volkow, Fowler, Wang, Ding, & Gatley, 2002). In addition, there are various forms of longer acting methylphenidate (i.e., Ritalin LA, Focalin, Concerta, Metadate CD), in which a controlled-release apparatus is implemented to circulate medication throughout a 12-hour period of time. As a result, the child may require only one dose of medication each day, which would be taken in the morning.

Another stimulant medication is a mixed salt derivative of amphetamine compounds, known as Adderall. At this time, no studies have specifically compared the efficacy of all of these medications. It is important to note that there is a slow buildup of this medication, which means that close supervision is required to find a therapeutic dose. Many children begin medication in early elementary school. The primary side effects can include a decrease in appetite and sleep disturbances. In addition, nausea, dizziness, and lightheadedness may occur. Very rarely, cardiac side effects, including irregular heart beat and high blood pressure, may occur; these side effects warrant immediate medical attention. Previous reports of methylphenidate having a negative impact on height have not been substantiated in the literature.

In individuals with DS and comorbid autism, there is no medication designed specifically to treat either disorder. As this particular population has lower cognitive ability, the risk of aggressive and self-injurious behavior is greater. Atypical antipsychotic medication may be prescribed to reduce aggressive behavior. Risperidone is an atypical antipsychotic medication that has been studied in children with autism alone and has shown efficacy in reducing stereotypic and aggressive behaviors. A recent report also noted that children who are on a 4-month treatment course of risperidone have a recurrence of self-injurious behaviors and aggression when a placebo is gradually introduced (McDougle et al., 2005). One major adverse effect of atypical antipsychotic medications is substantial weight gain due to increased appetite. One medication in particular, olanzapine (Zyprexa), may increase risk of hyperglycemia and diabetes mellitus (Newcomer and Haupt, 2006; Varma, Connolly, & Fulton, 2007).

Depression may occur in individuals as they reach adolescence or young adulthood. Physiologically, depression results from a primary imbalance of serotonin utilization by the brain, resulting in well-known symptoms. In individuals with depression, the first line of medical treatment is a class of medications known as selective serotonin reuptake inhibitors (SSRIs). Fluoxetine (Prozac) was the first of this group to receive attention, as it has been widely used in individuals with depression as well as anxiety. In children, there is limited research that demonstrates a beneficial outcome from SSRI treatment. Side effects can include gastrointestinal problems, dizziness, sleep disturbances, and suicidal ideation. The Food and Drug Administration (FDA) has issued a warning regarding recent cases in the United Kingdom that correlated adolescent suicide occurrence with SSRI treatment. In the United States, research indicates that SSRI therapy lowers the rate of suicide among children and adolescents in a population-based study (Gibbons, Hur, Bhaumik, & Mann, 2006).

Children and adolescents with DS experience variable psychiatric and behavioral diagnoses. Research supporting specific medications is limited, and most practitioners follow anecdotal evidence shared by their colleagues. There is not one particular medication that is completely successful. Children are unique in their response to medications and therefore may require multiple trials in the process of finding the appropriate treatment. When a behavioral diagnosis is involved, medication is warranted only if a child's ability to function is impacted in multiple settings, sufficient behavior modifications have been implemented, and the child is a danger to himself/herself or others.

## SUMMARY

DS is one of the most frequently occurring genetic conditions, and school personnel should therefore be well prepared to evaluate, intervene, and treat children with DS across the age span. Given the frequency of comorbid behavioral conditions, it is very important that professionals not simply attribute all aspects of a clinical presentation to DS alone but be prepared to assess and intervene for these other presenting conditions as well. Development and behavior, even within the context of DS, are dynamic, and some of these comorbid conditions may not present until later childhood or adolescence; thus, reevaluation is of paramount importance. There are numerous research-driven methods of assessment and intervention, and many resources exist to assist professionals in this regard.

## RESOURCES

### Books

Bruini, M. (2006). *Fine motor skills in children with Down syndrome: A guide for parents and professionals* (2nd ed.). Bethesda, MD: Woodbine House.

Kumin, L. (2003). *Early communication skills for children with Down syndrome: A guide for parents and professionals* (2nd ed.). Bethesda, MD: Woodbine House.

McGuire, D., & Chicoine, B. (2006). *Mental wellness in adults with Down syndrome: A guide to emotional and behavioral strengths and challenges.* Bethesda, MD: Woodbine House.

Miller, J. F., Leddy, M., & Leavitt, L. A. (Eds.). (1999). *Improving the communication of people with Down syndrome.* Baltimore: Brookes.

Pueschel, S. M. (2001). *A parent's guide to Down syndrome: Toward a brighter future.* Baltimore: Brookes.

Pueschel, S. M. (Ed.). (2006). *Adults with Down syndrome.* Baltimore: Brookes.

Stray-Gunderson, K. (Ed.). (1995). *Babies with Down syndrome: A new parent's guide* (2nd ed.). Bethesda, MD: Woodbine House.

Winders, P. C. (1997). *Gross motor skills in children with Down syndrome: A guide for parents and professionals.* Bethesda, MD: Woodbine House.

## Web Sites

The Arc of the United States

The Arc is the world's largest grassroots organization of and for people with intellectual and developmental disabilities devoted to promoting and improving supports and services for all people with intellectual and developmental disabilities across the life span. It focuses on helping families ensure that any person with a disability is afforded the rights, duties, and responsibilities of full participation as citizens in their community.

Web Site: www.thearc.org

Best Buddies International

Best Buddies is a nonprofit organization dedicated to enhancing the lives of people with intellectual disabilities by providing opportunities for one-to-one friendships and integrated employment.

Web Site: www.bestbuddies.org

Down Syndrome: Health Issues

This is a Web site that is monitored by a pediatrician who is a father of a child with DS. It provides information on the latest medical research and therapeutic interventions.

Web Site: www.ds-health.com

March of Dimes Birth Defects Foundation

The March of Dimes provides a range of information regarding genetic disorders and birth defects, working to improve the health of babies by preventing birth defects, premature birth, and infant mortality.

Web Site: www.marchofdimes.com

National Association for Down Syndrome (NADS)

NADS is the oldest organization in the country serving individuals with Down syndrome and their families; its mission is to ensure that all persons with Down syndrome have the opportunity to achieve their potential in all aspects of community life. It offers information, support, and advocacy in the form of conferences, products and publications, a Web site and an online discussion forum.

Web Site: www.nads.org

National Down Syndrome Congress (NDSC)
The mission of the NDSC is to provide information, advocacy, and support concerning all aspects of life for individuals with Down syndrome.

Web Site: www.ndsccenter.org

National Down Syndrome Society (NDDS)
The NDDS envisions a world in which all people with Down syndrome have the opportunity to realize their life aspirations, and it is committed to being the national leader in enhancing the quality of life and realizing the potential of all people with Down syndrome through national leadership in education, research, and advocacy.

Web Site: www.ndss.org

## REFERENCES


Accardo, P. J., & Capute, A. J. (2005). *The Capute Scales: Cognitive Adaptive Test/Clinical Linguistic and Auditory Milestone Scale.* Baltimore: Paul H. Brookes.

Baddeley A. (1992). Working memory. *Science, 255,* 556–559.

Bird, E. K., & Chapman, R. S. (1994). Sequential recall in individuals with Down syndrome. *Journal of Speech and Hearing Research, 37,* 1369–1380.

Blunden, S., Lushington, K., Lorenzen, B., Martin, J., & Kennedy, D. (2005). Neuropsychological and psychosocial function in children with a history of snoring or behavioral sleep problems. *Journal of Pediatrics, 146,* 780–786.

Capone, G., Goyal, P., Ares, W., & Lannigan, E. (2006). Neurobehavioral disorders in children, adolescents, and young adults with Down syndrome. *American Journal of Medical Genetics Part C: Seminar in Medical Genetics, 142,* 158–172.

Capone, G. T., Grados, M. A., Kaufmann, W. E., Bernad-Ripoll, S., & Jewell, A. (2005). Down syndrome and comorbid autism-spectrum disorder: Characterization using the Aberrant Behavior Checklist. *American Journal of Medical Genetics Part A, 134,* 373–380.

Carlesimo, G. A., Marotta, L., & Vicari, S. (1997). Long-term memory in mental retardation: Evidence for a specific impairment in subjects with Down's syndrome. *Neuropsychologia, 35,* 71–79.

Centers for Disease Control and Prevention. (2006). Improved national prevalence estimates for 18 selected major birth defects: United States, 1999–2001. *Morbidity and Mortality Weekly Report, 54,* 1301–1305.

Chapman, R. S., & Hesketh, L. J. (2001). Language, cognition, and short-term memory in individuals with Down syndrome. *Down's Syndrome, Research and Practice, 7,* 1–7.

Chapman, R. S., Seung, H. K., Schwartz, S. E., & Bird, E. K. (2000). Predicting language production in children and adolescents with Down syndrome: The role of comprehension. *Journal of Speech, Language, and Hearing Research, 43,* 340–350.

Cohen, W. I. (2006). Current dilemmas in Down syndrome clinical care: Celiac disease, thyroid disorders, and atlanto-axial instability. *American Journal of Medical Genetics Part C: Seminars in Medical Genetics, 142,* 141–148.

Committee on Genetics. (2001). Health supervision for children with Down syndrome. *Pediatrics, 107,* 442–449.

Connolly, B. H., Morgan, S. B., Russell, F. F., & Fulliton, W. L. (1993). A longitudinal study of children with Down syndrome who experienced early intervention programming. *Physical Therapy, 3,* 170–181.

Coppus, A., Evenhuis, H., Verberne, G. J., Visser, F., van Gool, P., Eikelenboom, P., et al. (2006). Dementia and mortality in persons with Down's syndrome. *Journal of Intellectual Disability Research, 50,* 768–777.

Dodd, K. J., & Shields, N. (2005). A systematic review of the outcomes of cardiovascular exercise programs for people with Down syndrome. *Archives of Physical Medicine and Rehabilitation, 86,* 2051–2058.

Dykens, E. M., Shah, B., Sagun, J., Beck, T., & King, B. H. (2002). Maladaptive behaviour in children and adolescents with Down's syndrome. *Journal of Intellectual Disability Research, 46,* 484–492.

Fallone, G., Owens, J. A., & Deane, J. (2002). Sleepiness in children and adolescents: Clinical implications. *Sleep Medicine Reviews, 6,* 287–306.

Gath, A., & Gumley, D. (1986). Behaviour problems in retarded children with special reference to Down's syndrome. *British Journal of Psychiatry, 149,* 156–161.

Ghaziuddin, M., Tsai, L. Y., & Ghaziuddin, N. (1992). Autism in Down's syndrome: Presentation and diagnosis. *Journal of Intellectual Disability Research, 36,* 449–456.

Gibbons, R. D., Hur, K., Bhaumik, D. K., & Mann, J. J. (2006). The relationship between antidepressant prescription rates and rate of early adolescent suicide. *American Journal of Psychiatry, 163,* 1898–1904.

Green, J. M., Dennis, J., & Bennets, L. A. (1989). Attention disorder in a group of young Down's syndrome children. *Journal of Mental Deficiency Research, 33,* 105–122.

Howlin, P., Wing, L., & Gould, J. (1995). The recognition of autism in children with Down syndrome: Implications for intervention and some speculations about pathology. *Developmental Medicine and Child Neurology, 37,* 406–414.

Jarrold, C., Baddeley, A. D., & Hewes, A. K. (2000). Verbal short-term memory deficits in Down syndrome: A consequence of problems in rehearsal? *Journal of Child Psychology and Psychiatry and Allied Disciplines, 41,* 233–244.

Kaufman, A. S., & Kaufman, N. L. (2006). *Kaufman Assessment Battery for Children* (2nd ed.). Bloomington, MN: Pearson Education.

Kent, L., Evans, J., Paul, M., & Sharp, M. (1999). Comorbidity of autistic spectrum disorders in children with Down syndrome. *Developmental Medicine and Child Neurology, 41,* 153–158.

Krinsky-McHale, S. J., Devenny, D. A., & Silverman, W. P. (2002). Changes in explicit memory associated with early dementia in adults with Down's syndrome. *Journal of Intellectual Disability Research, 46,* 198–208.

Lai, F., Kammann, E., Rebeck, G. W., Anderson, A., Chen, Y., & Nixon, R. A. (1999). APOE genotype and gender effects on Alzheimer disease in 100 adults with Down syndrome. *Neurology, 53,* 331–336.

Laws, G. (2004). Contributions of phonological memory, language comprehension and hearing to the expressive language of adolescents and young adults with Down syndrome. *Journal of Child Psychology and Psychiatry, 45,* 1085–1095.

Laws, G., & Gunn, D. (2004). Phonological memory as a predictor of language comprehension in Down syndrome: A five-year follow-up study. *Journal of Child Psychology and Psychiatry, 45,* 326–337.

Levanon, A., Tarasiuk, A., & Tal, A. (1999). Sleep characteristics in children with Down syndrome. *Journal of Pediatrics, 134,* 755–760.

Lott, I. T., Osann, K., Doran, E., & Nelson, L. (2002). Down syndrome and Alzheimer disease: Response to donepezil. *Archives of Neurology, 59,* 1133–1136.

Määttä, T., Tervo-Määttä, T., Taanila, A., Kaski, M., & Iivanainen, M. (2006). Mental health, behaviour and intellectual abilities of people with Down syndrome. *Down's Syndrome, Research and Practice, 11,* 37–43.

Mahoney, G., Robinson, C., & Fewell, R. R. (2001). The effects of early motor intervention on children with Down syndrome or cerebral palsy: A field-based study. *Journal of Developmental and Behavioral Pediatrics, 22,* 153–162.

Martínez-Frías, M. L., Pérez, B., Desviat, L. R., Castro, M., Leal, F., Rodríguez, L., et al. (2006). Maternal polymorphisms 677C-T and 1298A-C of MTHFR, and 66A-G MTRR genes: Is there any relationship between polymorphisms of the folate pathway, maternal homocysteine levels, and the risk for having a child with Down syndrome? *American Journal of Medical Genetics, 14,* 987–997.

McDougle, C. J., Scahill, L., Aman, M. G., McCracken, J. T., Tierney, E., Davies, M., et al. (2005) Risperidone for the core symptom domains of autism: Results from the study by the autism network of the Research Units on Pediatric Psychopharmacology. *American Journal of Psychiatry, 162,* 1142–1148.

Melyn, M. A., & White, D. T. (1973). Mental and developmental milestones of non-institutionalized Down's syndrome children. *Pediatrics, 52,* 542–545.

Miles, S., & Chapman, R. S. (2002). Narrative content as described by individuals with Down syndrome and typically developing children. *Journal of Speech, Language, and Hearing Research, 45,* 175–189.

Myers, B. A., & Pueschel, S. M. (1991). Psychiatric disorders in persons with Down syndrome. *Journal of Nervous and Mental Disease, 179,* 609–613.

Newborg, J., Stock, J. R., Wnek, L., Guidubaldi, J., & Svinicki, J. (1984). *Battelle Developmental Inventory.* Allen, TX: DLM/Teaching Resources.

Newcomer, J. W., & Haupt, D. W. (2006). The metabolic effects of antipsychotic medications. *Canadian Journal of Psychiatry, 51,* 480–491.

Ordonez, F. J., Rosety, M., & Rosety-Rodriguez, M. (2006). Influence of 12-week exercise training on fat mass percentage in adolescents with Down syndrome. *Medical Science Monitor, 12,* CR416–419.

Pearl, P. L., Weiss, R. E., & Stein, M. A. (2001). Medical mimics. Medical and neurological conditions simulating ADHD. *Annals of the New York Academy of Sciences, 931,* 97–112.

Pennington, B. F., Moon, J., Edgin, J., Stedron, J., & Nadel, L. (2003). The neuropsychology of Down syndrome: Evidence for hippocampal dysfunction. *Child Development, 74,* 75–93.

Pinter, J. D., Eliez, S., Schmitt, J. E., Capone, G. T., & Reiss, A. L. (2001). Neuroanatomy of Down's syndrome: A high-resolution MRI study. *American Journal of Psychiatry, 158,* 1659–1665.

Prasher, V. P. (1999). Down syndrome and thyroid disorders: A review. *Down's Syndrome, Research and Practice, 6,* 25–42.

Prasher, V. P., & Day, S. (1995). Brief report: Obsessive-compulsive disorder in adults with Down's syndrome. *Journal of Autism and Developmental Disorders, 25,* 453–458.

Rai, A. K., Singh, S., Mehta, S., Kumar, A., Pandey, L. K., & Raman, R. (2006). MTHFR C677T and A1298C polymorphisms are risk factors for Down's syndrome in Indian mothers. *Journal of Human Genetics, 51,* 278–283.

Raz, N., Torres, I. J., Briggs, S. D., Spencer, W. D., Thornton, A. E., Loken, W. J., et al. (1995). Selective neuroanatomic abnormalities in Down's syndrome and their cognitive correlates: Evidence from MRI morphometry. *Neurology, 45,* 356–366.

Reser, J. E. (2006). Evolutionary neuropathology and Down syndrome: An analysis of the etiological and phenotypical characteristics of Down syndrome suggests that it may represent an adaptive response to severe maternal deprivation. *Medical Hypotheses, 67,* 474–481.

Roubertoux, P. L., & Kerdelhue, B. (2006). Trisomy 21: From chromosomes to mental retardation. *Behavior Genetics, 36,* 346–354.

Scala, I., Granese, B., Sellitto, M., Salomè, S., Sammartino, A., Pepe, A., et al. (2006). Analysis of seven maternal polymorphisms of genes involved in homocysteine/folate metabolism and risk of Down syndrome offspring. *Genetics in Medicine, 8,* 409–416.

Spanò, M., Mercuri, E., Randò, T., Pantò, T., Gagliano, A., Henderson, S., et al. (1999). Motor and perceptual-motor competence in children with Down syndrome: Variation in performance with age. *European Journal of Paediatric Neurology, 3,* 7–13.

Sparrow, S. S., Balla, D. A., & Cicchetti, D. V. (1984). *Vineland Adaptive Behavior Scales.* Circle Pines, MN: American Guidance Service.

Stoel-Gammon, C. (2001). Down syndrome phonology: Developmental patterns and intervention strategies. *Down's Syndrome, Research and Practice, 7,* 93–100.

Torfs, C. P., & Christianson, R. E. (1998). Anomalies in Down syndrome individuals in a large population-based registry. *American Journal of Medical Genetics, 77,* 431–438.

Ulrich, D. A., Ulrich, B. D., Angulo-Kinzler, R. M., & Yun, J. (2001). Treadmill training of infants with Down syndrome: Evidence-based developmental outcomes. *Pediatrics, 108,* E84.

Uyanik, M., Bumin, G., & Kayihan, H. (2003). Comparison of different therapy approaches in children with Down syndrome. *Pediatrics International, 45,* 68–73.

van Trotsenburg, A. S., Vulsma, T., van Rosenburg-Marres, S. L., van Baar, A. L., Ridder, J. C., Heymans, H. S., et al. (2005). The effect of thyroxine treatment started in the neonatal period on development and growth of two-year-old Down syndrome children: A randomized clinical trial. *Journal of Clinical Endocrinology and Metabolism, 90,* 3304–3311.

Varma, M. K., Connolly, K., & Fulton B. (2007). Life-threatening hyperglycemia and acidosis related to olanzapine: A case report and review of the literature. *Journal of Intensive Care Medicine, 22,* 52–55.

Vicari, S. (2006). Motor development and neuropsychological patterns in persons with Down syndrome. *Behavior Genetics, 36,* 355–364.

Vicari, S., Marotta, L., & Carlesimo, G. A. (2004). Verbal short-term memory in Down's syndrome: An articulatory loop deficit? *Journal of Intellectual Disability Research, 48,* 80–92.

Volkow, N. D., Fowler, J. S., Wang, G., Ding, Y., & Gatley, S. J. (2002). Mechanism of action of methylphenidate: Insights from PET imaging studies. *Journal of Attention Disorders, 6*(Suppl. 1), S31–S43.

Waterhouse, L., Morris, R., Allen, D., Dunn, M., Fein, D., Feinstein, C., et al. (1996). Diagnosis and classification in autism. *Journal of Autism and Developmental Disorders, 26,* 59–86.

Wing, L., & Gould, J. (1979). Severe impairments of social interaction and associated abnormalities in children: Epidemiology and classification. *Journal of Autism and Developmental Disorders, 9,* 11–29.

CHAPTER SEVEN

# Encephalitis and Meningitis

Lauren S. Krivitzky, PhD

Encephalitis and meningitis both refer to conditions involving an acquired infection of the central nervous system (CNS). Encephalitis is a general term that refers to an inflammation of the brain, while meningitis refers to an inflammation of the meninges of the brain. The meninges are the three protective layers of the brain and spinal cord that develop during the prenatal period (see further discussion below). There are a few additional variants of these conditions. For example, when both the brain and spinal cord are inflamed, the condition is referred to as encephalomyelitis. In addition, when an individual with encephalitis also presents with meningeal involvement, the condition is often referred to as meningo-encephalitis.

## ENCEPHALITIS

### Description of the Disorder

Encephalitis is the result of a virus or other microorganism invading the brain and is acquired either prenatally or postnatally. For example, congenital rubella during early stages of pregnancy and congenital forms of herpes simplex can cause prenatal types of encephalitis (Palumbo, Davidson, Peloquin, & Gigliotti, 1995). Encephalitis can also be caused indirectly by vaccination for various childhood illnesses such as chicken pox or measles (Hynd & Willis, 1988).

A distinction is sometimes made between primary (or acute) and secondary (or chronic) encephalitis (National Institute of Neurological Disorders and Stroke [NINDS], 2004; Teeter & Semrud-Clikeman, 1997). Primary encephalitis, also known as acute viral encephalitis, is caused by a direct infection of the brain. In contrast, secondary encephalitis, also known as postinfectious encephalitis, results from either a previous viral infection or an immunization. Symptoms of secondary encephalitis often do not present until several weeks or months after the initial infection. Anderson, Northam, Hendy, and Wrennall (2001) describe four major forms of encephalitis, including acute viral encephalitis, postinfectious encephalomyelitis, chronic degenerative disease of the CNS, and chronic/slow CNS infections. Rasmussen's encephalitis is an example of a chronic degenerative CNS infection. The onset of this condition often occurs during childhood. Clinically, the disease typically causes intractable seizures and progressive neurological deterioration in one cerebral hemisphere. Finally, although many cases of encephalitis are considered sporadic, some infections occur as epidemics in a specific area, such as Japanese B encephalitis (Hokkanen & Launes, 2000).

In general, it is difficult to estimate precisely the incidence of encephalitis in the United States because reporting practices are unstandardized (Lazoff, 2005). Ho and Hirsch (1985) reported estimates between 1,300 and 4,300 cases annually in the United States. More recently, incidence rates have been reported individually for different types of encephalitis (Centers for Disease Control [CDC], 2005). For example, the incidence rate of arboviral encephalitis is reported to be quite variable from year to year, ranging from 150 to 3,000 cases per year. The incidence of the herpes simplex encephalitis is reported to be 0.2 cases per 100,000 (Lazoff, 2005). With regard to acute encephalitis, Koskiniemi and colleagues (1997) found the overall incidence to be 10.5 cases per 100,000 in children from 1 month to 15 years of age, with the highest numbers in children less than 1 year of age (18.4 per 100,000). Toltzis (2001) reported a mortality rate of 5% for encephalitis, although the rate varies depending on the specific type of encephalitis. Toltzis also estimated that approximately one-third of individuals with encephalitis (all forms) have some ongoing neurological or cognitive difficulties at the time of their discharge from the hospital.

## Causes, Related Medical Issues, and Treatment

The range of causes for encephalitis is quite varied. Viruses appear to account for a large proportion of cases (Ho & Hirsch, 1985). However, it should be noted that a large majority of cases have no known etiology. For example, different sources have estimated that half, or possibly as high as two-thirds, of cases of acute encephalitis have no known cause (Adler & Toor, 1984; Hokkanen & Launes, 2000). Most cases in the United States are caused by enteroviruses (i.e., small viruses made of ribonucleic acid [RNA] and protein such as the Coxsackie viruses and the poliovirus), the herpes simplex virus, animal bites (e.g., rabies virus), and arboviruses (i.e., viruses transmitted from infected animals or infected ticks, mosquitoes, or other insects). Weil and Levin (1995) have identified some of the various causes of encephalitis more globally, including measles, mumps, and rubella (30.4%); herpes viruses (24.1%); respiratory viruses (18.3%); microplasmal pneumonia (13.1%); enteroviruses (9.7%); postvaccination encephalitis (1%); and other causes (34.9%).

Individuals with encephalitis present with numerous types of symptoms, often depending on the type and severity of the illness. Fever, headache, vomiting, and fatigue are common. More subtle symptoms might include sleep difficulties and behavioral or mood changes (Hynd & Willis, 1988). Some types of encephalitis, such as herpes simplex virus type 1 and Rasmussen's encephalitis, present with seizure episodes. Focal neurological deficits can also occur in some types of encephalitis, such as language difficulties (i.e., aphasia), motor and gait disturbances (e.g., hemiparesis, ataxia), and cranial nerve palsies (Adler & Toor, 1984). More mild cases often present with flu-like symptoms.

Individuals with presumed encephalitis may go through many different types of medical testing (Teeter & Semrud-Clikeman, 1997). Samples of blood and cerebrospinal fluid (CSF) are often examined in an attempt to isolate the pathogen causing the illness. Electroencephalogram (EEG) is often used to assess brain wave activity and to detect seizure activity. Computerized tomography (CT) and magnetic resonance imaging (MRI) are used to look for signs of swelling (i.e., cerebral edema), any localized infection, and other signs of an inflammatory process.

There are a variety of possible associated medical issues in children with encephalitis, all of which depend on the severity and type of encephalitis. EEG changes are often seen in encephalitis and commonly include generalized slowing. Seizures may also occur during the acute stages of the illness and are often accompanied by spiking in the temporal lobes on EEG (Anderson et al., 2001). In addition, some children with encephalitis develop recurrent seizures. Other neurological consequences can also persist, including motor and speech difficulties.

The treatment for encephalitis depends on the cause and type identified. For example, some forms of encephalitis, such as that caused by the herpes simplex virus, can be treated with antiviral drugs such as acyclovir and ganciclovir. If seizures are an issue, anticonvulsant drugs may be prescribed to prevent future seizures. Corticosteroid drugs are used to prevent swelling and brain inflammation (NINDS, 2004). In Rasmussen's encephalitis, hemispherectomy (i.e., surgical removal of the affected hemisphere) often appears to slow down the neurological deterioration (Anderson et al., 2001). Patients with acute disseminated encephalomyelitis (ADEM) are treated with steroids.

## MENINGITIS

### Description of the Disorder

Meningitis refers to an inflammation of the meninges of the brain. The meninges are the three protective layers of the brain and spinal cord that develop during the prenatal period. They include the dura matter, a tough outer layer that is closest to the skull; the middle arachnoid matter; and the pia matter, a thin delicate layer that adheres directly to the surface of the brain. Between the different layers, there are spaces where CSF flows. These include the subdural space (between the dura and the arachnoid matter) and the subarachnoid space (between the arachnoid and pia matter). Together, the pia matter and the subarachnoid space are sometimes referred to as the leptomeninges, which is often the area that becomes inflamed in cases of meningitis (Hynd & Willis, 1988).

The most common causes of meningitis depend on the individual's age, although 95% of cases are reportedly caused by three primary agents: *Haemophilus influenzae* (Haemophilus meningitis), *Neisseria meningitides* (meningococcal meningitis), and *Streptococcus pneumoniae* (pneumococcal meningitis; Feigin, 1992). In neonates, the most common cause of meningitis is Group B Streptococcus, and women are now routinely screened for Strep B at the end of their pregnancies.

Prior to the development of a vaccine for bacterial meningitis, it was estimated that in children under 5 years of age, 30 to 70 children per 100,000 were infected per year (Feigin, 1992; Sell, 1987). Currently, the mortality rate for meningitis is estimated to be 10% overall (Davies & Rudd, 1994), although there is some variability depending on the cause. This is a dramatic improvement relative to the mortality rates in the 1950s (which were upwards of 90%) prior to the development of antibiotics. In addition, the development of a vaccine for *Haemophilus influenzae* type b meningitis in the 1980s greatly reduced the prevalence of meningitis in newborns. This caused the median age for development of meningitis to change from 15 months in 1985 to 25 years in 1995 (Adams et al., 1993; Peltola, Kilpi, & Antilla, 1992).

According to the NINDS (2004), pneumococcal meningitis is the most common type of meningitis. Approximately 6,000 cases are reported in the United States each year. Children under 2 years of age with compromised immune systems are at greatest risk for this type of meningitis. Meningococcal meningitis is the next most common, with about 2,600 cases identified in the United States per year. This form occurs most frequently in children ages 2 to 18 years of age, with the highest risk groups being children under 1 year of age, college students living in close quarters, and people with suppressed immune systems; 10% to 15% of these cases are fatal. Finally, Haemophilus meningitis used to be the most common form of bacterial meningitis. As mentioned above, rates of this type of meningitis have decreased dramatically since the discovery of the vaccine.

Viral and aseptic forms of meningitis are actually more common than bacterial meningitis but much less likely to result in death or disability (Anderson & Taylor, 2000). Meningitis is often caused by enteroviruses, which were described above under common causes of encephalitis. One study examining neuropsychological outcomes in both viral and bacterial meningitis noted worse overall outcomes (e.g., more deficits in working memory and other aspects of executive functions) for individuals with bacterial meningitis, although both groups were noted to show difficulties with memory and learning skills (Schmidt et al., 2006). Fungal infections can also cause meningitis. The most common cause of fungal meningitis is *Cryptococcus neoformans,* which is typically found in dirt and bird droppings (NINDS, 2004). Given these issues, the following discussions will generally refer to the bacterial forms of meningitis.

## Diagnosis, Related Medical Issues, and Treatment

Symptoms of meningitis may present either gradually (i.e., over the course of several days) or more acutely. When symptoms develop gradually, they are often nonspecific flu-like symptoms. In more acute cases, symptoms can develop over the course of several hours. The cardinal signs of acute meningitis include sudden fever, severe headaches (due to inflammation of the meningeal blood vessels), and nuchal rigidity (i.e., stiff neck). Nuchal rigidity refers to resistance to forward flexion in the neck (Hynd & Willis, 1988). In younger children, fever, lack of appetite, nausea/vomiting, irritability, jaundice, and respiratory problems are common (Snyder, 1994). Klein and Marcy (1990) conducted a meta-analysis of seven studies of children with meningitis (225 cases total). The most common presenting symptoms included hyperthermia, lethargy, anorexia or vomiting, respiratory distress, convulsions, irritability, jaundice, bulging fontanelle (i.e., outward curving of an infant's soft spot), diarrhea, and nuchal rigidity.

Acute neurological complications are common in children with meningitis. Two large studies examining these complications (Grimwood et al., 1995; Taylor, Schatschneider, & Rich, 1992) found relatively similar rates of these complications, which included seizures (24%–31% of sample), coma (13%–18%), hemiparesis (6%–9%), sensorineural hearing loss (6%–12%), cortical blindness (1%–2%), ataxia (2%–6%), and hydrocephalus (2% in both samples). One group also followed these children up to 12 years postillness (Anderson et al., 1997; Grimwood, Anderson, Anderson, Nolan, & Tan, 2000; Grimwood et al., 1995, 1996). At that time, 8.5% of the individuals had ongoing major sequelae, including seizures, severe hearing problems, spasticity, blindness, and intellectual impairment (IQ less than 70). Approximately 30% of the sample had what the authors termed "mild" sequelae, including fine motor problems, mild to moderate hearing problems, mild intellectual deficits (IQ ranging from 70 to 80), and behavioral difficulties.

In order to confirm a diagnosis of bacterial meningitis, it is important to look for the presence of bacteria in the CSF. This can be accomplished through a lumbar puncture. In bacterial meningitis, the CSF is generally cloudy, and there are elevated levels of protein and decreased glucose (Anderson & Taylor, 2000; Teeter & Semrud-Clikeman, 1997). The CSF can also be examined for the presence of blood or white blood cells; elevations would suggest the presence of an infection. In addition to the sampling of blood and CSF, several of the other techniques mentioned above (CT, MRI, and EEG) also may be utilized to clarify the diagnosis, particularly in more complex cases.

Bacterial forms of meningitis are typically treated with antibiotics. The treatment often starts with strong doses of general antibiotics followed by a several-week course of intravenous antibiotics in more severe cases. Corticosteroids are also used to treat brain swelling in meningitis and may be helpful in preventing hearing loss in some types of meningitis (Girgis et al., 1989; NINDS, 2004).

In contrast, viral meningitis cannot be treated with antibiotics, and patients may undergo treatments similar to those listed above for viral encephalitis. If the cause of the meningitis is determined to be a fungus, the individual is treated with an antifungal medication. For both meningitis and encephalitis, patients may also be treated with pain medications or sedatives in order to alleviate symptoms or make the person more comfortable (NINDS, 2004).

## Case Study

The following is the case of Jack, a 12-year-old, right-handed, African American male with an initial diagnosis of meningoencephalitis, which was later changed to acute disseminated encephalomyelitis. It should be noted that this case is somewhat atypical, as this child had a longer course of the illness, with recurrence, and also developed an additional complication from the infection that included involvement of the spinal cord, sometimes also referred to as transverse myelitis.

It is noteworthy that few large-scale studies have examined the outcome in children with encephalitis. The most widely studied group of encephalitis patients have been adults with HSV (herpes simplex) encephalitis. However, in the United States, this group accounts for only 5% to 10% of encephalitis cases, and they tend to have poorer outcomes. In fact, Hokkanen and Launes (2000) have noted that "little can be said about the cognitive profile in nonherpetic etiologies" (p. 162). There are more recent studies examining cognitive functioning in children and adults with bacterial meningitis (Anderson, Anderson, Grimwood, & Nolan, 2004; Schmidt et al., 2006). Findings from these studies will be incorporated below when appropriate.

## Relevant Medical History

Jack's medical history was generally unremarkable until he began to experience chest pain, headaches, and stomachache. He was initially treated for pneumonia, but his symptoms persisted and he developed blurred vision. He was subsequently admitted to the hospital for further workup. Initial scans of his brain were notable for a deep right frontal white matter area of low attenuation, cerebral white matter edema, and left parietal leptomeningeal enhancement. He was diagnosed with meningo-encephalitis (presumed to be from mycoplasma), treated with antibiotics, and discharged home. Jack remained medically stable for several months. However, he again presented to the hospital with a several-day history of headaches, emesis, and "wobbly walking." An MRI of the brain and spinal cord showed multiple enhancing white matter lesions in the corpus callosum and optic chiasm, which were reportedly worse than prior studies, and persistent T2 signal abnormalities in the spinal cord. At that time, he was diagnosed with a more chronic (postinfectious) form called multiphasic disseminated encephalomyelitis. It is of note that the precise incidence of encephalomyelitis is unknown but is estimated to account for 10% to 15% of the cases of acute-onset encephalitis (Moorthi, Schneider, & Dombovy, 1999).

Following the diagnosis, Jack was started on high-dose steroids. As mentioned above, a diagnosis of encephalomyelitis indicated that Jack's clinical presentation also included spinal cord involvement, which in his case involved decreased sensory and motor functions below the T-8 level of the spinal cord (i.e., below the waist). As a result, he experienced bowel and bladder incontinence. Given his functional deficits, he was transferred to a rehabilitation hospital for comprehensive inpatient rehabilitation, including physical therapy, occupational therapy, and speech/language therapy.

## Rehabilitation Course

Upon arrival at the rehabilitation hospital, Jack was fully oriented to person, place, time, and situation. He was initially very lethargic and presented with depressed mood and flat affect. He also presented with significant cognitive deficits in attention, speeded processing, and memory. Over the course of the next 2 months, he made significant gains in his cognitive status and was subsequently discharged from speech/language therapy. Although his motor skills improved, he continued to have decreased sensory and motor functions in his legs and required a wheelchair for mobility.

Because fewer individuals with encephalitis are admitted to rehabilitation units (in comparison to cases of stroke and brain injury), there is little group data assessing recovery in these patients. One study of eight individuals found that those with encephalitis made functional gains in motor and cognitive skills while on an inpatient rehabilitation unit, although their recovery was noted to be slower than that of individuals with traumatic brain injury and stroke (Moorthi et al., 1999). Two of the subjects in this cohort had diagnoses similar to Jack.

## Previous History

Jack's mother reported a complicated birth history; he was born prematurely (at 28 weeks gestation) and weighed approximately 2 pounds at birth. He remained in the hospital for about 1 month and required blood transfusions. Following his discharge home from the hospital, he was reported to have no other medical issues until his recent hospitalization. Developmentally, he achieved all speech/language and motor milestones within the normal time frame. Family medical and psychiatric histories were unremarkable.

Jack lives with his parents and younger brother. His mother reported no concerns with his behavior or mood prior to the hospitalization. She described him as a quiet child who had no difficulty making friends or getting along with others. Prior to the illness, Jack was in seventh grade in regular education classes. According to his school records, he was an above-average student, receiving all A's and B's on his report card. In addition, a review of standardized school testing that was completed a few months prior to his hospital admission revealed age-appropriate skills across all academic areas in comparison to national norms. Note that it is important to consider the child's premorbid functioning, as social and environmental factors are important predictors of outcome for all types of childhood infection (Kopp & Kralow, 1983).

## Behavioral Observations

Jack was seen for neuropsychological evaluation approximately 4 months following his admission to the rehabilitation hospital. He was evaluated in the 2 weeks prior to his discharge. Thus, testing was completed over the course of several 1- to 2-hour sessions, as opposed to over the course of 1 day. Throughout the evaluation, Jack was cooperative and displayed bright affect. His attention was generally well maintained in the one-to-one testing environment. He was generally slow to complete tasks (during all sessions), and his response style was cautious. His speech was well articulated, fluent, and appropriate in content. Vision and hearing appeared grossly within normal limits. Jack had difficulty with tasks requiring fine motor coordination, particularly with his right (dominant) hand. Overall, Jack appeared to put forth strong effort throughout the evaluation, and test results were considered to be a valid reflection of his neuropsychological functioning at the time of the evaluation. See Table 7.1 for a summary of the results of his evaluation.

## Evaluation Results

### *Intellectual Functioning*

Jack's intellectual abilities were found to be in the average range overall. He demonstrated relatively consistent (average) performance across measures of verbal reasoning, nonverbal reasoning, and auditory working memory. Processing speed was an area of relative weakness, falling into the low average range. It should be noted that most children with a history of encephalitis and meningitis present with average IQ scores; however, a higher percentage of children with these illnesses perform below the average range, and they typically perform below controls in studies (Anderson et al., 2004; Fellick et al., 2001; Rantala, Uhari, Saukkonen, & Sorri, 1991).

### *Academic Functioning*

With respect to basic academic skills, Jack's performance was consistently within age and grade expectations. Specifically, his performance was average across measures of single-word reading, spelling, and math computation. However, he had greater difficulty on a more complex paragraph-reading task in terms of both his reading fluency and reading

**TABLE 7.1 Neuropsychological Evaluation Results**

| Domain | Scaled Score | T Score | Standard Score |
|---|---|---|---|
| | Intellectual Functioning | | |
| WISC-IV Full Scale IQ | | | 99 |
| Verbal Comprehension | | | 98 |
| Perceptual Reasoning | | | 104 |
| Working Memory | | | 104 |
| Processing Speed | | | 85 |
| | Academic Achievement | | |
| WIAT-II Word Reading | | | 99 |
| Spelling | | | 97 |
| Numerical Operations | | | 97 |
| GORT-4 Oral Reading Quotient | | | 76 |
| Reading Comprehension | 6 | | |
| Reading Fluency | 6 | | |
| | Language | | |
| BNT | | | 120 |
| D-KEFS Verbal Fluency | | | |
| Letter Fluency | 7 | | |
| Category Fluency | 8 | | |
| | Visual-Spatial and Construction Skills | | |
| VMI-V VMI | | | 79 |
| Visual Perception | | | 91 |
| | Learning/Memory | | |
| CMS Stories Immediate | 6 | | |
| Stories Delayed | 6 | | |
| Dot Locations Total | 8 | | |
| Dot Locations Delayed | 9 | | |
| CVLT-C Total Trials 1-5 | | 33 | |
| Learning Slope | | | 78 |

**TABLE 7.1** *(Continued)*

| Domain | Scaled score | T Score | Standard Score |
|---|---|---|---|
| Short–Delay Free Recall | | | 78 |
| Short–Delay Cued Recall | | | 78 |
| Long–Delay Free Recall | | | 70 |
| Long–Delay Cued Recall | | | 70 |
| Discriminability | | | 85 |
| RCFT Immediate Recall | | 33 | |
| Delayed Recall | | 36 | |
| Recognition | | 46 | |
| Attention/Executive Functions | | | |
| D-KEFS Trail Making Test | | | |
| Visual Scanning | 6 | | |
| Number Sequencing | 6 | | |
| Letter Sequencing | 5 | | |
| Number-Letter Switching | 8 | | |
| D-KEFS Color Word Interference | | | |
| Color Naming | 6 | | |
| Word Reading | 6 | | |
| Inhibition | 5 | | |
| Inhibition-Switching | 6 | | |
| TOL Total Moves | | | 102 |
| Total Problem-Solving Time | | | 103 |
| Motor Skills | | | |
| GPT (preferred right) | | | <60 |
| (nonpreferred) | | | <60 |
| VMI-V Motor Coordination | | | 71 |
| Socioemotional Functioning | | | |
| BASC Self-Report | | | |
| Hyperactivity | | | 48 |

*Continued*

**TABLE 7.1** *(Continued)*

| Domain | Scaled Score | T Score | Standard Score |
|---|---|---|---|
| Aggression | | | 45 |
| Conduct Problems | | | 43 |
| Anxiety | | | 55 |
| Depression | | | 53 |
| Somatization | | | 58 |
| Withdrawal | | | 51 |
| Attention Problems | | | 56 |

*Note.* BASC, Behavior Assessment System for Children (Reynolds & Kamphaus, 1992); BNT, Boston Naming Test (Kaplan, Goodglass, Weintraub, & Segal, 1983); CMS, Children's Memory Scale (Cohen, 1997); CVLT-C, California Verbal Learning Test—Children's Version (Delis, Kramer, Kaplan, & Ober, 1994); D-KEFS, Delis-Kaplan Executive Function System (Delis, Kaplan, & Kramer, 2001); GORT-4, Gray Oral Reading Test—Fourth Edition (Wiederholt & Bryant, 2001); GPT, Grooved Pegboard Test (Trites, n.d.); RCFT, Rey Complex Figure Test and Recognition Trial (Meyers and Meyers, 1995); TOL, Tower of London—Drexel University (Culbertson & Zillmer, 2001); VMI-V, Beery-Buktenica Developmental Test of Visual-Motor Integration—Fifth Edition (Beery, Buktenica, & Beery, 2005); WIAT-II, Wechsler Individual Achievement Test—Second Edition (Wechsler, 2002); and WISC-IV, Wechsler Intelligence Scale for Children—Fourth Edition (Wechsler, 2003).

comprehension. In addition, Jack had difficulty with writing tasks due to his fine motor and speed difficulties. Of note, research has suggested that children with a history of meningitis are more than twice as likely as controls to require special education assistance (Anderson et al., 2004).

### *Verbal/Language Skills*

Jack's verbal/language skills were generally age appropriate, with a mild weakness in verbal fluency. Specifically, his verbal reasoning skills were average, and his ability to name pictures was above average. His verbal fluency skills (i.e., the ability to rapidly generate words by beginning letter or category) were low average to average.

### *Visual/Nonverbal Skills*

Jack's performance was also age appropriate on tasks measuring his visual/nonverbal abilities, with the exception of a weakness in visual construction. Specifically, he had no difficulty with motor-free nonverbal reasoning tasks and other measures requiring basic visual perception. However, he had greater difficulty on measures with more of a fine motor component, for example, ones requiring him to copy line drawings or trace within the lines. Jack's ability to construct a more complex geometric figure was also impaired and reflected his problems with visual construction and motor precision, although he was generally well organized in his approach to the drawing.

### *Memory and New Learning*

Jack's ability to learn and retain new information was variable. Initially, he did quite poorly on word-list learning across five learning trials, with moderate retention of information following an interference trial and a 20-minute delay. During this task, he displayed a slow learning curve and mildly improved performance with recognition (yes/no) cuing. His performance was slightly better, although still in the low average range, on a task requiring recall of verbally presented stories. With regard to visual memory, his performance on a measure of spatial learning and memory was average after three learning trials, with good retention after a 20-minute delay interval. His immediate and delayed recall of a complex figure were below average, although his performance improved significantly when he was presented with the information in a recognition format. It should be noted that memory deficits are seen more commonly in some types of encephalitis than in others. For example, difficulty with memory is a common sequela of HSV encephalitis (Hokkanen & Launes, 2000).

### *Attention and Executive Functions*

Jack exhibited variabe performance on tests of attention, working memory, and processing speed. Auditory working memory (i.e., the ability to hold and mentally manipulate information) was average on untimed measures. Sustained attention and impulse control also were within or above age expectations on a computerized measure of attention. In contrast, Jack's performance was below average across measures of speeded processing and attention tasks with a timed component. This included difficulties on tasks requiring pure cognitive processing speed (e.g., rapid naming, verbal fluency), cognitive inhibition, and psychomotor speed.

Jack demonstrated generally intact performance in the broader executive functions. Executive function is a cognitive domain that encompasses skills related to strategic, goal-directed behavior and self-regulation (e.g., problem solving, planning skills, organization, and impulse control). For example, his performance was solidly average across a tower task requiring planning and problem-solving efficiency, and he demonstrated good overall organization on a visual construction task requiring him to copy a complex geometric figure (although his drawing was notable for difficulties with motor precision). He also demonstrated good mental flexibility (e.g., switching between semantic categories or letters and numbers).

Although Jack had no significant difficulties with executive functions, it should be noted that children with encephalitis and meningitis often show some impairments in this domain. For example, Anderson and colleagues (2004) studied executive functioning in a group of long-term survivors of bacterial meningitis (12 years after acute illness). This study found that children with a history of meningitis were not severely impaired in executive functions but that their abilities were below developmental expectations. The authors noted that these children "took longer to complete tasks, made more errors, were less organized, and struggled with problem solving situations in both the verbal and spatial domains" (p. 76).

### *Sensory/Motor Skills*

Jack demonstrated significant weaknesses in his fine motor skills. He was slow and uncoordinated on a measure of fine motor dexterity and had difficulty with graphomotor coordination. Vision and hearing were functionally intact during the evaluation. Vision and hearing screenings at the hospital did not indicate any concerns.

### *Emotional and Behavioral Functioning*

Jack completed several self-report measures that assess emotional functioning. Results from his responses to a questionnaire indicated no clinically significant emotional or behavioral concerns. However, on a sentence completion task, his responses indicated wishes and concerns about his medical condition (e.g., I hope I *get better,* I wish that I *could walk*), concerns about school (e.g., I worry about *school*), and desires to go home from the hospital (e.g., I would like to *go home*). Jack's mother reported some concerns about his coping and adjustment, especially when she was not able to spend time at the hospital with him. At the time of this evaluation, Jack's mood and adjustment had shown significant improvement, particularly in the controlled hospital environment. Throughout his hospitalization, Jack received both individual and group psychotherapy to address these issues.

Although Jack did not present with significant behavioral difficulties, it should be noted that children with a history of meningitis and encephalitis are more likely to demonstrate behavioral difficulties than normal controls, including a higher likelihood of attention problems, oppositional behavior, and, in some cases, psychiatric problems (Fellick et al., 2001; Hokkanen & Launes, 2000). In addition, some research suggests that individuals with greater right-hemisphere disease have more behavioral difficulties, including a higher incidence of mood issues and depression (Gordon, Selnes, Hart, Hanley, & Whitly, 1990; Hokkanen et al., 1996). Behavioral difficulties and personality changes are more commonly seen in cases of HSV encephalitis.

## Summary of Findings

Overall, the results from Jack's neuropsychological evaluation indicated average overall intellectual functioning, along with many areas of strength (average to above-average skills) in basic academics (i.e., word reading, spelling, and math), picture naming, basic visual perception, sustained attention, working memory, and executive functioning (i.e., planning, organization, novel problem solving). New memory and learning skills were somewhat variable, with better performance noted when Jack was given a context for learning (e.g., a story versus a random list of words). Areas of more significant weakness were noted in Jack's motor and cognitive processing speed and select areas of attention (i.e., visual scanning, attention control). He demonstrated the greatest weakness in his fine motor skills, including problems with fine motor speed and dexterity, motor coordination, and visual construction. These fine motor issues also impacted his ability to complete functional academic tasks such as writing and drawing. Memory and speed issues appeared to affect his performance on a measure of reading comprehension.

Emotionally, Jack did not report any clinically significant concerns at the time of the evaluation, although he noted feelings of frustration related to his illness and hospitalization. In addition, throughout his hospitalization Jack displayed some evidence of sad mood and mild difficulties coping with his illness. It is important to note that Jack tended to internalize his feelings and required close support and monitoring of his mood when he returned to his home environment.

Overall, the deficits identified in the evaluation were relatively diffuse and felt to be attributable to Jack's neurological condition. Note that parent report, previous testing results, and academic records indicated that Jack's premorbid abilities were within age expectations. Thus, many of his scores likely represented a decline from his premorbid status. Certainly, his difficulties with speed, memory, and fine motor skills represented significant declines. Given that this evaluation was completed only a few months after the onset of his illness, it was felt that Jack would likely continue to recover over the next several months.

## INTERVENTIONS AND RECOMMENDATIONS

With regard to Jack's case, there were a few key areas to address: fine motor and visual-motor skills, speed of processing, memory and new learning, and emotional functioning. In the following sections, recommendations will be made to address these areas of weakness, which may not be relevant for every child with encephalitis or meningitis. Included are some additional recommendations that may not necessarily be relevant in this case but may be the types of strategies that would be helpful for other individuals with encephalitis.

### Motor Functioning

Students with significant fine motor difficulties often have trouble with note taking and other related academic tasks. It is important to examine individual students' schedules and determine where their fine motor problems may be an issue. In these cases, the following strategies are recommended:

1. The use of a note taker (scribe) is recommended as needed, so that the student can concentrate on the teacher's lectures without having to be concerned about keeping up with the notes. This can be another individual in the class who takes good notes. The student could obtain a copy of that individual's notes. Alternatively, the other student could take notes on carbon paper.
2. The student will likely benefit from being provided with teacher handouts of class notes or any overheads that were used during the class.
3. The student will benefit from using augmentative devices (i.e., a computer) for longer tests and writing assignments. Some students may require additional keyboard lessons and learning to use word prediction software.
4. Depending on the severity of the fine motor and visual-motor difficulties, the student may also require assistance with classes that require bimanual coordination or precise fine motor skills. For example, younger children may need assistance with skills such as cutting and pasting. Older students may require assistance in classes such as science, where they are required to use motor skills to perform experiments.

Students may also experience weaknesses with regard to gross motor issues that can impact their access to the school and limit their participation in activities. The following recommendations are provided to address these issues:

1. Students with significant mobility issues may require all of their classes to be wheelchair accessible. Some may need extra time between classes so that they will be able to maneuver their wheelchair when there are no other students in the hallway. The students may also require help with their materials.
2. Students with significant mobility issues may require special transportation to accommodate their wheelchair.
3. Students may benefit from an extra set of textbooks to keep at home. Keeping books at home alleviates the need for them to carry books back and forth, and it provides easy access to materials at home and in school. This modification is also helpful for students with memory difficulties.

## Speed of Processing

For students with slower processing speed, the following classroom modifications are provided:

1. Students with speed issues will benefit from relaxed time constraints. For example, as necessary, it may be beneficial to allow the student to complete lengthy assignments with extended (or unlimited) time, in particular, tasks that have a lengthy writing or reading component. Also consider amending the amount of work the student is required to do (including in-class assignments and homework).
2. Some students with processing speed deficits require more time to respond. It is important that these types of students be provided with adequate response time (sometimes up to 30 seconds) and be reminded to respond when there is a delay.
3. Note taking is often a significant issue for students with processing speed issues. Please see the above recommendations in the fine motor section for addressing note taking.

With regard to test taking, written examinations should also allow extra time to accommodate for difficulties with speed. Students should also be provided with additional time to organize their thoughts for essay questions and possibly also with scrap paper on which to jot down organizational notes. Students with speed issues may also need to receive these accommodations on statewide and standardized testing.

## Memory Functioning

A number of environmental accommodations can be made in order to prevent difficulties due to poor memory skills:

1. Students with memory difficulties will benefit from using a planner or notebook or electronic PDA for documenting daily assignments, appointments, and longer term projects. They often need someone to work with them on how to appropriately use such a device, and they benefit from someone checking their planner after each period to ensure that they are recording the appropriate information. This level of supervision can be decreased once they are able use the planner independently. Younger students (in kindergarten through third grade) might require someone to record assignments and to ensure that they take their planner home with them.
2. Older students (late middle school, high school) sometimes benefit from being allowed to tape-record lectures, so that they are able to go back and "fill in the gaps" for information they were unable to get the first time.
3. Some students benefit from carrying a small pocket-sized tape recorder in their pocket, so that they can easily record thoughts or reminders.

Teaching methods also may need modifying; information on helpful strategies is provided below:

1. Information should be presented in a multisensory fashion, to allow students to encode material in many different ways (e.g., verbal, visual, tactile, through modeling or demonstration).
2. Recall of simple facts and/or figural material may be achieved more easily when students verbally describe the information to themselves while studying or when this information is incorporated into stories, rhymes, songs, poems, or cartoons, which may make the information more meaningful and easier to encode and retrieve.
3. Instruction in mnemonic techniques, such as repetition, chunking, and visual imagery, also may help organize the information and facilitate later recall. Students with memory difficulties need frequent, distributed repetition and review of unfamiliar material over time.
4. New skills should be presented in close relationship to more familiar tasks or information so that they are linked to what the students already know.

5. Students with memory difficulties will benefit from the provision of simplified oral instructions, as well as written directions that they can refer to as needed.

Finally, test accommodations can be made in order to elicit the best performance from students with memory difficulties:

1. The amount of information that these students are tested on should be reduced or broken down into smaller amounts, so that they do not have just one or two large exams in a semester. This tends to be more of an issue for older students.
2. Students with memory difficulties should not be expected to take multiple examinations in 1 week. This is often a problem in middle school and high school, when several exams are crammed into a midterm or finals period.
3. As they may need more time to study for tests/quizzes, students with memory difficulties should be provided with adequate notice prior to the scheduling of an examination (i.e., no pop quizzes).
4. Alternative testing arrangements can help to circumvent difficulties with free retrieval of factual information. To test factual knowledge, multiple-choice or matching items are ideal. To test integration of information, oral examinations, for which the student is allowed to bring in a fact sheet or note card, would be best.
5. If the students have significant retrieval difficulties, they may need prompts, choices (i.e., is it this or that?), and cues (i.e., the first sound in the word). They should be graded on the content rather than the precision of their answers (e.g., they may "talk around" an answer rather than giving the exact word or answer).

## Emotional and Behavioral Functioning

Jack, the child in this case study, did not present with significant behavioral difficulties. Thus, recommendations regarding behavior management and personality changes are not included here. However, given that changes in personality and behavior do occur in children with encephalitis and meningitis, it is recommend that readers refer to the chapter on traumatic brain injury(TBI) in this text. Children with TBI often show behavioral and personality changes, and the recommendations provided regarding these issues are likely applicable to the types of issues seen in children with other acquired brain illnesses.

With regard to the current case, it was recommended that Jack's psychological functioning be closely monitored given that he was likely to be faced with new frustrations and issues related to his areas of weakness (e.g., physical changes in his body, mobility issues, possibly increased school difficulty). It was recommended that he be provided with the opportunity to participate in individual counseling with a mental health professional who would provide supportive therapy to address issues of concern. It also was recommended that he consider joining a local support group for individuals with spinal cord injuries.

## RESOURCES

### Books

Gordon, B., & Berger, L. (2003). *Intelligent memory: Improve the memory that makes you smarter.* New York: Viking Press.

Higbee, K. L. (2001). *Your memory: How it works and how to improve it* (2nd ed.). New York: Marlowe & Company.

Lash, M. (1992). *When your child goes to school after an injury.* Brick, NJ: Exceptional Parent.

Lorayne, H., & Lucas, J. (2000). *The memory book: The classic guide to improving your memory at work, at school, and at play* (Reissue ed.). New York: Ballantine Books.

Wolcott, G., Lash, M., & Pearson, S. (1995). *Signs and strategies for educating students with brain injuries: A practical guide for teachers and schools.* Houston, TX: HDI.

### Organizations and Web Sites

About Memory

This Web site provides many good resources and tips to improve memory.

Web Site: www.memory-key.com/MemoryGuide/memory_guide.htm

Centers for Disease Control (CDC)

The CDC is one of the best resources for health information. Information can be obtained by going to the Web site, typing in "encephalitis" or "meningitis," and clicking on the provided links.

Web Site: www.cdc.gov

Encephalitis Global

This Web site provides links to important resources and information, online support, and personal stories of survivors of encephalitis.

Web Site: www.encephalitisglobal.com

Encephalitis Society

The society offers support and resources, raises awareness, and encourages research.

Mailing Address: 7B Saville Street
Malton, North Yorkshire
YO17 7LL
United Kingdom
Web Site: www.encephalitis.info

Encephalitis Support Group

This is an e-mail support group for survivors of all types of encephalitis and their families, caregivers, and friends.

Web Site: groups.yahoo.com/group/encephgroup

Epilepsy Foundation

Although the Epilepsy Foundation is a good resource for epilepsy, it also provides information about Rasmussen's encephalitis. This information can be accessed by typing "Rasmussen's" into the search box and clicking on the provided links.

Mailing Address: 8301 Professional Place
Landover, Maryland 20785-7223
Phone Number: (800) 332-1000
Web Site: www.epilepsyfoundation.org

FightMeningitis.com

This Web site is strictly devoted to providing caregivers with information to understand and prevent meningitis.

Web Site: www.fightmeningitis.com

Kids Health

This is a good online resource for parents, children, and adolescents detailing information about many kinds of medical issues. Information for parents about encephalitis and meningitis can be obtained by clicking on "Parents" and then navigating to "Infections."

Web Site: www.kidshealth.org

LD Online

Although this Web site is best known for resources addressing difficulties related to learning disabilities and attention-deficit/hyperactivity disorder, there are many good resources to address memory difficulties. After going to the home page, type "memory" into the search box and click on the provided links.

Web Site: www.ldonline.org

Meningitis Foundation of America (MFA)

The MFA provides support, education, and research using donations provided by the public. Its Web site provides information about meningitis, national and international resources, and current press releases.

Mailing Address: 6610 Shadeland Station, Suite 200
Indianapolis, Indiana 46220
Phone Number: (800) 668-1129
Web Site: www.meningitisfoundationofamerica.org

National Information Center for Children and Youth With Disabilities

This organization provides information regarding disabilities, special education, and research-based information on effective educational practices.

Mailing Address: P.O. Box 1492
Washington, D.C. 20013-1492
Phone Number: (800) 695-0285
Web Site: www.nichcy.org

National Institute of Neurological Disorders and Stroke (NINDS)

NINDS has health information on a wide variety of topics. In order to access related information about encephalitis and meningitis, visit the Web site and click on the appropriate terms.

Web Site: www.ninds.nih.gov/disorders/disorder_index.htm

National Meningitis Association (NMA)

The NMA is a national nonprofit public charity whose primary goal is to educate about and increase awareness of meningococcal meningitis and meningococcal disease.

Mailing Address: 738 Robinson Farms Drive
Marietta, Georgia 30068
Phone Number: (866) 366-3662
Web Site: www.nmaus.org

## REFERENCES

Adams, W. G., Deaver, K. A., Cochi, S. L., Plikaytis, B. D., Zell, E. R., Broome, C. V., et al. (1993). Decline in childhood *Haemophilus Influenzae* type B (Hib) disease in the Hib vaccination era. *Journal of the American Medical Association, 269,* 221–226.

Adler, S. P., & Toor, S. (1984). Central nervous system infections. In J. M. Pellock & E. C. Meyer (Eds.), *Neurologic emergencies in infancy and childhood* (pp. 237–256). New York: Harper & Row.

Anderson, P., Anderson, V. A., Grimwood, K., Nolan, T., Catroppa, C., & Keir, E. (1997). Neuropsychological consequences of bacterial meningitis: A prospective study. *Journal of the International Neuropsychological Society, 3,* 47–48.

Anderson, V., Anderson, P., Grimwood, K., & Nolan, T. (2004). Cognitive and executive functioning 12 years after childhood bacterial meningitis: Effect of acute neurologic complications and age of onset. *Journal of Pediatric Psychology, 29,* 67–81.

Anderson, V. A., Northam, E., Hendy, J., & Wrennall, J. (2001). *Developmental neuropsychology: A clinical approach.* New York: Psychology Press.

Anderson, V. A., & Taylor, H. G. (2000). Meningitis. In K. O. Yeates, M. D. Ris, & H. G. Taylor (Eds.), *Pediatric neuropsychology: Research, theory and practice* (pp. 117–148). New York: Guilford Press.

Beery, K. E., Buktenica, N. A., & Beery, N. A. (2005). *Beery-Buktenica Developmental Test of Visual-Motor Integration* (5th ed.). Lutz, FL: Psychological Assessment Resources.

Centers for Disease Control (CDC). (2005). *CDC fact sheet: Arboviral encephalitis.* Retrieved June 21, 2007, from http://www.cdc.gov/ncidod/dvbid/arbor/arbofact.htm

Cohen, M. J. (1997). *Children's Memory Scale.* San Antonio, TX: The Psychological Corporation.

Culbertson, W. C., & Zillmer, E. A. (2001). *Tower of London—Drexel University.* North Tonawada, NY: Multi-Health Systems.

Davies, P. A., & Rudd, R. T. (1994). *Neonatal meningitis* (Clinics in Developmental Medicine, No. 132). Cambridge, England: Cambridge University Press.

Delis, D. C., Kaplan, E., & Kramer, J. H. (2001). *Delis-Kaplan Executive Function System.* San Antonio, TX: The Psychological Corporation.

Delis, D. C., Kramer, J. H., Kaplan, E., & Ober, B. A. (1994). *California Verbal Learning Test—Children's Version.* San Antonio, TX: The Psychological Corporation.

Feigin, R. D. (1992). Bacterial meningitis beyond the neonatal period. In R. D. Feigin & J. D. Cherry (Eds.), *Textbook of pediatric infectious diseases* (3rd ed., Vol. 1, pp. 401–428). Philadelphia: W. B. Saunders.

Fellick, J. M., Sills, J. A., Marzouk, O., Hart, C. A., Cooke, R.W.I., & Thomson, A.P.J. (2001). Neurodevelopmental outcome in meningococcal disease: A case-control study. *Archives of Disease in Childhood, 85,* 6–11.

Girgis, N. I., Farid, Z., Mikhail, I., Farray, I., Sultan, Y., & Kilpatrick, M. (1989). Dexamethasone treatment for bacterial meningitis in children and adults. *Pediatric Infectious Disease Journal, 8,* 848–851.

Gordon, B., Selnes, O. A., Hart, J., Hanley, D. F., & Whitly, R. J. (1990). Long term cognitive sequelae of acyclovir treated herpes simplex encephalitis. *Archives of Neurology, 47,* 646–647.

Grimwood, K., Anderson, P., Anderson, V. A., Nolan, T., & Tan, L. (2000). Twelve-year outcomes following bacterial meningitis: Further evidence for persisting effects. *Archives of Disease in Childhood, 83,* 111–116.

Grimwood, K., Anderson, V. A., Bond, L., Catroppa, C., Hore, R. L., Keir, E. H., et al. (1995). Adverse outcomes of bacterial meningitis in school-age survivors. *Pediatrics, 95,* 646–656.

Grimwood, K., Nolan, T., Bond, L., Anderson, V., Catroppa, C., & Keir, E. (1996). Risk factors for adverse outcomes in bacterial meningitis. *Journal of Pediatric Child Health, 32,* 457–462.

Ho, D. D., & Hirsch, M. S. (1985). Acute viral encephalitis. *Medical Clinics of North America, 69,* 415–429.

Hokkanen, L., & Launes, J. (2000). Cognitive outcome in acute sporadic encephalitis. *Neuropsychology Review, 10,* 151–167.

Hokkanen, L., Pontiainen, E., Valanne, L., Saknen, O., Iivanainen, H., & Launes, T. (1996). Cognitive impairment after acute encephalitis: Comparison of herpes simplex and other aetiologies. *Journal of Neurology, Neurosurgery, and Psychiatry, 61,* 478–484.

Hynd, G. W., & Willis, W. G. (Eds.). (1988). *Pediatric neuropsychology.* Boston: Allyn and Bacon.

Kaplan, E., Goodglass, H., Weintraub, S., & Segal, O. (1983). *Boston Naming Test.* Philadelphia: Lea & Febiger.

Klein, J. O., & Marcy, S. M. (1990). Bacterial sepsis and meningitis. In J. S. Remington & J. O. Klein (Eds.), *Infectious diseases of the fetus and newborn infant* (3rd ed., pp. 601–656). Philadelphia: W. B. Saunders.

Kopp, C., & Kralow, J. (1983). The developmentalist and study of biological residual in children after recovery from bacterial meningitis. *Archives of Pediatrics, 79,* 63–71.

Koskiniemi, M., Korppi, M., Mustonen, K., Rantala, H., Muttilainen, M., Herrgard, E., et al. (1997). Epidemiology of encephalitis in children: A prospective multi-center study. *European Journal of Pediatrics, 156,* 541–545.

Lazoff, M. (2005). *Encephalitis.* Retrieved April 13, 2007, from http://www.emedicine.com/EMERG/topic163.htm

Meyers, J. E., & Meyers, K. R. (1995). *Rey Complex Figure Test and Recognition Trial.* Odessa, FL: Psychological Assessment Resources.

Moorthi, S., Schneider, W. N., & Dombovy, M. L. (1999). Rehabilitation outcomes in encephalitis—A retrospective study 1990–1997. *Brain Injury, 13,* 139–146.

National Institute of Neurological Disorders and Stroke (NINDS). (2004). *NINDS meningitis and encephalitis fact sheet.* Retrieved April 13, 2007, from http://www.ninds.nih.gov/disorders/encephalitis_meningitis/detail_encephalitis_meningitis.htm

Palumbo, D. R., Davidson, P. W., Peloquin, L. J., & Gigliotti, F. (1995). Neuropsychological aspects of pediatric infectious diseases. In M. C. Roberts (Ed.), *Handbook of pediatric psychology* (2nd ed., pp. 342–361). New York: Guilford Press.

Peltola, H., Kilpi, T., & Antilla, M. (1992). Rapid disappearance of *Haemophilus influenzae* type b meningitis after routine childhood immunizations with conjugate vaccines. *Lancet, 340,* 592–594.

Rantala, H., Uhari, M., Saukkonen, A., & Sorri, M. (1991). Outcome after childhood encephalitis. *Developmental Medicine and Child Neurology, 33,* 858–867.

Reynolds, C. R., & Kamphaus, R. W. (1992). *Behavior Assessment System for Children.* Circle Pines, MN: American Guidance Service.

Schmidt, H., Heimann, B., Djukic, M., Fels, C., Wallesch, C. W., & Nau, R. (2006). Neuropsychological sequelae of bacterial and viral meningitis. *Brain, 129,* 333–345.

Sell, S. (1987). *Haemophilus influenzae* type B meningitis: Manifestations and long-term sequelae. *Pediatric Infectious Diseases, 6,* 775–778.

Snyder, N. D. (1994). Bacterial meningitis of infants and children. In K. Swaiman (Ed.), *Principles of neurology* (pp. 611–642). St. Louis, MO: Mosby.

Taylor, H. G., Schatschneider, C., & Rich, D. (1992). Sequelae of Haemophilus influenzae meningitis: Implications for the study of brain disease and development. In M. Tramontana and S. Hooper (Eds.), *Advances in child neuropsychology* (Vol. 1, pp. 50–108). New York: Springer-Verlag.

Teeter, P. A., & Semrud-Clikeman, M. (Eds.). (1997). *Child neuropsychology: Assessment and interventions for neurodevelopmental disorders.* Boston: Allyn and Bacon.

Toltzis, P. (2001). Infectious encephalitis. In H. B. Jenson & R. S. Baltimore (Eds.), *Pediatric infectious diseases: Principles and practice* (pp. 669–691). Norwalk, CT: Appleton & Lange.

Trites, R. (n.d.). *Grooved Pegboard Test.* Lafayette, IN: Lafayette Instruments.

Wechsler, D. (2002). *Wechsler Individualized Achievement Test* (2nd ed.). San Antonio, TX: The Psychological Corporation.

Wechsler, D. (2003). *Wechsler Intelligence Scale for Children* (4th ed.). San Antonio, TX: The Psychological Corporation.

Weil, M., & Levin, M. (1995). Infections of the nervous system. In J. Menkes (Ed.), *Textbook of child neurology* (pp. 379–509). Baltimore: Williams and Wilkins.

Wiederholt, J. L., & Bryant, B. R. (2001). *Gray Oral Reading Tests* (4th ed.). Austin, TX: Pro-Ed.

CHAPTER EIGHT

# Endocrinological Disorders

Shahal Rozenblatt, PhD

The endocrine system is composed of a diverse array of components whose functions are equally diverse, both in terms of function and dysfunction. The relationship between the ES and central nervous system (CNS) is comprised of multiple feedback loops (Blumenfeld, 2002; Hadley & Levine, 2006), so that disorders of the ES may initially present with neurological deficits and neurological deficits may be exacerbated by concomitant ES dysfunction (Goetz, 2003). As such, an understanding of the ES, its components, and the hormones involved is essential when working with children and adolescents, particularly within the context of dysfunction.

The purpose of this chapter is to introduce the reader to the anatomical and chemical substrates of the ES, their importance for the developmental process, and the consequences when the system malfunctions.

## DISORDERS OF THYROID FUNCTION

The thyroid gland is located in the front of the neck and typically weighs around 30 grams. Its role is to synthesize and secrete two essential hormones: triiodothyronine (T3) and tetraiodothyronine, or thyroxine, as it is more readily known (T4). Both hormones are synthesized from tyrosine

(Hadley & Levine, 2006). T3 and T4 are involved in the regulation of tissue metabolism. Production of T3 and T4 in the thyroid is regulated by the pituitary gland, specifically through secretion of thyroid-stimulating hormone (TSH), whose synthesis is in turn regulated by hypothalamic secretion of thyrotropin-releasing hormone (TRH; Straight, Bauer, & Ferry, 2003). In addition, there is a negative feedback loop wherein serum T4 regulates the release of TSH and TRH. In general, thyroid hormones are involved in the development of the CNS, maintenance of muscle mass, control of skeletal growth and differentiation, and the metabolism of carbohydrates, lipids, and vitamins (Porterfield & Hendrich, 1993; Zoeller, Bansal, & Parris, 2005). In their absence, physical and mental development is impaired.

Disorders of the thyroid gland can be divided into those that involve an underproduction of hormones (i.e., hypothyroidism) and those that involve an overproduction of hormones (i.e., hyperthyroidism), each with a distinct impact on physiological and, therefore, cognitive and behavioral functioning.

## Hypothyroidism

Hypothyroidism is the most common disorder of the thyroid gland in both children and adults and is twice as common in females as in males. It can be caused by dysfunction of the thyroid gland itself (primary hypothyroidism), a disturbance outside of the thyroid involving the pituitary or hypothalamus (central hypothyroidism), or resistance to thyroid hormone (Goetz, 2003). The prevalence of congenital forms of hypothyroidism (e.g., due to abnormal development or location/position of the organ) is 1 case per 3,500 in the U.S. population. Secondary and tertiary forms are rare (1 per 60,000 and 1 per 140,000 newborns worldwide, respectively; Straight et al., 2003). Thyroid dysfunction can develop as a result of destruction via viral or autoimmune damage, chronic inflammation with lymphocytic infiltration, cell death resulting from radiation damage, or defective hormone production. If left untreated in the newborn, hypothyroidism leads to profound growth failure and disrupted CNS development, the latter resulting in a condition called cretinism (Rovet & Hepworth, 2001). The age of onset of symptoms in children is unpredictable because initial increases in TSH may help compensate for insufficiency due to congenital malformations of the thyroid gland. Primary hypothyroidism is the most common form of hypothyroidism and most commonly affects women between the ages of 40 and 60 years (Goetz, 2003). Dysfunction of the hypothalamus or pituitary contributes to hypothyroidism in only 10% of cases.

Among the earliest signs of congenital hypothyroidism (CH) in the infant are prolonged gestation, increased birth weight, constipation, prolonged jaundice, poor feeding and management of secretions, hypothermia, decreased activity level, noisy respirations, and a hoarse cry (Postellon, Bourgeois, & Varma, 2006). The clinical features of the acquired form of hypothyroidism include goiter (i.e., a thyroid that appears "swollen" or "full," resulting in complaints of difficulty swallowing, hoarseness, or a feeling of pressure on the neck), slow growth with delayed bone maturation, mild increased weight in the torso area despite decreased appetite (moderate to severe weight gain/obesity is not characteristic of thyroid dysfunction and suggests the presence of other issues), lethargy and decreased energy, dry skin and puffiness, sleep disturbance (most typically obstructive sleep apnea), cold and heat intolerance, weight loss, tremors, and sexual pseudoprecocity (e.g., testicular enlargement in boys and early breast development and vaginal bleeding in girls; Straight et al., 2003).

Intellectual functioning in children with hypothyroidism has been an area of significant interest. In a review of the research literature, Derksen-Lubsen and Verkerk (1996) determined that there was a trend toward lower intelligence quotients (IQs) in children who were diagnosed and treated for CH. In fact, these children as a whole had IQ levels that were approximately 6 points below those of control participants.

Not all studies have demonstrated decrements in intellectual functioning between hypothyroid and euthyroid children (i.e., those with normal levels of circulating thyroid hormones). For example, Bongers-Schokking and De Muinck Keizer-Schrama (2005) found no differences in global IQ scores for children between 5 years 6 months and 7 years of age. However, they found that IQ correlated significantly with the level of treatment. For instance, children who received high levels of levothyroxine, a medication used in the treatment of hypothyroidism, tended to have higher IQ scores than children who received a lower level of the medication. Moreover, the children receiving high levels of levothyroxine had higher IQ scores even relative to control participants. Children who were treated with low or suboptimal levels of levothyroxine tended to have the lowest levels of IQ scores, albeit remaining in the average range.

Some researchers have attempted to clarify the issue of IQ and hypothyroidism by stratifying groups based on the level of severity of the condition. Kempers and colleagues (2006) evaluated the intellectual and motor development of young adults who were diagnosed with CH during the neonatal period. The patients were tested initially at 9.5 years of age and again at 21.5 years of age. The patients were divided into mild, moderate, and severe CH groups based on laboratory assays of T4. Intelligence scores did not differ significantly from testing at time 1 compared to testing at time 2, regardless of severity of CH; however, the severe CH group had significantly lower Full Scale, Verbal, and Performance IQ scores during each of the testing periods in comparison to those patients with moderate or mild levels of hypothyroidism. Results for the mild and moderate groups were fully within the average range, while results for the severe CH patients ranged from average to low average.

Recently, research has begun to focus on children who were diagnosed with compensated or subclinical hypothyroidism. This group of children tends to fall toward the lower end of the normal range for levels of free T4, and TSH is typically normal as well. Aijaz and colleagues (2006) found that this group of children did not differ from control participants in terms of verbal and nonverbal reasoning, suggesting that the severity of hypothyroidism, as with the work by Kempers and colleagues (2006), is likely the determining factor in level of intelligence.

Research on the neurocognitive functioning of individuals with primary hypothyroidism indicates multiple areas of deficit in addition to intelligence. Wekking and colleagues (2005), in a study of adults treated for CH in the Netherlands, found deficits in complex attention using the Paced Auditory Serial Addition Task (PASAT; Gronwall, 1977). The participants had greater difficulty with single-trial learning relative to the reference group on a measure of verbal memory (Rivermead Story Recall; Wilson, Cockburn, & Baddeley, 1985) but performed on par or better than the reference group when multiple practice trials were involved (California Verbal Learning Test [CVLT]; Delis, Kramer, Kaplan, & Ober, 1987). Using the Symptom Checklist 90 (SLC-90; Derogatis & Savits, 1999), Wekking and colleagues noted that their adult sample reported lower psychological well-being than the reference sample, including greater levels of depression, nervousness, and fatigue.

Pediatric research has noted a similar trend in terms of neurocognitive deficits. In their review of the research on patients who were treated early in development for CH, Derksen-Lubsen and Verkerk (1996) reported a trend toward lower scores on measures of intelligence and motor skills. Kempers and colleagues (2006) found that, in addition to lower IQ scores relative to matched controls, individuals diagnosed with CH via neonatal screening also evidenced motor deficits on tasks of manual dexterity, ball skill, and balance; they specifically noted that the deficits evidenced during childhood had not improved by the time the participants reached young adulthood. Zoeller and Rovet (2004) reviewed the clinical and experimental findings regarding the timing of thyroid action on brain development. They concluded that it is the level of thyroid hormone that is present in the fetus and neonatal system that determines the type of deficits that may be encountered. In general, delaying treatment was found to have a greater impact on visuomotor and language skill development, indicating that these areas of cognitive functioning are particularly sensitive to the level of thyroid hormone in the child's system. Summarizing across the various studies that were reviewed, Zoeller and colleagues (2005) concluded that prenatal thyroid hormone loss contributes to deficits in visual processing and motor and visuomotor abilities. Deficiencies occurring during the early neonatal period are associated with impaired visuospatial abilities, whereas insufficiency that occurs somewhat later during postnatal development is associated with sensorimotor and language impairments. Even later during infancy, thyroid hormone deficits are associated with language, fine motor, auditory processing, attention, and memory deficits.

Animal models have lent some support for the conclusions noted above. For example, Friedhoff, Miller, Armour, Schweitzer, and Mohan (2000) found a gender difference in rats with prenatal hypothyroidism, in that females were more sensitive than males, resulting in learning problems. Furthermore, animals that were treated for thyroid insufficiency differed from those that were exposed to thyroid hormone insufficiency throughout the perinatal period. Animals that were treated tended to exhibit learning deficits and increased motor activity, whereas those that were exposed to chronic thyroid hormone insufficiency exhibited reduced motor activity. This finding suggests a link between the level of thyroid hormone and the development of symptoms often associated with attention-deficit/hyperactivity disorder (ADHD). In fact, Rovet and Hepworth (2001) found that adolescent participants with CH struggled on measures that required them to maintain their focus and inhibit inappropriate responses on a measure of continuous performance. More severe cases of CH were associated with additional difficulties, including requiring more practice trials in order to encode verbal information, thereby affecting learning ability. Rovet and Hepworth also found that relative to the control participants, the clinical sample demonstrated a higher rate of commission errors (i.e., responding to the incorrect stimulus) on a measure of continuous performance and tended to work at a slower rate than controls on a measure of scanning speed. In contrast, clinical participants were not significantly slower when required to maintain two sets of competing data in mind. Finally, the hypothyroid adolescents were less accurate and more prone to perseverative errors on the Wisconsin Card Sorting Test (WCST; Heaton, 1981), indicating decreased executive functioning.

Not all research points to deficits as a result of hypothyroidism. Wu, Flowers, Tudiver, Wilson, and Punyasavatsut (2006) conducted a study in which they examined academic functioning in a group of children diagnosed with subclinical forms of hypo- and hyperthyroidism relative to euthyroid controls. They found that the children with subclinical hypothyroidism actually performed better than the other two groups in terms of arithmetic and reading skills on a measure of academic achievement (Wide Range Achievement Test, Revised; Jastak & Wilkinson, 1984) and also obtained higher scores on a measure of visuomotor integration (Block Design of the Wechsler Intelligence Scale for Children, Revised; Wechsler, 1974).

The presence of mental health–related issues in children and adults with hypothyroidism is undisputed, but the research is relatively scant, which points to the lack of sufficient interaction between mental health practitioners (psychologists and psychiatrists) and the field of endocrinology. The most common mental health–related issues that have been the target of research are associated with depression and anxiety. Goetz (2003) reported CNS features in individuals with hypothyroidism that included forgetfulness, inattention, apathy, and slowing of speech, movement, and mentation, all of which are frequently associated with mood disorders (American Psychiatric Association, 2000). In a study of 89 adult participants with subclinical hypothyroidism, Jorde, Waterloo, Storhaug, and colleagues (2006) found an association between lower levels of T4 and the presence of depressive symptoms, which tended to remit with institution of proper treatment. Similarly, Wekking and colleagues (2005) found that adults with CH tended to report lower levels of well-being relative to euthyroid controls.

Storch and colleagues (2004) looked at the psychological correlates of peer victimization in children with endocrine disorders and found that acts such as bullying were positively related to child reports of depression, social anxiety, and loneliness and parent reports of externalizing symptoms. Regarding psychological variables, the authors found that 7.5% of the children in their sample reported clinically significant depressive symptoms on the Children's Depression Inventory (CDI; Kovacs, 1992), 5.7% reported clinically significant levels of loneliness on the Asher Loneliness Scale (Asher, Hymel, & Renshaw, 1984), and 19.8% of the youth reported elevated levels of social anxiety using the Social Anxiety Scale for Children—Revised (LaGreca & Stone, 1993).

### *Hashimoto's Thyroiditis*

Hashimoto's thyroiditis (HT) is part of the spectrum of autoimmune thyroid disorders (AITDs). It is characterized by the destruction of thyroid gland cells through the action of various cell- and antibody-mediated mechanisms (Odeke & Nagelberg, 2006) that are beyond the scope of this chapter. In HT, the thyroid is typically goitrous or atrophic (i.e., decreased in size) but may be normal in size. Patients often present with antibodies to various thyroid antigens, most commonly antithyroid peroxidase or antithyroglobulin, and less frequently with TSH receptor-blocking antibodies. There is also a small group of individuals who are antibody negative. Regardless of which mechanism or combination thereof the patient presents with, the result of HT is inadequate production and secretion of T3 and T4.

Both internationally and in the United States, HT remains the most common cause of hypothyroidism in individuals older than 6 years of age. In one epidemiological study of children, Rallison and colleagues (cited in Radetti et al., 2006) found that 1.2% of the sample met diagnostic criteria for HT, with increased prevalence in children with Turner's syndrome, celiac disease, and diabetes mellitus. Prevalence data based on gender in children were not reported; however, in adults the prevalence is 3.5 per 1,000 women and 0.8 per 1,000 men, with women being 10 to 15 times more likely to present with the disorder. The medical picture of HT is in line with other forms of hypothyroidism already noted above.

Although HT is the most common cause of acquired hypothyroidism, there is surprisingly little data on cognitive functioning. However, studies have been conducted that associate HT with severe mental health–related issues. For example, in a review of the clinical profile of individuals with HT, Odeke and Nagelberg (2006) described the possibility of psychosis, depression, dementia, memory loss, and lack of energy as complicating features. Degner, Meller, Bleich, Schlautmann, and Rüther (2001) found that 6.1% of a large sample of inpatients with various diagnoses, including major depression and psychotic disorders, exhibited some type of thyroid dysfunction. Less than 1% of their sample met criteria for HT, but of the 20 patients who did, 11 were diagnosed with major depression, 5 with bipolar disorder, 3 with schizoaffective disorder, and 1 with schizophrenia. Several words of caution are required regarding these findings. First, this was a correlational study, and the fact that many of the psychiatric patients presented with thyroid dysfunction does not imply a causal relationship. Second, the research was done using psychiatric inpatients whose conditions are more severe than those of a typical mental health patient, let alone someone whose symptoms are due to thyroid dysfunction. Lastly, caution should be used when attempting to generalize from adult-based findings to children.

The research on HT in children has focused on a condition referred to as Hashimoto's encephalopathy. Encephalopathy is a complication of HT that is a function of neurological deterioration, either acutely or insidiously, and that is generally treatable and at least partially reversible with the use of steroids. It can manifest as a stroke-like event, with acute seizures, confusion, or a decline in cognitive functioning (Chong, Rowland, & Utiger, 2003; Watemberg, Willis, & Pellock, 2000). The condition is typically found in adults but has been reported in children. A single case report was provided by Watemberg and colleagues, who described a 9-year-old girl who was brought to an emergency room with generalized tonic-clonic seizures that were followed by confusion and agitation. She was followed for approximately 6 months and demonstrated a pattern of relapse and partial recovery (she did not return to premorbid baseline in terms of maturity level or academics). These findings are in line with other case reports of both children and adults that were reviewed by Watemberg and colleagues, but further research is necessary in this area.

More extreme deficiency or even absence of thyroid hormones results in a condition known as cretinism. The major symptoms of cretinism are failure of skeletal growth and maturation, as well as marked retardation in the development of intellect (Hadley & Levine, 2006). Review of the literature on this extreme type of hypothyroidism reveals that even in endemic areas where nutrition and health care are less developed, the rates are fairly low. Jalil, Mia, and Ali (1997) conducted an epidemiological study of the prevalence rates of cretinism in individuals ranging in age from 2 to 45 years in two areas of Bangladesh, one that was hyperendemic and one that was not endemic for cretinism. The prevalence rate for cretinism in the hyperendemic area was 0.6%, whereas there were no cases of cretinism in the nonendemic area. Actual prevalence rates in the United States are not available in the literature, but the condition is most commonly found in those regions of the world where iodine deficiency is a problem. This is not the case in the United States, as there are many ways of obtaining the necessary levels of iodine, including from iodized salt.

### *Summary*

The impact of hypothyroidism on the human body is multifarious, but continued work and collaboration between the medical and mental health fields will provide a clearer and more complete picture, particularly in children. In terms of neurocognitive functioning, those working with children who have either congenital or acquired hypothyroid conditions need to attend to the possibility of decreased performance on IQ testing, deficits in motor skills, problems encoding verbal information, and attention problems, such as maintaining focus, inhibiting responses, and demonstrating cognitive flexibility. Mental health issues also are problematic for this group of patients in terms of depressive symptoms, anxiety, and, in the case of encephalopathy associated with HT, confusion, agitation, memory deficits, and seizures. It is also important to keep in mind that the types of deficits that arise depend on when the hypothyroid condition developed and that the more severe the condition, the more extensive the deficits. Furthermore, it is necessary to remember that not all children with hypothyroidism will manifest all of these deficits, and no consensus has been reached yet about the types of deficits.

## Hyperthyroidism

Hyperthyroidism occurs when the thyroid gland produces excessive thyroid hormones. Recall that thyroid hormones affect mitochondrial oxidative capacity, protein synthesis and degradation, tissue sensitivity to neurotransmitters, muscle fiber growth and development, and capillary growth (Goetz, 2003). The clinical manifestations of thyroid overactivity include weight loss despite adequate appetite; insomnia; fatigue; palpitations; heat intolerance and sweating; diarrhea; deterioration of fine motor skills, particularly handwriting; muscle weakness; and eye symptoms (Fenton, Gold, & Sadeghi-Nejad, 2006).

Hyperthyroidism in children is a relatively rare occurrence, and 95% of childhood cases of hyperthyroidism are the result of Graves' disease. As such, the prevalence rate of Graves' disease, which is 0.02% in childhood, approximates the general frequency of hyperthyroidism in children but accounts for only 5% of the total cases of Graves' disease in the general population (Fenton et al., 2006). The prognosis for children with Graves' disease is generally quite good but can be considerably worse when it occurs in very young children or during the neonatal period. Children who experience the disease at a much younger stage are more prone to prematurity, airway obstruction, and heart failure, which increases their mortality rate to as high as 16% (Fenton et al.). The age of peak incidence is between 10 and 15 years, with 3 to 6 females for every male with the disease.

Because the vast majority of cases of childhood hyperthyroidism are due to Graves' disease, more research has been conducted on this specific disorder than on other types of hyperthyroidism. The following discussion will therefore focus on the neurocognitive and psychological components of Graves' disease, which is an immune-mediated disorder that results from the production of thyroid-stimulating immunoglobulins (TSI) by stimulated B lymphocytes. TSI binds to the TSH receptor to mimic the action of TSH, thereby stimulating thyroid growth and hormone overproduction (Ferry & Levitsky, 2006; Goetz, 2003).

The research on Graves' disease in children is quite limited, and therefore a significant portion of the data presented below is based on studies with adults. Segni, Leonardi, Mazzoncini, Pucarelli, and Pasquino (1999) found that children with hyperthyroidism were more likely to exhibit behavioral disturbances including decreased attention span, difficulties with concentration, hyperactivity, sleep problems, tachycardia (i.e., cardiac arrhythmia involving rapid heart rate), tremor, and weight loss despite appropriate appetite. Several studies of adults with Graves' disease have garnered evidence of frontal lobe involvement as characterized by executive dysfunction. Tremont, Somerville, and Stern (2000) reported results from the Rey-Osterrieth Complex Figure Test (RCFT; Meyers & Meyers, 1995), finding that adults with Graves' hyperthyroidism had poorer performance relative to euthyroid controls. Tremont and colleagues reported the results of single photon emission computed tomography (SPECT) on female patients with Graves' disease. For two of the patients, the investigators found hypoperfusion (i.e., less blood flow and hence lower glucose metabolism) that was prominent in the frontal lobes and the anterior temporal regions, while findings for the third patient were in the normal range. Both of the patients with abnormal SPECT findings demonstrated deficits on neuropsychological measures of verbal learning, figural fluency, and visual construction. The patient with normal SPECT findings did not reveal such deficits. Fukui, Hasegawa, and Takenaka (2001) reported the SPECT findings for a 67-year-old man who experienced progressive impairment of attention, memory, construction skills, and behavior with concomitant hand tremor and weight loss over a 2-year period. SPECT findings pointed to hypoperfusion bilaterally in the temporoparietal regions. Subsequent treatment with methimazole resulted in improved memory and construction abilities.

Stern and colleagues (1996) surveyed the neuropsychiatric complaints of adults with Graves' disease. Respondents reported significant issues with memory, attention, planning, and productivity. Trzepacz, McCue, Klein, Levey, and Greenhouse (1988) examined the psychiatric and neuropsychological sequelae of patients with untreated Graves' disease. Although they surveyed only a small number of participants (13 adults), more than half met criteria for major depressive disorder and generalized anxiety disorder compared to fewer other hospitalized medical patients. On neuropsychological testing, the participants were found to have mild deficits in attention, memory, and complex problem solving.

Not all studies have found the presence of neuropsychological deficits. Vogel and colleagues (2007) evaluated a sample of 31 consecutively referred patients who had been newly diagnosed with Graves' disease. They found higher ratings on psychiatric measures prior to treatment but no differences on neuropsychological test performance. They further reported that thyroid levels did not correlate with neuropsychological test findings or psychiatric ratings. After reaching a euthyroid state, previously reported psychiatric and cognitive impairments decreased significantly.

*Summary*

Graves' disease is the most common cause of hyperthyroidism in children, accounting for 95% of cases, but the condition is generally rare. As such, it is not surprising that research is scant on this age group. The studies reviewed indicated that both timing and severity of the disorder impact how significant the clinical manifestation will be. The prognosis for hyperthyroidism, including Graves' disease, is generally quite good in children, but when it occurs at a very young age or during the neonatal period, severe complications such as airway obstruction and congestive heart failure can occur, significantly increasing mortality rates.

The primary deficits exhibited by individuals with Graves' disease on neuropsychological measures indicate the presence of executive dysfunction. Specifically, Graves' disease appears to be associated with greater impairment in attention, including the ability to sustain attention and inhibit behaviors. Problems with memory also have been noted based on both the administration of memory tests and self-reports of impairment. These results suggest that individuals with Graves' disease are likely to require more time and effort in order to learn and consolidate new information. Planning and organizational skills are affected in these individuals as well, which can result in a work product that is less well developed than should be the case. Unlike the findings for hypothyroidism, decrements in intellectual functioning were not reported in individuals with hyperthyroid conditions. However, the psychological and neuropsychiatric sequelae, including the presence of high levels of depressive features and anxiety, do overlap with hypothyroidism.

## DISORDERS OF THE ADRENAL GLANDS

The adrenal glands are located adjacent to the upper surface of each kidney and typically weigh between 3.5 and 4.5 grams (Hadley & Levine, 2006). In many mammals, the adrenal glands are composed of steroidogenic and chromaffin tissue. Steroidogenic tissue, as the name implies, is the primary site where glucocorticoids, such as cortisol, are produced. The secretion of cortisol is effected by stimulation of the hypothalamic-pituitary-adrenal (HPA) axis, whereby the hypothalamus secretes cortisol-releasing hormone (CRH), which, in turn, stimulates the pituitary, resulting in the release of adrenocorticotropic hormone (ACTH). ACTH then works to cause the release of cortisol from the adrenal glands. The level of cortisol serves as part of a negative feedback loop, signaling the hypothalamic-pituitary component of the HPA to cease production of stimulating hormones (Blumenfeld, 2002). Chromaffin tissue is the area where mineralocorticoids, such as aldosterone, are produced. The steroidogenic tissue forms a cortical mass around the chromaffin tissue and is therefore often referred to as the adrenal cortex, whereas the chromaffin tissue is referred to as the adrenal medulla (Hadley & Levine, 2006). As with the thyroid, adrenal dysfunction can result in either hypo- or hyperadrenalism.

## Hypoadrenalism

Hypoadrenalism is also known as adrenal insufficiency (AI). Classic AI is caused by Addison's disease, which was first described in the 19th century by British physician Thomas Addison. In its primary form, Addison's disease results from bilateral destruction of the adrenal glands. In its secondary form, AI results from hypothalamic or pituitary dysfunction (Goetz, 2003). In either case, AI is characterized by pigmentation of the skin and mucous membranes, nausea, vomiting, weight loss, muscle weakness, lethargy, and a tendency to faint (Victor & Ropper, 2001). In children, hypoglycemia also is present (Wilson & Speiser, 2006).

Primary AI is rare. A more likely cause is iatrogenic, central AI, but the exact prevalence is unknown. AI secondary to congenital adrenal hyperplasia (CAH) occurs in 1 per 16,000 infants. Autoimmune AI is more common in females than in males and in adults than in children. AI due to adrenoleukodystrophy occurs almost exclusively in males due to its X-linked inheritance, whereas secondary insufficiency is equally prevalent in males and females (Wilson & Speiser, 2006).

According to the American Academy of Pediatrics, Section on Endocrinology and Committee on Genetics (2000), cognitive functioning in children with disorders of hyposecretion of adrenal hormones has not been well studied, particularly in terms of neuropsychological functioning. Mercado, Wilson, Cheng, Wei, and New (1995) provided a preliminary report based on maternal accounts of children's cognitive and behavioral functioning using a standardized questionnaire. They did not find significant differences in behavioral or cognitive ratings for children at risk for CAH who were either treated or not with prenatal dexamethasone. However, the authors did find what they called "neurologically silent" white matter abnormalities and temporal lobe atrophy in both children and adults with CAH. Using an abbreviated version of the Wechsler Intelligence Scale for Children (Donders, 1997) and subtests of A Developmental Neuropsychological Assessment (NEPSY; Korkman, Kirk, & Kemp, 1998), Hirvikoski and colleagues (2007) evaluated a group of prenatally treated 7- to 17-year-old children. Although trends toward lower verbal processing speed were found in children with CAH who were treated prenatally with dexamethasone, these differences did not hold up following statistical correction.

Chrousos (2004) reviewed the expected neurocognitive manifestations of Addison's disease, listing the following: lack of energy (i.e., asthenia), depression, memory dysfunction, executive dysfunction, hyperalgesia (i.e., hypersensitivity to pain), fatigue, and poor sleep quality. The primary adrenal hormone involved is posited to be cortisol, as it is involved in hippocampal function and also fluctuates across the sleep cycle (for a review of the literature and potential mechanisms of action, see Payne & Nadel, 2004). Blair, Granger, and Razza (2005) studied the relationship between cortisol reactivity and executive function in preschool children attending a Head Start program. They found that moderate elevation of cortisol, followed by downregulation, was positively associated with executive functions such as cognitive flexibility and self-regulation. In rats that had their adrenal glands removed, the physiological response of the dentate gyrus of the hippocampus to stimulation was found to be attenuated (Hadley & Levine, 2006). These results lend indirect support to the relationship between hypofunction of the adrenal glands and deficits in memory and executive function.

## Hyperadrenalism

The clinical components of Cushing's disease were first described by American neurosurgeon H. W. Cushing in 1932. The features included truncal obesity, reddish-purple cutaneous striae (i.e., irregular areas of skin that look like bands), dryness and pigmentation of the skin, fragility of skin blood vessels, excessive facial hair, baldness, cyanosis and mottling of the skin and extremities, osteoporosis, muscle weakness, and hypertension (Victor & Ropper, 2001). The cause of Cushing's disease is a pituitary microadenoma (i.e., a tumor that is less than 1 centimeter in size) that produces ACTH, which, in turn, stimulates the adrenal glands. These tumors are often referred to as *basophils* because of their affinity for specific stains that give them a purplish or blue appearance. Basophils are further classified by the type of hormone they secrete. For example, the tumors involved in Cushing's disease are corticotrophic because their cells secrete ACTH. When the combination of symptoms reported above is due to a primary adrenal tumor, ectopic production of ACTH by other tumors (e.g., lung carcinoma), or prolonged administration of glucocorticoids (e.g., prednisone), the term *Cushing's syndrome* is appropriate (Adler & Dipp, 2006; Victor & Ropper, 2001).

The majority of cases of Cushing's syndrome are due to exogenous glucocorticoids such as those used in the treatment of inflammation or infection. The annual incidence of endogenous Cushing's syndrome has been estimated at 13 cases per million individuals, of which approximately 70% are due to Cushing's disease, 15% to ectopic ACTH secretion, and 15% to primary adrenal tumor. The female-to-male ratio is 5:1, and the peak incidence of Cushing's syndrome occurs in persons aged 25 to 40 years. Ectopic ACTH secretion occurs later in life, usually due to lung cancer (Adler & Dipp, 2006).

The impact of excess glucocorticoid exposure on the brain is quite significant, particularly in light of the fact that the brain continues to develop throughout childhood and adolescence. Those areas of the brain most sensitive to the impact of corticosteroids include the hippocampus, prefrontal cortex (PFC), and amygdala (Romeo & McEwen, 2006). In their review of the animal literature, Romeo and McEwen highlighted the impact of corticosterone, which is the animal analog of cortisol, on the rat brain, including the hippocampus, PFC, and amygdala. The hippocampus is a brain region that is critical for learning and memory consolidation (Mesulam, 2000). Prolonged exposure to corticosterone resulted in a reduction of the branching of the apical dendrites of the CA3 region of the hippocampus, with the outcome being spatial memory impairment. These results were reversed when the animals were placed in a relatively stress-free environment (which included reduction of the level and time of exposure to corticosterone) or when antidepressant medication was administered (Romeo & McEwen).

The PFC is involved in executive functioning, emotion regulation, and fear extinction (Sotres-Bayon, Cain, & LeDoux, 2006). Romeo and McEwen (2006) reported that in adult rats, stress due to chronic restraint (i.e., 6 hours per day for a period of 3 weeks) resulted in reductions in both apical dendritic branching and spine density of the medial prefrontal cortical pyramidal neurons, including the areas of anterior cingulate cortex and prelimbic area. In contrast to the medial PFC, the orbitofrontal cortex showed growth as a result of repeated stress. PFC atrophy due to stress-induced remodeling is associated with impairment of the ability to shift attention set and inhibit impulses that are not appropriate to the context (Liston et al., 2006; Mesulam, 2000).

In contrast to the impact of stress on the morphology of the hippocampus and PFC, adult rats showed dendritic hypertrophy in the basolateral but not the central nucleus of the amygdala. These animals exhibited what were described as elevated anxiety-like behaviors that persisted even after 3 weeks of stress-free recovery (Vyas, Pillai, & Chattarji, 2004).

In line with the animal model described above, Chrousos (2004) reported the following neurocognitive findings in his review of the clinical sequelae of Cushing's syndrome and glucocorticoid hypersensitivity: anxiety, insomnia, depression, memory dysfunction, and executive dysfunction. Furthermore, Arnaldi and colleagues (2003) reported that between 50% and 80% of patients with Cushing's syndrome met diagnostic criteria for major depression. Moreover, children with hypersecretion of cortisol were reported to exhibit an elevated level of obsessive-compulsive features. In a study of 48 adults diagnosed with Cushing's disease, Starkman, Giordani, Berent, Schork, and Schteingart (2001) found that their patient group had lower verbal IQ scores than nonpatient controls; the difference was statistically significant. What is more, verbal learning and memory were significantly lower in the patient group, including delayed recall of verbal material. In contrast to the deficits noted on the verbal components of memory tasks, memory for visual material was not significantly different between the patients and control participants. Patients with Cushing's disease were also significantly more depressed than control participants.

Arnaldi and colleagues (2003) further reported that many of the psychological features associated with Cushing's syndrome remitted after normalization of cortisol levels, typically with surgery to remove the adrenal glands. However, some data suggest that problems with social, psychological, and cognitive functioning continue to plague many patients despite normal cortisol levels. At the time of diagnosis and 1 year after normalization of cortisol levels, Merke and colleagues (2005) performed clinical, cognitive, and psychological testing, as well as magnetic resonance brain imaging (MRI) on 11 children with Cushing's syndrome ranging in age from 8 to 16 years. The authors reported no significant differences in IQ between the two groups, and no psychopathology was identified at baseline. However, baseline neuroimaging indicated that children with Cushing's syndrome had significantly smaller cerebral volumes, enlarged ventricles, and a smaller amygdala. Hippocampal volume also was smaller in the patient group, but this difference did not reach statistical significance. The posttreatment evaluation revealed significant reversal of cerebral atrophy marked by an increase in total cerebral volume and decrease in ventricular volume. Despite the physiological reversal of atrophy, the children with Cushing's syndrome experienced a significant decline in Full Scale IQ, which fell from a standard score of 112 (±19 points) to 98 (±14 points) at 1 year. Also noted was a decline in school performance without any associated psychopathology. The reasons for the decline in performance are not clear, but Merke and colleagues posit the possible impact of prior excess cortisol, surgery, and a relative cortisol deficiency subsequent to treatment. In terms of IQ scores, one also needs to consider regression toward the mean as a potential factor, as the children in this group scored in the high average range relative to normative data (Healy & Goldstein, 1978).

*Mental Health and the HPA Axis*

The importance of the HPA axis in our mental health is becoming ever clearer. This section provides a brief summary of the research on the role of the HPA axis in a variety of disorders that are frequently encountered by mental health professionals. Lopez, Vazquez, Chalmers, and Watson (1997) reviewed the HPA axis's role in the regulation of serotonin receptors, specifically in terms of the implications for the neurobiology of suicide. The primary hypothesis is that 5-HT receptor changes that have been observed in individuals who committed suicide may be worsened by or a direct result of HPA overactivity. In support of their hypothesis, Lopez and colleagues cited a number of lines of research. First, in terms of animal models, they reported the well-known finding that chronic unpredictable stress leads to high levels of corticosteroid production. Second, chronic stress results in specific changes to 5-HT receptor sites, with general increases in cortical receptor sites but decreases in hippocampal regions. Moreover, chronic administration of antidepressant medication prevents many of the changes in 5-HT receptors that have been observed to result from stress, and the medication also reverses overactivity of the HPA axis. Although not conclusive in and of itself, this review highlights the potential role of HPA axis in depression and suicidal behavior.

According to the *Diagnostic and Statistical Manual of Mental Disorders—Fourth Edition, Text Revision* (*DSM-IV-TR*; American Psychiatric Association, 2000), posttraumatic stress disorder (PTSD) requires a person to have experienced or witnessed some type of event that results in a threat to the physical integrity of the self or others. This results in intense fear, helplessness, or horror. The traumatic event is persistently reexperienced, resulting in avoidance of stimuli associated with the trauma and persistent symptoms of increased arousal that were not present before the trauma. Yehuda (1997) reviewed the literature on the relationship between the HPA axis and PTSD. In contrast to the typical finding that cortisol levels are elevated in individuals who are experiencing stress, participants with PTSD, whether soldiers, victims of child abuse, or women who were raped, have lower levels of cortisol in comparison to individuals who have suffered similar traumatic events but who do not meet diagnostic criteria for PTSD. In addition to lower levels of circulating cortisol, the PTSD patients also had a higher number of glucocorticoid receptors and increased sensitivity to the dexamethasone suppression test (dexamethasone is a chemical that suppresses the release of ACTH from the pituitary and CRF from the hypothalamus) and metyrapone stimulation test (metyrapone is used to prevent adrenal steroidogenesis by blocking the conversion of cortisol from its precursor,

11-deoxycortisol, thereby resulting in a disruption of the negative feedback cycle between the adrenal glands and pituitary). Yehuda suggested that these findings point to the presence of enhanced negative feedback of the HPA in PTSD patients due to increased receptor sensitivity to glucocorticoids.

### *Summary*

Although Cushing's syndrome and Cushing's disease are less common in children than in adults, the cognitive and psychological consequences are quite significant. Current data, based on a combination of animal models, research on adult humans, and research on children and adolescents, point to several neurocognitive sequelae of hypersecretion of cortisol. Executive dysfunction is likely, including effects on working memory, attention, and self-regulation, probably as a consequence of hypercortisolism's influence on the frontal lobes. Changes in hippocampal volume have been noted to affect verbal learning and memory in humans and visuospatial learning in animals. Anxiety-related symptoms were demonstrated in both human participants and animals; humans also demonstrated elevated levels of depression and obsessive-compulsive features, the latter being noted only in children. In addition, it is important to note that despite the physiological improvements in cortisol level and reversal of the brain atrophy following treatment, both adults and children continued to exhibit psychological and cognitive problems.

Research on psychiatric disorders points to the prominent role played by the HPA axis, particularly in anxiety, depression, and PTSD. Therefore, any complete evaluation should look at mood and anxiety-related issues in individuals with disorders of the adrenal glands.

## DISORDERS OF THE PARATHYROID (PT)

Humans typically have four PT glands located on the posterior region of the thyroid gland. The PT is composed of two primary cell types, *chief* cells (responsible for secretion of parathyroid hormone [PTH]) and *oxyphil* cells (whose function is unknown; Hadley & Levine, 2006). PTH, along with aldosterone, is one of two hormones that are necessary for life. It is responsible for controlling calcium ion ($Ca^{2+}$) homeostasis. $Ca^{2+}$ is an essential component of multiple physiological functions including bone structure, blood clotting, maintenance of the transmembrane potential of cells, and cell replication. As with other hormones, the level of PTH secreted by the PT is controlled by circulating levels of $Ca^{2+}$ (Hadley & Levine).

Disorders of the PT can involve either hyper- or hyposecretion of PTH, which are called hyperparathyroidism and hypoparathyroidism, respectively. According to Klein (2006), hyperparathyroidism involves the proliferation of PTH-secreting cells (chief cells) in one or more of the PT glands. The cause of hypersecretion can be genetic mutation, which is termed primary hyperparathyroidism, or a variety of underlying conditions that cause secondary forms of the disorder. These can include renal failure, hypocalcemia (i.e., abnormally low calcium levels), and high serum phosphorus levels. The exact mechanisms that result in hypersecretion of PTH remain uncertain. In adults, the prevalence of primary hyperparathyroidism is reported to be 1 in 500–1,000 individuals. The prevalence in children is unknown (Klein). Morbidity is most frequently due to hypercalcemia that results in bradycardia (i.e., abnormally slow heart rate) and heart block as well as dehydration. The male-to-female ratio is 1:3, with the majority of cases occurring after the age of 30 years (Klein).

Clinically, patients with hyperparathyroidism generally present as asymptomatic, and elevated levels of PTH are discovered incidentally. When symptoms are present, they are specific to hypercalcemia and include muscle weakness, depression, increased sleepiness, nausea and vomiting, acute abdominal pain, constipation, and polydipsia (i.e., chronic excessive thirst; Klein, 2006). Psychiatric and neurological manifestations can also include delirium, psychosis, anxiety, and neuromuscular irritability and muscle spasms (Velasco, Manshadi, Breen, & Lippmann, 1999). Jorde, Waterloo, Saleh, Haug, and Svartberg (2006) assessed the neuropsychological functioning of adult patients and found a decrease in executive functioning relative to normal controls on tasks of processing speed, word fluency, and attention. The hyperparathyroid group also had higher depression ratings. Similar findings were obtained by Dotzenrath and colleagues (2006) in terms of neuropsychiatric and cognitive changes after surgery for primary hyperparathyroidism.

Hypoparathyroidism is a condition in which deficient amounts of PTH are secreted by the PT glands. The condition can be either inherited or acquired; it has the net effect of decreasing serum calcium levels and increasing serum phosphate levels. The condition results in loss of both the direct and indirect effects of PTH on bone, kidney, and gut. The clinical features of hypocalcemia include muscle aches, facial twitching, carpopedal spasm (i.e., involuntary contractions of the hands and feet), stridor (i.e., high-pitched breathing due to narrowed airways), seizures, and syncope (i.e., temporary loss of consciousness). The disorder is also frequently associated with chromosomal defects such as DiGeorge anomaly and velocardiofacial syndrome, both involving 22q11 deletions (Thornton, Kelly, & Willcutts, 2006). The incidence of idiopathic (i.e., arising from an unknown cause) hypoparathyroidism has not been determined in the United States, and the rates of hypoparathyroidism due to thyroid surgery depend on the extent of tissue excision. Hypoparathyroidism tends to present in newborns but can manifest at any age; it is equally prevalent in males and females (Thornton et al., 2006).

In a review of the literature, Velasco and colleagues (1999) described the psychological and cognitive features of hypoparathyroidism as including delirium, cognitive impairment, psychosis, depression, and anxiety. They report that this symptom picture is more common in instances of surgically induced hypoparathyroidism.

### Summary

Hyperparathyroidism is a condition that rarely affects children and is more likely to manifest in adults over the age of 30. In contrast, hypoparathyroidism is frequently found in children, particularly in newborns, where it is usually a congenital condition comorbid with other genetic disorders. Hypoparathyroidism can also result from surgical treatment for thyroid disorders, whereby the PT glands are damaged and/or removed due to their close proximity to the thyroid. Although the pediatric neuropsychological literature on this topic is scant, based on the available data, assessment for mental health–related issues such as depression and anxiety is recommended, and cognitive testing should involve tasks that measure executive functioning, including attention, processing speed, and verbal fluency.

## CLINICAL CASE

The following is a brief synopsis of the case of an adolescent, John, who was 12 years 8 months old at the time of evaluation. He was diagnosed with the DiGeorge anomaly, tetralogy of Fallot, and Hashimoto's thyroiditis with resulting hypothyroidism. In line with the tetralogy of Fallot, John presented with atrial and ventricular septal defects and an overriding aortic arch (i.e., aortic arch that is incorrectly situated) that was corrected at 5 days of age. A hernia was surgically repaired when he was 2 years old, and he had surgery for cleft palate at 5 years of age. The cleft palate contributed to delays in language acquisition and led to articulation problems. John also had hypotonia (i.e., muscle weakness), as a result of which he did not begin to walk until 16 months of age. He continues to receive physical therapy. John has not suffered head trauma or seizures and does not present with other medical issues. He was diagnosed with ADHD, Combined Type, during a neuropsychological evaluation completed at

7 years of age and was subsequently treated with Focalin by a developmental pediatrician. Hearing and vision were within normal limits.

Although John's appetite was normal, he is very picky about the foods he will eat. He also has significant social difficulties that result from limited eye contact, poor inflection and volume of speech, inadequate understanding of social cues, and a highly immature presentation (e.g., he collects Webkins).

John has been evaluated on multiple occasions. The Kaufman Assessment Battery for Children (K-ABC; Kaufman & Kaufman, 1983) was administered to John when he was 3 and 6 years old, with resulting Mental Processing Composite scores of 112 (79th percentile) and 101 (53rd percentile), respectively. The Wechsler Intelligence Scale for Children—Third Edition (WISC-III; Wechsler, 1991) was administered when John was 8 years old, with Full Scale IQ, Verbal IQ, and Performance IQ scores of 95 (37th percentile). Table 8.1 demonstrates how his IQ scores, based on the Wechsler Intelligence Scale for Children—Fourth Edition (WISC-IV; Wechsler, 2003), have changed over the years.

It is clear that John's intellectual functioning has declined steadily from the age of 3, when John demonstrated high-average intelligence, to the most recent evaluation. The one exception to the general decline was noted on the Perceptual Reasoning index, where his performance was average.

Assessment of academic achievement using the Wechsler Individual Achievement Test—Second Edition (WIAT-II; Wechsler, 2001) indicated that word decoding and reading comprehension were in the borderline and deficient range, respectively; arithmetic problem solving and word problems were deficient as was spelling, but the writing component

**TABLE 8.1 Standard Scores from the Wechsler Intelligence Scale for Children—Fourth Edition at 10, 11, and 12 years of Age**

| | Age at Testing | | |
|---|---|---|---|
| Index | 10 | 11 | 12 |
| Full Scale IQ | 91 | 72 | 76 |
| Verbal Comprehension | 95 | 71 | 75 |
| Perceptual Reasoning | 94 | 84 | 98 |
| Working Memory | 97 | 83 | 68 |
| Processing Speed | 88 | 73 | 80 |

could not be completed due to John's high level of frustration with this section.

Memory was assessed using the California Verbal Learning Test—Children's Version (CVLT-C; Delis, Kramer, Kaplan, & Ober, 1994). Results pointed to significant impairment in John's ability to learn the list and also in immediate and delayed recall, as well as delayed recognition. Regarding executive functioning, problems with sustained attention were noted, as was limited impulse control (Conners' Continuous Performance Test—Second Edition; Conners, 2000). Problem solving and strategic thinking, however, were average (Tower of London, Drexel Version; Culbertson & Zillmer, 2000).

Parent and teacher rating scales (Child Behavior Checklist, Teacher Report Form [Achenbach, 1991]; Behavior Rating Instrument of Executive Functioning [Gioia, Isquith, Guy, & Kenworthy, 2000]) were completed. Both sets of ratings pointed to multiple areas of concern. With regard to social skills, John was described as a child who is highly immature in his interactions with peers. He does not understand social conventions, including the nuances involved in interpersonal interactions. He struggles to control his emotions, resulting in inappropriate behaviors at home and in school, and is often unable to follow multistep or complex instructions without receiving significant guidance and support from an adult. His ability to monitor and modulate his reactions to situations is limited and often results in meltdowns. On the other hand, only minor problems were reported with regard to attention on the behavior ratings.

The Adaptive Behavior Assessment System—Second Edition (Harrison & Oakland, 2003) was administered to assess how well John is able to function on a daily basis. Areas of strength were noted in terms of John's ability to take care of his own health and safety needs, indicating that he matches his peers in his understanding of general safety rules and his handling of dangerous items. He does not have any problems following the rules of games and activities and has a varied number of interests.

The deficits that John demonstrated during the neuropsychological evaluation indicate the presence of an attention disorder as well as learning deficits. This combination of findings is in line with the common cognitive, emotional, and behavioral presentations of individuals diagnosed with Hashimoto's thyroiditis and subsequent hypothyroidism. Common issues include a decline in intellectual functioning, impaired attention, and issues with memory. As should also be clear, the clinical picture is complicated by the presence of the DiGeorge anomaly, which is often associated with mental retardation and other cognitive deficits. Although no clear connection exists between tetralogy of Fallot and cognitive or emotional functioning, the brain is so dependent on a steady supply of oxygen that the impact that this defect may have had on John's CNS cannot be discounted.

As a rule of thumb, it is useful to understand the impact that a specific endocrine disorder can have on functioning, but given that disorders do not occur in isolation of other factors, the use of a broad-based battery is quite useful. In this case, although John's presentation is in line with the literature on Hashimoto's thyroiditis and hypothyroidism, one cannot definitively say that these conditions are the causal factors. The use of a broad-based approach can provide a better understanding of the individual's areas of strength and weakness so that a more effective intervention plan can be put in place.

## CONCLUSION

As can readily be seen, the endocrine system and its constituent components are highly complex in terms of their function and involvement with other body systems. Regarding the CNS, we have seen that the endocrine system participates, whether directly or indirectly, in cognition, including intellectual functioning, memory, attention, and executive functions. It also plays a significant role in emotion regulation and mobilization and has been implicated in psychosis, depression, and anxiety disorders including PTSD and obsessive-compulsive symptoms.

Given the diverse role of the endocrine system and the variable impact that it can have on homeostasis when its function is disordered, it is important that the evaluation of children and adolescents focus on a broad-based battery (Russell, Russell, & Hill, 2005). This will enable the evaluator to develop a clear and comprehensive picture of the child or adolescent, enabling the development and implementation of necessary services.

While this chapter attempts to provide a thorough description of the neuropsychological components of endocrinological disorders, it is certainly not complete. Multiple subject areas had to be omitted due to space considerations, including the involvement of the endocrine system in other disorders including velocardiofacial syndrome, Down syndrome, DiGeorge anomaly, and others with which endocrine issues are often comorbid. Further research and collaborative efforts between medical and psychological professionals are also necessary if a better and more complete understanding of the role of the endocrine system in the cognitive and emotional development of children and adolescents is desired.

## RESOURCES

Advanced Psychological Assessment, P.C.

This is the author's Web site, which provides information about neuropsychology and neuropsychological assessment, as well as a wide variety of disorders that range from ADHD and learning disorders to brain tumors and epilepsy, their diagnosis and treatment, and their impact on cognitive, emotional, and interpersonal functioning.

Web Site: www.advancedpsy.com

American Thyroid Association

This organization is comprised of professionals who are involved in research on and treatment of thyroid disorders. Information is available for the public and professionals.

Web Site: www.thyroid.org

Cushing's Support and Research Foundation

This group provides information and support for patients and their families, increases awareness and educates the public about Cushing's disease and Cushing's syndrome, and raises and distributes funds for Cushing's disease and Cushing's syndrome research.

Web Site: www.csrf.org

Directory of Endocrine and Metabolic Diseases Organizations

This directory will allow individuals to obtain a list of additional resources on a wide variety of endocrinological issues, both for informational purposes and advocacy.

Web Site: http://endocrine.niddk.nih.gov/resources/organizations.htm

eMedicine World Medical Library

This comprehensive Web site provides peer-reviewed articles on a wide variety of medical and psychological disorders.

Web Site: www.emedicine.com

National Institutes of Health

The NIH provides information about a wide variety of medical and psychological diseases and disorders, including resources for individuals.

Web Site: www.nih.gov

## REFERENCES

Achenbach, T. M. (1991). *Manual for the Child Behavior Checklist/4–18 and 1991 profile.* Burlington: University of Vermont.

Adler, G., & Dipp, S. L. (2006). *Cushing syndrome.* Retrieved June 19, 2007, from http://www.emedicine.com/med/topic485.htm

Aijaz, N. J., Flaherty, E. M., Preston, T., Bracken, S. S., Lane, A. H., & Wilson, T. A. (2006). Neurocognitive function in children with compensated hypothyroidism: Lack of short term effects on or off thyroxin [Electronic version]. *Biomed Central Endocrine Disorders, 6.* Retrieved June 19, 2007, from http://www.biomedcentral.com/1472–6823/6/2

American Academy of Pediatrics, Section on Endocrinology and Committee on Genetics. (2000). Technical report: Congenital adrenal hyperplasia. *Pediatrics, 106,* 1511.

American Psychiatric Association. (2000). *Diagnostic and statistical manual of mental disorders* (4th ed., text revision). Washington, DC: Author.

Arnaldi, G., Angeli, A., Atkinson, A. B., Bertagna, X., Cavagnini, F., Chrousos, G. P., et al. (2003). Diagnosis and complications of Cushing's syndrome: A consensus statement. *Journal of Clinical Endocrinology and Metabolism, 88,* 5593–5602.

Asher, S. R., Hymel, S., & Renshaw, P. D. (1984). Loneliness in children. *Child Development, 55,* 1456.

Blair, C., Granger, D., & Razza, R. P. (2005). Cortisol reactivity is positively related to executive function in preschool children attending Head Start. *Child Development, 76,* 554–567.

Blumenfeld, H. (2002). *Neuroanatomy through clinical cases.* Sunderland, MA: Sinauer Associates.

Bongers-Schokking, J. J., & De Muinck Keizer-Schrama, S. M. P. F. (2005). Influence of timing and dose of thyroid hormone replacement on mental, psychomotor, and behavioral development in children with congenital hypothyroidism. *Journal of Pediatrics, 147,* 768–774.

Chong, J. Y., Rowland, L. P., & Utiger, R. D. (2003). Hashimoto encephalopathy: Syndrome or myth? *Archives of Neurology, 60,* 164–171.

Chrousos, G. P. (2004). Is 11Beta-hydroxysteroid dehydrogenase type 1 a good therapeutic target for blockade of glucocorticoid actions? *Proceedings of the National Academy of Sciences, 101,* 6329–6330.

Conners, K. (2000). *Conners' Continuous Performance Test—Second Edition for Windows.* North Tonawanda, NY: Multi-Health Systems.

Culbertson, W. C., & Zillmer, E. A. (2000). *Tower of London, Drexel Version* (2nd ed.). Lutz, FL: Psychological Assessment Resources.

Degner, D., Meller, J., Bleich, S., Schlautmann, V., & Rüther, E. (2001). Affective disorders associated with autoimmune thyroiditis. *Journal of Neuropsychiatry and Clinical Neurosciences, 13,* 532–533.

Delis, D. C., Kramer, J., Kaplan, E., & Ober, B. A. (1987). *California Verbal Learning Test (CVLT) manual.* San Antonio, TX: The Psychological Corporation.

Delis, D. C., Kramer, J., Kaplan, E., & Ober, B. A. (1994). *California Verbal Learning Test—Children's Version (CVLT-C) manual.* San Antonio, TX: The Psychological Corporation.

Derksen-Lubsen, G., & Verkerk, P. H. (1996). Neuropsychologic development in early treated congenital hypothyroidism: Analysis of literature data. *Pediatric Research, 39,* 561–566.

Derogatis, L. R., & Savits, K. L. (1999). The SCL-90, brief symptom inventory, and matching clinical rating scales. In M. E. Maruish (Ed.), *The use of psychological testing for treatment planning and outcome assessment* (2nd ed.). Mahwah, NJ: Lawrence Erlbaum.

Donders, J. (1997). A short form of WISC-III for clinical use. *Psychological Assessment, 9,* 15–20.

Dotzenrath, C. M., Kaetsch A. K., Pfingsten, H., Cupisti, K., Weyerbrock, N., Vossough, A., et al. (2006). Neuropsychiatric and cognitive changes after surgery for primary hyperparathyroidism. *World Journal of Surgery, 30,* 680–685.

Fenton, C. L., Gold, J. G., & Sadeghi-Nejad, A. (2006). *Hyperthyroidism.* Retrieved July 4, 2007, from http://www.emedicine.com/med/topic1099.htm

Ferry, R. J., & Levitsky, L. L. (2006). *Graves' disease.* Retrieved July 19, 2007, from http://www.emedicine.com/ped/topic899.htm

Friedhoff, A. J., Miller, J. C., Armour, M., Schweitzer, J. W., & Mohan, S. (2000). Role of maternal biochemistry in fetal brain development: Effect of maternal thyroidectomy on behaviour and biogenic amine metabolism in rat progeny. *International Journal of Neuropsychopharmacology, 3,* 89–97.

Fukui, T., Hasegawa, Y., & Takenaka, H. (2001). Hyperthyroid dementia: Clinicoradiological findings and response to treatment. *Journal of the Neurological Sciences, 184,* 81–88.

Gioia, G. A., Isquith, P. K., Guy, S. C., & Kenworthy, L. (2000). *The Behavior Rating Inventory of Executive Function professional manual.* Odessa, FL: Psychological Assessment Resources.

Goetz, C. G. (2003). *Textbook of clinical neurology* (2nd ed.). Philadelphia: W. B. Saunders.

Gronwall, D. M. A. (1977). Paced auditory serial-addition task: A measure of recovery from concussion. *Perceptual and Motor Skills, 44,* 367–373.

Hadley, M. E., & Levine, J. E. (2006). *Endocrinology* (6th ed.). Upper Saddle River, NJ: Pearson.

Harrison, P. L., & Oakland T. (2003). *Adaptive Behavior Assessment System* (2nd ed.). San Antonio, TX: Harcourt Assessment.

Healy, M. J. R., & Goldstein, H. (1978). Regression to the mean. *Annals of Human Biology, 5,* 277–280.

Heaton, R. (1981). *Wisconsin Card Sorting Test.* Odessa, FL: Psychological Assessment Resources.

Hirvikoski, T., Nordenström, A., Lindholm, T., Lindblad, F., Ritzén, E. M., Wedell, A., et al. (2007). Cognitive functions in children at risk for congenital adrenal hyperplasia treated prenatally with dexamethasone. *Journal of Clinical Endocrinology and Metabolism, 92,* 542–548.

Jalil, M. Q., Mia, M. J., & Ali, S. M. (1997). Epidemiological study of endemic cretinism in a hyperendemic area. *Bangladesh Medical Research Council Bulletin, 23,* 34–37.

Jastak, S., & Wilkinson, G. S. (1984). *The Wide Range Achievement Test administration manual* (rev. ed.). Indianapolis, IN: Jastak Associates.

Jorde, R., Waterloo, K., Saleh, F., Haug, E., & Svartberg, J. (2006). Neuropsychological function in relation to serum parathyroid hormone and serum 25–hydroxyvitamin D levels: The Tromso study. *Journal of Neurology, 253,* 464–470.

Jorde, R., Waterloo, K., Storhaug, H., Nyrnes, A., Sundsfjord, J., & Jenssen, T. G. (2006). Neuropsychological function and symptoms in subjects with subclinical hypothyroidism and the effect of thyroxine treatment. *Journal of Endocrinology and Metabolism, 91,* 145–153.

Kaufman, A. S., & Kaufman, N. L. (1983). *Kaufman Assessment Battery for Children administration and scoring manual.* Circle Pines, MN: American Guidance Service.

Kempers, M. J. E., van der Sluijs Veer, L., Nijhuis-van der Sanden, M. W. G., Kooistra, L., Wiedijk, B. M., Faber, I., et al. (2006). Intellectual and motor development of young adults with congenital hypothyroidism diagnosed by neonatal screening. *Journal of Clinical Endocrinology and Metabolism, 91,* 418–424.

Klein, G. L. (2006). *Hyperparathyroidism.* Retrieved July 11, 2007, from http://www.emedicine.com/ped/topic1086.htm

Korkman, M., Kirk, U., & Kemp, S. (1998). *NEPSY: A Developmental Neuropsychological Test.* San Antonio, TX: The Psychological Corporation.

Kovacs, M. (1992). *The Children's Depression Inventory manual.* Toronto: Multi-Health Systems.

LaGreca, A. M., & Stone, W. L. (1993). Social Anxiety Scale for Children—Revised: Factor structure and concurrent validity. *Journal of Clinical Child Psychology, 22,* 17–27.

Liston, C., Miller, M. M., Goldwater, D. S., Radley, J. J., Rocher, A. B., Hof, P. R., et al. (2006). Stress-induced alterations in prefrontal cortical dendritic morphology predict selective impairments in perceptual attentional set-shifting. *Journal of Neuroscience, 26,* 7870–7874.

Lopez, J. F., Vazquez, D. M., Chalmers, D. T., & Watson, S. J. (1997). Regulation of 5-HT receptors and the hypothalamic-pituitary-adrenal axis: Implications for the neurobiology of suicide. *Annals of the New York Academy of Sciences, 836,* 106–134.

Mercado, A. B., Wilson, R. C., Cheng, K. C., Wei, J. Q., & New, M. I. (1995). Prenatal treatment and diagnosis of congenital adrenal hyperplasia owing to steroid 21-hydroxylase deficiency. *Journal of Clinical Endocrinology and Metabolism, 80,* 2014–2020.

Merke, D. P., Giedd, J. N., Keil, M. F., Mehlinger, S. L., Wiggs, E. A., Holzer, S., et al. (2005). Children experience cognitive decline despite reversal of brain atrophy one year after resolution of Cushing syndrome. *Journal of Clinical Endocrinology and Metabolism, 90,* 2531–2536.

Mesulam, M. M. (2000). Behavioral neuroanatomy: Large-scale networks, association cortex, frontal syndromes, the limbic system, and hemispheric specialization. In M. M. Mesulam (Ed.), *Principles of behavioral and cognitive neurology* (2nd ed., pp. 1–120). New York: Oxford University Press.

Meyers, J. E., & Meyers, K. R. (1995). *Rey Complex Figure Test and Recognition Trial.* Odessa, FL: Psychological Assessment Resources.

Odeke, S., & Nagelberg, S. B. (2006). *Hashimoto thyroiditis.* Retrieved July 11, 2007, from http://www.emedicine.com/med/topic949.htm

Payne, J. D., & Nadel, L. (2004). Sleep, dreams, and memory consolidation: The role of the stress hormone cortisol. *Learning and Memory, 11,* 671–678.

Porterfield, S. P., & Hendrich, C. E. (1993). The role of thyroid hormones in prenatal and neonatal neurological development: Current perspectives. *Endocrine Reviews, 14,* 94–106.

Postellon, D., Bourgeois, M. J., & Varma, S. (2006). *Congenital hypothyroidism.* Retrieved July 11, 2007, from http://www.emedicine.com/ped/topic501.htm

Radetti, G., Gottardi, E., Bona, G., Corrias, A., Salardi, S., & Loche, S. (2006). The natural history of euthyroid Hashimoto's thyroiditis in children. *Journal of Pediatrics, 149,* 827–832.

Romeo, R. D., & McEwen, B. S. (2006). Stress and the adolescent brain. *Annals of the New York Academy of Sciences, 1094,* 202–214.

Rovet, J. F., & Hepworth, S. (2001). Attention problems in adolescents with congenital hypothyroidism: A multicomponential analysis. *Journal of the International Neuropsychological Society, 7,* 734–744.

Russell, E. W., Russell, S. L. K., & Hill, B. D. (2005). The fundamental psychometric status of neuropsychological batteries. *Archives of Clinical Neuropsychology, 20,* 785–794.

Segni, M., Leonardi, E., Mazzoncini, B., Pucarelli, I., & Pasquino, A. M. (1999). Special features of Graves' disease in early childhood. *Thyroid, 9,* 871–877.

Sotres-Bayon, F., Cain, C. K., & LeDoux, J. E. (2006). Brain mechanisms of fear extinction: Historical perspectives on the contribution of prefrontal cortex. *Biological Psychiatry, 60,* 329–336.

Starkman, M. N., Giordani, B., Berent, S., Schork, M. A., & Schteingart, D. E. (2001). Elevated cortisol levels in Cushing's disease are associated with cognitive decrements. *Psychosomatic Medicine, 63,* 985–993.

Stern, R. A., Robinson, B., Thorner, A. R., Arruda, J. E., Prohaska, M. L., & Prange, A. J., Jr. (1996). A survey study of neuropsychiatric complaints in patients with Graves' disease. *Journal of Neuropsychiatry and Clinical Neuroscience, 8,* 181–185.

Storch, E. A., Lewin, A. B., Silverstein, J. H., Heidgerken, A. D., Strawser, M. S., Baumeister, A., et al. (2004). Social-psychological correlates of peer victimization in children with endocrine disorders. *Journal of Pediatrics, 145,* 784–789.

Straight, A. M., Bauer, A. J., & Ferry, R. J. (2003). *Hypothyroidism.* Retrieved June 8, 2007, from http://www.emedicine.com/ped/topic1141.htm

Thornton, P. S., Kelly, A., & Willcutts, M. (2006). *Hypoparathyroidism.* Retrieved July 11, 2007, from http://www.emedicine.com/ped/topic1125.htm

Tremont, G., Somerville, J. A., & Stern, R. A. (2000). Neuropsychological performance in Graves' hyperthyroidism: Evidence of executive dysfunction [Abstract]. *Archives of Clinical Neuropsychology, 15,* 665–666.

Trzepacz, P. T., McCue, M., Klein, I., Levey, G. S., & Greenhouse, J. (1988). A psychiatric and neuropsychological study of patients with untreated Graves' disease. *General Hospital Psychiatry, 10,* 49–55.

Velasco, P. J., Manshadi, M., Breen, K., & Lippmann, S. (1999). Psychiatric aspects of parathyroid disease. *Psychosomatics, 40,* 486–490.

Victor, M., & Ropper, A. H. (2001). *Principles of neurology* (7th ed.). New York: McGraw Hill.

Vogel, A., Elberling, T. V., Hording, M., Dock, J., Rasmussen, A. K., Feldt-Rasmussen, U., et al. (2007). Affective symptoms and cognitive functions in the acute phase of Graves' thyrotoxicosis. *Psychoneuroendocrinology, 32,* 36–43.

Vyas, A., Pillai, A. G., & Chattarji, S. (2004). Recovery after chronic stress fails to reverse amygdaloid neuronal hypertrophy and enhanced anxiety-like behavior. *Neuroscience, 128,* 667–673.

Watemberg, N., Willis, D., & Pellock, J. M. (2000). Encephalopathy as the presenting symptom of Hashimoto's thyroiditis. *Journal of Child Neurology, 15,* 66–69.

Wechsler, D. (1974). *Wechsler Intelligence Scale for Children* (rev. ed.). New York: The Psychological Corporation.

Wechsler, D. (1991). *Wechsler Intelligence Scale for Children*(3rd ed.). San Antonio, TX: The Psychological Corporation.

Wechsler, D. (2001). *Wechsler Individual Achievement Test*(2nd ed.). San Antonio, TX: The Psychological Corporation.

Wechsler, D. (2003). *Wechsler Intelligence Scale for Children*(4th ed.). San Antonio, TX: The Psychological Corporation.

Wekking, E. M., Appelhof, B. C., Fliers, E., Schene, A. H., Huyser, J., Tijssen, J. G. P., et al. (2005). Cognitive functioning and well-being in euthyroid patients on thyroxine replacement therapy for primary hypothyroidism. *European Journal of Endocrinology, 153,* 747–753.

Wilson, B., Cockburn, J., & Baddeley, A. D. (1985). *The Rivermead Behavioural Memory Test.* Bury St. Edmunds, England: Thames Valley Test Company.

Wilson, T. A., & Speiser, P. (2006). *Adrenal insufficiency.* Retrieved June 19, 2007, from http://www.emedicine.com/ped/topic47.htm

Wu, T., Flowers, J. W., Tudiver, F., Wilson, J. L., & Punyasavatsut, N. (2006). Subclinical thyroid disorders and cognitive performance among adolescents in the United States [Electronic version]. *Biomed Central Pediatrics, 6.* Retrieved June 19, 2007, from http://www.biomedcentral.com/1471–2431/6/12

Yehuda, R. (1997). Sensitization of the hypothalamic-pituitary-adrenal axis in posttraumatic stress disorder. *Annals of the New York Academy of Science, 821,* 57–75.

Zoeller, R. T., Bansal, R., & Parris, C. (2005). Bisphenol-A, an environmental contaminant that acts as a thyroid hormone receptor antagonist in vitro, increases serum thyroxine, and alters RC3/neurogranin expression in the developing rat brain. *Endocrinology, 146,* 607–612.

Zoeller, R. T., & Rovet, J. (2004). Timing of thyroid hormone action in the developing brain: Clinical observations and experimental findings. *Journal of Neuroendocrinology, 16,* 809–818.

# CHAPTER NINE

# Epilepsy

Kristy S. Hagar, PhD

## DESCRIPTION OF THE DISORDER

### Incidence and Prevalence

Epilepsy is one of the most common neurological disorders in children, affecting approximately 0.5% to 1% of children through the age of 16 years (Pellock, 2004b). Between 20,000 and 45,000 children are diagnosed annually with newly recognized seizures, with the median age of onset between 5 and 6 years of age (Shinnar & Pellock, 2002).

An epileptic seizure is defined as "a clinical manifestation presumed to result from abnormal and excessive discharge of a set of neurons in the brain," according to the Commission on Epidemiology and Prognosis, International League Against Epilepsy (CEP/ILAE, 1993, p. 593). Epilepsy, or seizure disorder, is defined as two or more unprovoked seizures more than 24 hours apart in a child over 1 month of age. Children within their first year of life are at the highest risk of developing epilepsy (Shinnar & Pellock, 2002). A single or isolated seizure and febrile seizures (i.e., a seizure occurring in childhood associated with fever) are not considered for a diagnosis of epilepsy (CEP/ILAE).

## Etiology and Underlying Causes

A seizure occurs when there is atypical electrical activity in the brain, and seizure types are classified by location (i.e., where the excessive or abnormal electrical discharges are presumed to be occurring in the brain) and semiology (i.e., the observable clinical behavior that results from the abnormal discharges). The nerve cells in the brain communicate with each other using electrical discharges or "firing," resulting in a release of neurotransmitters that are either excitatory (i.e., resulting in an increased likelihood that another cell will fire) or inhibitory (i.e., resulting in a decreased likelihood of a cell firing). In normal brain functioning, there is cooperation and balance between the excitatory and inhibitory neurons. For example, moving a finger is the result of a coordinated, purposeful firing of multiple motor neurons with both excitatory and inhibitory neurotransmitters playing a role. In contrast, a seizure occurs when this balance is disrupted, that is, when the electrical activity in the brain is excessive or abnormal. Depending on the area where these neurons fire, usually repeatedly, there can be a disruption in consciousness, changes in movement (e.g., arms or legs stiffening or jerking), and/or sensory changes (e.g., tingling, burning sensation) as a result of this atypical and unintended discharge of neurons.

As noted above, seizures are classified by where the abnormal activity is believed to be occurring in the brain as well as by the clinical manifestation of the seizure. The CEP/ILAE established guidelines for epidemiological studies of epilepsy in 1993. Within this document, seizure classifications were established that continue to be widely accepted and used for clinical description and epidemiological research (CEP/ILAE, 1993; Shinnar & Pellock, 2002). The first tier of classification is based on localization, which describes where the abnormal discharges are occurring in the brain.

*Generalized seizures* involve the whole brain, as there is no indication of a specific focal onset. Generalized seizures can be convulsive (i.e., tonic, tonic-clonic), nonconvulsive (termed *absence seizures*), or myoclonic. Absence seizures, formerly called petit mal seizures, present with very subtle symptoms, such as staring and unresponsiveness (Freeman, Vining, & Pillas, 1997). Absence seizures are usually brief, lasting 15 to 30 seconds, and sometimes present with very subtle or unnoticeable physical changes such as a change in facial expression (Ahmed & Varghese, 2006). *Partial seizures* are diagnosed when evidence suggests that a specific part of the brain is affected. Partial seizures are further classified into simple partial (consciousness is not impaired, but physical or sensory symptoms are noted) or complex partial seizures (impairment of consciousness is evident, and there is a disruption of motor movement or sensation). Sometimes a partial seizure spreads to other parts of the brain, and in this case the additional term *secondarily generalized* is included in the description of the seizure (CEP/ILAE, 1993; National Society for Epilepsy [NSE], 1999b).

Certain factors can increase the risk of developing seizures, as a result of known or suspected central nervous system (CNS) disruption. These factors could include conditions such as infection, stroke, or trauma (CEP/ILAE, 1993). *Symptomatic* seizures are seizures that result from a known CNS dysfunction. Conditions such as mental retardation and cerebral palsy, although sometimes not directly linked to a known physical cause, are also associated with an increased risk for seizures.

In many cases, the cause of epileptic seizures is unknown. In these cases, the term *cryptogenic etiology* is used. Seizures or seizure syndromes are described as *idiopathic* if particular clinical features are evident but no clear antecedent or event can be identified (Shinnar & Pellock, 2002).

Within the description of seizure types, it is important to relay information regarding nonepileptic events. Nonepileptic events (NEE) are common in the pediatric population and can occur in children and adolescents with or without epilepsy (Pakalnis, Paolicchi, & Gilles, 2000; Paolicchi, 2002). A large number of NEE events can appear to be epileptic in nature and may be difficult to differentiate from true epileptic events, especially in children or teens with complex medical and physical conditions or cognitive delays (Paolicchi). Pseudoseizures, also known as psychogenic seizures, appear epileptic in nature but are not accompanied by abnormal electrical activity in the brain (Freeman et al., 1997). Underlying psychological disorders, psychosocial stress, and family stress are often attributed causes of pseudoseizures, and therefore treatment must focus on alleviating these underlying stressors in order to obtain improvement of symptoms (Pakalnis et al.; Paolicchi).

## DIAGNOSING EPILEPSY

Epilepsy must be diagnosed by a physician. Although many types of tests may assist in determining the clinical picture of the presence or type of epilepsy, the diagnosis remains a clinical decision based on a variety of data. A careful history of the patient is required, as well as detailed information regarding the events that appear to be seizure activity. Often, an electroencephalogram (EEG) is obtained to assist the physician in the diagnosis. An EEG records the brain's electrical activity by means of electrodes placed on various points across the skull. The electrodes recognize the small electrical impulses and then record and map their location in various areas of the brain. The EEG also records unusual or atypical activity that may then be analyzed by the physician to assist with diagnosis. It is important to note, however, that an EEG is only one clinical tool the physician will utilize, and a negative EEG does not necessarily refute the presence of seizures or seizure syndromes (NSE, 1999a).

## FACTORS AFFECTING NEUROPSYCHOLOGICAL OUTCOME

Many variables affect neuropsychological outcome for children with epilepsy. It has been commonly reported in the literature that children with epilepsy are at greater risk for academic underachievement (Dunn & Austin, 1999; Fastenau et al., 2004; Sabbagh, Soria, Escolano, Bulteau, & Dellatolas, 2006) and vocational difficulties into adulthood (Shinnar & Pellock, 2002). Although many longitudinal studies with children have focused predominantly on intellectual abilities (Dodrill, 2004), some studies have described neuropsychological deficits in this population including executive dysfunction (Culhane-Shelburne, Chapieski, Hiscock, & Glaze, 2002), impaired discourse processing (Caplan et al., 2006), memory difficulties (Koop, Fastenau, Dunn, & Austin, 2005), slower psychomotor speed (Fastenau et al.), and lower academic performance (McNelis, Dunn, Johnson, Austin, & Perkins, 2007).

### Other Variables Affecting Outcome

Children and teens who experience a chronic medical condition are often at higher risk of adjustment difficulties. Research on the emotional and behavioral presentation of children and adolescents with epilepsy indicates that they often exhibit comorbid psychiatric and/or behavioral difficulties (Pellock, 2004b). Plioplys (2003) found that depression is common but often unrecognized in children and adolescents with epilepsy, and successful development may be negatively impacted by the chronic nature of both depression and epilepsy. Caplan and colleagues (2005) found a high rate of anxiety disorder or affective disorder diagnoses (33%) among pediatric epilepsy patients, as well as an alarming rate of suicidal ideation/plan (20%). Williams and colleagues (2003) studied children and adolescents with epilepsy and discovered mild to moderate symptoms of anxiety in 18% of the patients assessed; polytherapy (i.e., multiple AEDs prescribed for seizure control) was related to increased anxious symptoms. Miller, Palermo, and Grewe (2003) observed that children who were on polytherapy for epilepsy were at greater risk for lower health-related quality of life (HRQOL) compared to healthy children. Family functioning and support can also impact coping with epilepsy. Fastenau and colleagues

(2004) observed that academic achievement in children and teens with epilepsy was affected not only by neuropsychological deficits but also by a disruptive or unsupportive home environment.

## RELATED MEDICAL ISSUES

For children and adolescents with epilepsy, etiological factors as well as treatment factors may further influence their overall presentation and functioning. Children who have other medical risk factors in addition to seizures, such as mental retardation, cerebral palsy, or certain genetic syndromes, are at higher risk of behavioral, academic, and social difficulties compared to children without these additional medical risks (Besag, 2004; Dunn & Austin, 1999; Pellock, 2004b).

Medication to control seizures also may impact behavioral or neurocognitive functioning, and children may be particularly susceptible to cognitive side effects of antiepileptic medications due to their introduction during critical phases of neurodevelopment (Ortinski & Meador, 2004). Managing pediatric patients' seizures with only one medication is optimal and desirable (Pellock, 2004a), and some experience good control of seizures on only one medication. However, approximately 25% to 30% of patients may be refractory to drug treatment (Bebin, 2002) and/or require polytherapy that may increase their risk of poor adjustment (Miller et al., 2003). Loring and Meador (2004) noted that effects of antiepileptic drugs (AEDs) have been studied relatively infrequently in children, despite concerns reflected in the adult literature that AEDs can result in cognitive impairment. For children, studies that have assessed the side effects of AEDs have often investigated the impact on global intelligence, which may not reflect subtle neurocognitive changes. However, of the AEDs studied in children, phenobarbital, which is considered an older, traditional AED, may negatively impact overall intelligence. The authors suggest that poorer cognitive functioning may be related to the drug's effect on processing efficiency and attention. In addition, the literature is lacking with regard to well-designed studies of children prescribed the newer AEDs and the longitudinal effects of these medications over several years of schooling (Bebin).

## RESULTS FROM NEUROPSYCHOLOGICAL EVALUATION

The following case study is presented to illustrate the emotional, cognitive, and academic concerns that can arise in children and adolescents with seizure disorder. As noted above, seizure types can vary significantly, as can the individual's responsiveness to treatment (i.e., monotherapy vs. polytherapy). Additional factors, such as academic support, family functioning, and physical and mental health, can contribute to the risk factors for any child with a chronic illness or disease, particularly when the CNS is affected.

## Background and Demographic Information

Nora, age 14 years, was diagnosed with seizure disorder (complex partial seizures) at 5 years of age. Her early developmental history was unremarkable. She was the product of a normal pregnancy and delivery, and no postnatal problems were reported. Language development was reportedly normal, but motor milestones were delayed (e.g., walking at 14 months, difficulty grasping toys). At the time of the evaluation, Nora's parents continued to describe her fine and gross motor coordination as delayed compared to peers and to her older and younger siblings.

Nora was receiving Depakote at the time of the evaluation but continued to have breakthrough seizures periodically (i.e., once or twice per month). She attended the ninth grade at a suburban public high school and was enrolled in special education under the eligibility of Other Health Impairment (OHI). She received instruction in the regular education classroom with opportunity to attend Content Mastery (i.e., academic support through a special education classroom, generally after material is presented in the regular classroom setting). The family has moved twice since Nora was in kindergarten, and her parents reported no significant disruption in academic instruction or support services across Nora's years of schooling.

On a recent visit to the pediatric neurologist, Nora's parents reported concerns about her ability to succeed in high school and even some concern about post–high school employment, which prompted the neurologist to refer Nora for neuropsychological evaluation. Nora had been periodically assessed through the school system as part of her special education eligibility but had never undergone neuropsychological evaluation.

## Behavioral Observations

Nora presented to the neuropsychology clinic with her mother and father. She was casually dressed, but her grooming was slightly disheveled. She greeted the examiner appropriately and had no difficulty separating from her parents to participate in testing. Nora was assessed during a single assessment session, with a 1-hour break for lunch. During the assessment (approximately 5 hours long), no unusual behavior or seizure-like activity was observed. When questioned, Nora reported that she did not have any seizures during the evaluation.

Her eye contact was appropriate. Nora occasionally initiated conversation, but overall she presented as a quiet, reserved adolescent. She did not appear anxious in the testing environment, and her attention and concentration were generally age appropriate. Nora was not fidgety or overly active during the testing session. She benefited from occasional breaks and returned to tasks without difficulty. Rapport was easily established. The results of the evaluation were deemed to be an accurate reflection of Nora's skills and abilities.

## Test Results

Data from the administered tests are listed in Tables 9.1, 9.2, and 9.3. Nora's performance on the Wechsler Intelligence Scale for Children—Fourth Edition (Wechsler, 2003), resulted in a Full Scale IQ (FSIQ) in the lower end of the average range (30th percentile). Her verbal comprehension skills were in the upper end of the average range (70th percentile), and her perceptual reasoning skills were solidly in the average range. In contrast, Nora's working memory was low average overall (18th percentile), and her processing speed, as measured by the two paper-pencil tasks was borderline low (5th percentile). It is important to note that Nora's lower score on the Processing Speed index was solely due to slower completion of items compared to peers, as Nora made no errors on either task (Coding and Symbol Search). Because of the high degree of variability across the four index scores, a General Ability index (GAI) score was calculated. The GAI is a composite score based on the Verbal Comprehension index (VCI) and Perceptual Reasoning index (PRI) scores; it does not include the Working Memory index (WMI) or Processing Speed index (PSI) (Raiford, Weiss, Rolfus, & Coalson, 2005). In Nora's case, the PSI was substantially (and statistically) lower compared to the VCI and PRI, therefore resulting in an FSIQ that was markedly depressed by the PSI score. The GAI can serve as a substitute for the FSIQ in these circumstances and assist in determining an ability-achievement discrepancy. In Nora's case, the GAI was also used to account for the effect of slower motor processing speed. Nora's performance resulted in a GAI score that was solidly in the average range (63rd percentile).

Additional neuropsychological measures included memory, visual-motor integration, motor speed, and academic achievement. Nora generally exhibited average to slightly above-average verbal and visual memory skills, as measured by the Children's Memory Scale (Cohen, 1997) and the California Verbal Learning Test—Children's Version (Delis, Kramer, Kaplan, & Ober, 1994). She appeared to benefit from time to organize and store information into memory in both the verbal and visual domains. Nora's visual-motor integration skills, as measured by the Beery-Buktenica Developmental Test of Visual-Motor Integration—Fifth Edition (Beery, Buktenica, & Beery, 2004), were average for her age. On a pegboard task that measures fine motor speed and coordination (Tiffin, 1968), Nora's performance was significantly below average for her dominant (right) hand and below average for her left hand.

On the Woodcock-Johnson Tests of Achievement—Third Edition (WJ-III; Woodcock, McGrew, & Mather, 2001), Nora demonstrated average to above-average academic skills in reading, math calculations, and spelling but substantially weaker fluency in these same areas. Although academic fluency is not used to determine a specific learning disability, this result is consistent with other neuropsychological testing indicating weaker motor and processing skills that substantially impact Nora's ability to produce information in an efficient and timely manner.

Ratings of Nora's behavior at home and at school, as evaluated on the Parent Rating Scale of the Behavior Assessment System for Children—Second Edition (Reynolds & Kamphaus, 2004), revealed concerns regarding anxious symptoms, withdrawal, learning problems, and some attention problems. Nora's rating of her own behavior did not reveal any significant concerns. On the Behavior Rating Inventory of Executive Function (Gioia, Isquith, Guy, & Kenworthy, 2000), Nora's teachers and parents reported difficulties with regard to Nora's planning and organization skills, working memory, and ability to monitor her behavior.

## Interventions

The following recommendations were generated from the neuropsychological assessment of Nora's skills and abilities. However, these recommendations could be considered in a broader context of benefiting many children and adolescents with epilepsy in the academic setting:

- Assess Nora on her accuracy and thoroughness rather than number of items completed (e.g., allow extra time or reduce items if time is limited). She might struggle to complete assignments or tests that require fine motor speed and coordination and/or efficient processing speed (i.e., filling out score sheets or test booklets). Providing assistance by allowing Nora to briefly mark the items, then having a peer or teacher fill items in appropriately to be read by a scanner, is suggested. Allowing her to answer orally could also be considered.
- Given the weaknesses noted in processing speed, motor speed, and fluency, it is recommended that Nora should not be withheld from

**TABLE 9.1 Neuropsychological Testing Data**

| Scale | Scaled Score | T Score | Standard Score |
|---|---|---|---|
| Wechsler Intelligence Scale for Children—Fourth Edition | | | |
| Full Scale IQ | | | 92 |
| General Ability index | | | 105 |
| Verbal Comprehension index | | | 108 |
| Perceptual Reasoning index | | | 100 |
| Working Memory index | | | 86 |
| Processing Speed index | | | 75 |
| Woodcock-Johnson Tests of Achievement—Third Edition | | | |
| Letter-Word Identification | | | 105 |
| Reading Fluency | | | 83 |
| Calculation | | | 90 |
| Math Fluency | | | 60 |
| Spelling | | | 119 |
| Writing Fluency | | | 74 |
| California Verbal Learning Test—Children's Version | | | |
| List A Total Trials 1–5 | | 49 | |
| List A Trial 1 Free Recall | | 55 | |
| List A Trial 5 Free Recall | | 50 | |
| List B Free Recall | | 45 | |
| List A Short-Delay Free Recall | | 50 | |
| List A Short-Delay Cued Recall | | 50 | |
| List A Long-Delay Free Recall | | 50 | |
| List A Long-Delay Cued Recall | | 50 | |
| Recognition | | 50 | |

*Continued*

**TABLE 9.1** *(Continued)*

| Scale | Scaled Score | T Score | Standard Score |
|---|---|---|---|
| | Children's Memory Scale | | |
| Stories—Immediate | 10 | | |
| Stories—Delayed | 12 | | |
| Stories—Delayed Recognition | 14 | | |
| Faces—Immediate | 11 | | |
| Faces—Delayed | 13 | | |
| | Purdue Pegboard Test | | |
| Preferred hand (right) | | | 77 |
| Nonpreferred hand (left) | | | 87 |
| | Beery-Buktenica Developmental Test of Visual-Motor Integration—Fifth Edition | | |
| VMI | | | 99 |
| Visual Perception | | | 97 |
| Motor Coordination | | | 92 |

**TABLE 9.2 T Scores From Parent and Teacher Ratings of Behavioral and Emotional Functioning**

| Scale | Parent | Teacher |
|---|---|---|
| | Behavior Assessment System for Children—Second Edition | |
| Externalizing Problems | 54 | 55 |
| Hyperactivity | 67 | 58 |
| Aggression | 43 | 52 |
| Conduct Problems | 51 | 54 |
| Internalizing Problems | 70 | 63 |
| Anxiety | 76 | 56 |
| Depression | 69 | 53 |

**TABLE 9.2** *(Continued)*

| Scale | Parent | Teacher |
|---|---|---|
| Somatization | 55 | 72 |
| Behavioral Symptoms Index | 72 | 56 |
| Atypicality | 63 | 51 |
| Withdrawal | 83 | 47 |
| Attention Problems | 75 | 66 |
| School Problems | | 70 |
| Learning Problems | | 71 |
| Adaptive Skills | 35 | 46 |
| Adaptability | 43 | 54 |
| Social Skills | 38 | 46 |
| Leadership | 40 | 47 |
| Activities of Daily Living | 40 | |
| Functional Communication | 40 | 46 |
| Study Skills | | 41 |
| Behavior Rating Inventory of Executive Function | | |
| Behavioral Regulation Index | 58 | 57 |
| Inhibit | 58 | 57 |
| Shift | 81 | 60 |
| Emotional Control | 77 | 51 |
| Metacognition Index | 68 | 71 |
| Initiate | 68 | 63 |
| Working Memory | 73 | 71 |
| Plan/Organize | 70 | 68 |
| Organization of Materials | 46 | 70 |
| Monitor | 66 | 71 |
| General Executive Composite | 72 | 67 |

**TABLE 9.3 T Scores From Self-Report Ratings of Emotional and Behavioral Functioning**

| Scale | BASC-II SRP |
|---|---|
| School Problems | 54 |
| Attitude to School | 45 |
| Attitude to Teachers | 52 |
| Internalizing Problems | 46 |
| Anxiety | 51 |
| Depression | 48 |
| Sense of Inadequacy | 52 |
| Inattention/Hyperactivity | 51 |
| Attention Problems | 45 |
| Hyperactivity | 57 |
| Emotional Symptoms Index | 48 |
| Atypicality | 41 |
| Locus of Control | 50 |
| Social Stress | 47 |
| Personal Adjustment | 53 |
| Relations With Parents | 54 |
| Interpersonal Relations | 48 |
| Self-Esteem | 61 |
| Self-Reliance | 45 |

*Note.* BASC-II SRP, Behavior Assessment System for Children—Second Edition, Self-Report (Reynolds & Kamphaus, 2004).

preferred activities to finish schoolwork. Schoolwork that is sent home in addition to homework can also easily become overwhelming. Adjusting Nora's schoolwork and homework load in consideration of her slower processing skills is suggested, so that it amounts to no more than 1 to 1.5 hours of homework nightly. Examples include completing only the even or odd items on worksheets and reducing reading assignments into numbers of paragraphs, pages, or chapters to complete, targeting perhaps two-thirds completion.

- Nora appeared to benefit significantly from time to consolidate information into memory. Avoid on-the-spot questioning, and allow

Nora time to encode the information efficiently. If she is questioned during class discussions, provide some cues if she seems to have difficulty retrieving an answer from memory. This strategy can also be used if Nora demonstrates word-finding difficulties, which may be exacerbated by anxiety if she feels pressured to respond but cannot find the right words or information she wants to relay.

- Difficulties with working memory (reported as a struggle for Nora by teachers and parents and noted during testing) can often be addressed by providing short breaks, even just for a minute or two. Short breaks for Nora might be self-initiated or teacher initiated and could include a stretch break, a walk to the pencil sharpener, or reviewing work with the teacher.
- Copying or note taking, which requires brief memorization of the material, is also strongly impacted by difficulties with working memory. Classroom instructions, even simple one- or two-step procedures, tax working memory and may be more difficult for Nora to complete accurately. Repeat verbal directions, and check for understanding. As verbal comprehension skills are a strength for Nora, provide copies of notes on the board or overhead so as to allow her the best chance to listen to the lecture rather than being bogged down by having to multitask with efficient writing or copying (a significant learning weakness) and listening at the same time.
- A consistent weakness in academic fluency was noted in the current evaluation across several academic domains. Allow additional time for reading and writing assignments, and/or reduce material that Nora must learn or process in a short period of time. It will be important, however, to make sure that Nora is tested only on material she has been exposed to if assignments are reduced.
- Encourage success through small steps. Break down a task or assignment into steps, and keep track of each section until the project is completed. A checklist on the refrigerator is often great for something like this at home, and Nora might benefit from a small notepad or sticky notes inside her school binder to keep track of assignments, projects, and so on.
- Due to the higher level of anxiety reported in the home setting, it is recommended that Nora and her family consider psychotherapeutic support to teach Nora effective coping and anxiety-reducing strategies. Continued communication between Nora's parents, her school, and her neurologist will also be of utmost importance to provide the best care for Nora.
- Enrolling Nora in extracurricular activities, such as classes through a parks and recreation department, may provide opportunities for social interactions outside of the school setting. Volunteering,

which might also require one or both of her parents to volunteer with her, depending on the setting, is also an excellent way to meet other people and interact in the community.

In addition to specific academic or environmental interventions that are tailored to each individual child, some additional medical interventions are often recommended in the treatment of epilepsy. One of the interventions that has been used since the 1920s is the ketogenic diet (Freeman et al., 1997). The ketogenic diet consists of a high fat, adequate protein, and low carbohydrate meal plan that has experienced a renewal of interest over the last decade (Freeman, Kossoff, & Hartman, 2007). The mechanism of action is not entirely clear (Kraphohl, Deutinger, & Kömürcü, 2007), but this diet has demonstrated efficacy in reducing some types of seizures in children and allows significant decreases or elimination of antiepileptic medications (Hemingway, Freeman, Pillas, & Pyzik, 2001). The ketogenic diet, although requiring adherence and close monitoring, is often a less invasive intervention to initially attempt with intractable epilepsy, and it has demonstrated effectiveness even after the diet is discontinued (Martinez, Pyzik, & Kossoff, 2007). Many centers admit children for observation when initiating the diet, and close monitoring by neurologists, pediatricians, and dieticians is required to determine the response to the diet and possible adverse effects (Freeman et al., 2007). For those patients for whom the diet does not effectively reduce seizures, other interventions such as epilepsy surgery or vagus nerve stimulation (VNS) are available (Hemingway et al.; Kang, Kim, Kim, & Kim, 2005).

VNS is another intervention that is often used to treat epilepsy in conjunction with anticonvulsant medications (Kossoff et al., 2007), as an option for children with drug-resistant seizures (Benifla, Rutka, Logan, & Donner, 2006) and/or for patients who are not candidates for epilepsy surgery (McHugh et al., 2007; Saneto et al., 2006). The vagus nerve is 1 of 12 cranial nerves; it originates in the medulla in the CNS (Kraphohl et al., 2007). Electrical stimulation of the vagus nerve has been shown to have an effect on brain activity, and Zabara (1985) posited that VNS had the potential to control epileptic seizures. Although the exact mechanism of how VNS affects seizure control is unknown, it appears to affect blood flow to different regions of the brain that are correlated with reduced seizure activity (Benifla et al.; McHugh et al.) and/or stimulate neurons that help modulate cortical excitability (Li & Mogul, 2007).

For some patients, epilepsy surgery may be a treatment option when medications and/or other interventions are ineffective in controlling seizure activity. Uncontrolled epilepsy can result in significant risks for emotional, behavioral, social, and cognitive functioning (Smith, Elliott, & Lach,

2004), and therefore surgery to remove abnormal tissue in order to reduce or eliminate seizure activity is the intervention of choice for some children with intractable epilepsy and their families (Freeman et al., 1997).

Several types of epilepsy surgery can be performed depending on the type of seizures and the identified area of abnormal electrical activity (Freeman et al., 1997). Corpus callosotomy is an operation that cuts the tissue connecting the right and left hemispheres; it can be effective in reducing the frequency of specific (i.e., generalized tonic-clonic or atonic) seizures (Freeman et al., 1997; Nei, O'Connor, Liporace, & Sperling, 2006). A hemispherectomy removes all or part of one side of the brain, and focal excision removes a limited area of brain tissue that has been identified as triggering seizure activity (Freeman et al., 1997). While many factors influence outcome following epilepsy surgery, in many cases children who have undergone epilepsy surgery do not demonstrate a decline in overall cognitive ability (Sherman et al., 2003), although memory problems or other cognitive issues that were present prior to surgery may persist (Smith, Elliott, & Lach, 2006; Turanh, Yalnizoğlu, Genç-Açikgöz, Akalan, & Topçu, 2006).

For children who have undergone epilepsy surgery and who may or may not continue on antiepileptic medications, some general considerations and accommodations can often be helpful in the school setting. Some accommodations may be very specific for a child who has undergone hemispherectomy, as they will have hemianopsia (i.e., loss of the visual field opposite to the hemisphere that was removed) and experience difficulties related to the traditional hemispheric functions of the removed hemisphere. For example, children who have undergone left hemispherectomy may experience expressive and receptive language deficits and therefore may benefit from repetition of instructions, small group instruction, checking for understanding, and simplification of directions, instructions, or requests to one or two steps. Children who have had complete or partial removal of their right hemisphere may experience visual-perceptual deficits, spatial awareness difficulties, and some social deficits. Accommodations such as extended time for copying and drawing, reduction of visually "busy" material, and copies of notes and diagrams that are placed on a chalkboard or overhead projector can be very beneficial.

## CONCLUSION

In summary, children and adolescents with epilepsy are a very heterogenous group, and each individual's presentation may be influenced by the type and severity of epilepsy, the number of antiepileptic medications required to control the epilepsy, and the additional medical interventions that may have been implemented (i.e., epilepsy surgery), as well as overall cognitive, behavioral, and social abilities that are as diverse as in the general population. For any student with a medical condition, particularly those conditions that can have such a profound effect on the CNS as epilepsy, close academic monitoring is critical. Additional supports and services in school and the community, and coordination between school, parents, and medical personnel, can help ensure a positive educational experience for children and adolescents whose lives are impacted by epilepsy.

## RESOURCES

### Books

Blackburn, L. B. (2003). *Growing up with epilepsy: A practical guide for parents*. New York: Demos Vermande Medical Publishing.

Freeman, J. M., Vining, E. P. G., & Pillas, D. J. (1997). *Seizures and epilepsy in childhood: A guide for parents* (2nd ed.). Baltimore: Johns Hopkins Press.

Goldstein, S., & Reynolds, C. (Eds.). (1999). *Handbook of neurodevelopmental and genetic disorders in children*. New York: Guilford Press.

Gosselin, K. (2002). *Taking seizure disorders to school: A story about epilepsy*. Plainview, NY: JayJo Books.

Phelps, L. (1998). *Health-related disorders in children and adolescents: A guidebook for understanding and educating*. Washington, DC: American Psychological Corporation.

### Organizations and Web Sites

The Charlie Foundation

The Charlie Foundation is a Web site designed for families and professionals to provide information and raise awareness about the ketogenic diet in the treatment of epilepsy.

Web Site: www.charliefoundation.org/

Epilepsy Foundation of America

The Epilepsy Foundation of America Web site provides information, advocacy, and community resources for families living with epilepsy.

Web Site: www.epilepsyfoundation.org/

International League Against Epilepsy

The International League Against Epilepsy (ILAE) is an association of physicians and other health care professionals who strive to provide the best quality care to patients with epilepsy and to promote research, education, and training.

Web Site: www.ilae-epilepsy.org/

National Institute of Neurological Disorders and Stroke (NINDS)

The NINDS is affiliated with the National Institutes of Health. Their mission is to reduce the burden of neurological disease by providing research funding, coordinating and conducting research, and providing information.

Web Site: www.ninds.nih.gov/

## REFERENCES


Ahmed, R., & Varghese, T. (2006). Unusual presentation of absence seizures: A case report. *Journal of Pediatric Neurology, 4,* 45–47.

Bebin, M. (2002). Pediatric partial and generalized seizures. *Journal of Child Neurology, 17,* S65–S69.

Beery, K. E., Buktenica, N. A., & Beery, N. A. (2004). *Beery-Buktenica Developmental Test of Visual-Motor Integration* (5th ed.). Bloomington, MN: Pearson Assessments.

Benifla, M., Rutka, J. T., Logan, W., & Donner, E. J. (2006). Vagal nerve stimulation for refractory epilepsy in children: Indications and experience at The Hospital for Sick Children. *Child's Nervous System, 22,* 1018–1026.

Besag, F.M.C. (2004). Behavioral aspects of pediatric epilepsy syndromes. *Epilepsy and Behavior, 5,* S3–S13.

Caplan, R., Siddarth, P., Bailey, C. E., Lanphier, E. K., Gurbani, S., Shields, W. D., et al. (2006). Thought disorder: A developmental disability in pediatric epilepsy. *Epilepsy and Behavior, 8,* 726–735.

Caplan, R., Siddarth, P., Gurbani, S., Hanson, R., Sankar, R., & Shields, W. D. (2005). Depression and anxiety disorders in pediatric epilepsy. *Epilepsia, 46,* 720–730.

Cohen, M. (1997). *Children's Memory Scale.* San Antonio, TX: The Psychological Corporation.

Commission on Epidemiology and Prognosis, International League Against Epilepsy (CEP/ILAE). (1993). Guidelines for epidemiologic studies on epilepsy. *Epilepsia, 34,* 592–596.

Culhane-Shelburne, K., Chapieski, L., Hiscock, M., & Glaze, D. (2002). Executive functions in children with frontal and temporal lobe epilepsy. *Journal of the International Neuropsychological Society, 8,* 623–632.

Delis, D. C., Kramer, J. H., Kaplan, E., & Ober, B. A. (1994). *California Verbal Learning Test—Children's Version.* San Antonio, TX: The Psychological Corporation.

Dodrill, C. B. (2004). Neuropsychological effects of seizures. *Epilepsy and Behavior, 5,* S21–S24.

Dunn, D. W., & Austin, J. K. (1999). Behavioral issues in pediatric epilepsy. *Neurology, 53,* S96–S100.

Fastenau, P. S., Shen, J., Dunn, D. W., Perkins, S. M., Hermann, B. P., & Austin, J. K. (2004). Neuropsychological predictors of academic underachievement in pediatric epilepsy: Moderating roles of demographic, seizure, and psychosocial variables. *Epilepsia, 45,* 1261–1272.

Freeman, J. M., Kossoff, E. H., & Hartman, A. L. (2007). The ketogenic diet: One decade later. *Pediatrics, 119,* 535–543.

Freeman, J. M., Vining, E.P.G., & Pillas, D. J. (1997). *Seizures and epilepsy in childhood: A guide for parents* (2nd ed.). Baltimore: Johns Hopkins Press.

Gioia, G. A., Isquith, P. K., Guy, S. C., & Kenworthy, L. (2000). *Behavior Rating Inventory of Executive Function.* Odessa, FL: Psychological Assessment Resources.

Hemingway, C., Freeman, J. M., Pillas, D. J., & Pyzik, P. L. (2001). The ketogenic diet: A 3- to 6-year follow-up of 150 children enrolled prospectively. *Pediatrics, 108,* 898–905.

Kang, H. C., Kim, Y. J., Kim, D. W., & Kim, H. D. (2005). Efficacy and safety of the ketogenic diet for intractable childhood epilepsy: Korean multicentric experience. *Epilepsia, 46,* 272–279.

Koop, J. I., Fastenau, P. S., Dunn, D. W., & Austin, J. K. (2005). Neuropsychological correlates of electroencephalograms in children with epilepsy. *Epilepsy Research, 64,* 49–62.

Kossoff, E. H., Pyzik, P. L., Rubenstein, J. E., Bergqvist, C., Buchhalter, J. R., Donner, E. J., et al. (2007). Combined ketogenic diet and vagus nerve stimulation: Rational polytherapy? *Epilepsia, 48,* 77–81.

Kraphohl, B. D., Deutinger, M., & Kömürcü, F. (2007). Vagus nerve stimulation: Treatment modality for epilepsy. *Medsurg Nursing, 16,* 39–44.

Li, Y., & Mogul, D. J. (2007). Electrical control of epileptic seizures. *Journal of Clinical Neurophysiology, 24,* 197–204.

Loring, D. W., & Meador, K. J. (2004). Cognitive side effects of antiepileptic drugs in children. *Neurology, 62,* 872–877.

Martinez, C. C., Pyzik, P. L., & Kossoff, E. H. (2007). Discontinuing the ketogenic diet in seizure-free children: Recurrence and risk factors. *Epilepsia, 48,* 187–190.

McHugh, J. C., Singh, H. W., Phillips, J., Murphy, K., Doherty, C. P., & Delanty, N. (2007). Outcome measurement after vagal nerve stimulation therapy: Proposal of a new classification. *Epilepsia, 48,* 375–378.

McNelis, A. M., Dunn, D. W., Johnson, C. S., Austin, J. K., & Perkins, S. M. (2007). Academic performance in children with new-onset seizures and asthma: A prospective study. *Epilepsy and Behavior, 10,* 311–318.

Miller, V., Palermo, T. M., & Grewe, S. D. (2003). Quality of life in pediatric epilepsy: Demographic and disease-related predictors and comparison with healthy controls. *Epilepsy and Behavior, 4,* 36–42.

National Society for Epilepsy (NSE). (1999a). *Diagnosing epilepsy.* Retrieved May 5, 2007, from http://www.epilepsynse.org.uk/

National Society for Epilepsy (NSE). (1999b). *Seizures.* Retrieved May 5, 2007, from http://www.epilepsynse.org.uk/

Nei, M., O'Connor, M., Liporace, J., & Sperling, M. R. (2006). Refractory generalized seizures: Response to corpus callosotomy and vagal nerve stimulation. *Epilepsia, 47,* 115–122.

Ortinski, P., & Meador, K. J. (2004). Cognitive side effects of antiepileptic drugs. *Epilepsy and Behavior, 5,* S60–S65.

Pakalnis, A., Paolicchi, J., & Gilles, E. (2000). Psychogenic status epilepticus in children: Psychiatric and other risk factors. *Neurology, 54,* 969–970.

Paolicchi, J. M. (2002). The spectrum of nonepileptic events in children. *Epilepsia, 43,* 60–64.

Pellock, J. M. (2004a). The challenge of neuropsychiatric issues in pediatric epilepsy. *Journal of Child Neurology, 19,* S1–S5.

Pellock, J. M. (2004b). Defining the problem: Psychiatric and behavioral comorbidity in children and adolescents with epilepsy. *Epilepsy and Behavior, 5,* S3–S9.

Plioplys, S. (2003). Depression in children and adolescents with epilepsy. *Epilepsy and Behavior, 4,* S39–S45.

Raiford, S. E., Weiss, L. G., Rolfus, E., & Coalson, D. (2005). *WISC-IV General Ability Index, Technical Report #4.* San Antonio, TX: Harcourt Assessment.

Reynolds, C. R., & Kamphaus, R. W. (2004). *Behavior Assessment Scale for Children* (2nd ed). Circle Pines, MN: AGS Publishing.

Sabbagh, S. E., Soria, C., Escolano, S., Bulteau, C., & Dellatolas, G. (2006). Impact of epilepsy characteristics and behavioral problems on school placement in children. *Epilepsy and Behavior, 9,* 573–578.

Saneto, R. P., Sotero de Menezes, M. A., Ojemann, J. G., Bournival, B. D., Murphy, P. J., Cook, W. B., et al. (2006). Vagus nerve stimulation for intractable seizures in children. *Pediatric Neurology, 35,* 323–326.

Sherman, E. M. S., Slick, D. J., Connolly, M. B., Steinbok, P., Martin, R., Strauss, E., et al. (2003). Reexamining the effects of epilepsy surgery on IQ in children: Use of regression-based change scores. *Journal of the International Neuropsychological Society, 9,* 879–886.

Shinnar, S., & Pellock, J. M. (2002). Update on the epidemiology and prognosis of pediatric epilepsy. *Journal of Child Neurology, 17,* S4–S17.

Smith, M. L., Elliott, I. M., & Lach, L. (2004). Cognitive, psychosocial, and family function one year after pediatric epilepsy surgery. *Epilepsia, 45,* 650–660.

Smith, M. L., Elliott, I. M., & Lach, L. (2006). Memory outcome after pediatric epilepsy surgery: Objective and subjective perspectives. *Child Neuropsychology, 12,* 151–164.

Tiffin, J. (1968). *Purdue Pegboard examiner's manual.* Rosemont, IL: London House.

Turanh, G., Yalnizoğlu, D., Genç-Açikgöz, D., Akalan, N., & Topçu, M. (2006). Outcome and long term follow-up after corpus callosotomy in childhood onset intractable epilepsy. *Child's Nervous System, 22,* 1322–1327.

Wechsler, D. (2003). *Wechsler Intelligence Scale for Children* (4th ed.). San Antonio, TX: Harcourt Assessment.

Woodcock, R. W., McGrew, K. S., & Mather, N. (2001). *Woodcock-Johnson Tests of Achievement* (3rd ed.). Rolling Meadows, IL: Riverside.

Williams, J., Steel, C., Sharp, G. B., DelosReyes, E., Phillips, T., Bates, S., et al. (2003). Anxiety in children with epilepsy. *Epilepsy and Behavior, 4,* 729–732.

Zabara, J. (1985). Time course of seizure control to brief, repetitive stimuli. *Epilepsia, 26,* 518.

CHAPTER TEN

# Fetal Alcohol Spectrum Disorders

Karin S. Walsh, PsyD, and Emily F. Law, MA

Joey is a 4-year 4-month-old African American male who presents with impaired attention, poor impulse control, delayed language acquisition, and difficulty with behavior management. Joey attends a home-based day care, where his behaviors have become increasingly problematic. He is prescribed Adderall for attention, as well as Pulmicort and albuterol for asthma.

Joey was exposed to alcohol, heroin, and cocaine in utero. He was born 4 weeks prematurely and weighed 2 pounds 6 ounces. He experienced numerous complications after birth, including cocaine and heroin addiction and withdrawal as well as respiratory disease. He required treatment in the neonatal intensive care unit (NICU) for 2 months for various medical complications. Following his hospitalization, he was discharged to foster care. Joey's early motor and language milestones were significantly delayed; he did not speak or walk until he was approximately 2 years old. His medical history is significant for asthma and strabismus (i.e., a misalignment of the eyes), which was treated surgically. Fetal alcohol syndrome (FAS) was identified soon after birth, as he has the classic physical features of FAS and a confirmed history of maternal alcohol use during pregnancy.

Joey was identified for early intervention services and received occupational, physical, and speech therapies sporadically during his first

3 years of life. An early assessment at 3 years of age documented significant speech/language delays, but he did not receive intervention at that time. Behavioral dysregulation became increasingly apparent and disruptive as Joey grew older, including specific concerns with aggression, poor frustration tolerance, and poor social functioning. Joey was involved in a behavioral therapy program for a brief period, but the intervention was of limited success. He was previously diagnosed with a nonspecified mood disorder and Attention-Deficit/Hyperactivity Disorder (ADHD)—Combined Type. The stimulant medication that he was prescribed has been of some benefit in controlling these behaviors.

Joey currently attends day care with five other children. He was identified for a Head Start preschool when he was 4 years of age; however, he was not financially eligible to attend. Significant difficulties have surfaced in day care, as the other children are fearful of, and overwhelmed by, Joey's behavior. His behaviors are so significant that they prohibit his involvement in any extracurricular activities. He has subsequently had difficulty establishing and maintaining relationships with both peers and authority figures.

## DESCRIPTION OF THE DISORDER

Prenatal exposure to alcohol is associated with a variety of negative outcomes referred to as fetal alcohol syndrome (FAS), fetal alcohol effects (FAE), and alcohol-related neurodevelopmental disorder (ARND). According to guidelines established by the Research Society on Alcoholism (Sokol & Clarren, 1989), FAS is diagnosed when signs of abnormality in each of the following three categories are present: (a) prenatal and/or perinatal growth retardation (i.e., weight, height, and/or head circumference below the 10th percentile when corrected for gestational age); (b) central nervous system (CNS) involvement (i.e., signs of neurological abnormality, developmental delay, or intellectual impairment); and (c) characteristic facial dysmorphology, including microphthalmia (i.e., abnormally small eyes), short palpebral fissures (i.e., small opening between the eyelids), poorly developed philtrum (i.e., flattening of the vertical ridges between the nose and mouth; see Figure 10.1), thin upper lip, underdeveloped ears (i.e., "railroad track" appearance; see Figure 10.2), epicanthal folds (i.e., folds at inner eye), flattening of the maxillary area (i.e., underdeveloped mid-face area [Wattendorf & Muenke, 2005]; see Figure 10.3), and fifth digit clinodactyly (i.e., deformed fifth finger; see Figure 10.4). The partial expression of these symptoms has traditionally been known as FAE and has more recently been labeled ARND. A history of confirmed prenatal exposure to alcohol is typically essential in diagnosing teratogenic alcohol effects. However, it is possible to diagnose the full syndrome without confirmed maternal drinking if the characteristic clinical expression is complete.

The most recent estimate of the worldwide incidence rate of FAS is 0.97 per 1,000 live births (Abel, 1995). The United States has one of the highest incidence rates worldwide at 1.95 per 1,000 live births, compared to only 0.08 per 1,000 in Europe (Abel, 1998a). FAS has been observed across socioeconomic status (SES) and ethnic groups; however, children living in poverty are more likely to be affected. In the United States, lower SES, African American, and Native American populations have 10 times the prevalence rates compared to middle SES White groups (Abel, 1995). An estimated 2,000 children are born with FAS each year in the United States, and FAS-related expenditures are estimated at $250 million per year (Abel, 1998b).

Early identification of FAS has been cited as an important role for school psychologists and school personnel (Phelps, 1995; Phelps & Grabowski, 1993). While FAS is difficult to diagnose, a referral to the pediatric neuropsychologist or other appropriate professional (e.g., developmental pediatrician) can assist in such early identification and in the development of an appropriate educational and treatment plan for that child. Major obstacles to FAS diagnosis include changes in the constellation of FAS facial features as the child ages (making them particularly difficult to recognize in newborns and adults), variations in the severity of symptoms across individuals, reliance on maternal report for alcohol consumption during pregnancy, and lack of diagnostic agreement for the less severe variations of the syndrome (Aase, 1994). FAS is relatively rare, and therefore it is unlikely that the majority of school psychologists have received substantial training and supervision in identifying the physical and neurocognitive features of FAS (Smith & Graden, 1998). School psychologists and other school personnel will likely need to consult with experts in developmental disabilities upon encountering suspected cases of FAS (see Resources below).

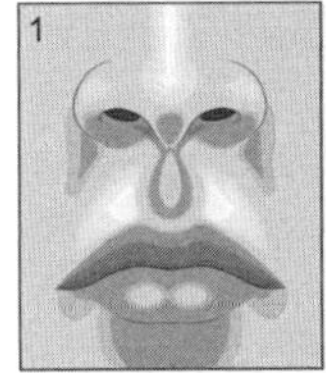

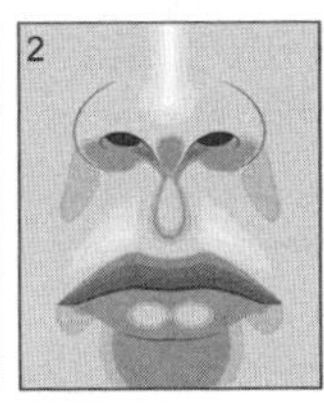

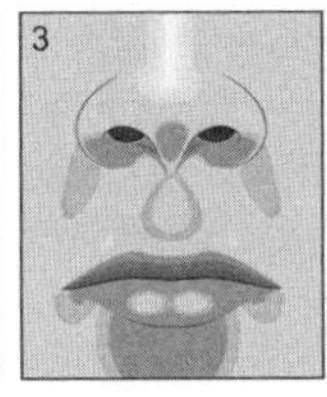

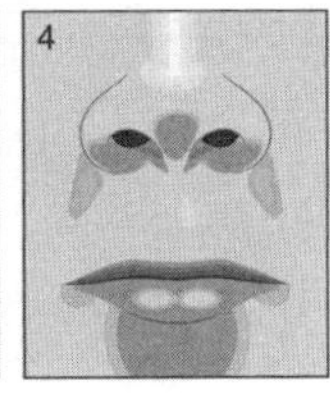

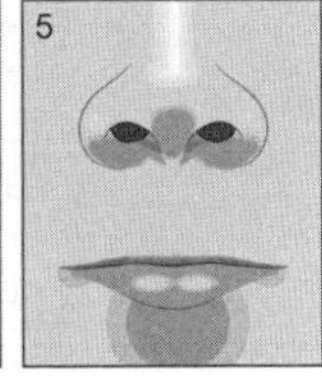


FIGURE 10-1 Philtrum guide: Full range of definition in philtrum.
Permission to reprint obtained from Darryl Leja, National Human Genome Research Institute, National Institutes of Health, 50 South Drive, Room 5523, Bethesda, Maryland 20892-8002.

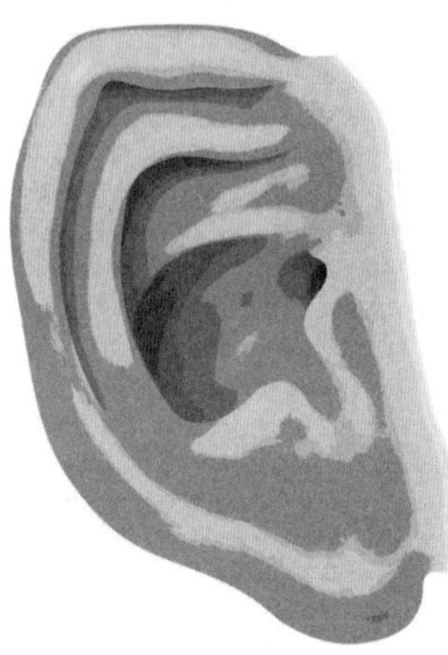

FIGURE 10.2 "Railroad track" ear deformity.

Permission to reprint obtained from Darryl Leja, National Human Genome Research Institute, National Institutes of Health, 50 South Drive, Room 5523, Bethesda, Maryland 20892-8002.

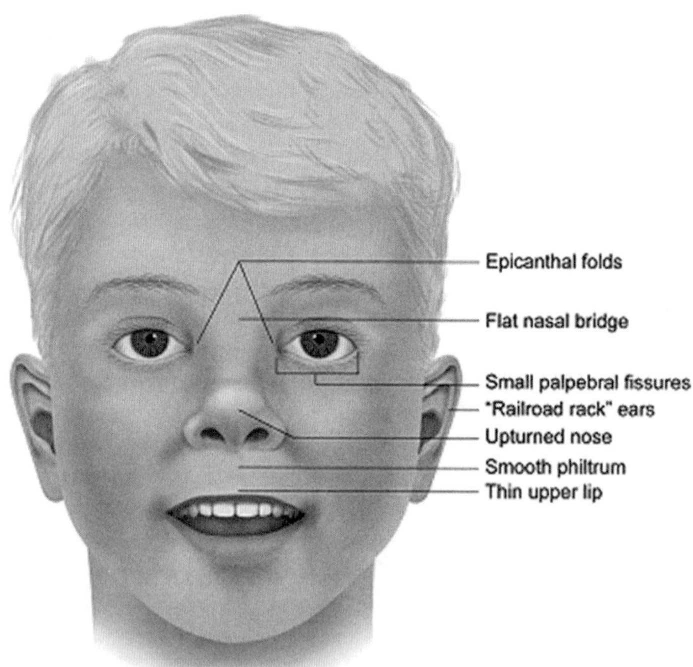


FIGURE 10.3 Typical facial features observed in FAS.

Permission to reprint obtained from Darryl Leja, National Human Genome Research Institute, National Institutes of Health, 50 South Drive, Room 5523, Bethesda, Maryland 20892-8002.

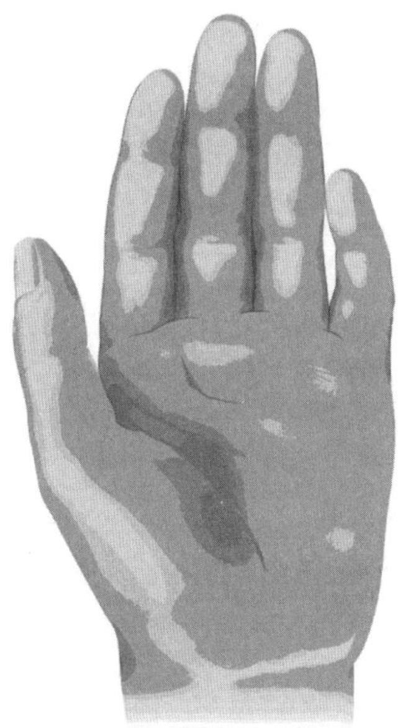

FIGURE 10.4 Characteristic fifth finger clinodactyly.
Permission to reprint obtained from Darryl Leja, National Human Genome Research Institute, National Institutes of Health, 50 South Drive, Room 5523, Bethesda, Maryland 20892-8002.

Alcohol can have significant effects on the development of the CNS by interfering with neurotransmitter production, cell development, cell migration, and brain growth throughout gestation (Phelps, 2005). Considerable damage can occur well before the mother is aware she is pregnant, as early as the 11th day after conception (Johnson, Swayze, Sato, & Andreasen, 1996). Sustained exposure to alcohol in the womb often results in significant cortical abnormalities, affecting the basal ganglia, cerebellum, and corpus callosum preferentially (Phelps, 2005). Damage to these brain regions is associated with impairments in motor functioning, processing speed, and integration of information, as well as impaired attention and emerging executive function skills. A compromised corpus callosum hinders the communication between the cortical hemispheres, which often results in rather "disconnected" performance. FAS is the leading cause of mild mental retardation in children, over and above Down syndrome and fragile X syndrome (Streissguth et al., 1991). Significant sequelae include delays in language and motor development, hypotonia (i.e., low muscle tone), conductive hearing loss, and visual deficits.

The toxicity of alcohol to the fetus is dose dependent, and different profiles of alcohol-related birth defects are associated with varying exposure levels at critical periods in fetal development (Roebuck, Mattson, & Riley, 1998). Diversity in FAS symptomatology is also attributed to differences in how quickly mothers and infants metabolize alcohol, as well as genetic differences in vulnerability of the CNS to alcohol (Driscoll, Streissguth, & Riley, 1990; Streissguth & Dehaene, 1993). Therefore, no single pattern of brain malformations and associated symptomatology is related to prenatal exposure to alcohol. School psychologists and other school personnel can play an important role in helping parents, teachers, and administrators understand that each child exposed to alcohol prenatally will likely demonstrate a different pattern of strengths and weaknesses and require varying levels of support within the academic setting (Smith & Graden, 1998).

## COMORBID FACTORS

In addition to the facial abnormalities and atypical growth patterns characteristic of fetal alcohol spectrum disorders (FASD), a number of other factors impact the child's developing CNS and result in altered neurocognitive and neuroemotional abilities. In addition to alcohol, many children with FAS have been exposed to other toxic substances prenatally (e.g., heroin, cocaine, etc.). The likelihood of premature birth increases when cocaine is being used, as the substance itself has the potential to induce labor (Singer et al., 2002). Substance use during pregnancy is often associated with poor prenatal care and nutrition, which may further impact fetal development. Some of these issues may continue after the child is born, including poor nutrition, exposure to high stress environments, and/or deprivation. Each of these factors alone can alter brain development and further impact the CNS of the child already compromised by exposure to alcohol in utero, although discussion of this topic is beyond the scope of this chapter (Als et al., 2004). Clearly, these children often have complex histories including physiological and environmental insults during the prenatal and perinatal periods that impact the developing brain and, subsequently, the child's neurocognitive and socioemotional functioning.

## CASE CONTINUATION

Considering the information provided above, a continuation of Joey's case is provided to elaborate the residual impact of various described physiological and environmental insults on the child's functioning across environments.

The following observations were made during a neuropsychological evaluation with Joey when he was 4 years old. A number of physical and behavioral characteristics associated with fetal alcohol effects were immediately evident. Facial features indicative of prenatal exposure to alcohol, including a smooth philtrum (i.e., area between the upper lip and nose), a thin upper lip, wide-set eyes, and ear deformities were evident. His stature was consistent with his age, although his head circumference was underdeveloped (i.e., microcephaly), which was confirmed upon measurement. This is not uncommon in children who have been exposed to significant levels of toxic substances (i.e., alcohol) and is indicative of atypical brain development.

Joey exhibited some concerning behaviors that put him at significant safety risk, including a lack of apprehension toward strangers and willingness to accompany strangers without hesitation. He also demonstrated a lack of appreciation for typical social boundaries and immediately exhibited a physical closeness with those around him that was not typical for a child his age. Notably, he was socially connected and was interested in interacting and sharing with the adults who surrounded him.

Joey responded well to reinforcement, although his behaviors were highly perseverative or repetitious. He was echolalic and often repeated the last two words he heard, indicating the significance of his language impairments. Although he was not oppositional, it was difficult to redirect him to task during these times, and he required repeated prompts to do so. Joey demonstrated a clear desire to comply with instructions and work to the best of his abilities, and he responded appropriately to redirection.

Joey was highly distractible and required a significant amount of external structure including physical (e.g., touching of hands and face to focus attention, physically moving him into position) and verbal (e.g., "look," "come here") prompts. He generally responded well to increased structure and physical prompts. However, even with this level of external structure an apparent reduction in hyperactivity as the result of his medication, Joey was able to sit and focus on a task for only a few minutes at a time, provided he was interested in the task and appeared to comprehend it. He clearly expressed his displeasure when he became frustrated with a task, and he attempted to engage in escape behavior by saying he had to use the restroom.

Evidence of Joey's language impairments emerged immediately. A clear difference was apparent in behavior during verbal and nonverbal tasks. While he was easy to engage and elicit responses from during less verbally mediated tasks, he was more difficult to engage during highly verbal tasks. There was concern regarding language comprehension, as he required repetition, restating, and modeling to complete several tasks. His ability to express himself was also notably impaired. He often repeated what others had said and rarely generated well-formed independent communication.

Motor difficulties were also evident. He demonstrated a lack of lateral dominance for writing (i.e., he alternated between left and right hands), and he used an immature, fisted grip. Although he ambulated independently, his gait was observed to be wide set and ataxic (i.e., poorly coordinated).

### Assessment Results

The results of Joey's neuropsychological evaluation indicated neurocognitive functioning at a 24-month age equivalent across developmental domains, which is indicative of a greater than 50% delay in development. Impairments in global intellect, language, motor skills, attention, and processing abilities were demonstrated. His adaptive skills were also significantly impaired. As a result, his ability to obtain preacademic skills was significantly impaired.

A number of positive characteristics were also identified, including Joey's ability to spontaneously interact playfully with others, although this required monitoring. He also responded well to positive praise and reinforcement and to consistent structure and limit setting. He further demonstrated an impressive ability to accommodate to change.

Nonetheless, Joey demonstrated a pattern of congenitally based global neurocognitive impairments consistent with a diagnosis of mild mental retardation (see Table 10.1), the most likely cause of which was his exposure to alcohol in utero, although a number of factors likely contributed to his neurological and neurocognitive development. His impairments across domains are consistent with this level of mental retardation, and therefore the difficulties he exhibits across the various domains do not constitute individual diagnoses (i.e., ADHD). Further, although Joey demonstrated some behaviors that may appear to be consistent with a pervasive developmental disorder (PDD; i.e., perseverative behavior, poor social connectedness, language impairments, etc.), these behaviors are often observed in children with mental retardation. In addition, he demonstrated appropriate interest in social interactions with the adults who surrounded him, and there was no evidence of stereotypical behavior nor of rigid interests or activities.

## INTERVENTIONS

Fetal alcohol exposure is a serious public health problem that deserves considerable attention. However, currently there are no empirically based

**TABLE 10.1 Neuropsychological Testing Data**

| | Scaled Score | T Score | Standard Score |
|---|---|---|---|
| Intellectual Functioning | | | |
| DAS Global | | 61 | |
| Verbal | | 65 | |
| Nonverbal | | 61 | |
| Adaptive Functioning | | | |
| ABAS-II Global | | | 35 |
| Communication | 3 | | |
| Community Use | 5 | | |
| Functional Pre-Academics | 5 | | |
| Home Living | 3 | | |
| Health and Safety | 5 | | |
| Leisure | 2 | | |
| Self-Care | 3 | | |
| Self-Direction | 4 | | |
| Social | 1 | | |
| Motor | 4 | | |
| Learning/Memory | | | |
| SB Bead Memory | | | 90 |
| DAS | | | |
| Recall of Objects—Immediate | | 28 | |
| Recall of Objects—Delayed | | 33 | |
| Recognition of Pictures | | 29 | |
| Language Functioning | | | |
| PPVT-III | | | 78 |

*Continued*

**TABLE 10.1** *(Continued)*

| | Scaled Score | T Score | Standard Score |
|---|---|---|---|
| DAS Verbal Comprehension | | 22 | |
| Naming Vocabulary | | 31 | |
| **Visual-Motor/Fine Motor Functioning** | | | |
| DAS Picture Similarities | | 40 | |
| Pattern Construction (Standard) | | 25 | |
| Copying | | 32 | |
| WRAVMA Drawing | | | 88 |
| Pegboard (preferred right) | | | 67 |
| Pegboard (nonpreferred) | | | 82 |
| **Preacademic Skills** | | | |
| BBCS-R School Readiness Composite | 5 | | |
| **Socioemotional Functioning** | | | |
| CBCL (Parent) | | | |
| Hyperactivity | | 71 | |
| Aggression | | 82 | |
| Conduct Problems | | 77 | |
| Anxiety | | 54 | |
| Depression | | 63 | |
| Somatization | | 53 | |
| Withdrawal | | 63 | |
| Attention Problems | | 77 | |

*Note.* ABAS-II, Adaptive Behavior Assessment System—Second Edition (Harrison & Oakland, 2003); BBCS-R, Bracken Basic Concept Scales—Revised (Bracken, 2006); CBCL, Child Behavior Checklist (Achenbach, 1991); DAS, Differential Ability Scales (Elliott, 1990); PPVT-III, Peabody Picture Vocabulary Test—Third Edition (Dunn & Dunn, 1997); SB, Stanford-Binet Intelligence Scale—Third Edition (Terman & Merrill, 1960); and WRAVMA, Wide Range Assessment of Visual Motor Abilities (Adams & Sheslow, 1995).

interventions for children impacted by such exposure and their families (Phelps, 2005). Schools and communities have a unique opportunity to provide appropriate remediation and shelter for these children in order to minimize potential victimization, dependent living, unemployment, psychopathology, and homelessness in adulthood (Streissguth et al., 1991; Streissguth, Barr, Kogan, & Bookstein, 1997). To combat the deleterious effects of prenatal alcohol exposure, the following three-pronged approach is widely recommended: (a) prevention of prenatal substance use through middle school and high school educational programming, (b) early diagnosis and comprehensive preschool interventions for FAS/FAE/ARND infants and their families, and (c) provision of appropriate multilevel and multidisciplinary special education services from infancy through young adulthood for all qualified youth (Olson, 2002; Phelps, 1995, 2005; Streissguth et al., 1997). In addition, alcohol treatment and recovery support, respite care for parents, family crisis services, post-adoption support services, and consistent long-term support for families are often needed to maintain stable and nurturing home environments (Olson).

An accurate alcohol-related diagnosis can have many benefits, including an explanation for the child's cognitive and behavioral difficulties as well as facilitation of realistic expectations of the child (Olson, 2002). Because there is no specific pattern of impairments among children with FAS and related disorders, educational programming should be based on each child's unique pattern of strengths and weaknesses, which can be identified through a developmental or neuropsychological evaluation. It is important to collect clear and consistent data about the utility and effectiveness of the curriculum and teaching techniques used for the child with FAS, altering the interventions and supports accordingly. Clearly defined short- and long-term academic goals that are uniquely tailored to the child's strengths and limitations, as well as routine objective assessment of specific target goals, should be clearly outlined in an individualized education program (IEP). Regular meetings with parents can help to ensure that goals are being targeted both in the home and school settings.

In addition to social and educational interventions, environmental and family factors must be considered during the assessment and intervention process. Living in a stable and nurturing home is the strongest protective factor against secondary disabilities among adolescents and adults with FAS, which include mental health problems, disrupted school experiences, trouble with the law, and drug and alcohol abuse (Streissguth et al., 1997). The home environments of children with FAS are often unstable due to continued alcohol abuse by a biological parent, which may result in impaired parenting skills, strained parent–child relations, and major disruptions in caregiving. Repeated moves and disruptions associated with foster care or institutionalization are also significant factors in a child's success or failure (Streissguth et al., 1991). Family factors must be continually evaluated as part of an ecological approach to assessment and intervention with children exposed to alcohol and their families.

## Preschool Children

Given his relatively early diagnosis, Joey and his family would benefit from intensive preschool and home-based interventions targeting cognitive, speech and language, orthopedic, and behavioral impairments. Enrollment in a special education preschool in order to provide accommodations for all areas of disability is essential. Similar to other young children with FAS, Joey demonstrated deficits in language acquisition and fine motor skill development. He would benefit from intensive speech and language services to address and intervene in his language development. Occupational and physical therapy services would be recommended as well to assist him in developing functional fine motor skills as well as improving balance and coordination, which will be necessary in the academic environment. Given his combination of motor impairments and impulsivity, Joey will require constant supervision for learning and safety purposes. He would benefit from being enrolled in a classroom with a limited student-to-teacher ratio (i.e., 5:1). This level of programming would not only enhance his academic progress and accommodate his unique needs but would also enhance his social development; it has been demonstrated that children with varying levels of mental retardation benefit significantly from interactions with typically developing peers (Guralnick, Connor, Hammond, Gottman, & Kinnish, 1996; Guralnick & Groom, 1988).

Joey's curriculum should focus on repetition, pairing verbal with visual information when teaching, as well as a slowed pace of teaching with increased external cues to assist in his acquisition of new information and skills. His teachers may consider using his perseveration (i.e., tendencies to focus on particular aspects of his environment) as learning opportunities. For example, his teachers and parents might focus on a particular area of interest and expand on it as a learning format. A balance between fostering perseverative tendencies to take advantage of learning opportunities and encouraging a wider variety of interests is required, as perseveration can become maladaptive.

Joey demonstrated significant difficulty with sustained attention, impulsivity, and hyperactivity and could typically sustain his attention for only 2 to 3 minutes at a time. Preschoolers with FAS may work most successfully when learning periods are limited to brief intensive sessions with frequent sensory breaks and physical activity. Individuals working with Joey should say his name and use body language (e.g., make eye contact, stand close to him) to ensure that they have his attention prior to giving verbal instructions. Joey will need repetition and clarification of task instructions as well as reminders to stay on task for extended periods of time, and multistep instructions should be broken down into smaller components. Transitions should be minimized or highly regulated so that Joey knows what to expect, and he should be given time to acclimate before moving on to novel learning tasks. Joey demonstrated that he works well in a one-to-one format featuring frequent positive prompting and encouragement. The provision of consistency and structure will enhance the learning process for children with FAS like Joey, and clear expectations for behavior and reinforcement of appropriate responses are strongly recommended (Phelps, 1995).

Children with FAS often demonstrate a lack of developmentally appropriate apprehension with adult strangers (Phelps & Grabowski, 1993). These children may benefit from practicing basic safety skills with their parents, teachers, and therapists. It is important that these children have an opportunity to demonstrate these skills in closely supervised situations within the community so they can be redirected as needed. Preschool children with FAS may also benefit from an identification bracelet if their ability to convey vital personal information (e.g., address, phone number, etc.) is limited (see Resources below).

## School-Age Children and Adolescents

School-age children with FAS typically demonstrate difficulties with short-term memory, information processing, problem solving, organization, behavioral compliance, and ADHD symptomatology (i.e., hyperactivity, impulsivity, distractibility, inattentiveness; Phelps, 1995). As children with FASD grow older, continued coordination between the school, family, and community-based services is essential. The majority of school-age children with FAS will likely require a resource room or a self-contained placement to best accommodate their varied educational needs (Streissguth et al., 1991). Similar to interventions designed for preschool children with FAS, structure, consistency, brief presentations, variety, and repetition continue to be key strategies to teach and maximize learning in school-age children with FAS (Tanner-Halverson, 1997). In addition, social skills training in school settings or through structured extracurricular activities may enhance the child's ability to establish and maintain peer relations (Olson, 2002). Continued use of ecologically based, intervention-oriented assessments and multidisciplinary intervention teams is highly recommended (Smith & Graden, 1998).

Psychostimulants may be necessary to treat inattention, disinhibition, and hyperactivity in school-age children with FAS and related disorders (Phelps, 1995). Given the wide variability of CNS dysfunction associated with prenatal alcohol exposure, medication dosage and type will require consistent monitoring and adjustments (Snyder, Nanson, Snyder, & Block, 1997). Notably, medication for children with FAS must be considered as one component of a multimodal intervention that also includes behavior management and parent training (Snyder et al.). Many children with FAS present with attention and executive function deficits, and as they mature, their motoric overactivity decreases while attention and executive functioning difficulties remain (Streissguth et al., 1991). For alcohol-affected adolescents and adults, medication (if prescribed) must serve as only one part of a comprehensive multimodal intervention plan (Snyder et al.).

In addition to attention and executive function difficulties, adolescents with FAS and related disorders may demonstrate continued cognitive deficits, impaired academic performance, poor judgment, lack of self-direction, and difficulty perceiving social cues (Phelps, 1995). Interventions designed for adolescents with FAS and related conditions must support them in their normal developmental tasks (e.g., developing friendships, establishing autonomy) in a way that ensures their safety while allowing some experimentation and testing of adult rules (Olson, 2002). As youth with FAS and related disorders enter high school, vocational counseling, job training, and the development of adaptive living skills become essential (Phelps, 1995). School psychologists and other school personnel can play an important role in facilitating vocational counseling and job training, as the behavior problems commonly seen in adolescents with FAS may make them unsuitable for traditional vocational training programs (Streissguth et al., 1991). In addition, high school students with FAS may benefit from social skills training to foster peer relations and help them behave in a socially appropriate manner (Olson, 2002).

Services that may facilitate the transition to adulthood for adolescents with FAS include group homes for individuals who have mental illness and/or are involved with the legal system but are not significantly mentally retarded, specialized therapy for inappropriate sexual behavior, and parenting support programs for alcohol-affected parents (Olson, 2002). Individuals with FAS and related disorders may qualify for supplemental security income (SSI) and may be eligible for services under their respective state's Division of Developmental Disabilities (DDD). Supplemental security income is a federal income supplement program designed to help disabled people who have little or no income by providing monetary support to meet basic needs for food, clothing, and shelter. DDD is a state-run organization responsible for determining eligibility and authorizing paid services for individuals with a developmental disability as defined by state law. DDD services vary by state and may include case management, employment, day program services, housing, social and recreational activities, and medical and mental health care.

When facilitating an individual's transition from adolescence to adulthood, school psychologists and school personnel may encounter difficulties related to restricted access to services, as the varied disabilities associated with FAS and related disorders often do not conform to current system guidelines for SSI funding, DDD eligibility, and entry into special education or vocational rehabilitation programs (Olson, 2002; Streissguth et al., 1991). In addition to playing an important role in developing transition programs for adolescents with FAS, school personnel should consider working on a policy level to change eligibility criteria for existing services for individuals with FAS and related conditions.

## CONCLUSION

Youth of all ages with FAS and related disorders are in need of early identification and intervention due to the risk of school failure and other long-term functional disruptions including homelessness, psychopathology, and substance abuse. Effective prevention programs (e.g., school-based substance use prevention programs, prenatal counseling, and substance use treatment) and multimodal intervention programs tailored to each individual's needs throughout the life span are essential. As a member of a multidisciplinary assessment and intervention team, school personnel (psychologists, counselors, teachers, etc.) can play a crucial role in coordinating interdisciplinary services for these individuals and their families. By facilitating suitable interventions, school personnel can substantially improve expected long-term outcomes for children and adolescents suffering the consequences of prenatal exposure to alcohol.

## RESOURCES

### Books

Dorris, M. (1989). *The broken cord.* New York: HarperCollins.

Kleinfeld, J., Morse, B., & Wescott, S. (Eds.). (2000). *Fantastic Antone grows up: Adolescents and adults with fetal alcohol syndrome.* Fairbanks: University of Alaska Press.

Kleinfeld, J., & Wescott, S. (Eds.). (1993). *Fantastic Antone succeeds: Experiences in educating children with fetal alcohol syndrome.* Fairbanks: University of Alaska Press.

Malbin, D. (1993). *Fetal alcohol syndrome, fetal alcohol effects: Strategies for professionals.* Center City, MN: Hazelden Publishing and Educational Services.

Streissguth, A. (1997). *Fetal alcohol syndrome: A guide for families and communities.* Baltimore: Brookes.

Streissguth, A., & Kanter, J. (Eds.). (1997). *The challenge of fetal alcohol syndrome: Overcoming secondary disabilities.* Seattle: University of Washington Press.

## Organizations and Web Sites

The Arc of the United States

The Arc of the United States is a national nonprofit group with state and local chapters in most states that provide advocacy and other services for families and children affected by developmental disabilities. The Arc's Web site provides links to chapters with FAS projects and state-by-state information for families needing services for their children.

Mailing Address: 1010 Wayne Avenue, Suite 650
Silver Spring, Maryland 20910
Phone Number: (301) 565-3842
Web Site: www.thearc.org

Civitas

Civitas is the communication group that produces a public engagement campaign that provides important information about what young children need every day to ensure quality early learning. It provides materials designed to support parents as their child's first teacher.

Mailing Address: 2210 West North Avenue
Chicago, Illinois 60647
Phone Number: (312) 226-6700
Web Site: www.civitas.org/

Family Empowerment Network (FEN): Supporting Families Affected by FAS/FAE

FEN is a national resource, referral, and support organization for families affected by FAS and FAE.

Mailing Address: 777 South Mills Street
Madison, Wisconsin 53715
Phone Number: (800) 462-5254
Web Site: www.fammed.wisc.edu/fen

Fetal Alcohol Syndrome Diagnostic and Prevention Network (FAS DPN)

The Washington State FAS DPN is a network of five community-based clinics in Washington State linked by the core clinical/research/

training clinic at the Center on Human Development and Disability at the University of Washington in Seattle, Washington. The FAS DPN mission is to encourage FAS prevention through screening, diagnosis, intervention, research, and training.

Web Site: depts.washington.edu/fasdpn

Fetal Alcohol Syndrome Family Resource Institute (FASFRI)

FASFRI is a nonprofit organization that provides referrals and support in finding help, parent support and advocacy, as well as information for parents of children affected by FAS.

Web Site: www.fetalalcoholsyndrome.org/index.html

National Center on Birth Defects and Developmental Disabilities

This organization is supported by the Department of Health and Human Services within the Centers for Disease Control and Prevention (CDC).

Mailing Address: NCBDDD, CDC
1600 Clifton Road, Mail-Stop E-86
Atlanta, Georgia 30333
Phone Number: (800) CDC-INFO
Web Site: www.cdc.gov/ncbddd/fas

National Organization on Fetal Alcohol Syndrome (NOFAS)

NOFAS is a nonprofit organization dedicated to improving the quality of life for those individuals and families affected by alcohol-related birth defects. Its Web site provides FAS resources, information on parenting strategies, and a national/state directory of providers and support groups. The Web site also contains a directory that lists diagnostic clinics, support groups, and family members willing to be contacted.

Mailing Address: 900 17th Street, NW, Suite 910
Washington, D.C. 20006
Phone Number: (800) 66-NOFAS
Web Site: www.nofas.org

State Department of Health

Your respective State Department of Health may have information on the diagnosis of FAS, referrals to clinics in your area, and applying for services from your state's Division of Developmental Disabilities. You can find its phone number in your phone book in the state/local government section listed under Department of Health.

Web Site: www.fda.gov/oca/sthealth.htm

Substance Abuse and Mental Health Services Administration (SAMHSA)
The SAMHSA FASD Center for Excellence is a federal initiative devoted to preventing and treating FASD. This Web site provides information and resources about FASD, as well as materials individuals can use to raise awareness about FASD.

| | |
|---|---|
| Mailing Address: | SAMHSA FASD Center for Excellence<br>2101 Gaither Road, Suite 600<br>Rockville, Maryland 20850 |
| Phone Number: | (866) STOP-FAS |
| Web Site: | fascenter.samhsa.gov |

## REFERENCES


Aase, J. M. (1994). Clinical recognition of FAS: Difficulties of detection and diagnosis. *Alcohol Health and Research World, 18,* 5–9.

Abel, E. L. (1995). An update on the incidence of FAS: FAS is not an equal opportunity birth defect. *Neurotoxicology and Teratology, 17,* 437–443.

Abel, E. L. (1998a). Fetal alcohol syndrome: The American paradox. *Alcohol and Alcoholism, 33,* 195–201.

Abel, E. L. (1998b). Prevention of alcohol abuse-related birth effects I: Public education efforts. *Alcohol and Alcoholism, 33,* 411–416.

Achenbach, T. M. (1991). *Integrative Guide to the 1991 CBCL/4–18, YSR, and TRF Profiles.* Burlington: University of Vermont, Department of Psychology.

Adams, W., & Sheslow, D. (1995). *Wide Range Assessment of Visual Motor Abilities.* Lutz, FL: Psychological Assessment Resources.

Als, H., Duffy, F. H., McAnulty, G. B., Rivkin, M. J., Vajapeyam, S., Mulkern, R. V., et al. (2004). Early experience alters brain function and structure. *Pediatrics, 113,* 846–857.

Bracken, B. A. (2006). *Bracken Basic Concept Scale* (3rd ed.). San Antonio, TX: Harcourt Assessment.

Driscoll, C. D., Streissguth, A. P., & Riley, E. P. (1990). Prenatal alcohol exposure: Comparability of effects in humans and animal models. *Neurotoxicology and Teratology, 12,* 231–237.

Dunn, L. M., & Dunn, L. M. (1997). *Examiner's manual for the Peabody Picture Vocabulary Test* (3rd ed.). Circle Pines, MN: American Guidance Service.

Elliott, C. D. (1990). *Differential Ability Scales: Administration and scoring manual.* San Antonio, TX: The Psychological Corporation.

Guralnick, M. J., Connor, R. T., Hammond, M., Gottman, J. M., & Kinnish, K. (1996). Immediate effects of mainstreamed settings on the social interactions and social integration of preschool children. *American Journal on Mental Retardation, 100,* 359–377.

Guralnick, M. J., & Groom, J. M. (1988). Peer interactions in mainstreamed and specialized classrooms: A comparative analysis. *Exceptional Children, 54,* 415–425.

Harrison, P. L., & Oakland, T. (2003). *Adaptive Behavior Assessment System* (2nd ed.). San Antonio, TX: The Psychological Corporation.

Johnson, V. P., Swayze, V. W., Sato, Y., & Andreasen, N. C. (1996). Fetal alcohol syndrome: Craniofacial and central nervous system manifestations. *American Journal of Medical Genetics, 61,* 329–339.

Olson, H. C. (2002). Helping children with fetal alcohol syndrome and related conditions: A clinician's overview. In R. J. McMahon & R. D. Peters (Eds.), *The effects of parental dysfunction on children* (pp. 147–178). New York: Kluwer Academic/Plenum.

Phelps, L. (1995). Psychoeducational outcomes of fetal alcohol syndrome: Diagnostic features and psychoeducational risk factors. *School Psychology Review, 24,* 200–212.

Phelps, L. (2005). Fetal alcohol syndrome: Neuropsychological outcomes, psychoeducational implications, and prevention models. In R. C. D'Amato, E. Fletcher-Janzen, & C. R. Reynolds (Eds.), *Handbook of school neuropsychology* (pp. 561–573). New Jersey: John Wiley & Sons.

Phelps, L., & Grabowski, J. (1993). Fetal alcohol syndrome: Diagnostic features and psychoeducational risk factors. *School Psychology Quarterly, 7,* 112–128.

Roebuck, T. M., Mattson, S. N., & Riley, E. P. (1998). A review of the neuroanatomical findings in children with fetal alcohol syndrome or prenatal exposure to alcohol. *Alcoholism: Clinical and Experimental Research, 22,* 339–344.

Singer, L. T., Arendt, R., Minnes, S., Farkas, K., Salvator, A., Kirchner, H. L., et al. (2002). Cognitive and motor outcomes of cocaine-exposed infants. *Journal of the American Medical Association, 287,* 1952–1960.

Smith, J. J., & Graden, J. L. (1998). Fetal alcohol syndrome. In L. Phelps (Ed.), *Health-related disorders in children and adolescents: A guidebook for understanding and educating* (pp. 291–298). Washington, DC: American Psychological Association.

Snyder, J., Nanson, J., Snyder, R., & Block, G. (1997). A study of stimulant medication in children with FAS. In A. Streissguth & J. Kanter (Eds.), *The challenge of fetal alcohol syndrome: Overcoming secondary disabilities* (pp. 64–77). Seattle: University of Washington Press.

Sokol, R. J., & Clarren, S. K. (1989). Guidelines for use of terminology describing the impact of prenatal alcohol on the offspring. *Alcoholism: Clinical and Experimental Research, 13,* 597–598.

Streissguth, A. P., Asae, J. M., Clarren, S. K., Randels, S. P., LaDue, R. A., & Smith, D. F. (1991). Fetal alcohol syndrome in adolescents and adults. *Journal of the American Medical Association, 265,* 1961–1967.

Streissguth, A. P., Barr, H., Kogan, J., & Bookstein, F. (1997). Primary and secondary disabilities in fetal alcohol syndrome. In A. P. Streissguth & J. Kanter (Eds.), *The challenge of fetal alcohol syndrome: Overcoming secondary disabilities* (pp. 25–39). Seattle: University of Washington Press.

Streissguth, A. P., & Dehaene, P. (1993). Fetal alcohol syndrome in twins of alcoholic mothers: Concordance of diagnosis and IQ. *American Journal of Medical Genetics, 47,* 857–861.

Tanner-Halverson, P. (1997). A demonstration classroom for young children with FAS. In A. P. Streissguth & J. Kanter (Eds.), *The challenge of fetal alcohol syndrome: Overcoming secondary disabilities* (pp. 78–88). Seattle: University of Washington Press.

Terman, L. M., & Merrill, M. A. (1960). *Stanford-Binet Intelligence Scale: Manual for the third revision.* Boston: Houghton Mifflin.

Wattendorf, D. J., & Muenke, M. (2005). Fetal alcohol spectrum disorders. *American Family Physician, 72,* 279–282.

CHAPTER ELEVEN

# HIV/AIDS

Jillian C. Schneider, PhD, and
Karin S. Walsh, PsyD

Robert, an 11-year 3-month-old African American male, was born prematurely to a mother who was positive for human immunodeficiency virus (HIV) and who used illicit substances while pregnant. Upon evaluation, he presented with impaired attention, concerns regarding his social relationships, and emotional and behavioral management difficulties. Robert is enrolled in the fifth grade, where these concerns have become increasingly problematic, interfering with his academic progress. He is prescribed multiple medications to manage the symptoms of his HIV, including nucleoside analogue reverse transcriptase inhibitors (NRTIs; Epivir, Retrovir, and Ziagen) as well as desmopressin acetate (to control frequent urination) and NordiFlex (growth hormone).

Robert tested positive for HIV at birth and required medical intervention for drug addiction due to his biological mother's use of illicit substances while pregnant. His early development and medical history were consistent with a static encephalopathic course of HIV (i.e., nonprogressive cognitive and motor impairment). His attainment of early motor and language milestones was significantly delayed, and he had substantial orthopedic impairments (Legg-Calvé-Perthes disease), left eye amblyopia (i.e., decreased vision), growth retardation, and microcephaly (i.e., small head circumference).

Robert's early home environment was unstable, and early neglect was suspected. He was left on a doorstep as an infant and did not have regular contact with his biological mother or father. His biological mother is currently deceased, and information regarding Robert's biological father is unknown. After being discovered on a doorstep, Robert was placed in a group home until he was 2 years old. At that time, he was placed with his current adoptive family, with whom he has lived consistently over the past 9 years. Although Robert has a good relationship with his adoptive parents, he has more difficulty getting along with the children in his extended family. He also has difficulty getting along with his classmates at school. Robert is occasionally teased by his peers, which results in frustration and maladaptive behaviors (e.g., verbal and physical aggression).

Robert is in the fifth grade and receives special education services in an inclusion program. Significant difficulties with attention (e.g., sustained attention, task persistence, task completion) and processing speed have been present since kindergarten but have worsened over the past several years. Additionally, concerns regarding Robert's emotional and behavioral dysregulation have become increasingly apparent and disruptive, including specific concerns with motivation to perform in class, defiance related to school work, poor frustration tolerance, and verbal and physical aggression toward others.

## DESCRIPTION OF THE DISORDER

Acquired immunodeficiency syndrome (AIDS) was first described in the literature in 1981 as an unusual form of pneumonia (i.e., pneumocystis carinii) found in previously healthy men who were gay or who used substances intravenously. Currently, AIDS, and the virus that causes the disorder, HIV, is considered to be a much broader disease affecting men, women, and children alike (Spiegel & Bonwit, 2002). It is widely understood that HIV can be transmitted through heterosexual as well as homosexual contact, through blood products, and from mother to child. The focus of this chapter will be on pediatric HIV/AIDS and the impact of vertically acquired (i.e., mother-to-child) HIV/AIDS on neuropsychological and neurobehavioral development. Horizontal acquisition is notably more uncommon (approximately 7% of pediatric HIV cases), and these children tend to have different neuropsychological profiles than those children with the more common vertically acquired disease (Pulsifer & Aylward, 2000).

### Incidence and Prevalence

In 2005, approximately 15,000 children and adolescents living in the United States were infected with either HIV or AIDS (Centers for Disease Control and Prevention [CDC], 2005), and most of these individuals were either African American or Hispanic, with the majority residing in metropolitan areas (CDC, 1998). Today, the majority (91%) of HIV-infected children acquired the disease from their mothers before or during birth, or through breastfeeding (i.e., vertical transmission; Lindegren, Steinberg, & Byers, 2000; Llorente, LoPresti, & Satz, 1997; Pulsifer & Aylward, 2000; Spiegel & Bonwit, 2002; Wolters, Brouwers, & Perez, 1999). With advances in research and treatment, a diagnosis of HIV/AIDS no longer means imminent death. In fact, many children with vertically acquired HIV infection and AIDS are now surviving into middle childhood, early adolescence, and beyond (American Academy of Pediatrics, 1999; Howland et al., 2000). According to the American Academy of Pediatrics (1999), the median life span for children with vertically acquired HIV infection has been reported to be between 8.6 and 13 years; between 36% and 61% of infants with vertically acquired HIV are expected to survive to the age of 13 years.

## Disease Classification

The CDC (1992) classifies children and adolescents with HIV/AIDS into three distinct groups based on T-cell count (i.e., white blood cells that contribute to the immune system response) and disease-related symptoms corresponding to the stage of illness, as can be seen in Table 11.1.

Notably, for younger children (less than 13 years of age), the degree of immune system compromise required to determine illness stage is based on the child's age (i.e., under 12 months, 1 to 5 years, 6 to 12 years) as well as symptom presentation (i.e., asymptomatic, mildly symptomatic, moderately symptomatic, severely symptomatic; CDC, 1994).

## Disease Progression

The progression of HIV infection to AIDS varies from child to child, with the median age of progression for children with vertically acquired HIV being 1.75 years of age (Pulsifer & Aylward, 2000). In addition, the age of onset of first symptoms (e.g., delayed milestones, opportunistic infections, cognitive impairment) appears to be related to the progression of the illness in children who acquired HIV through vertical transmission (Pulsifer & Aylward, 2000). Three general patterns of disease progression, based on the rate of active virus replication, have been observed in children and adolescents: (a) rapid progression; (b) steady, subacute progression; and (c) static progression (Report of the NIH panel to define principles of therapy of HIV infection, 1998). According to the National Pediatric and Family HIV Resource Center (1999), 20% of children progress rapidly from HIV to AIDS, 60% demonstrate a steady progression, and 20% have a slow progression.

**TABLE 11.1 Stages of HIV Illness**

| Stage | Characteristics | T-Cell Count |
|---|---|---|
| AIDS | Presence of an AIDS-defining opportunistic infection such as recurrent pneumonia, cytomegalovirus disease, or encephalopathy | Current or prior T-cell count below 200 |
| Symptomatic HIV | Presence of non-AIDS-defining illnesses such as splenomegaly (i.e., enlarged spleen), dermatitis, or recurrent or persistent upper respiratory infection | Current T-cell count above 200 |
| Asymptomatic HIV | No serious illness | Current T-cell count above 200 |

*Note.* This table has been adapted from Reger, Welsh, Razani, Martin, and Boone (2002).

HIV infection is associated with central nervous system (CNS) involvement (e.g., developmental delay, impaired cognition, language impairments, and motor difficulties) and changes in neurobehavioral status, particularly in advanced stages of the illness (Bornstein et al., 1992; Wolters et al., 1999). The degree and rate of CNS compromise is related to disease progression. Rapid progression is often characterized by severe and pervasive neuropsychological dysfunction (e.g., delayed acquisition of milestones, failure to thrive, intellectual impairment, motor dysfunction, language impairment, adaptive skills compromise) secondary to encephalopathy (Epstein et al., 1985; Llorente et al., 1997). Encephalopathy is often used in describing compromised CNS functioning related to HIV infection in children, although the term is also used loosely to refer to a decline in motor or mental status secondary to CNS disease process or involvement (e.g., cerebral atrophy, severe white matter degeneration; Brouwers et al., 1990). Children with rapidly progressing HIV often experience an onset of symptoms prior to their first birthday and often die before reaching their fifth birthday (Pulsifer & Aylward, 2000). Children who experience a steady disease progression may experience CNS compromise; however, the rate of encephalopathy is slower than for those with rapid progression (Llorente et al.). Developmental milestones are generally acquired at a slower pace compared to uninfected children, and intellectual functioning and motor skills are often impaired, although not to the degree observed in children with rapid progression (Belman et al., 1989; Pulsifer & Aylward). Finally, children with static disease progression demonstrate a steady acquisition of cognitive and motor skills, although not necessarily at a pace consistent with that of their typically developing peers (Pulsifer & Aylward), and their cognitive impairments are more subtle and less debilitating (Belman et al., 1985).

## Infections

Children with compromised immune systems are continuously at risk for developing infections. In addition to being at greater risk for developing life-threatening illnesses from common childhood viral (e.g., measles, chickenpox) and bacterial (e.g., sepsis, meningitis, pneumonia) infections (Burroughs & Edelson, 1991; Spiegel & Bonwit, 2002), HIV-infected children are at risk for opportunistic infections or illnesses that almost never occur in individuals with uncompromised immune systems (e.g., cytomegalovirus, toxoplasmosis of the brain, cryptococcal meningitis; National Institute of Allergy and Infectious Disease [NIAID], 2004; Spiegel & Bonwit, 2002), as well as more serious neurological complications (e.g., stroke, brain tumor; Brouwers, Moss, Wolters, & Schmitt, 1994; Wolters, et al., 1999). It is important to remain vigilant for signs of compromised immune functioning (e.g., recurring illnesses, opportunistic infections), as they are treatable and in some cases preventable.

## Medication and Adherence to Treatment

Although there is no cure for HIV/AIDS, advances in treatment, through the use of highly active antiretroviral therapy (HAART), have slowed the progression of HIV infection to AIDS (Palella et al., 1998) and improved neurodevelopment, cognitive functioning, and behavior in children and adolescents with HIV (Brouwers et al., 1990; Moss et al., 1994). HAART medications work to reduce viral loads to undetectable levels and maintain remission without interruption (American Psychiatric Association [APA], 2000). These drugs typically work by minimizing the virus replication process and by reducing the destruction of CD4+ cells, allowing the immune system to function more adequately, thereby slowing the progression of the disease (Koenig & Bachanas, 2006). Although these medications work to suppress replication, recent evidence suggests that they do not eradicate HIV from all parts of the body, particularly the lymphoid tissue and the brain (APA, 2000).

When taken properly, HAART can markedly slow the progression of HIV, thereby decreasing illness and death (Palella et al., 1998). However, as for children and adolescents with any chronic illness, treatment adherence is particularly challenging. Adherence is of the utmost concern with antiretroviral treatment because the regimens are strict and even minor deviations can result in viral resistance and permanent loss of efficacy for existing medications (APA, 2000). According to Paterson and colleagues (2000), HAART requires near perfect (95%) adherence to be effective, and when adherence drops below this level, there is less chance that the viral load will be properly controlled.

Adherence is difficult for several reasons, including the medication regimen (i.e., timing of doses, number of different medications), associated side effects, disclosure of medical status to schools and significant others to allow for support of the regimen, developmental level, and psychosocial factors. The medication schedules are often complex, requiring multiple medications to be taken at various times throughout the day, and most must be coordinated around complex dietary considerations for maximum efficacy (e.g., dietary fat restrictions, timing around meals). For example, it is not uncommon for an individual to be prescribed 15 to 20 different pills per day (Steele & Grauer, 2003). In addition, many medications have an unpleasant taste or may be formulated in sizes that are difficult to swallow (Steele & Grauer). Further, HAART can cause debilitating side effects including nausea, diarrhea, and significant fatigue. What makes adherence more challenging is that these medications are often prescribed prior to the onset of symptoms of HIV disease, and the child may feel more ill after the initiation of HAART than before starting it (Walsh, Horne, Dalton, Burgess, & Gazzard, 2001). Regarding disclosure, concerns exist that taking medications in public can possibly reveal HIV status. As such, children and adolescents may attempt to conceal the fact that they are taking medications. Developmentally, teens often feel invincible and immortal and may not realize the long-term consequences of poor adherence (La Greca, 1990).

## Disclosure

One of the most important and difficult decisions children with HIV and their families must make is whether to disclose HIV status to the school. The decision to inform school personnel of a child's HIV status is often associated with significant anxiety for the family, who must weigh the potential benefits of disclosure against the fear of discrimination or loss of privacy (Cohen et al., 1997). Because medical management of HIV plays such a large part in controlling the disease and sequelae, confidentiality becomes increasingly difficult to maintain as the disease progresses. In one study, the administration of medication in school was a strong predictor of whether the school was informed of the diagnosis. Families who chose not to disclose HIV status to school personnel had to arrange complex medication schedules to avoid administration during school hours (Cohen et al.).

In some cases, the infected child may not know about his or her HIV status. In most cases, the average age at disclosure is 8 years (Cohen et al., 1997). According to one study, over two-thirds of children ages 5 through 10 had not been told about their HIV status, whereas 1 in 20 children over 10 years old were not aware of their status (Cohen et al.). In the same study, approximately half (47%) of families had informed someone in the school of their child's disease status (Cohen et al.), and when disclosure occurred, school nurses (88%), principals (62%), and classroom teachers (47%), in that order, were the most likely to be informed about the child's status.

## COMORBID DISORDERS

In addition to the effects of HIV/AIDS on the developing brain, other factors, such as prenatal exposure to teratogenic (i.e., toxic) substances and poor prenatal care and nutrition, impact fetal brain development. For example, prenatal exposure to alcohol is associated with dysmorphology (i.e., congenital malformations such as small eye openings, thin upper lip, and flat or absent groove between nose and upper lip), growth retardation, and CNS impairment (i.e., intellectual impairment, developmental delay, neurological abnormality; Sokol & Clarren, 1989). Substance use and related environmental factors (e.g., impoverished environment, neglect, unstable living arrangements) may continue after the child is born, further contributing to the potential for atypical neurological development as well as social, emotional, and behavioral dysregulation. Impoverished environmental conditions can also disrupt the normal development of the CNS in children exposed to these conditions (Als et al., 2004), resulting in significant cognitive and behavioral dysfunction. A full discussion of these factors and their contribution to an already compromised neurological system is beyond the scope of this chapter.

## CASE CONTINUATION

In light of the information outlined above, a continuation of Robert's case is provided to elaborate on the residual impact of these physiological and environmental insults on the child's functioning across environments.

### Assessment Results

In the context of evaluating Robert, several notable behavioral observations were made. He was small in stature, and clear evidence of microcephaly (i.e., small head circumference) was noted, which contributed to him appearing younger than his chronological age. While Robert's motivation was consistent and appropriate, his ability to sustain attention was highly variable, and he was prone to impulsive responses and disinhibition. However, the highly structured and supportive assessment environment was beneficial in assisting with these difficulties. Robert's cognitive processing speed and motor reaction time were impaired, and he often required additional time to complete tasks. In addition, difficulties with executive function skills were evident, most notably surrounding working memory, especially on tasks that were more lengthy and complex. There was no qualitative evidence of communication difficulties, although some problems with fine motor control and dexterity were apparent, as were some gross motor alterations, specifically with gait, balance, and coordination.

Consistent with qualitative observations, Robert's neuropsychological profile was most notable for significant impairments in processing speed, attention and executive functions (e.g., working memory, self-monitoring, inhibitory control), and motor skills. Academically, his most notable impairment was in mathematics. These impairments are associated with his HIV and are consistent with the diagnosis of Cognitive Disorder Not Otherwise Specified (NOS) (see Table 11.2 for specific test scores). His impairments across domains suggest disrupted white matter, especially in the frontal and subcortical (i.e., basal ganglia) regions of the brain, as these regions are the substrates for processing speed, attention, executive functions, and motor abilities. Robert's atypical cortical development (as evidenced by his significant microcephaly), which is likely the result of his prenatal exposure to teratogenic substances, possible early neglect, and the natural course of his HIV, is consistent with the neuropsychological impairments demonstrated in his profile, as the regions associated with such impairments are the most susceptible to insult.

As with other children with HIV, Robert's language skills were demonstrated to be age appropriate, and he was able to communicate effectively, although he required extra time to formulate his thoughts and ideas due to slow processing abilities.

## INTERVENTIONS AND RESOURCES

An increasing number of children with vertically acquired HIV/AIDS are attending our national schools (Crocker, 1994). However, no empirically based guidelines or interventions have been established to assist children and families impacted by the disease. As described in detail above, HIV/AIDS is a complex medial condition, affecting multiple aspects of a child's life (e.g., medical, academic, socioemotional), and each of these facets must be considered when designing a curriculum for educating

**TABLE 11.2 Neuropsychological Testing Data**

| | Scaled Score | T Score | Standard Score |
|---|---|---|---|
| | Intellectual Functioning | | |
| DAS Global | | | 78 |
| Verbal | | | 84 |
| Nonverbal | | | 78 |
| | Adaptive Functioning | | |
| ABAS-II Global | | | 56 |
| Communication | 3 | | |
| Community Use | 1 | | |
| Functional Academics | 4 | | |
| Home Living | 2 | | |
| Health and Safety | 4 | | |
| Leisure | 5 | | |
| Self-Care | 4 | | |
| Self-Direction | 1 | | |
| Social | 1 | | |
| | Attention/Executive Functioning | | |
| TEA-Ch Score! | 5 | | |
| TEA-Ch Creature Counting | 8 | | |
| DAS Recall of Digits | | 44 | |
| D-KEFS Trails Visual Scanning | 7 | | |
| Trails Number Sequencing | 3 | | |
| Trails Letter Sequencing | 1 | | |
| Trails Number-Letter Switching | 1 | | |
| Trails Motor Speed | 3 | | |
| Tower Test Total Achievement | 9 | | |
| Tower Test Move Accuracy | 8 | | |
| Tower Test Rule Violations | 7 | | |

*Continued*

**TABLE 11.2** *(Continued)*

| | Scaled Score | T Score | Standard Score |
|---|---|---|---|
| BRIEF (Parent) | | | |
| Inhibit | | 50 | |
| Shift | | 63 | |
| Emotional Control | | 51 | |
| Initiate | | 62 | |
| Working Memory | | 80 | |
| Plan/Organize | | 67 | |
| Organization of Materials | | 63 | |
| Monitor | | 51 | |
| Learning /Memory | | | |
| CMS Stories Immediate | 3 | | |
| Stories Delay | 4 | | |
| Stories Delayed Recognition | 7 | | |
| Faces Immediate | 9 | | |
| Faces Delayed | 8 | | |
| DAS Recall of Objects—Immediate | | 29 | |
| Recall of Objects—Delayed | | 20 | |
| Language Functioning | | | |
| CELF-IV Concepts and Directions | 5 | | |
| CELF-IV Formulated Sentences | 7 | | |
| Fine Motor Functioning | | | |
| Grooved Pegboard (Left Hand) | | | 100 |
| Grooved Pegboard (Right Hand) | | | 96 |
| Hand Dynamometer (Left Hand) | | | <50 |
| Hand Dynamometer (Right Hand) | | | <50 |

**TABLE 11.2** *(Continued)*

| | Scaled Score | T Score | Standard Score |
|---|---|---|---|
| Academic skills | | | |
| WJ-III Letter-Word Identification | | | 96 |
| Calculation | | | 53 |
| Spelling | | | 88 |
| Applied Problems | | | 67 |
| Socioemotional Functioning | | | |
| BASC-2 (Parent) | | | |
| Hyperactivity | | 50 | |
| Aggression | | 62 | |
| Conduct Problems | | 84 | |
| Anxiety | | 38 | |
| Depression | | 53 | |
| Somatization | | 42 | |
| Atypicality | | 73 | |
| Withdrawal | | 69 | |
| Attention Problems | | 69 | |

*Note.* ABAS-II, Adaptive Behavior Assessment System—Second Edition (Harrison & Oakland, 2003); BASC-2, Behavior Assessment System for Children—Second Edition (Reynolds & Kamphaus, 2004); BRIEF, Behavior Rating Inventory of Executive Function (Gioia, Isquith, Guy, & Kenworthy, 2000); CELF-IV, Clinical Evaluation of Language Fundamentals—Fourth Edition (Semel, Wigg, & Secord, 2003); CMS, Children's Memory Scale (Cohen, 1997); DAS, Differential Ability Scales (Elliott, 1990); D-KEFS, Delis-Kaplan Executive Function System (Delis, Kaplan, & Kramer, 2001); TEA-Ch, Test of Everyday Attention for Children (Manly, Robertson, Anderson, & Nimmo-Smith, 1999); and WJ-III, Woodcock-Johnson Tests of Achievement – Third Edition (Woodcock, McGrew, & Mather, 2001).

children with HIV/AIDS. Schools and communities have the unique opportunity to not only provide educational support when needed, but also make school a safe and supportive environment by providing counseling; educating students, staff, and other members of the community about the virus; and reducing the stigma associated with the medical condition (Jones, 2006). The following guidelines are offered to combat the deleterious effects associated with HIV/AIDS:

1. Serial neuropsychological assessments should be completed to identify specific cognitive impairments and academic weaknesses, and

appropriate remediation and/or accommodations should be implemented (Llorente et al., 1997).

2. Confidentiality of HIV status should be maintained at all times and disclosed to members of the educational staff only with parental/guardian consent (Bogden, Vega-Matos, & Ascroft, 2001).
3. Procedures for medication administration should be outlined, taking precautions to ensure confidentiality (Fair, Garner-Edwards, & McLees-Lane, 2006).
4. Environmental risks (i.e., viral/bacterial or infectious disease outbreaks) should be communicated to families as early as possible so that appropriate treatment can be instituted (Jones, 2006; Spiegel & Mayers, 1991).
5. A mentor or counselor should be identified to assist/counsel students and their families through difficult situations (e.g., dying/death, teasing/bullying, depression, academic failure, etc.; Jones, 2006).
6. Staff education and in-service training should be offered and should include reliable information regarding transmission, prevention, civil rights, mental health, cognitive functioning, and death/bereavement.
7. Developmentally appropriate information regarding HIV/AIDS should be disseminated to students, delivered by trained teachers, health educators, or nurses, with the goal of influencing students' knowledge, feelings, attitudes, behavior, and acceptance with regard to people with HIV (Crocker, 1994).

Although impairments in intellectual functioning, attention, expressive language, motor skills, and behavior/adaptive skills have been readily observed in children with HIV, it is important to appreciate the degree of heterogeneity in the pediatric HIV/AIDS population (Llorente et al., 1997). Therefore, educational accommodations and placement should be determined on a case-by-case basis, via neuropsychological assessment, and continuously monitored to assess for ongoing appropriateness. It is important to keep in mind that even asymptomatic children and adolescents can demonstrate subtle neurocognitive deficits that can be identified through neuropsychological evaluations (Brouwers et al., 1994). Therefore, neuropsychological evaluations are considered an invaluable tool in early identification of such alterations. Specific goals for remediation and accommodation that are tailored to the student's strengths and weaknesses should be developed and outlined in an individualized education plan (IEP). These goals should be regularly reevaluated and updated as needed. Regular meetings with the child's parents/guardians should be conducted to help ensure that goals are being targeted both at home and school.

Environmental and family factors also contribute to a child's functioning and must be considered during the assessment and intervention process. All individuals with HIV/AIDS may face stressors associated with stigma, secrecy, frequent medical contacts, possible hospitalizations, and school absence. In addition, it is not uncommon for some children with HIV/AIDS to live in impoverished environments and/or unstable living arrangements and have to cope with the chronic illness or death of a parent. Given these stressors, it is not surprising that children and adolescents with HIV/AIDS are at high risk for social, emotional, and behavioral problems (Pulsifer & Aylward, 2000). Thus, environmental and family factors must be assessed continuously as part of an ecological approach to assessment and intervention.

## Academic Placement

As described above, accurate assessment of a child's neurocognitive profile and potential areas of impairment is essential for determining appropriate intervention and academic placement. Teaching should be tailored to the student's developmental level and pace, taking his or her strengths and weaknesses into consideration.

1. Children who demonstrate specific cognitive and academic weaknesses, such as Robert, should be considered for special education services under the Other Health Impairment (OHI) or Multiple Disabilities classification incorporating OHI and other relevant categories (e.g., Specific Learning Disability, Speech/Language Impairment, etc.). Students will benefit from interventions tailored to their unique strengths and weaknesses. For example, Robert would benefit from teaching strategies focused on executive functions, classroom interventions aimed to support attentional weaknesses, pull-out services for mathematics, and occupational therapy (OT) to address motor impairments.
2. Students with global cognitive impairments should be considered for special education services under the classification of Multiple Disabilities incorporating OHI and Mental Retardation. These students may perform best in highly structured, self-contained educational settings with a low student-to-teacher ratio (e.g., 5:1) that afford individualized (i.e., one-to-one) and/or small group support for prominent cognitive, language, motor, and behavioral needs. Additional pull-out services for OT and speech/language therapy may be necessary. Also, these children often benefit from extended school year (ESY) services to facilitate retention. This is especially true of children with an encephalopathic disease course, where regression is a risk.

## Processing Speed

Students with impaired processing abilities, such as Robert, often exhibit a significant disruption in their ability to process and respond to incoming information efficiently and effectively. Diminished processing speed not only exacerbates the appearance of attentional deficits but may also result in a loss of task-oriented behavior. In addition, such impairments may limit the amount of information a student can learn and retain at one time, and these children can easily fall behind. Further, compromised processing speed negatively impacts performance across academic domains including fluency and reading comprehension. Robert and other students with impaired processing abilities would benefit from the following accommodations:

1. Provision of additional time on all tasks, including tests and in-class assignments.
2. Modified homework assignments, which may include shortened assignments or altered projects.
3. Individualized support in order to monitor the student's progress and make adjustments accordingly. These students will often require repetition, as they have difficulty maintaining the pace of the instruction.

## Attention

Attention and executive functions are often compromised in even seemingly asymptomatic individuals (Brouwers, Moss, Wolters, Eddy, & Pizzo, 1989; Llorente et al., 1997), and difficulties in these areas become even more evident in the later stages of HIV (Wolters et al., 1999). Impaired attention often reduces an individual's availability for learning and, as such, interferes significantly with functional abilities across settings. The following recommendations can be useful in addressing such difficulties:

1. Increase the structure and support in the environment. Children with attentional weaknesses tend to perform best in highly structured environments. This may include having a set schedule and consistent patterns throughout the day, as the child will learn what to expect and when, which will minimize off-task behavior.
2. Preferential seating toward the front of the classroom, close to the teacher, and away from distracters (e.g., open doors and windows, disruptive classmates) can be beneficial. This will allow for monitoring of on-task behavior and the provision of subtle prompts (e.g., nonverbal signal, moving closer to the student, speaking to the student) to reengage the students.

3. Taking tests in a quiet environment that is free from distractions can also be beneficial. If auditory stimuli interfere with the ability to function, providing the students with earplugs to wear can help to facilitate attention to task.
4. Children and adolescents will benefit from brief breaks throughout the school day that allow them periodic out-of-seat movement (e.g., stretch time, taking notes to the office, getting a drink of water, bathroom breaks). This is an excellent way to support attention.
5. Older children and adolescents are encouraged to record lectures to review later and to compare their classroom notes with those of another classmate.
6. A homework diary to keep track of daily homework assignments may be beneficial. Teachers should work closely with their students to ensure that assignments are written down properly. Older children and adolescents are also encouraged to use a daily planner/organizer to keep track of daily activities, commitments, and study time.
7. Reinforcing on-task and appropriate behavior will promote appropriate future behavior in preschool. Children respond best when consequences and rewards are provided immediately and when positive behavior is reinforced consistently across environments. Extrinsic motivators, such as rewards (e.g., verbal praise, a smile, classroom privileges, line leading, passing out materials, free time), should be provided for completing assignments and behaving appropriately. It will be important to work with behavioral therapists to determine which reinforcers work best for each student.

## Executive Functioning

Executive functioning skills include initiation of problem solving, working memory, planning and organization, inhibitory control, and cognitive flexibility. The following recommendations are provided to address weaknesses in each of these areas (adapted from Gioia et al., 2000).

### *Initiation*

Slow initiation of problem solving can impact a child's ability to complete tasks in a timely manner. Although it may be difficult to decrease a child's response time, the following modifications may assist the child in completing work more efficiently:

1. Increasing support (prompting, modeling), structure (preplanning), and building routines can assist with initiation difficulties. This will increase the automaticity of various practices.

2. Creating checklists or "cookbooks" for certain activities can provide the student with the tools to get started, as the initial steps are already established, minimizing the demands on his/her ability to generate the strategy.
3. Children with initiation difficulties often feel overwhelmed, which can increase nervousness and worry surrounding performance, further limiting his/her ability to initiate the task. Helping the student break work or tasks down into manageable steps can reduce this problem.
4. Hands-on, active learning models often support difficulties with initiation, and attempts to utilize such teaching strategies can be beneficial.

*Working Memory*

Weaknesses in auditory and verbal working memory may be misinterpreted as inattention or poor receptive language. Although these deficits may be difficulty to remediate, accommodations can assist children in completing tasks.

1. Pre-teaching and organizational strategies can be highly beneficial for students with working memory difficulties. Exposing these students to information and tasks can minimize the impact of working memory abilities on their overall performance.
2. Avoiding open-ended questions (e.g., short-answer or essay questions) and utilizing recognition paradigms (e.g., true/false, multiple choice) is suggested. If open-ended questions are used, follow-up questions in the form of more structured questions (i.e., when, what, where, etc.) are also recommended to allow for a more accurate assessment of the students' knowledge.
3. Encourage self-talk or verbal mediation during tasks, as this is often beneficial for students who have difficulty holding information in mind during work periods.
4. Teaching mnemonic devices can be helpful in learning and recall for these students.

*Planning and Organization*

Without a plan to complete a complex task, students may waste time unnecessarily. Providing them with structure to set goals and determine progress is very important.

1. Encourage the student to participate in setting a goal for the activity or task, and ask him/her to predict the outcome. Assist

the student in planning and organizing approaches toward the stated goal.

2. Assist the students in getting an extra set of all textbooks to keep at home to minimize the impact of organizational difficulties, as these students tend to have difficulty remembering what materials are necessary for task completion.
3. Planning and organizing long-term projects or assignments tend to be particularly difficult for many of these students, and it can be beneficial to assist them by assigning the project in discrete segments, with interspersed deadlines.
4. Providing a consultation period with the teacher at the beginning of the day to help organize the day can be highly beneficial for these students.

### *Inhibitory Control*

It is very difficult for some children to inhibit impulsive behavior. Providing techniques that they can learn to increase response time will positively affect overall performance:

1. Teach response-delay techniques, such as counting to five before responding. Developing a visual cue (such as a stop sign) that can prompt the student to wait before responding can be helpful. Including the student in the development of such a cue will increase the likelihood of its success.
2. Ask the student to verbalize a plan prior to beginning work. This will provide a time buffer that may minimize impulsive responding and result in more accurate and efficient work.
3. Small group activities can be beneficial in providing the student with models and cues for focused and well-controlled behaviors.
4. Minimize involvement in unstructured activities, as these will increase the likelihood of impulsive behavior.

### *Cognitive Shifting and Flexibility*

As children age, greater demands are placed on their ability to shift between tasks and demonstrate cognitive flexibility. Not all children acquire these skills without training, and the following recommendations may assist in this process:

1. Increasing the consistency in the student's schedule can be beneficial in providing a predictable environment, which will foster

flexibility and shifting skills. Children with difficulty shifting can be expected to struggle with inconsistency and minimal structure.

2. Consider the provision of visual cues, such as organizers, schedules, or calendar boards, so the student can view the daily schedule and prepare for changes and shifts.
3. Establishing "routines for a change in routine" can be beneficial, in setting an alternative approach when the typical schedule is altered.
4. Attempt to minimize the presentation of multiple tasks or instructions at once, as students with difficulty shifting will struggle to manage such information or work.
5. Providing a "two-minute warning" is one of the most effective strategies for helping students who have difficulty shifting transition into alternate activities.

## Motor Functioning

Motor deficits are common in children with Robert's history. In fact, motor skills tend to be most vulnerable to disease progression due to the impact of HIV/AIDS on the basil ganglia (Fowler, 1994). Specific motor impairments typically include abnormalities in gait, strength, coordination, and muscle tone (Belman, 1994), most of which were observed with Robert. Recommendations to address motor weaknesses are outlined below:

1. Occupational and physical therapy are recommended to assist with motor impairments, in order to develop functional fine motor skills and balance and coordination that will be necessary in the academic environment. The therapists may also explore the use of devices to assist with writing (e.g., computer, slant board, etc.) and other activities that place high demands on motor functioning.
2. Graphomotor difficulties can lead to significant fatigue, which will exacerbate the student's already compromised processing and attentional systems, leaving him/her with fewer resources to learn and function adequately within the classroom. This also puts the student at greater risk of frustration and the use of maladaptive behaviors to cope with these experiences.
3. Students with compromised motor speed may benefit from reduced motor demands in the classroom. For example, students should not be required to handwrite assignments unless handwriting is the primary objective of the lesson. Instead, students should be allowed to type or dictate their responses.

4. In addition, students with graphomotor impairments would benefit from listening without having to take notes. Students should be allowed to tape-record lessons, annotate handouts, or photocopy notes from a classmate.

## Socioemotional and Behavior Management

Given the medical, social, and environmental stressors associated with HIV/AIDS, children and adolescents with the HIV virus are at significant risk for emotional and behavioral difficulties. In addition to the typical stressors associated with HIV/AIDS (e.g., stigma, complex medication regimen, frequent medical contacts, etc.), cognitive and academic impairments can result in significant emotional and behavioral sequelae. The student's emotional and behavioral functioning should be closely monitored and addressed when necessary. Specific recommendations are offered below:

1. Students living with HIV/AIDS will benefit from individual and group therapy. A supportive environment (e.g., teachers, counselors) is essential for children and adolescents living with HIV/AIDS.
2. In order to support the establishment of a positive academic experience, the formation of a relationship with a trusted mentor (i.e., school psychologist, counselor, teacher, etc.) within the school may be beneficial. The student would benefit from regular/unlimited access to mental health services within the academic environment.
3. Children and adolescents coping with HIV/AIDS may require assistance, through therapy, to learn novel coping mechanisms for addressing frustrating situations (e.g., teasing, rejection, academic failure). Students will benefit from learning a repertoire of coping skills to access when these feelings emerge. For example, teach and use concrete strategies for identifying and intervening with intense emotions, such as a "thermometer" for measuring the emotion, with specific interventions associated with various ratings.
4. Identify and manage antecedents to maladaptive behavior. This can be accomplished through a functional behavior assessment (FBA) and subsequent behavioral interventions.
5. Model appropriate emotional modulation and behavior. This may include talking through situations that provoke negative emotions and explaining how the feelings are being dealt with appropriately.

6. Provide cool-off periods when necessary, where the child can leave the stressful situation and have time to calm down. The student may be taught simple relaxation techniques by the counselor, such as diaphragmatic breathing or visualization, to use during these times.

## CONCLUSION

Youth of all ages with HIV/AIDS are in need of early identification and intervention. Manifestations of HIV-related CNS disease are variable and may range from subtle weaknesses in one or two domains, such as attention and motor skills, to global cognitive impairment. In addition, social, emotional, and behavioral dysregulation are common in children and adolescents with HIV/AIDS (Pulsifer & Aylward, 2000). Effective prevention programs (e.g., school-based education, prenatal counseling) and multimodal intervention programs that are tailored to meet the unique needs of each HIV-infected individual are essential. School personnel are in the unique position to play a crucial role in coordinating interdisciplinary services for individuals with HIV and their families. By facilitating suitable interventions, school personnel can substantially improve expected long-term outcomes for children and adolescents with HIV/AIDS.

## RESOURCES

### Books

Algozzine, R. F., & Ysseldyke, J. E. (1996). *Teaching students with medical, physical, and multiple disabilities: A practical guide for every teacher (A practical approach to special education for every teacher).* Thousand Oaks, CA: Corwin Press.

Bartlett, J. G., & Finkbeiner, A. K. (2001). *The guide to living with HIV infection: Developed at the Johns Hopkins AIDS Clinic.* Baltimore: Johns Hopkins University Press.

Best, A., Wiener, L. S., & Pizzo, P. A. (1996). *Be a friend: Children who live with HIV speak.* Morton Grove, IL: Albert Whitman & Company.

Forbes, A. (1997). *AIDS Awareness Library.* New York: Rosen.

Lyon, M. E., & D'Angelo, L. J. (Eds.). (2006). *Teenagers, HIV, and AIDS: Insights from youths living with the virus (Sex, love, and psychology).* Westport, CT: Praeger.

Merrifield, M. (1998). *Come sit by me* (2nd ed.). Markham, Ontario, Canada: Fitzhenry & Whiteside.

Roberts, J., & Cairns, K. (1999). *School children with HIV/AIDS: Quality of life experience in public schools.* Calgary, Alberta, Canada: Detselig Enterprises.

Shore, K. (2006). *Special kids problem solver: Ready-to-use interventions for helping all students with academic, behavioral and physical problems.* Paramus, NJ: Prentice Hall.

Wiener, L. S., & Pizzo, P. A. (1994). *Be a friend: Children who live with HIV speak.* Washington, DC: Magination Press.

## Organizations and Web Sites

AIDS Alliance for Children, Youth, & Families

This is a nonprofit group dedicated to addressing the concerns of children, women, and families affected by HIV/AIDS.

Mailing Address: 1600 K Street NW, Suite 200
Washington, D.C. 20006
Phone Number: (888) 917-AIDS
Web Site: www.aids-alliance.org

AVERT

This group provides AIDS and HIV information, including information about HIV/AIDS infection, HIV testing, prevention, global and African information, AIDS treatment, statistics, and personal stories.

Mailing Address: 4 Brighton Road
Horsham, West Sussex
RH13 5BA
United Kingdom
Web Site: www.avert.org

The Body

This organization provides extensive information and resources about HIV/AIDS.

Web Site: www.thebody.com

Centers for Disease Control and Prevention (CDC) National AIDS Clearinghouse

The CDC National Prevention Information Network (NPIN) provides information regarding the most recent activities, news, or publications about HIV/AIDS prevention, the current state of the epidemic in the United States, and the current CDC guidelines and recommendations for the detection, treatment, and care of HIV/AIDS.

Phone Number: (800) 458-5231
Web Site: www.cdcnpin.org

Child Welfare Information Gateway

Child Welfare Information Gateway promotes the safety, permanency, and well-being of families by connecting child welfare, adoption, and related professionals as well as concerned citizens to timely, essential information.

Mailing Address: 1250 Maryland Avenue SW
Washington, D.C. 20024

Phone Number: (800) 394-3366
Web Site: www.childwelfare.gov

Elizabeth Glaser Pediatric AIDS Foundation

The Elizabeth Glaser Pediatric AIDS Foundation is an organization dedicated to identifying, funding, and conducting basic pediatric HIV/AIDS research.

Phone Number: (888) 499-HOPE
Web Site: www.pedaids.org

National Institute of Health Office of AIDS Research (OAR)

The NIH OAR is responsible for the scientific, budgetary, legislative, and policy elements of the NIH AIDS research program.

Web Site: www.oar.nih.gov

National Pediatric AIDS Network (NPAN)

The NPAN provides information about HIV/AIDS from preconception through adolescents.

Mailing Address: P.O. Box 1032
Boulder, Colorado 80306
Phone Number: (800) 646-1001
Web Site: www.npan.org

Positive Life

This Web site provides information in an effort to improve the quality of life for youth as it pertains to HIV/AIDS.

Web Site: www.positivelife.net

Ryan White Foundation

This Web site provides stories told by Ryan White and his family about their personal struggles dealing with HIV.

Web Site: ryanwhite.com

Youth and HIV

This organization provides information about the global HIV/AIDS epidemic.

Web Site: youthandhiv.org

## REFERENCES

Als, H., Duffy, F. H., McAnulty, G. B., Rivkin, M. J., Vajapeyam, S., Mulkern, R. V., et al. (2004). Early experience alters brain function and structure. *Pediatrics, 113,* 846–857.

American Academy of Pediatrics. (1999). Disclosure of illness status to children and adolescents with HIV infection. *Pediatrics, 103,* 164–166.

American Psychiatric Association (APA). (2000). Practice guidelines for the treatment of patients with HIV/AIDS. *American Journal of Psychiatry, 157,* 1–62.

Belman, A. L. (1994). HIV-1-associated CNS disease in infants and children. In R. W. Price & S. W. Perry (Eds.), *HIV, AIDS, and the brain* (pp. 289–310). New York: Raven Press.

Belman, A. L., Diamond, G., Park, Y., Nozyce, M., Douglas, C., Cabot, T., et al. (1989). Perinatal HIV infection: A prospective longitudinal study of the initial CNS signs. *Neurology, 39,* S278–S279.

Belman, A. L., Ultmann, M. H., Horoupian, D., Novick, B., Spiro, A. J., Rubinstein, A., et al. (1985). Neurological complications in infants and children with acquired immune deficiency syndrome. *Annals of Neurology, 18,* 560–566.

Bogden, J. F., Vega-Matos, C. A., & Ascroft, J. (2001). *Someone at school has AIDS: A complete guide to education policies concerning HIV infection.* Alexandria, VA: National Association of State Boards of Education.

Bornstein, R. A., Nasrallah, H. A., Para, M. F., Whitacre, C. C., Rosenberger, P., Fass, R. J., et al. (1992). Neuropsychological performance in asymptomatic HIV infection. *Journal of Neuropsychiatry and Clinical Neurosciences, 4,* 336–394.

Brouwers, P., Moss, H., Wolters, P., Eddy, J., Balis, F., Poplack, D., et al. (1990). Effect of continuous infusion zidovudine therapy on neuropsychological functioning in children with symptomatic human immunodeficiency virus infection. *Journal of Pediatrics, 117,* 980–985.

Brouwers, P., Moss, H., Wolters, P., Eddy, J., & Pizzo, P. (1989). Neuropsychological profile of children with symptomatic HIV infection prior to antiretroviral therapy [Abstract]. *Proceedings from the V International Conference on AIDS, 1,* 316.

Brouwers, P., Moss, H., Wolters, P., & Schmitt, F. A. (1994). Developmental deficits and behavioral change in pediatric AIDS. In I. Grant & A. Martin (Eds.), *Neuropsychology of HIV infections* (pp. 310–338). New York: Oxford University Press.

Burroughs, M. H., & Edelson, P. J. (1991). Medical care of the HIV-infected child. *Pediatric Clinics of North America, 38,* 45–67.

Centers for Disease Control and Prevention (CDC). (1992). 1993 revised classification system for HIV infection and expanded surveillance case definition for AIDS among adolescents and adults. *Morbidity and Mortality Weekly Report, 41,* 1–19.

Centers for Disease Control and Prevention (CDC). (1994). 1994 revised classification system for human immunodeficiency virus infection in children less than 13 years of age. *Morbidity and Mortality Weekly Report, 43,* 1–10.

Centers for Disease Control and Prevention (CDC). (1998). *HIV/AIDS Surveillance Report, 10*(2), 1–43.

Centers for Disease Control and Prevention (CDC). (2005). *HIV/AIDS Surveillance Report, 17,* 1–54.

Cohen, J., Reddington, C., Jacobs, D., Meade, R., Picard, D., Singelton, K., et al. (1997). School-related issues among HIV-infected children. *Pediatrics, 100,* 8–12.

Cohen, M. J. (1997). *Children's Memory Scale.* New York: The Psychological Corporation.

Crocker, A. C. (1994). Supports for children with HIV infection in school: Best practices guidelines. *Journal of School Health, 64,* 32–38.

Delis, D., Kaplan, E., & Kramer, J. (2001). *The Delis-Kaplan Executive Function System: Examiner's manual.* San Antonio, TX: The Psychological Corporation.

Elliott, C. D. (1990). *Differential Ability Scales: Administration and scoring manual.* San Antonio, TX: The Psychological Corporation.

Epstein, L. G., Sharer, L. R., Joshi, V. V., Fogas, M. M., Koenigsberger, M. R., & Oleske, J. M. (1985). Progressive encephalopathy in children with acquired immune deficiency syndrome. *Annals of Neurology, 17,* 488–496.

Fair, C., Garner-Edwards, D., & McLees-Lane, M. (2006). Assessment of HIV-related school policy in North Carolina. *Journal of HIV/AIDS and Social Services: Research, Practice, and Social Policy, 4,* 47–63.

Fowler, M. G. (1994). Pediatric HIV infection: Neurologic and neuropsychological findings. *Acta Paediatrica, Supplement, 400, 59–62.*

Gioia, G. A., Isquith, P. K., Guy, S. C., & Kenworthy, L. (2000). *The Behavior Rating Inventory of Executive Function professional manual.* Odessa, FL: Psychological Assessment Resources.

Harrison, P. L., & Oakland, T. (2003). *Adaptive Behavior Assessment System* (2nd ed.). San Antonio, TX: The Psychological Corporation.

Howland, L. C., Gortmaker, S. L., Mofenson, L. M., Spino, C., Gardner, J. D., Gorski, H., et al. (2000). Effects of negative life events on immune suppression in children and youth infected with human immunodeficiency virus type 1. *Pediatrics, 106,* 540–546.

Jones, R. (2006). *Living with HIV/AIDS: Students tell their stories of stigma, courage, and resilience.* Alexandria, VA: National School Boards Association.

Koenig, L. J., & Bachanas, P. J. (2006). Adherence to medications for HIV: Teens say "Too many, too big, too often." In M. E. Lyon & L. J. D'Angelo (Eds.), *Teenagers, HIV, and AIDS: Insights from youths living with the virus (Sex, love, and psychology)* (pp. 45–65). Westport, CT: Praeger.

La Greca, A. M. (1990). Issues in adherence with pediatric regimens. *Journal of Pediatric Psychology, 15,* 423–436.

Lindegren, M. L., Steinberg, S., & Byers, R. H. (2000). Epidemiology of HIV/AIDS in children. *Pediatric Clinical Neuropsychology in America, 47,* 1–20.

Llorente, A. M., LoPresti, C. M., & Satz, P. (1997). Neuropsychological and neurobehavioral sequelae associated with pediatric HIV infection. In C. Reynolds & E. Fletcher-Janzen (Eds.), *Handbook of clinical child neuropsychology* (2nd ed., pp. 634–650). New York: Plenum Press.

Manly, T., Robertson, I. H., Anderson, V., & Nimmo-Smith, I. (1999). *The Test of Everyday Attention for Children: Manual.* Bury St. Edmunds, England: Thames Valley Test Company.

Moss, H. A., Brouwers, P., Wolters, P. L., Wiener, L., Hersh, S., & Pizzo, P. A. (1994). The development of a Q-sort behavioral rating procedure for pediatric HIV patients. *Journal of Pediatric Psychology, 19,* 27–46.

National Institute of Allergy and Infectious Disease (NIAID). (2004). *HIV infection in infants and children, NIAID fact sheet.* Bethesda, MD: National Institutes of Health, U.S. Department of Health and Human Services. Retrieved April 19, 2007, from http://www.niaid.nih.gov/factsheets/hivchildren.htm

National Pediatric and Family HIV Resource Center. (1999). *Infants, children, and HIV: Just the facts.* Retrieved April 1, 2007, from http://www.thebody.com/content/art5973.html

Palella, F. J., Delaney, K. M., Moorman, A. C., Loveless, M. O., Fuhrer, J., Satten, G., et al. (1998). Declining morbidity and mortality among patients with advanced human immunodeficiency virus infection. *New England Journal of Medicine, 338,* 853–860.

Paterson, D. L., Swindells, S., Mohr, J., Brester, M., Vergis, E., Squier, C., et al. (2000). Adherence to protease inhibitory therapy and outcomes in patients with HIV infection. *Annals of Internal Medicine, 133,* 21–30.

Pulsifer, M. B., & Aylward, E. H. (2000). Human immunodeficiency virus. In K. O. Yeates, M. D. Ris, & H. G. Taylor (Eds.), *Pediatric neuropsychology: Research, theory, and practice* (pp. 381–402). New York: Guilford Press.

Reger, M., Welsh, R., Razani, J., Martin, D. J., & Boone, K. B. (2002). A meta-analysis of the neuropsychological sequelae of HIV infection. *Journal of the International Neuropsychology Society, 8,* 410–424.

Report of the NIH Panel to define principles of therapy of HIV infection. (1998). *Annals of Internal Medicine, 128,* 1057–1078.

Reynolds, C., & Kamphaus, R. W. (2004). *Behavior Assessment System for Children, Parent Rating Scale* (2nd ed.). Circle Pines, MN: American Guidance Services.

Semel, E., Wigg, E. H., & Secord, W. A. (2003). *Clinical Evaluation of Language Fundamentals* (4th ed.). San Antonio, TX: The Psychological Corporation.

Sokol, R. J., & Clarren, S. K. (1989). Guidelines for use of terminology describing the impact of prenatal alcohol on the offspring. *Alcoholism: Clinical and Experimental Research, 13,* 597–598.

Spiegel, H. M., & Bonwit, A. M. (2002). HIV infection in children. In M. Batshaw (Ed.), *Children with disabilities* (5th ed., pp. 123–139). Washington, DC: Brookes.

Spiegel, H., & Mayers, A. (1991). Psychosocial aspects of AIDS in children and adolescents. *Pediatric Clinics of North America, 38,* 153–167.

Steele, R. G., & Grauer, D. (2003). Adherence to antiretroviral therapy for pediatric HIV infection: Review of the literature and recommendations for research. *Clinical Child and Family Psychology Review, 6,* 17–30.

Walsh, C., Horne, R., Dalton, M., Burgess, A. P., & Gazzard, B. G. (2001). Reasons for non-adherence to antiretroviral therapy: Patients' perspectives provide evidence of multiple causes. *AIDS Care, 13,* 709–720.

Wolters, P. L., Brouwers, P., & Perez, L. A. (1999). Pediatric HIV infection. In R. T. Brown (Ed.), *Cognitive aspects of chronic illness in children* (pp. 105–141). New York: Guilford Press.

Woodcock, R. W., McGrew, K. S., & Mather, N. (2001). *Woodcock-Johnson Tests of Achievement* (3rd ed.). Rolling Meadows, IL: Riverside.

CHAPTER TWELVE

# Hydrocephalus

Peter L. Stavinoha, PhD, and
Sarah Schnoebelen, PhD

## DESCRIPTION OF THE DISORDER

The term *hydrocephalus* comes from the Greek words *hydro*, meaning water, and *cephalus*, meaning head, and describes the excessive accumulation of cerebrospinal fluid (CSF) in the brain. It generally is defined as occurring when there is dilation in some part of the ventricle system secondary to an increase in CSF (Young & Young, 1997). In order to understand the mechanisms that lead to hydrocephalus, a basic understanding of the ventricular system in the brain is necessary. The ventricular system is composed of four hollow cavities (i.e., ventricles) interconnected by channels (i.e., foramen), through which CSF circulates. CSF is a colorless, clear fluid that is produced by a structure called the choroid plexus, located in the ventricles. CSF has several important functions, including protecting the brain by cushioning it from shock, delivering nutrients, removing waste products, and transmitting biochemicals that regulate overall functioning of the central nervous system. Hydrocephalus can be present congenitally (i.e., at birth) or acquired, and a variety of medical conditions occurring at multiple points of development may result in hydrocephalus. Therefore, hydrocephalus itself is not considered to be a specific disease entity.

## Symptoms

Presenting symptoms secondary to increased intracranial pressure (ICP) caused by excessive CSF vary based on age and etiology. Infants tolerate CSF pressure differently than adults as the sutures connecting the bones of the skull have not yet closed and can expand to accommodate the increasing CSF. Therefore, among the most common symptoms of hydrocephalus in infants is an atypically large head size or unusual acceleration in head growth. Other indicators include vomiting, sleepiness, irritability, and seizures. There may also be a downward deviation of the eyes, often referred to as "sunsetting." Older children are more likely to experience headache, vomiting, nausea, papilledema (i.e., swelling of the optic nerve), blurred vision, and diplopia (i.e., double vision), as well as the sunsetting described above. Disturbances in balance, coordination, and gait, as well as urinary incontinence and lethargy, are often noted. Furthermore, personality and cognitive changes may occur (National Institute of Neurological Disorders and Stroke [NINDS], 2005).

## Incidence, Prevalence, and Etiology

There are two primary types of hydrocephalus, obstructive (noncommunicating) and communicating. In obstructive hydrocephalus, a blockage of CSF drainage occurs at some point in the ventricle system. Many disorders associated with neural tube deficits, such as spina bifida, are associated with obstructive hydrocephalus. Furthermore, obstructive hydrocephalus may be present in cases of brain tumor, especially brain stem or posterior fossa tumors, as well as aqueductal stenosis, which is the narrowing of the cerebral aqueduct connecting the third and fourth ventricles. In communicating hydrocephalus, the blockage of CSF flow occurs after the CSF leaves the ventricles or, alternatively, secondary to an increased production of CSF or a reduction of normal absorption of CSF. For example, some tumors, such as choroid plexus papillomas and choroid plexus carcinomas, result in excessive secretion of CSF (Eisenberg, McComb, & Lorenzo, 1974; Ghatak & McWhorter, 1976). In children, communicating hydrocephalus accounts for approximately 30% of the cases; the remaining cases are obstructive (Menkes & Till, 1995).

In addition, two other terms have commonly been utilized to describe hydrocephalus. *Arrested hydrocephalus* refers to cases in which, after a period of increased ICP, equilibrium has been established in the ventricular system, either surgically or spontaneously, and no further accumulation of CSF occurs (Menkes & Till, 1995). Terms such as *compensated* or *nonprogressive* hydrocephalus also are often utilized to describe this situation (Fletcher, Dennis, & Northrup, 2000). *Normal pressure hydrocephalus* is another term seen in the literature. Although historically thought to be present primarily in elderly patients and associated with dementia, gait problems, and incontinence, some authors argue that a better description of this term is *chronic hydrocephalus*, indicative of an active but slowly progressing process that is also present in childhood (Bret, Guyotat, & Chazal, 2002). When all causes of hydrocephalus are considered, the prevalence of this condition is estimated to be approximately 1 in every 500 children (NINDS, 2005).

## Medical Conditions Associated With Hydrocephalus

### *Congenital Cases*

For those children who are identified as hydrocephalic in infancy, common etiologies include neural tube defects, Dandy-Walker syndrome, and aqueductal stenosis (Fletcher et al., 2000). The most frequently encountered neural tube defect is spina bifida meningomyelocele. *Spina bifida* refers to any congenital condition in which the bones of the spine are not properly closed. The most severe type of spina bifida is meningomyelocele, in which the spinal cord protrudes through the spinal column. Hydrocephalus is present in at least 75% of children diagnosed with this condition (Reigel & Rotenstein, 1994), generally secondary to the Chiari Type II malformation (i.e., a structural malformation marked by reduced size of the indented space in the skull in which the cerebellum resides, which results in the downward displacement of part of the cerebellum and brain stem into the spinal cavity, which subsequently obstructs the flow of CSF). Additional information about spina bifida can be obtained by reading the respective chapter in this volume.

Dandy-Walker syndrome is another congenital brain malformation thought to be due to neural tube closure failure and also is frequently associated with hydrocephalus (Menkes & Till, 1995). This condition is rare, with an estimated incidence of 1 per 25,000 to 35,000 births (Hirsch, Pierre-Kahn, Renier, Sainte-Rose, & Hoppe-Hirsch, 1984). Dandy-Walker syndrome is characterized by full or partial agenesis (i.e., failure or lack of development) of the cerebellar vermis, dilation of the fourth ventricle, and enlargement of the posterior fossa. Full or partial agenesis of the corpus callosum also is frequently present. Approximately 75% to 80% of children with this condition develop hydrocephalus (Menkes & Till).

### *Acquired Cases*

Prematurity and very low birth weight are risk factors for intraventricular hemorrhage (i.e., bleeding inside or around the ventricles), which can occur with varying degrees of severity. In some cases, the blood products filling the ventricles may cause blockage of CSF. Infections, such as meningitis, also can produce communicating hydrocephalus as a result of the buildup of fluids. Trauma, either accidental or nonaccidental (e.g., shaken baby syndrome), may result in hydrocephalus. In these cases, hematomas (i.e., collection of blood secondary to hemorrhage) may compress the cerebral aqueduct or other areas of the ventricular system (Karasawa et al., 1997). As indicated previously, a rare type of tumor, the choroid plexus papilloma, which generally occurs in young children (Pencalet et al., 1998), may result in hydrocephalus. In these cases, overproduction of CSF is often observed (Eisenberg et al., 1974; Ghatak & McWhorter, 1976), and, on occasion, blockage of the ventricle system occurs secondary to the direct impact of the tumor mass (Pencalet et al.).

## Treatment

Although medications are occasionally used in a temporary fashion in an attempt to decrease edema or CSF production, progressive hydrocephalus often requires neurosurgery. Shunting is a neurosurgical technique utilized to bypass the obstruction of CSF and allow for fluid draining and a reduction and maintenance of ICP. A common procedure used in pediatric cases is the ventriculoperitoneal shunt (commonly referred to as a VPS or VP shunt), which involves the placement of a catheter from the lateral ventricle to the peritoneal (i.e., abdominal) cavity (Drake & Iantosca, 2001). A valve controls the flow of CSF. One of the primary risks associated with shunt placement is infection, which is generally reported to occur in approximately 10% of all shunt procedures (Duhaime, 2006). Furthermore, a high percentage of children require shunt revisions due to infection, disconnection, or blockage, with nearly two-thirds of the sample in a Swedish study requiring at least one additional procedure (Persson, Hagberg, & Uvebrant, 2005). Endoscopic third ventriculostomy (ETV) is a newer technique that involves surgically creating a small hole in the floor of the third ventricle, which allows for CSF to be diverted away from the obstruction.

## Factors Affecting Neuropsychological Outcome

Hydrocephalus produces diffuse damage in both cortical and subcortical regions (Erickson, Baron, & Fantie, 2001), although there is some suggestion that the more posterior regions of the brain may be affected to a greater degree in childhood hydrocephalus (Fletcher, McCauley, et al., 1996) because the occipital horns, located at the posterior portion of the lateral ventricles, may dilate at a faster rate than other parts of the system (Brann, Qualls, Wells, & Papile, 1991) and result in compression and, ultimately, gray matter death (Fletcher, McCauley, et al.). The gray matter of the brain is composed of the nerve cell bodies, whereas white matter is formed by the myelinated axons of the neurons, which allow for transmission of impulses between neurons. A recent imaging study using diffusion tensor imaging (DTI), a technique that measures the characteristics of white matter, was suggestive of compression of white matter tracts in the brain in acute hydrocephalus (Assaf, Ben-Sira, Constantini, Chang, & Beni-Adani, 2006).

As has been highlighted in the literature, much of the research done in children with hydrocephalus has included participants with congenital forms of the condition, such as spina bifida myelomeningocele, or has utilized heterogeneous groups in which a variety of etiologies are represented (Erickson et al., 2001). Therefore, some caution must be taken in reviewing the literature and generalizing the findings to cases of hydrocephalus with different etiologies. In addition, the course and outcome of hydrocephalus are influenced by factors such as age of onset, length of time of increased ICP, and the rate at which ICP rises, as well as the presence of any other brain abnormalities (Menkes & Till, 1995). For example, research suggests that infants demonstrate more rapid neurological decline than do older children, who face a slower progression (Pollack, Pang, Albright, & Krieger, 1992). Furthermore, it is generally thought that acute hydrocephalus, which is identified and treated immediately, may result in limited neurocognitive morbidity (Ris & Noll, 1994).

For the purposes of this chapter, the most commonly reported neurocognitive deficits in school-age children will be outlined; however, as indicated above, a number of factors are thought to shape the neurocognitive profile of any given child based on their specific presentation. For more comprehensive treatment of neurocognitive deficits in this population and various influencing factors, such as age and etiology, the reader is referred to the review by Erickson and colleagues (2001).

## Common Neuropsychological Findings

Many children with hydrocephalus obtain overall IQ scores in the average range on standardized testing; however, the scores appear to be skewed downward, with many children performing in the low average range and a higher-than-expected percentage of children scoring in the below-average range (e.g., Friedrich, Lovejoy, Shaffer, Shurtleff, & Beilke, 1991; Hirsch, 1992; McCullough & Balzer-Martin, 1982; McLone, Czyzewski, Raimondi, & Sommers, 1982), although the level of intellectual functioning may depend on the etiology of the hydrocephalus. Perhaps the most frequently cited neurocognitive finding in children with hydrocephalus is a profile of better developed verbal than nonverbal reasoning abilities (e.g., Dennis et al., 1981; Donders, Rourke, & Canady, 1991; Fletcher et al., 1992; Ito et al., 1997; Riva et al., 1994; Wills, 1993). Such a pattern has been attributed to the effect of greater involvement of the posterior brain, the region that is associated with visual-spatial functioning, as well as the diffuse white matter deficits described above. However, as noted by Fletcher and colleagues (2000), studies reporting group averages do not tell the whole story, as some research suggests that reliance on the verbal-performance distinction correctly categorizes only half of the cases of treated hydrocephalus and that such a discrepancy may not be a consistent finding over time for many children (Brookshire et al., 1995).

Although the finding of relatively preserved verbal skills on standardized intelligence measures may suggest that language functioning is intact in children with hydrocephalus, subtle deficits do appear to exist. Some of these children have been portrayed as exhibiting "cocktail party" speech (coined by Hadenius, Hagberg, Hyttnes-Bensch, & Sjogren, 1962, as cited in Tew, 1979). This language pattern has been characterized by fluent, well-articulated speech but superficial usage of words and evidence of a lack of understanding of some words or phrases. Children with hydrocephalus have been found to display poor comprehension of both written language (Barnes & Dennis, 1992) and oral language (Barnes & Dennis, 1998), and Barnes and Dennis note that these difficulties are not a result of generalized linguistic deficits but rather represent a particular difficulty in determining meaning from context. Specifically, making inferences based on reading material is difficult for these children, as is the interpretation of novel idioms (Barnes & Dennis, 1998; Dennis & Barnes, 1993). Therefore, children with hydrocephalus may exhibit intact basic vocabulary and word-reading skills but struggle with higher order aspects of language comprehension and inferential reasoning. Although they may demonstrate good verbal fluency, the actual amount of content they produce in written or oral discourse may be below average (Barnes & Dennis, 1998).

Associated with the commonly observed deficits on nonverbal intellectual tasks are visual-perceptual and visual-motor integration problems (e.g., Brookshire et al., 1995; Donders et al., 1991; Fletcher et al., 1992, 1997; Friedrich et al., 1991; Sandler, Macias, & Brown, 1993). Furthermore, a variety of simple motor deficits have been observed in this population (Hetherington & Dennis, 1999). Therefore, visual-spatial deficits are likely to be observed in tasks with and without a motor demand. Considering that these basic deficits are coupled with fine motor difficulties, everyday academic tasks, such as handwriting, may be impaired. As indicated above, imaging research has suggested that the posterior areas of the brain may be more affected in hydrocephalus than the anterior regions, and imaging studies have observed relationships between relatively greater CSF accumulation in the posterior brain regions and poorer performance on nonverbal and motor measures (Fletcher, McCauley, et al., 1996). A recent study examining visual-perceptual deficits in children with hydrocephalus and spina bifida found that these children demonstrated greater difficulties on "action-based" visual tasks such as mental rotation and figure-ground discrimination than "object-based" tasks such as facial recognition and line orientation (Dennis, Fletcher, Rogers, Hetherington, & Francis, 2002). The authors suggested that such deficits may make it difficult for children with hydrocephalus to build "situation models," which, in turn, may contribute to the observed language difficulties secondary to inefficiencies in creating a mental representation, or model, of what they are reading or hearing in order to make an appropriate inference.

Other neuropsychological functions, including memory, attention, executive functioning, and processing speed, also have been studied in this population. Although earlier research revealed a pattern of conflicting results regarding performance on memory tests (for a review, see Wills, 1993), more recent studies have found deficits in verbal learning and memory (Yeates, Enrile, Loss, Blumenstein, & Delis, 1995), as well as more pervasive encoding and retrieval deficits across measures of verbal and nonverbal memory (Scott et al., 1998) in children with shunted hydrocephalus. Problems with working memory, or the ability to hold information "on line" in one's mind while performing some operation or manipulation with that information, also have been observed (Boyer, Yeates, & Enrile, 2006).

Attentional difficulties have frequently been reported in children with hydrocephalus (Brewer, Fletcher, Hiscock, & Davidson, 2001; Fletcher, Brookshire, et al., 1996; Loss, Yeates, & Enrile, 1998), and these difficulties sometimes appear to persist even when tasks minimizing motor requirements are utilized (Brewer et al., 2001), although this is not a universal finding (Fletcher, Brookshire, et al.). In particular, difficulties in the focusing or orientating of attention, functions thought to be mediated by posterior brain networks, as opposed to the sustaining of attention, have been observed (Brewer et al.). A recent study found that attention-deficit/hyperactivity disorder (ADHD) tends to occur in slightly more than 30% of children with spina bifida and hydrocephalus, a much higher percentage than that found in the general population (Burmeister et al., 2005). The presentation of these children was observed to be marked in general by inattentiveness, distractibility, and disorganization as opposed to impulsivity and hyperactivity (Burmeister et al.).

Problems with executive functioning, the group of skills and processes that allow an individual to set an appropriate goal, develop organized plans for goal achievement, implement these plans and evaluate their effectiveness, and switch strategy as necessary, have been reported, although the impairment does not appear to be uniform across all types of executive functioning. Research suggests that children with hydrocephalus may have difficulty forming concepts, maintaining set, and solving problems (Fletcher, Brookshire, et al., 1996). On self- and parent-report behavioral rating scales measuring executive functioning in "real life," adolescents and their parents endorsed executive dysfunction (Mahone, Zabel, Levey, Verda, & Kinsman, 2002). Some researchers have suggested that the particular profile of executive functioning assets and deficits is consistent with problems with arousal and orientation of attention due to posterior brain involvement as opposed to executive deficits (e.g., perseveration) commonly detected in individuals with frontal lobe injuries (Burmeister et al., 2005; Fletcher, Brookshire, et al., 1996). Furthermore, deficits in information processing speed have been described in children and adolescents presenting with hydrocephalus (e.g., Boyer et al., 2006; Jacobs, Northam, & Anderson, 2001).

In general, the assessment of academic skills in this population has consistently indicated difficulties in arithmetic, and it has been observed that children with hydrocephalus may be more likely to make math procedural errors (e.g., Ayr, Yeates, & Enrile, 2005; Barnes et al., 2002). Furthermore, although basic word recognition and word-decoding skills are often preserved in individuals with hydrocephalus, as indicated previously, reading comprehension is frequently impaired (Barnes & Dennis, 1992). In many ways, the particular profile of strengths and weaknesses described above is consistent with descriptions of the syndrome of nonverbal learning disability, which is characterized by problems with visual-spatial processing, nonverbal reasoning, math skills, visual-motor and fine motor functioning, and often social skills but relatively preserved auditory memory, verbal reasoning, word decoding, and spelling. Using the criteria of assets and deficits outlined by Rourke (1995), Yeates, Loss, Colvin, and Enrile (2003) determined that about half of the participants in their sample of children with myelomeningocele and hydrocephalus demonstrated a neurocognitive profile consistent with the description of a nonverbal learning disorder. The authors noted that, when considered as a group, individuals with hydrocephalus appear to exhibit many characteristics consistent with the nonverbal learning disability syndrome, although social and pragmatic language were not directly measured. However, the specific profiles of individual children with hydrocephalus are quite heterogeneous. As with any population, clinicians are warned to be cautious in making generalizations about specific neurocognitive profiles based on diagnosis alone. Therefore, comprehensive assessment to determine the individual child's pattern of strengths and weaknesses is essential.

Some previous research has indicated that many children with hydrocephalus who do not meet criteria for mental retardation do not present with significant behavioral problems (Fernell, Gillberg, & von Wendt, 1991a). However, other studies have suggested higher rates of behavior difficulties in this population compared to typically developing children (e.g., Fletcher et al., 1995; Lindquist, Carlsson, Persson, & Uvebrant, 2006; Williams & Lyttle, 1998). Nonetheless, no specific psychiatric profile has been noted in children with hydrocephalus (Donders, Rourke, & Canady, 1992). As would be expected, behavioral problems are more likely to exist in the presence of impaired cognitive functioning (Fernell et al., 1991a; Lindquist et al.), and complicating conditions such as cerebral palsy and epilepsy also have been observed to increase the likelihood of behavioral difficulties (Lindquist et al.). Higher rates of autistic symptomatology also have been reported in children with hydrocephalus compared to the general population (Fernell, Gilberg, & von Wendt, 1991b; Lindquist et al.), with higher rates of autistic features observed in those children presenting with greater severity of brain damage (Fernell et al., 1991b). Furthermore, behavioral problems have been observed to be more significant in adolescents than in younger children (Holler, Fennell, Crosson, Boggs, & Mickle, 1995).

## RELATED MEDICAL ISSUES

As indicated at the beginning of this chapter, hydrocephalus is not a diagnostic entity in and of itself but is present in a variety of medical conditions, many of which, such as brain tumor, spina bifida, and traumatic brain injury, are discussed elsewhere in this volume. As the majority of children with spina bifida exhibit hydrocephalus, it is worth noting that these children frequently have related physical issues, including weakness or paralysis and incontinence, and we refer the interested reader to the specific chapter in this volume covering spina bifida. Certainly, it is important to note that for those children who have undergone shunt placement, the potential for complications, including mechanical failure, obstruction, infection, and the need for revision, exists. Therefore, children with hydrocephalus should receive regular medical monitoring, and if symptoms of hydrocephalus reappear, immediate medical attention is recommended.

## RESULTS FROM NEUROPSYCHOLOGICAL EVALUATION

As noted above, aqueductal stenosis is the congenital obstruction of the aqueduct of Sylvius, the channel that connects the third and fourth ventricles. As this is the most common type of congenital obstructive hydrocephalus, a case of aqueductal stenosis is presented below. As with any type of brain injury, numerous factors impact the child's current functional success and eventual functional outcome. The case below illustrates a number of common findings in cases of hydrocephalus, though cases of hydrocephalus vary widely in terms of educational needs, neuropsychological findings, and social and emotional functioning. This again emphasizes the need for comprehensive, individualized evaluation of functioning as well as ongoing monitoring of functioning in order to address changing needs stemming from new developmental challenges and medical changes related to hydrocephalus.

## Background and Demographic Information

At the time of evaluation, Joseph, a right-handed White boy, had recently turned 12 years old and had recently completed fifth grade. He was diagnosed with aqueductal stenosis with associated hydrocephalus during infancy, and he had a VP shunt placed shortly after birth. Since that time, repeated magnetic resonance imaging (MRI) scans revealed enlarged ventricles bilaterally consistent with his hydrocephalus. Joseph underwent surgery to revise his shunt on two different occasions due to shunt malfunction. Each shunt malfunction surgery was preceded by an increase in headaches and eventually nausea, common markers of increased ICP.

Joseph began school in a prekindergarten program at a small private Christian school. His mother reported that he seemed to function well in that environment, and she noted that teachers never raised any significant concerns about Joseph's academic or cognitive development. Due to a recent move, Joseph changed schools and attended fifth grade in a regular education public school program. He initially made a relatively smooth transition into his new classroom setting. However, by the end of the first semester, his teachers had significant concerns with regard to his classroom performance. Specifically, teachers reported slow completion of work, difficulty understanding and completing assignments, poor organization, difficulty with handwriting, and particular difficulty with math performance. Joseph's parents indicated that he seemed to be spending a great deal of time completing homework assignments each evening, to the point of significant fatigue. He was a conscientious student who was adamant that he needed to complete his homework, though he typically required a great deal of assistance and supervision. Joseph's parents were somewhat confused by the level of difficulty that teachers were reporting during fifth grade, particularly given that no concerns were raised by teachers while he attended the small private school. It seemed apparent that Joseph had been informally provided with a great deal of support and flexibility with regard to curriculum and work expectations at the private school, but this was not effectively documented or communicated to his parents.

Because of concerns raised during the first semester, a student support team meeting was convened shortly after winter break. It was determined that Joseph exhibited a level of educational need that warranted evaluation for possible special education services. A neuropsychological evaluation had been suggested to Joseph's parents several years earlier by his neurosurgeon, but his parents had put this off because of their perception that Joseph seemed to be performing fairly well at school. Given the concerns raised by staff at Joseph's new school, his parents opted to pursue a neuropsychological evaluation as part of his special education eligibility determination.

Joseph's mother acknowledged that she has always been overprotective with him and has long harbored concerns about his ability to interact with others his age. Joseph was described as socially immature and reportedly got along much better with children younger than himself. He had difficulty reading social cues, and he consistently got stuck on conversation topics that were not of interest to classmates. Joseph's teacher indicated that she had to monitor him closely in the classroom and on the playground to ensure that he was not teased or picked on excessively. She frequently let Joseph stay in the classroom with her during recess, an arrangement that he seemed to enjoy. Same-age peers quickly lost patience with Joseph, though his mother reported that his social immaturity seemed to be well tolerated in the private school setting. At the time of the evaluation, his social difficulties had become more prominent, as Joseph was more frequently teased and left out than he was in his previous school placement. Due to the shunt placement, Joseph was prohibited from participating in many typical athletic team activities during his childhood, and he avoided unstructured active play with peers. Since the family's move, Joseph had had difficulty establishing stable friendships with others, aside from routinely playing with two younger children in the neighborhood.

Joseph was described as typically in a good mood. Since the move, his mother reported that he frequently complained of loneliness. No difficulties with sleep or appetite were reported. Joseph's mother echoed teacher concerns about Joseph's capacity to organize his belongings, though she acknowledged that she has always been quick to step in and take care of things for him. No significant concerns were raised with regard to attention, concentration, or activity level. In the past, Joseph occasionally complained of headaches and nausea, and these reports have typically been precursors to the need for shunt revision. Otherwise, Joseph did not typically complain of physical ailments and was rarely sick.

## Behavioral Observations

Joseph was accompanied to the evaluation by his mother. He demonstrated no difficulty separating from her in order to participate in the testing activities. Conversational speech was fluent, grammatically intact, and free from word-finding difficulties. In fact, Joseph was quite talkative over the course of evaluation and seemed to enjoy the one-to-one attention inherent to the testing situation. Consistent with parent and teacher report, Joseph appeared socially immature and was frequently silly. Joseph seemed eager to interact and converse with the examiner, and at times he had to be prompted back to the task at hand. He acknowledged that he did not have many friends at his new school, and he reported that the work has been very hard in comparison to his previous private school placement. Attention, concentration, and activity level were observed to be within normal limits in this one-to-one setting. Joseph was mildly clumsy with his hands during evaluation (e.g., dropping his pencil, knocking materials off the table on a couple of occasions), though no other obvious gross or fine motor difficulties were observed. Joseph appeared interested in performing well on each of the activities presented to him, and he seemed to put forth very good effort. As noted above, he occasionally required prompting to work on a task instead of socializing with the examiner, and he responded very favorably to these cues and prompts. Overall, it was felt that results of testing provided a reliable and valid sample of Joseph's level of functioning in the measured domains.

## Test Results

Test scores are summarized in Tables 12.1 and 12.2. Findings revealed that Joseph was experiencing a number of common late effects of hydrocephalus. In particular, although his composite IQ fell in the low average range, his neurocognitive pattern was characterized by a significant discrepancy between verbal information processing abilities and nonverbal abilities. Within Joseph's verbal performance, a trend suggests increasing difficulty with verbal information processing as demands become more abstract. In addition to difficulties with visual-spatial processing, Joseph exhibited a significant weakness in speed of information processing, a common finding in cases of long-standing hydrocephalus. Auditory working memory deteriorated with increasing complexity of information, though Joseph's overall verbal memory capacity was largely normal and commensurate with his verbal/language-based cognitive ability. In contrast, visual memory was an area of weakness for Joseph, again congruent with his lower functioning across tasks tapping visual-spatial cognitive functioning. Visual-motor skill was low average, and Joseph had difficulty with both visual-perceptual functions and bilateral motor dexterity. His performance on tasks requiring executive functions was suggestive of difficulty with both abstract concept formation and cognitive flexibility. Joseph tended to have difficulty generating appropriate problem-solving strategies and benefiting from feedback in order to modify his problem-solving approach.

Academically, Joseph exhibited core academic skill development that was, in general, at average to low average in reading, written expression, and math. Among individual subtests, the findings were again relatively typical for children who have experienced long-standing hydrocephalus. Specifically, Joseph's strongest performances tended to be on language-based tasks that were amenable to rote memory (e.g., sight word recognition and written spelling). Joseph's weakest performances were on tasks tapping basic math calculation as well as speed of completion of academic tasks. Difficulties with processing speed and academic fluency were in keeping with both parent and teacher reports that Joseph takes a very long time to complete many academic activities. Clearly Joseph had worked hard to maintain his academic performance in light of his significant difficulties with nonverbal information processing, processing speed, and executive functions. It is likely that Joseph had relied on his good rote verbal memory to perform adequately on many academic tasks, though current curriculum demands seemed to be exceeding his cognitive capacity as tasks had begun to require much more in the way of abstract thinking, synthesis, and information organization.

Results of behavior rating scales reinforced parent and teacher perceptions of Joseph's difficulties with social integration both at home and in his classroom setting. According to his caregivers' responses, Joseph exhibited strong social desire but had difficulty reading and responding to social cues, to the point that he came across as socially awkward. Within a middle school peer group, Joseph was experiencing less tolerance than he was accustomed to in his earlier elementary school years. It is noteworthy that Joseph acknowledged his social difficulties, both during an interview as well as on a self-report rating scale. Finally, although Joseph did not endorse issues related to anxiety, his parent and teacher both rated him as exhibiting anxious and depressed behavior. Joseph had a desire to do well and a desire to please, and his current educational placement was such that his significant effort was yielding mediocre results at best. As such, Joseph was likely experiencing anxious and depressed symptoms in response to the poor fit between him and the environmental demands, and the relatively recent stressor of the family's move and change of school also likely contributed to this behavior pattern in Joseph.

**TABLE 12.1 Neuropsychological Testing Data**

| Scale | Scaled Score | T-Score | Standard Score |
|---|---|---|---|
| Wechsler Intelligence Scale for Children—Fourth Edition | | | |
| Full Scale IQ | | | 86 |
| Verbal Comprehension Index | | | 102 |
| Perceptual Reasoning Index | | | 82 |
| Working Memory Index | | | 88 |
| Processing Speed Index | | | 80 |
| Woodcock-Johnson Tests of Achievement—Third Edition | | | |
| Letter-Word Identification | | | 102 |
| Reading Fluency | | | 88 |
| Passage Comprehension | | | 95 |
| Calculation | | | 85 |
| Math Fluency | | | 90 |
| Applied Problems | | | 90 |
| Spelling | | | 109 |
| Writing Fluency | | | 83 |
| Writing Samples | | | 98 |
| California Verbal Learning Test—Children's Version | | | |
| List A Total Trials 1–5 | | 49 | |
| List A Trial 1 Free Recall | | 45 | |
| List A Trial 5 Free Recall | | 55 | |
| List B Free Recall | | 35 | |
| List A Short-Delay Free Recall | | 55 | |
| List A Short-Delay Cued Recall | | 50 | |
| List A Long-Delay Free Recall | | 60 | |
| List A Long-Delay Cued Recall | | 55 | |
| Recognition | | 55 | |
| Children's Memory Scale | | | |
| Stories—Immediate | 10 | | |
| Stories—Delayed | 9 | | |

**TABLE 12.1** *(Continued)*

| Scale | Scaled Score | T-Score | Standard Score |
|---|---|---|---|
| Stories—Delayed Recognition | 9 | | |
| Dot Locations— Learning | 6 | | |
| Dot Locations— Total Score | 5 | | |
| Dot Locations— Long Delay | 6 | | |
| Faces—Immediate | 7 | | |
| Faces—Delayed | 6 | | |
| Wisconsin Card Sorting Test | | | |
| Total Errors | | | 68 |
| Perseverative Responses | | | 72 |
| Perseverative Errors | | | 69 |
| Nonperseverative Errors | | | 76 |
| Judgment of Line Orientation | | | |
| JLO | | | 57 |
| Grooved Pegboard Test | | | |
| Preferred Hand (right) | | | 65 |
| Non-preferred Hand (left) | | | 53 |
| Beery-Buktenica Developmental Test of Visual-Motor Integration—Fifth Edition | | | |
| VMI | | | 82 |

*Note.* Beery-Buktenica Developmental Test of Visual-Motor Integration—Fifth Edition (VMI-V; Beery, Buktenica, & Beery, 2004); Judgment of Line Orientation (JLO; Benton, Hamsher, Varney, & Spreen, 1983); Children's Memory Scale (CMS; Cohen, 1997); California Verbal Learning Test—Children's Version (CVLT-C; Delis, Kramer, Kaplan, & Ober, 1994); Wisconsin Card Sorting Test (WCST; Grant & Berg, 1993); Grooved Pegboard Test (Trites, n.d.); Wechsler Intelligence Scale for Children—Fourth Edition (WISC-IV; Wechsler, 2003); Woodcock-Johnson Tests of Achievement—Third Edition (WJ-III; Woodcock, McGrew, & Mather, 2001).

**TABLE 12.2 T Scores From Behavioral and Emotional Testing**

| Scale | CBCL | TRF | YSR |
|---|---|---|---|
| Total Problems | 59 | 60 | 50 |
| Social Problems | 70 | 72 | 66 |
| Thought Problems | 55 | 57 | 50 |
| Attention Problems | 62 | 54 | 57 |
| Externalizing Problems | 43 | 49 | 46 |
| Rule-Breaking Behavior | 50 | 50 | 50 |
| Aggressive Behavior | 50 | 52 | 52 |
| Internalizing Problems | 63 | 68 | 51 |
| Anxious/Depressed | 68 | 73 | 54 |
| Withdrawn/Depressed | 60 | 62 | 54 |
| Somatic Complaints | 50 | 58 | 51 |

*Note.* CBCL, Child Behavior Checklist, Parent Form (Achenbach, 2001a); TRF, Teacher Report Form (Achenbach, 2001b); YSR, Youth Self-Report (Achenbach, 2001c).

## INTERVENTIONS

During an extensive feedback conference with Joseph's parents as well as consultation with staff at school, a number of recommendations were made to address the prominent issues Joseph presented in terms of difficulties at school, underlying neurocognitive weaknesses, and difficulties with social interaction and emotional adjustment. Although no prescribed set of interventions is applicable to every student who has experienced hydrocephalus, the interventions for Joseph's case address a variety of issues that are common to students who have experienced long-standing hydrocephalus.

Because Joseph's weak classroom performance was a primary reason for evaluation, the first recommendation was for appropriate educational placement and planning based on recognition of Joseph's significant educational need. As in Joseph's case, many students with hydrocephalus do not exhibit a typical discrepancy between IQ and the results of academic achievement tests that are commonly used to identify students with specific learning disabilities. Instead, educational need is defined by Joseph's track record of difficulty in the classroom that is well documented by his teacher, as well as the fact that he exhibited neurocognitive deficits that are consistent with the late effects of hydrocephalus and that correlate directly with

Joseph's most significant areas of educational need. It was recommended that the multidisciplinary special education evaluation team consider Joseph's eligibility for special services under the handicapping condition of Other Health Impairment (OHI), as this code most appropriately captures the link between Joseph's deficits and the corresponding medical etiology.

Assuming special education eligibility, it was recommended that Joseph's individual education plan (IEP) provide for modifications and accommodations to address prominent areas of need. For example, Joseph had been spending an inordinate amount of time doing his homework, in part because of slow processing speed and other neurocognitive deficits, as well as his desire to please and his perception that he must complete anything assigned to him. A reduction in the amount of homework assigned to Joseph was recommended, to be carried out through shortened assignments, availability of classroom support to assist with completion of assignments during the school day, and a limit on the time that Joseph would be permitted to spend on homework each night.

Availability of review and reinstruction services also was recommended to be incorporated into the IEP. In Joseph's case, the most appropriate method for operationalizing this was a period each day during which Joseph would be pulled out of his regular classroom and would have access to a special education teacher. In other settings, this intervention could be carried out within the regular education classroom, keeping in mind that the distractions of a regular classroom may hinder the student's ability to benefit from this intervention.

A number of strategies were suggested that could be incorporated into the IEP to address issues related to visual-spatial information processing weakness. For example, Joseph exhibited a strength in his verbal memory and verbal cognitive ability overall, particularly in comparison to below-average nonverbal, visual-spatial memory and cognitive ability. Rehearsing information out loud in order to better digest and remember it was recommended in order to take advantage of Joseph's strengths. This oral rehearsal technique might include reading or reciting information aloud as a primary study method for remembering information later. Subsequently, oral testing procedures could be judiciously utilized by students with significant handwriting deficits, which are relatively common in students who have experienced hydrocephalus.

Compensatory methods for organizing and dividing visual information also were recommended. For example, Joseph could be instructed in the use of a highlight pen to "grid" a worksheet into smaller, more manageable parts. A highlight pen could also be used to mark problems or questions as they are completed in order to avoid skipping lines or problems on the worksheet. In addition, the use of place markers or spacers would provide a method by which a complex visual stimulus such as a worksheet or page of text could be reduced to a more manageable amount of information.

Although it was not recommended at the time, assistive technology, such as the use of a calculator in math class, was discussed as potentially necessary for Joseph in the future. Given his significant weakness with visual-spatial information processing, it was anticipated that Joseph would experience increasing difficulty in math as the math curriculum became more abstract, and independent use of compensatory devices such as a calculator was encouraged. Embedded in the process of educational planning should be strategies to help the student develop greater levels of self-reliance, independence, and self-advocacy.

Organizational assistance was recommended as part of the IEP due to Joseph's difficulty with executive functions and organization in particular. It was recommended that Joseph receive direct instruction and modeling in the use of organizational strategies, and it was also suggested that he receive ongoing support, such as a daily check-in with a teacher who could verify that his materials were in order (e.g., that he has his assignments together, that he has materials needed to complete homework, etc.).

Because of difficulties with fine motor function, and handwriting difficulties in particular, it was recommended that Joseph undergo evaluation by the school's occupational therapist in order to determine whether direct occupational therapy or consultation services would be warranted. Handwriting difficulties are common in children with hydrocephalus, and deficits in processing speed compound this weakness. It was recommended that Joseph have access to copies of teacher or peer notes and that he not be required to copy large amounts of information from the board. The combination of slow speed and fine motor difficulties can result in the student spending an inordinate amount of energy on mundane tasks such as handwriting and copying, often at the expense of energy for more important cognitive and educational activities.

In addition, the school staff were encouraged to identify relevant social skills interventions or groups within the school environment in which Joseph could participate to address his social deficits. In part, it was important to address Joseph's social needs through direct intervention, and it was also important to identify groups in which he could participate that could provide him with a positive social outlet. It was recommended that direct counseling with Joseph be considered if, after implementation of an appropriate IEP and related services, he continued to exhibit symptoms of anxiety or depression in the school environment.

Joseph's parents were encouraged to seek additional information about the late effects of hydrocephalus and to seek support for themselves given the emotional strain that can be created by raising a child with special needs. In Joseph's case, his parents had not been fully aware of the extent of his neurocognitive deficits until he enrolled in a public school and was faced with a more demanding and fast-paced curriculum. In order to facilitate their adjustment and provide support, several additional consultation appointments were scheduled with the neuropsychologist in order to address ongoing issues with the design and implementation of the IEP, as well as to provide Joseph's parents with additional education about the late neurocognitive effects of hydrocephalus.

Finally, neuropsychological reevaluation was recommended prior to Joseph's transition to high school. Certainly, it is important to update the profile of neurocognitive strengths and weaknesses in a student who has documented brain injury. In addition, given that Joseph's parents had only recently been confronted with the educational implications of his long-standing hydrocephalus, it was important to offer the family a level of support and guidance to help them become prudent advocates for their child's interests. They need a thorough understanding of the child's neurocognitive strengths and liabilities, as well as a thorough understanding of the full range of educational and community program options available to help the student eventually live and work as independently as he or she is capable.

## RESOURCES

### Books


Bellush, T. R. (2004). *All about me (and my shunt)*. Victoria, British Columbia, Canada: Trafford.

Icon Health Publications. (2002). *The official parent's sourcebook on hydrocephalus: A revised and updated directory for the Internet age*. San Diego: Author.

Toporek, C., & Robinson, K. (1999). *Hydrocephalus: A guide for patients, families, and friends*. Sebastopol, CA: Patient-Centered Guides.


### Organizations and Web Sites

Guardians of Hydrocephalus Research Foundation

The Guardians of Hydrocephalus Research Foundation is a non-profit organization with the goal of aiding children with hydrocephalus who require medical procedures and special equipment. The foundation also works to provide information to the public and support research.

Mailing Address: 2618 Avenue Z<br>Brooklyn, New York 11235-2023<br>Phone Number: (718) 743-4473<br>Web Site: ghrf.Homestead.com/ghrf.html

Hydrocephalus Association

The Hydrocephalus Association provides support, education, and advocacy for individuals and families affected by hydrocephalus, as well as professionals involved in the care of individuals with hydrocephalus.

| | |
|---|---|
| Mailing Address: | 870 Market Street<br>San Francisco, California 94102 |
| Phone Number: | (888) 598-3789 |
| Web Site: | www.hydroassoc.org |

National Hydrocephalus Foundation

The National Hydrocephalus Foundation exists to disseminate information about the condition, facilitate communication among affected individuals and families, increase public awareness of the condition, and support and promote research about hydrocephalus.

| | |
|---|---|
| Mailing Address: | 12413 Centralia Road<br>Lakewood, California 90715-1623 |
| Phone Number: | (888) 857-3434 |
| Web Site: | nhfonline.org |

## REFERENCES


Achenbach, T. (2001a). *Child Behavior Checklist.* Burlington: Achenbach System of Empirically Based Assessment, University of Vermont.

Achenbach, T. (2001b). *Teacher's Report Form.* Burlington: Achenbach System of Empirically Based Assessment, University of Vermont.

Achenbach, T. (2001c). *Youth Self Report.* Burlington: Achenbach System of Empirically Based Assessment, University of Vermont.

Assaf, Y., Ben-Sira, L., Constantini, S., Chang, L. C., & Beni-Adani, L. (2006). Diffusion tensor imaging in hydrocephalus: Initial experience. *American Journal of Neuroradiology, 27,* 1717–1724.

Ayr, L. K., Yeates, K. O., & Enrile, B. G. (2005). Arithmetic skills and their cognitive correlates in children with acquired and congenital brain disorder. *Journal of the International Neuropsychological Society, 11,* 249–262.

Barnes, M. A., & Dennis, M. (1992). Reading in children and adolescents after early onset hydrocephalus and in normally developing age peers: Phonological analysis, word recognition, word comprehension, and passage comprehension skill. *Journal of Pediatric Psychology, 17,* 445–465.

Barnes, M. A., & Dennis, M. (1998). Discourse after early-onset hydrocephalus: Core deficits in children of average intelligence. *Brain and Language, 61,* 309–334.

Barnes, M. A., Pengelly, S., Dennis, M., Wilkinson, M., Rogers, T., & Faulkner, H. (2002). Mathematics skills in good readers with hydrocephalus. *Journal of the International Neuropsychological Society, 8,* 72–82.

Beery, K. E., Buktenica, N. A., & Beery, N. A. (2004). *Beery-Buktenica Developmental Test of Visual-Motor Integration* (5th ed.). Bloomington, MN: Pearson Assessments.

Benton, A. L., Hamsher, K., Varney, N. R., & Spreen, O. (1983). *Judgment of Line Orientation*. New York: Oxford University Press.

Boyer, K. M., Yeates, K. O., & Enrile, B. G. (2006). Working memory and information processing speed in children with myelomeningocele and shunted hydrocephalus: Analysis of the Children's Paced Auditory Serial Addition Test. *Journal of the International Neuropsychological Society, 12,* 305–313.

Brann, B. S., IV, Qualls, C., Wells, L., & Papile, L. (1991). Asymmetric growth of the lateral cerebral ventricle in infants with posthemorrhagic ventricular dilation. *Journal of Pediatrics, 118,* 108–112.

Bret, P., Guyotat, J., & Chazal, J. (2002). Is normal pressure hydrocephalus a valid concept in 2002? A reappraisal in five questions and proposal for a new designation of the syndrome as "chronic hydrocephalus." *Journal of Neurology, Neurosurgery, and Psychiatry, 73,* 9–12.

Brewer, V. R., Fletcher, J. M., Hiscock, M., & Davidson, K. C. (2001). Attention processes in children with shunted hydrocephalus versus attention deficit-hyperactivity disorder. *Neuropsychology, 15,* 185–198.

Brookshire, B. L., Fletcher, J. M., Bohan, T. P., Landry, S. H., Davidson, K. C., & Francis, D. J. (1995). Verbal and nonverbal skill discrepancies in children with hydrocephalus: A five-year longitudinal follow-up. *Journal of Pediatric Psychology, 20,* 785–800.

Burmeister, H., Hannay, J., Copeland, K., Fletcher, J. M., Boudousquie, A., & Dennis, M. (2005). Attention problems and executive functions in children with spina bifida and hydrocephalus. *Child Neuropsychology, 11,* 265–283.

Cohen, M. (1997). *Children's Memory Scale*. San Antonio, TX: Harcourt Assessment.

Delis, D. C., Kramer, J. H., Kaplan, E., & Ober, B. A. (1994). *California Verbal Learning Test—Children's Version*. San Antonio, TX: The Psychological Corporation.

Dennis, M., & Barnes, M. A. (1993). Oral discourse after early-onset hydrocephalus: Linguistic ambiguity, figurative language, and script-based inferences. *Journal of Pediatric Psychology, 18,* 639–652.

Dennis, M., Fitz, C. R., Netley, C. T., Sugar, J., Derek, C. F., Harwood-Nash, M. B., et al. (1981). The intelligence of hydrocephalic children. *Archives of Neurology, 38,* 607–615.

Dennis, M., Fletcher, J. M., Rogers, T., Hetherington, R., & Francis, D. J. (2002). Object-based and action-based visual perception in children with spina bifida and hydrocephalus. *Journal of the International Neuropsychological Society, 8,* 95–106.

Donders, J., Rourke, B. P., & Canady, A. I. (1991). Neuropsychological functioning of hydrocephalic children. *Journal of Clinical and Experimental Neuropsychology, 13,* 607–613.

Donders, J., Rourke, B. P., & Canady, A. I. (1992). Emotional adjustment of children with hydrocephalus and of their parents. *Journal of Child Neurology, 7,* 375–380.

Drake, J. M., & Iantosca, M. R. (2001). Management of pediatric hydrocephalus with shunts. In D. G. McLone (Ed.), *Pediatric neurosurgery: Surgery of the developing nervous system* (4th ed., pp. 505–525). Philadelphia: W. B. Saunders.

Duhaime, A. C. (2006). Evaluation and management of shunt infections in children with hydrocephalus. *Clinical Pediatrics, 45,* 705–713.

Eisenberg, H. M., McComb, J. G., & Lorenzo, A. W. (1974). Cerebrospinal fluid overproduction and hydrocephalus associated with choroids plexus papilloma. *Journal of Neurosurgery, 40,* 381–385.

Erickson, K., Baron, I. S., & Fantie, B. D. (2001). Neuropsychological functioning in early hydrocephalus: Review from a developmental perspective. *Child Neuropsychology, 7,* 199–299.

Fernell, E., Gillberg, C., & von Wendt, L. (1991a). Behavioural problems in children with infantile hydrocephalus. *Developmental Medicine and Child Neurology, 33,* 388–395.

Fernell, E., Gillberg, C., & von Wendt, L. (1991b). Autistic symptoms in children with infantile hydrocephalus. *Acta Paediatrica Scandinavia, 80,* 451–457.

Fletcher, J. M., Brookshire, B. L., Landry, S. H., Bohan, T. P., Davidson, K. C., Francis, D. J., et al. (1995). Behavioral adjustment of children with hydrocephalus: Relationships with etiology, neurological, and family status. *Journal of Pediatric Psychology, 20,* 109–125.

Fletcher, J. M., Brookshire, B. L., Landry, S. H., Bohan, T. P., Davidson, K. C., Francis, D. J., et al. (1996). Attentional skills and executive functions in children with early hydrocephalus. *Developmental Neuropsychology, 12,* 53–76.

Fletcher, J. M., Dennis, M., & Northrup, H. (2000). Hydrocephalus. In K. O. Yeates, M. D. Ris, & H. G. Taylor (Eds.), *Pediatric neuropsychology: Research, theory, and practice* (pp. 25–46). New York: Guilford Press.

Fletcher, J. M., Francis, D. J., Thompson, N. M., Brookshire, B. L., Bohan, T. P., Landry, S. H., et al. (1992). Verbal and nonverbal skill discrepancies in hydrocephalic children. *Journal of Clinical and Experimental Neuropsychology, 14,* 593–609.

Fletcher, J. M., Landry, S. H., Bohan, T. P., Davidson, K. C., Brookshire, B. L., & Lachar, D. (1997). Effects of intraventricular hemorrhage and hydrocephalus on the long-term neurobehavioral development of preterm very-low-birthweight infants. *Developmental Medicine and Child Neurology, 39,* 596–606.

Fletcher, J. M., McCauley, S. R., Brandt, M. E., Bohan, T. P., Kramer, L. A., Francis, D. J., et al. (1996). Regional brain tissue composition in children with hydrocephalus: Relationships with cognitive development. *Archives of Neurology, 53,* 549–557.

Friedrich, W. N., Lovejoy, M. C., Shaffer, J., Shurtleff, D. B., & Beilke, R. L. (1991). Cognitive abilities and achievement status of children with myelomeningocele: A contemporary sample. *Journal of Pediatric Psychology, 16,* 423–428.

Ghatak, N. R., & McWhorter, J. M. (1976). Ultrastructural evidence for CSF production by a choroids plexus papilloma. *Journal of Neurosurgery, 45,* 409–415.

Grant, D. A., & Berg, E. A. (1993). *Wisconsin Card Sorting Test.* San Antonio, TX: The Psychological Corporation.

Hadenius, A. M., Hagberg, B., Hyttnes-Bensch, K., & Sjogren, I. (1962). The natural prognosis of infantile hydrocephalus. *Acta Paediatrica (Uppsala), 51,* 117–118.

Hetherington, R., & Dennis, M. (1999). Motor function profile in children with early onset hydrocephalus. *Developmental Neuropsychology, 15,* 25–51.

Hirsch, J. F. (1992). Surgery of hydrocephalus: Past, present and future. *Acta Neurochirurgica, 116,* 155–160.

Hirsch, J. F., Pierre-Kahn, A., Renier, D., Sainte-Rose, C., & Hoppe-Hirsch, E. (1984). The Dandy-Walker malformation: A review of 40 cases. *Journal of Neurosurgery, 61,* 515–522.

Holler, K. A., Fennell, E. B., Crosson, B., Boggs, S. R., & Mickle, J. P. (1995). Neuropsychological and adaptive functioning in younger versus older children shunted for early hydrocephalus. *Child Neuropsychology, 1,* 63–73.

Ito, J., Saijo, H., Araki, A., Tanaka, H., Tasaki, T., Cho, K., et al. (1997). Neuroradiological assessment of visuoperceptual disturbance in children with spina bifida and hydrocephalus. *Developmental Medicine and Child Neurology, 39,* 385–392.

Jacobs, R., Northam, E., & Anderson, V. (2001). Cognitive outcome in children with myelomeningocele and perinatal hydrocephalus: A longitudinal perspective. *Journal of Developmental and Physical Disabilities, 13,* 389–405.

Karasawa, H., Furuya, H., Naito, H., Sugiyama, K., Ueno, J., & Kin, H. (1997). Acute hydrocephalus in posterior fossa injury. *Journal of Neurosurgery, 86,* 629–632.

Lindquist, B., Carlsson, G., Persson, E.-K., & Uvebrant, P. (2006). Behavioral problems and autism in children with hydrocephalus. *European Child and Adolescent Psychiatry, 15,* 214–219.

Loss, N., Yeates, K. O., & Enrile, B. G. (1998). Attention in children with myelomeningocele. *Child Neuropsychology, 4,* 7–20.

Mahone, E. M., Zabel, T. A., Levey, E., Verda, M., & Kinsman, S. (2002). Parent and self-report ratings of executive function in adolescents with myelomeningocele and hydrocephalus. *Child Neuropsychology, 8,* 258–270.

McCullough, D. C., & Balzer-Martin, L. A. (1982). Current prognosis in overt neonatal hydrocephalus. *Journal of Neurosurgery, 57,* 378–383.

McLone, D. G., Czyzewski, D., Raimondi, A. J., & Sommers, R. C. (1982). Central nervous system infections as a limiting factor in the intelligence of children with myelomeningocele. *Pediatrics, 70,* 338–342.

Menkes, J. H., & Till, K. (1995). Malformations of the central nervous system. In J. H. Menkes (Ed.), *Textbook of child neurology* (5th ed., pp. 240–324). Baltimore: Williams & Wilkins.

National Institute of Neurological Disorders and Stroke [NINDS]. (2005, August). *Hydrocephalus fact sheet* (NIH Publication No. 05-385). Retrieved March 5, 2007, from http://www.ninds.nih.gov/disorders/hydrocephalus/detail_hydrocephalus.htm

Pencalet, P., Sainte-Rose, C., Lellouch-Tubiana, A., Kalifa, C., Brunelle, F., Sgouros, S., et al. (1998). Papillomas and carcinomas of the choroid plexus in children. *Journal of Neurosurgery, 88,* 521–528.

Persson, E. K., Hagberg, G., & Uvebrant, P. (2005). Hydrocephalus prevalence and outcome in a population-based cohort of children born in 1989–1998. *Acta Paediatrica, 94,* 726–732.

Pollack, I. F., Pang, D., Albright, A. L., & Krieger, D. (1992). Outcome following hindbrain decompression of symptomatic Chiari malformations in children previously treated with myelomeningocele closure and shunts. *Journal of Neurosurgery, 77,* 881–888.

Reigel, D. H., & Rotenstein, D. (1994). Spina bifida. In W. R. Creek (Ed.), *Pediatric neurosurgery* (3rd ed., pp. 51–76). Philadelphia: W. B. Saunders.

Ris, M. D., & Noll, R. B. (1994). Long-term neurobehavioral outcome in pediatric brain-tumor patients: Review and methodological critique. *Journal of Clinical and Experimental Neuropsychology, 16,* 21–42.

Riva, D., Milani, N., Giorgi, C., Pantaleoni, C., Zorzi, C., & Devoti, M. (1994). Intelligence outcome in children with shunted hydrocephalus of different etiology. *Child's Nervous System, 10,* 70–73.

Rourke, B. P. (1995). Introduction: The NLD syndrome and the white matter model. In B. P. Rourke (Ed.), *Syndrome of nonverbal learning disabilities: Neurodevelopmental manifestations* (pp. 1–26). New York: Guilford Press.

Sandler, A. D., Macias, M., & Brown, T. T. (1993). The drawings of children with spina bifida: Developmental correlations and interpretations. *European Journal of Pediatric Surgery 3*(Suppl. 1), 25–27.

Scott, M. A., Fletcher, J. M., Brookshire, B. L., Davison, K. C., Landry, S. H., Bohan, T. C., et al. (1998). Memory functions in children with early hydrocephalus. *Neurospychology, 12,* 578–589.

Tew, B. (1979). The "cocktail party syndrome" in children with hydrocephalus and spina bifida. *British Journal of Disorders of Communication, 14,* 89–101.

Trites, R. (n.d.). *Grooved Pegboard Test.* Lafayette, IN: Lafayette Instruments.

Wechsler, D. (2003). *Wechsler Intelligence Scale for Children* (4th ed.). San Antonio, TX: The Psychological Corporation.

Williams, J., & Lyttle, S. (1998). Mother and teacher reports of behaviour and perceived self-competence of children with hydrocephalus. *European Journal of Pediatric Surgery, 8*(Suppl. 1), 5–9.

Wills, K. E. (1993). Neuropsychological functioning in children with spina bifida and/or hydrocephalus. *Journal of Clinical Child Psychology, 22,* 247–265.

Woodcock, R. W., McGrew, K. S., & Mather, N. (2001). *Woodcock-Johnson Tests of Achievement* (3rd ed.). Rolling Meadows, IL: Riverside.

Yeates, K. O., Enrile, B. G., Loss, N., Blumenstein, E., & Delis, D. C. (1995). Verbal learning and memory in children with myelomeningocele. *Journal of Pediatric Psychology, 20,* 801–815.

Yeates, K. O., Loss, N., Colvin, A. N., & Enrile, B. G. (2003). Do children with myelomeningocele and hydrocephalus display nonverbal learning disabilities? An empirical approach to classification. *Journal of the International Neuropsychological Society, 9,* 653–662.

Young, P. A., & Young, P. H. (1997). *Basic clinical neuroanatomy.* Philadelphia: Williams & Wilkins.

CHAPTER THIRTEEN

# Lead Exposure

Bonny J. Forrest, JD, PhD

In recent years, the median blood lead concentration in the United States has decreased from 15 μg/dL (micrograms per deciliter) a generation ago to approximately 2 μg/dL in 1999. However promising that decrease, it does not mean that the threat to children's well-being is over. For several reasons, the struggle to prevent lead poisoning and, if it occurs, to mitigate its effects remains critically important.

First, among children of color and children living in poverty, the rates of blood lead concentration continue to be elevated above the median (Shannon et al., 2005).

Second, it is far from clear that a "safe" level of exposure to lead exists. Although the Centers for Disease Control (CDC) and the World Health Organization (WHO, 1995) define a blood concentration of 10 μg/dL or greater as concerning, no threshold level has been documented below which lead has no effect on children's cognitive ability, and government agencies have reinforced the possibility that any amount of lead exposure is unsafe. For example, in 1998 the Centers for Medicare and Medicaid Services (cited in Agency for Toxic Substances and Disease Registry, 1999) issued a revised policy statement describing negative associations between blood lead levels below 10 μg/dL and intelligence. More recently, various researchers have called for the reassessment of the 10 μg/dL levels (Lanphear et al., 2005).

Third, the cognitive and behavioral effects of lead exposure in early childhood, which can be profound, are difficult to treat. Unfortunately, attempts at removing the lead (including chelation therapy) have resulted in few improvements in cognitive, behavioral, or neuropsychological functioning. Although steps can be taken to help affected children learn and function in the classroom, prevention of initial and repeated exposure remains the best practice for combating childhood lead poisoning.

Given these findings, it is particularly important to prevent exposure to lead and, if exposure occurs, to identify it as early as possible. Ideally, that identification would come through medical screening, but not all children receive adequate screening. For example, the 1998 statement by the Centers for Medicare and Medicaid Services (cited in Agency for Toxic Substances and Disease Registry, 1999) noted that Medicaid-eligible children are screened for lead exposure at unacceptably low rates. As a result, teachers are critical in the fight to eliminate lead poisoning—an entirely preventable health problem—because they can educate parents and students about the dangers of lead exposure and work with families to encourage screening and avoid additional exposure. In addition, they can help to identify the effects of lead in their students. The symptoms of lead poisoning can be difficult to distinguish, however, because some of them—poor attention or language difficulties, for example—can look like other learning issues that are not caused by lead exposure.

The purpose of this chapter is to describe some of the behavioral and academic issues frequently associated with lead exposure, at both low and greater levels, so that school personnel may be prompted to ask themselves whether a child's difficulties in the educational environment, whatever form they take, may be attributable to lead exposure. The chapter discusses the symptoms of lead poisoning, related medical issues, typical neuropsychological test performances (illustrated by the cases of two children affected by different levels of lead exposure), and common classroom and medical interventions. It also provides a list of additional resources.

## SOURCES OF LEAD EXPOSURE

From 1976 to 1980, before federal legislation removed lead from gasoline and decreased emissions from other environmental sources, children in the United States between the ages of 1 and 5 had median blood lead concentrations of 15 μg/dL. From 1988 to 1991, the median was 3.6 μg/dL, and in 1999 the median had decreased to 1.9 μg/dL. Unfortunately, children of color and children living in poverty continue to experience higher concentrations. Although lead exposure can come from a variety of environmental sources, the greatest cause of lead poisoning in children is ingestion of dust and chips from surfaces that are deteriorating, especially in older homes where lead paint remains. For example, in 1998, in the over 16 million homes in the United States with children younger than 6 years of age, 25% of those children had elevated lead levels. More recently, lead in drinking water from older lead pipes has been identified as a problem in a number of major metropolitan areas.

## DESCRIPTION OF THE DISORDER

### Overview

Although animal models exist that show the effects of even low-level lead exposure, the exact mechanisms by which lead affects cognition and behavior remain poorly understood. It is, however, well established that lead can cause permanent learning difficulties in children, especially children under 6 years of age, who are generally more sensitive than adults to lead's damaging effects. Although lead affects virtually every system in the body, it is particularly harmful to the developing brain and nervous system of young children. No amount of lead in the body has been identified as safe; however, the effects of lead depend on its level in the blood. In children, very high levels can cause deafness, blindness, coma, convulsions, and even death. Moderate levels, too, can harm the brain and nervous system, kidneys, and liver. Even very low levels are associated with learning difficulties in the classroom.

Although the symptoms of lead poisoning are often quite striking, they are also somewhat diffuse and can be associated with a number of causes. Children with lead poisoning may not present as being "sick." Even if they do show some signs of lead poisoning, these symptoms can often be mistaken for other more common problems, such as the flu. Early symptoms of lead exposure may include sluggishness or restlessness, headache, stomachache, constipation, irritability, and poor appetite. As more lead accumulates, children may become clumsy and weak, and they may lose previously learned skills. More severe symptoms may include vomiting, loss of sight or hearing, seizures, and variable levels of consciousness. Children who are not lead poisoned also may show some of these symptoms, and many of the symptoms of lead poisoning may indicate other health conditions or learning and behavior problems. However, if lead poisoning is suspected, the child should be referred immediately to a medical professional for testing. A professional can determine whether a child has been lead poisoned through a simple test that measures the amount of lead in the child's blood. Children who have been exposed need to be repeatedly retested for elevated blood lead levels over time.

## Lead Exposure Research: An Introduction

Research into the effects of lead exposure at low levels began in the 1970s with the Herbert Needleman study of schoolchildren in Chelsea and Somerville, Massachusetts (Needleman et al., 1979). That study addressed many of the methodological problems of previous investigations. It took into account the potential effects of causes other than lead exposure and used statistical methods that more precisely separated out the factors uniquely attributable to lead. The authors reported a difference in IQ of approximately 4.5 points between groups of children with "high" and "low" tooth lead.

Subsequent studies have expanded our understanding of the pre- and perinatal effects of low-level lead exposure. Low-level fetal lead exposure has been associated with delays in mental and motor development in infants (Bellinger, Leviton, Waternaux, Needleman, & Rabinowitz, 1987; Dietrich et al., 1987; Wigg et al., 1988). Although some follow-up studies found these deficits to be transitory, one study found highly significant inverse associations between prenatal maternal blood lead concentrations and children's mental development at 4 years of age (Wasserman et al., 1994). Another recent study also suggests that prenatal exposure has latent effects on certain neuropsychological functions, including attention and the ability to construct a design from visual input (Ris, Dietrich, Succop, Berger, & Bornschein, 2004).

In children exposed to lead after birth, less noticeable effects on the central nervous system (CNS) are frequently observed. Although the CDC recommends the reduction of lead levels to under 10 μg/dL in order to be safe, it is fairly well established that no amount of lead exposure is good for children. In most cases, blood concentrations of lead peak at approximately 2 years of age; in addition, because of the susceptibility of infants to the effects of lead, even those levels considered to be safe can be associated with lower intelligence scores.

### *General Intelligence*

In studies of intelligence that sample adequate numbers of children and adjust for other variables that could affect intelligence, a relationship between low-level lead exposure and decreased IQ has been unequivocally demonstrated (Bellinger & Dietrich, 1994; Needleman & Gatsonis, 1990; Pocock, Smith, & Baghurst, 1994; Schwartz, 1994a; WHO, 1995). Estimates of the size of lead's effect on IQ have varied somewhat, but recent meta-analyses (large analyses of all relevant studies) have set the effect size at about 0.25 IQ points per 1 µg/dL of lead in the blood, meaning that for every µg/dL increase in blood lead, IQ will drop approximately one-quarter of a point (Schwartz, 1994b).

### *Academic Achievement*

More recently, there have been reports of measurable lead effects on academic performance that occurred at blood levels well below the current CDC guideline of 10 µg/dL (Ris et al., 2004). For example, reading scores have been found to be inversely related to lead levels below 10 µg/dL (Lanphear, Dietrich, Auinger, & Cox, 2000). Some evidence also exists that the negative effects of lead exposure on children's functioning (e.g., reading and intelligence) may actually be greater at lower lead concentrations (Dudek & Merecz, 1997; Schwartz, 1994a).

Teachers also have reported that lead exposure affects other aspects of brain and behavior functions that are important in the classroom. They report that children with elevated lead levels are more inattentive, hyperactive, and disorganized and are less able to follow directions. Additional studies have shown lower graduation rates and greater absentee rates (Shannon et al., 2005). Increased aggression and delinquency have also been linked to increased lead exposure (Shannon et al.). More subtle effects on hearing and balance are also reported (Shannon et al.).

### *Neuropsychological Functioning*

The developing CNS is especially sensitive to toxicant exposure. Neuropsychological testing is specifically designed to assess CNS functioning and cognitive development. Although most studies assessing low-level postnatal exposure have relied only on standardized measures of intelligence rather than neuropsychological measures, the available data on the effects of low-level exposure on neuropsychological functions suggest that it negatively affects performance on tests of motor, visuospatial, visuoconstructional, and higher abstract and executive regulatory reasoning abilities (Baghurst et al., 1992, 1995; Dietrich, 2000; Dietrich, Berger, & Succop, 1993; Dietrich, Succop, Berger, & Keith; 1992; Stiles & Bellinger, 1993; Winneke, Brockhaus, Ewers, Kramer, & Neuf, 1990; Yeates, Ris, & Taylor, 2000). One recent study documented motor, attention, and visuoconstruction deficits that persisted into adolescence for children exposed both prenatally and postnatally to low lead levels (Ris et al., 2004). Using functional magnetic resonance imaging, a more recent study documented the long-lasting impact of lead exposure on language function (Yuan et al., 2006).

These patterns may not be identical in all children exposed to lead. Some researchers contend that because children are exposed to lead at different times in their development (and, therefore, their neuronal systems are exposed differentially), they will more typically exhibit different patterns of neuropsychological performance than a single signature pattern (Lidsky & Schneider, 2006). However, as the cases described below indicate, there are likely to be some similarities in the symptoms exhibited.

### *Symptoms in the Classroom*

In school, children with lead poisoning may exhibit what appear to be, on the surface, general learning difficulties or poor overall performance. More specifically, they may fail to finish their assignments, have a low tolerance for frustration, be easily distractible, or have difficulty staying seated and concentrating. They may also call out in class or otherwise be disruptive.

These behavioral problems are symptoms of lead poisoning and by-products of difficulties in brain functioning in a variety of domains, including attention, executive function, and speech and language. As a result, in comparison with other children, children who have been exposed to lead are much more likely to have reading difficulties, poor vocabulary, attention problems, poor fine motor coordination, greater school absenteeism, and lower class ranking (Shannon et al., 2005). They are also more likely to drop out of high school. And because the behaviors often represent difficulties in how the brain processes information, the problems associated with lead poisoning remain long after childhood.

## NEUROPSYCHOLOGICAL EVALUATION OF TWO CHILDREN

The following test results from two representative cases can help school personnel understand the range of symptoms exhibited by children exposed to lead, including the underlying causes of the symptoms. These cases illustrate the effects of lead poisoning at two levels. As stated previously, although the effects of lead poisoning vary, some similarities exist. For example, most children with lead exposure suffer attentional difficulties. At higher levels these symptoms are likely to be more pronounced, with greater deficits in higher order functions such as organization and planning. Difficulties with motor skills also are frequently reported across levels.

The first case documents the effects of lead exposure within the lower range (a high of approximately 6 μg/dL) for Ray. The second case documents the findings for Loretta, who had a blood lead level of 33 μg/dL, within the range considered to be unsafe by the CDC and WHO (1995). The cases help illustrate that, even at low levels, lead can create attention and language difficulties and that, at higher levels, it can significantly interfere with a child's ability to learn in the classroom. At the time of testing, both children were 8 years old.

## Test Results

### *Summary*

Both children exhibited the hallmark symptoms of lead poisoning, including problems with language, motor abilities, and attention. Attention is one component of broader executive function abilities, and both children also exhibited several other executive deficits, including poor organizational and planning abilities and persistence with ineffective learning strategies. Expressive language, the currency that children use to communicate in the classroom, was more affected than receptive abilities. In addition, the more complex information became, the more difficulties appeared with neuropsychological performance in general, and with executive functions in particular. In the more extreme case of lead exposure, although Loretta's cognitive deficits were similar to those experienced by Ray, her ability to pay attention was so poor that it impaired every aspect of her performance on tests. Similarly, her language deficits were more serious.

### *General Intelligence*

The children had intelligence levels at the borderline levels. Specific scores on intelligence and language tests are set forth in Table 13.1.

### *Academic Achievement*

Each of the children completed selected achievement subtests of the Woodcock-Johnson Tests of Achievement—Third Edition (WJ-III; Woodcock, McGrew, & Mather, 2001). In sharp contrast to their below-average performances on the Wechsler Intelligence Scale for Children—Fourth Edition (WISC-IV; Wechsler, 2003), their scores on most of the WJ-III subtests fell solidly in the average range. However, reading and writing tasks (extensions of language skills and also heavily influenced by attention) were more difficult for both children. In addition, each of the children appeared to exert a great deal of effort on these tasks.

**TABLE 13.1 Selected Composite Standard Scores**

| | Ray | Loretta |
|---|---|---|
| WISC-IV | | |
| Verbal Comprehension Index | 65 | 74 |
| Perceptual Reasoning Index | 78 | 86 |
| Working Memory Index | 87 | 75 |
| Processing Speed Index | 99 | 87 |
| Full Scale IQ | 74 | 73 |
| CASL | | |
| Antonyms | 94 | 75 |
| Syntax Construction | 72 | 70 |
| Paragraph Comprehension | 99 | 114 |
| Nonliteral Language | 74 | 83 |
| Pragmatic Judgment | 75 | 81 |

*Note.* CASL, Comprehensive Assessment of Spoken Language (Carrow-Woolfolk, 1999); WISC-IV, Wechsler Intelligence Scale for Children – Fourth Edition (Wechsler, 2003).

### *Specific Neuropsychological Functions*

Comprehensive neuropsychological assessment evaluates behavior comprehensively as it relates to CNS function. The testing performances of the two children are described generally by function, highlighting the most significant results for each child.

*Attention and Concentration.* As expected, each of the children displayed variability in their attentiveness. For instance, Ray's ability to sustain attention, concentrate, and exert mental control was in the low average range on the WISC-IV, and he performed better than only 18% of his age-mates. As a result of these difficulties, Ray frequently missed directions in the classroom, but because of his poor language abilities, he was unable to speak up and ask for assistance. Similarly, Loretta displayed poor attentiveness and hyperactivity but with more extreme levels of difficulty. On the WISC-IV, Loretta's ability to sustain attention, concentrate, and exert mental control was in the borderline range, and she performed better than only 6% of her age-mates. This was true even though she was on medication designed to improve her attention and concentration. During testing Loretta was unable to sit still most of the time, and a portion of the WJ-III that assessed a child's ability to quickly compose simple sentences had to be discontinued because she was unable to retain the instructions. These difficulties mirror her similar experiences in the classroom. Loretta was unable to sit still during lessons, and she was frequently in trouble for her inability to attend to class materials and her disruption of lectures.

*Executive Functioning.* The executive system is essentially a system of self-governance, self-monitoring, and self-regulation. It provides us with the ability to organize and plan, initiate and maintain activity, learn from past mistakes, and change our behavior to conform to environmental demands. Both Ray and Loretta exhibited anomalies of the executive system, performing well on some tests of executive ability but not on others. More specifically, they had difficulties with working memory and with tasks that required the organization and manipulation of complex visual and verbal material.

Not surprisingly, Loretta had greater difficulties with her executive system. Although she was able to produce simple verbal material by meaningful categories (e.g., certain letters of the alphabet or animals) on a test of verbal fluency, her performances dropped dramatically when information became more complex, either verbally or visually. For example, she had great difficulty organizing and copying complex visuospatial information and performed in the bottom 1% of children in a test that involved copying a complex figure. In the classroom, these difficulties meant that when Loretta had to copy and organize large quantities of information, she was hopelessly frustrated and unable to follow through on the teacher's directions.

*Language Functioning.* Both children had significant language difficulties, although Loretta's problems were again more severe. In conversations with the examiner, Ray's speech was generally good, but he had difficulties with his expressive language abilities, especially in unstructured tasks. Testing of Ray's language abilities revealed that his oral language functioning was in the low range, with his overall score on the Comprehensive Assessment of Speech and Language (CASL; Carro Woolfolk, 1999) falling in the borderline range. The specifics of his performance on the CASL are illuminating. The test was developed in order to assess both language knowledge and performance according to four categories of performance (lexical/semantic, syntactic, supralinguistic, and pragmatic) and three processing systems (oral expression, comprehension and expression, and retrieval). Although Ray scored in the average range on a test to measure his ability to identify words that are opposite in meaning, he performed in the borderline range on a test designed to better understand a person's syntactic abilities by assessing the ability to use the morphosyntactic rules of language to formulate and produce sentences.

By contrast, on another test of syntactic ability that relied on auditory comprehension instead of expression, Ray's score fell solidly in the average range. His score fell to the borderline ranges on tests primarily assessing comprehension but requiring oral expression. On a test requiring primarily expression with a smaller comprehension component, his performance also fell in the borderline range. These results suggested relative difficulty accessing and expressing complex semantic linguistic stores.

Language was an area of great difficulty for Loretta as well. In conversations with the examiner, her speech was halting and lacking in rhythm and structure. Her articulation was very poor, and at times her speech was very difficult to understand. Not surprisingly, testing of Loretta's language abilities revealed that her oral language functioning was in the low range. On the CASL, her overall score was in the low average range, with several areas in the borderline range. As did Ray, Loretta had difficulty accessing and expressing complex semantic linguistic stores. Overall, a mild discrepancy existed between the expression and retrieval systems that may also be related to difficulties with the phoneme-grapheme components of comprehension.

Each of the children's poor language skills resulted in poor academic performance. Ray asked for help infrequently and was perceived as shy by both his teacher and his classmates. When Loretta spoke up in the classroom, her teacher had great difficulty understanding her at the most basic level.

*Memory.* With regard to memory functions in general, both children performed essentially within the normal ranges on tests of simple visual memory. As was evident, however, from their performances on the WISC-IV and other measures requiring them to process information quickly or pay greater attention, their performance on any domain was poorer when the particular task in that domain required fast or complex processing. This was particularly true in the assessment of their memory abilities. For example, Ray performed in the impaired range on a test of his ability to recall a figure he had just drawn (the immediate delay trial of the figure-drawing test). Ray's initial drawing was organized (unlike Loretta's), but after a short delay he was unable to recall the figure, and he required a greater time to consolidate this information from his working memory, as evidenced by a much better performance after a 30-minute delay. Although children at this age typically do worse at 3 minutes than at 30, Ray's performance was outside what is typical for a child his age.

Ray's difficulties appear to arise from his working memory. Working memory is sometimes thought of as a synonym for short-term memory. However, the two terms have slightly different meanings. Working memory emphasizes the active, task-based nature of the memory store; it is implicated particularly in carrying out complex cognitive tasks. The classic example is complicated mental arithmetic, in which a person must hold the results of previous calculations in working memory while he or she works on the next stage. The working memory contains two complementary systems for storing information, the articulatory loop and the visuospatial scratchpad. (Both systems are linked to the so-called central executive system, a more active system that actually performs the short-term memory task.) Ray appears to have difficulty with both working memory systems when information is complex. However, he also appears to have slightly greater difficulty on even simple verbal tasks, compared to his performance on nonverbal tasks. In the classroom, this difficulty frequently manifests in an inability to recall multistep directions given orally by Ray's teachers.

*Motor Functioning.* Both children performed normally with both hands on a test requiring fine motor speed, accuracy, and dexterity. However, on a test assessing the ability to control motor performance when drawing, Ray scored in the borderline range, and Loretta scored in the low average range. Similarly, Ray has great difficulty writing. He formed letters and sentences only with a great deal of effort and had to "shake out" his hand frequently during writing tasks. The few writing samples he provided during the examination also exhibited dysgraphia (i.e., poor writing abilities) and great difficulty with printing. Loretta had great difficulty with handwriting as well. Because both children were in classrooms that "graded" handwriting abilities, these motor difficulties contributed significantly to their increased frustration in school.

*Visuospatial Functioning.* Each child's basic visuospatial abilities were within normal limits, with scores ranging from average to high average. On tests requiring that they draw or copy a simple visual stimulus example, they performed reasonably well. Consistent with their performances on other tests, however, their performance was impaired when the information became more complex. This indicated that they had good visuospatial abilities but that their working memory difficulties impeded their performances on more complex visuospatial tasks.

*Emotional Functioning and Personality.* Scores on instruments that capture others' perceptions of the children's performance and behavior, as well as their own perception, reflect numerous clinically significant difficulties for each of the children, including anxiety, depression, and perfectionism. In particular, both of the children seemed very sad and anxious during testing. For example, they asked repeatedly if they were stupid and became teary eyed at several points during the sessions. On numerous occasions they asked about their performances and whether they were getting things "right."

## INTERVENTIONS

As a first step, preventing continuing exposure is critical. School personnel can turn to the pages at the end of this chapter for a list of organizations from which information about prevention (as well as other topics) can be obtained.

### Medical Interventions

Chelation therapy can be used to speed the process by which the body rids itself of lead. At the simplest level, chelation uses chemical substances to bind to the lead in the blood stream and thereby cause that lead to be excreted through normal bodily processes (i.e., urination). The word *chelate* refers to the ability to form tightly bound associations with metal ions. In chelation, ligands (i.e., ions that attach to other ions) attach to a central metal ion. When a ligand attaches itself to a central metal ion with the use of two or more additional atoms, the result is referred to as a chelating group and the resulting ring is a metal "chelate." This binding removes the metal ions from circulation and promotes removal of any metal bound to enzymes and other tissue components. The metal chelate complexes, which are water soluble, are then excreted in the urine (Ettinger, n.d.).

Chelation therapy increases the rate of lead excretion in the short term by as much as 25 to 30 times. In the absence of treatment, after removal from exposure, blood lead concentrations decline rapidly at first but thereafter continue to decline only slowly over a period of months or years. Although lead chelation reduces blood lead concentrations rapidly, the levels may rebound within weeks to months after treatment. As a result, repeated courses of treatment are often required. The persistence of elevated lead levels is believed to occur because the majority of lead concentrates in bone, where a variety of factors (e.g., growth spurts) can result in re-release of lead into the blood stream. With or without treatment, children with higher initial blood lead levels have been shown to have greater declines compared to children with lower blood lead level initially (Ettinger, n.d.).

## Educational Interventions

The cognitive effects of lead exposure persist long after the toxins have been removed from the environment and the CNS. Consequently, these children's difficulties in school are likely to become more pronounced as greater demands are made on them academically, and the effects of lead exposure are likely to follow them well into adulthood. Although no studies have assessed the effectiveness of educational interventions specifically for those already exposed to lead, interventions geared toward children with similar symptoms and cognitive issues may help affected children to catch up and progress in their development. These interventions are listed below.

### *Assistive Technology*

In the home, provision of specialized computer software (and a computer) that focuses on reading, math, and writing abilities may be helpful. At school, a laptop computer may be necessary as the curriculum becomes more difficult, in part to reduce handwriting requirements that tax motor skills.

### *Classroom Support*

Several things may be helpful in order to increase classroom support for these students. These may include:

- A counselor to monitor progress.
- Tutoring after school and during the summer.
- A one-on-one aide to assist in school and at home.
- At college, an assistant for note taking and other accommodations appropriate to the environment.
- For attentional issues, a structured environment with short, frequent periods of learning.
- Full assessments of speech and language issues, followed by interventions designed to meet individual strengths and weaknesses.

### *Other Forms of Support*

Depending on the specific needs of each student, other methods of intervention, accommodation, and support may be needed:

- Occupational therapy for motor difficulties.
- Enrollment in a commercial program for children with reading difficulties (e.g., Fast ForWord or Lindamood Bell).

- As children get older, access to vocational and rehabilitation counselors, as their cognitive difficulties will likely affect their career choices.

## Additional Evaluations and Other Specialized Guidance

- Comprehensive pediatric neurological and psychopharmacological consultations.
- A comprehensive speech and language evaluation and supplemental neuropsychological assessments.
- A behavioral specialist to assist the family in setting up a behavioral support system.
- Nutritional counseling to monitor the amount of iron and calcium intake (inadequate amounts can increase the negative effects of ingested lead).

## Actions Teachers Can Take to Educate Families About Lead Exposure

School personnel, especially classroom teachers, can do many things to help educate children and their families about the risks of lead exposure. Initially, teachers can instruct preschool and kindergarten students on how to prevent lead exposure. For example, young students should be advised not to chew on painted surfaces, toys, or crayons, or eat paint chips. They can be taught to routinely wash their hands with soap and water before eating, before bedtime, and after playing. Helping students understand that eating healthy meals and snacks that contain calcium, iron, and vitamin C (milk, orange juice, dark green vegetables, meat, beans, etc.) will ensure that they are getting enough vitamins. Many of these issues about lead poisoning can be taught in 1st through 12th grades during health and environmental classes. Teachers may want to include a take-home assignment about lead exposure to discuss with parents and to promote the school-to-home learning connection.

Many Internet sites contain model curriculums for teaching children of various ages about lead and its hazardous effects. A simple Google search using "teachers and lead poisoning" yields a multitude of creative choices. The resource list below includes some of the best sources of information.

# CONCLUSION

The ongoing effort to prevent exposure to lead remains vitally important. As part of that effort, teachers and other school personnel can play a key role by helping to educate parents about lead hazards and the consequences of lead exposure. As long as lead remains in a child's environment, however, screening children for exposure, and effective medical and educational intervention for those who have been exposed, will also be of critical importance. School personnel can be on the front lines in identifying children who may have been exposed to lead and in advocating for them to receive a thorough medical evaluation and, if necessary, for steps to be taken to remove the source of lead from their environment. Finally, school personnel are best placed to work with other experts to design educational interventions that are tailored to a child's individual education needs, interventions that can not only help with classroom performance but also create a better life for the child as he or she becomes an adult.

## RESOURCES

### Books

Kessel, I., & O'Connor, J. T. (2001). *Getting the lead out: The complete resource for preventing and coping with lead poisoning* (rev. ed.). Cambridge, MA: Perseus.

This book explains the nature and sources of lead poisoning, discusses the basic measures for minimizing the associated risks, explains the physical and emotional effects of lead poisoning, and gives readers the information they will need to identify symptoms of poisoning in their children as well as lists of resources addressing each special need that may emerge due to exposure.

Livingston, D. (1997). *Maintaining a lead safe home* (3rd ed.). N.p.: Community Resources.

This book is a do-it-yourself manual for home owners and property managers; it provides step-by-step instructions and detailed illustrations of affordable solutions to lead-based paint problems.

Stapleton, R. M. (1995). *Lead is a silent hazard.* New York: Walker & Company.

This book is written by a former CBS news producer who decided to have his baby son tested for lead after researching a segment on the effects of lead poisoning on children.

### Organizations and Web Sites

Agency for Toxic Substances and Disease Registry

An agency of the U.S. Department of Health and Human Services. The Web site gives general information about lead poisoning and other toxic substances.

Web Site: www.atsdr.cdc.gov/index.html

Childhood Lead Poisoning and Prevention Program

This program is located within the U.S. Centers for Disease Control and Prevention (CDC), National Center for Environmental Health.

It provides information to state and local health departments and facts for public knowledge.

Web Site: www.cdc.gov/nceh/lead/lead.htm

Coalition to End Childhood Lead Poisoning
This is a national nonprofit organization that has information directed to parents for prevention and treatment of child lead poisoning.

Web Site: www.leadsafe.org/index.htm

Community Lead Education and Reduction Corps (CLEAR Corps)
This Web site provides information on research, risk assessment, and abatement.

Mailing Address: 1416 Sulphur Spring Road
Baltimore, Maryland 21227
Phone Number: (410) 247-3339
Web Site: www.clearcorps.org

Consumer Protection Safety Commission
The Web site of this federal department offers information on lead in consumer products and aims to increase awareness of paint and chemical stripper hazards.

Web Site: www.cpsc.gov

Department of Housing and Urban Development (HUD)
The Web site of this federal department offers printable guidelines and information on lead hazard control in English and Spanish. It also has a Web page dedicated to information for parents.

Web Site: www.hud.gov/offices/lead

Environmental Defense Fund (EDF)
By typing "lead" into the search box, readers can access publications such as "Hour of Lead" (a brief history of lead poisoning in the United States), "What You Should Know About Lead in China Dishes," and other publications on environmental toxins.

Web Site: www.environmentaldefense.org

Environmental Protection Agency (EPA)
The Web site of this federal department offers a page about lead with information, brochures, technical issues relevant to the federal lead program, and U.S. regulations. Within the main EPA Web site, the National Lead Information Clearinghouse provides the general public and professionals with information about lead hazards and their prevention. The National Lead Information Center provides information on laboratories across the country that test paint for lead contamination.

Phone Number: (800) 424-LEAD
Web Sites: www.epa.gov/lead
www.epa.gov/lead/pubs/nlic.htm

Food and Drug Administration

By typing "lead poison" into the search box on the Web site of this federal department, readers can find suggestions against childhood lead poisoning and products that contain lead.

Web Site: www.fda.gov

Lead Listing Service

This Web site provides a state-by-state listing of companies providing lead services, including lead-based paint inspection, risk assessment, and abatement contracting.

Web Site: www.leadlisting.org

MedlinePlus Information on Lead Poisoning

This information is from the National Library of Medicine at the National Institutes of Health. It provides articles from federal departments, e.g., the EPA, OSHA, and HUD.

Web Site: www.nlm.nih.gov/medlineplus/leadpoisoning.html

National Environmental Training Association (NETA)

This organization offers a one-day training course on the maintenance of lead-based paint. The course, which was developed under a grant from HUD and EPA, provides basic training for multifamily maintenance staff in how to deal with lead paint safely during repair and repainting projects. The trainer's package includes a detailed instructor's manual, overhead transparencies, and a 9-part video. Each trainee receives a laminated planning tool. The course is available for $129 through NETA at 602-956-6099 or HUD User at 800-245-2691.

National Institute of Environmental Health Sciences (NIEHS)

The link below will take the reader to the "Alphabetical Index of Health Topics" page. It offers some articles about lead's effects on children and family members.

Web Site: www.niehs.nih.gov/external/faq/alpha-l.htm

National Safety Council (NSC)

The NSC Web site lists government, tribal, and independent organizations that provide information on lead poisoning, including a link to material suitable for children.

Web Sites: www.nsc.org/issues/lead/
www.nsc.org/ehc/nlic/kidspage.htm

Occupational Safety and Health Administration (OSHA)

The U.S. Department of Labor's OSHA provides information on its Web site regarding the identification and evaluation procedures, the health effects of lead, and additional information.

Web Site: www.osha.gov/SLTC/lead/index.html

United Parents Against Lead (UPAL)

UPAL is comprised of parents of lead-poisoned kids. The UPAL Web site provides information and referrals to families on a state, local, and national level.

Phone Number: (773) 324-7824
Web Site: www.upal.org

## REFERENCES


Agency for Toxic Substances and Disease Registry. (1999). Toxicological profile for lead (update). Atlanta, GA: U.S. Department of Health and Human Services.

Baghurst, P., McMichael, A., Tong, S., Wigg, N., Vimpani, G., & Robertson, E. (1995). Exposure to environmental lead and visual-motor integration at age 7 years: The Port Pirie Cohort Study. *Epidemiology, 6,* 104–109.

Baghurst, P., McMichael, A., Wigg, N., Vimpani, G., Robertson, E., Roberts, R., et al. (1992). Environmental exposure to lead and children's intelligence at the age of seven years. *New England Journal of Medicine, 327,* 1279–1284.

Bellinger, D., & Dietrich, K. (1994). Low level lead exposure and cognitive function in children. *Pediatric Annals, 23,* 600–605.

Bellinger, D., Leviton, A., Waternaux, C., Needleman, H., & Rabinowitz, M. (1987). Longitudinal analyses of prenatal and postnatal lead exposure and early cognitive development. *New England Journal of Medicine, 316,* 1037–1043.

Carrow-Woolfolk, E. (1999). *Comprehensive Assessment of Spoken Language.* Bloomington, MN: Pearson Assessments.

Dietrich, K. (2000). Environmental neurotoxicants and psychological development. In K. Yeates, M. Ris, & H. Taylor (Eds.), *Pediatric neuropsychology: Research, theory, and practice* (pp. 206–234). New York: Guilford Press.

Dietrich, K., Berger, O., & Succop, P. (1993). Lead exposure and the motor developmental status of urban six-year-old children in the Cincinnati Prospective Study. *Pediatrics, 91,* 301–307.

Dietrich, K., Krafft, K., Bornschein, R., Hammond, P., Berger, O., Succop, P., et al. (1987). Low-level fetal lead exposure effect on neurobehavioral development in early infancy. *Pediatrics, 80,* 721–730.

Dietrich, K., Succop, P., Berger, O., & Keith, R. (1992). Lead exposure and the central auditory processing abilities and cognitive development of urban children: The Cincinnati Lead Study cohort at age 5 years. *Neurotoxicology and Teratology, 14,* 51–56.

Dudek, B., & Merecz, D. (1997). Impairment of psychological functions in children environmentally exposed to lead. *International Journal of Occupational Medicine and Environmental Health, 10,* 37–46.

Ettinger, A. S. (n.d.). *Chelation therapy for childhood lead poisoning: Does excretion equal efficacy?* Retrieved July 21, 2007, from http://www.hsph.harvard.edu/Organizations/DDIL/chelation.htm

Lanphear, B., Dietrich, K., Auinger, P., & Cox, C. (2000). Cognitive deficits associated with blood lead concentrations, 10 microg/dL in US children and adolescents. *Public Health Reports, 115,* 521–529.

Lanphear, B., Hornung, R., Khoury, J., Yolton, K., Baghurst, P., Bellinger, D., et al. (2005). Low-level environmental lead exposure and children's intellectual function: An international pooled analysis. *Environmental Health Perspectives, 113,* 894–899.

Lidsky, T., & Schneider, J. (2006). Adverse effects of childhood lead poisoning: The clinical neuropsychological perspective. *Environmental Research, 100,* 284–293.

Needleman, H., & Gatsonis, C. (1990). Low level lead exposure the IQ of children. *Journal of the American Medical Association, 263,* 673–678.

Needleman, H., Gunnow, C., Leviton, A., Reed, R., Peresie, H., Maher, C., et al. (1979). Deficits in psychological and classroom performance of children with elevated dentine lead levels. *New England Journal of Medicine, 300,* 689–695.

Pocock, S., Smith, M., & Baghurst, P. (1994). Environmental lead and children's intelligence: A systematic review of the epidemiological evidence. *British Medical Journal, 309,* 1189–1187.

Ris, M., Dietrich, K., Succop, P., Berger, O., & Bornschein, R. (2004). Early exposure to lead and neuropsychological outcome in adolescence. *Journal of the International Neuropsychological Society, 10,* 261–270.

Schwartz, J. (1994a). Low level lead exposure and children's IQ: A meta-analysis and search for a threshold. *Environmental Research, 65,* 42–55.

Schwartz, J. (1994b). Societal benefits of reducing lead exposure. *Environmental Research, 66,* 105–124.

Shannon, M., Best, D., Binns, H., Kim, J., Mazur, L., Weil, W., et al. (2005). Lead exposure in children: Detection, prevention and management. *Pediatrics, 116,* 1036–1046.

Stiles, K., & Bellinger, D. (1993). Neuropsychological correlates of low-level lead exposure in school-age children: A prospective study. *Neurotoxicology and Teratology, 15,* 27–35.

Wasserman, G., Graziano, J., Factor-Litvak, P., Popovac, D., Morina, N., Musabegovic, A., et al. (1994). Consequences of lead exposure and iron supplementation on childhood development at age 4 years. *Neurotoxicology and Teratology, 16,* 233–244.

Wechsler, D. (2003). *Wechsler Intelligence Scale for Children* (4th ed.). San Antonio, TX: The Psychological Corporation.

Wigg, N., Vimpani, F., McMichael, A., Baghurst, P., Robertson, S., & Roberts, R. (1988). Port Pirie cohort study: Childhood blood lead and neuropsychological development at age two years. *Journal of Epidemiology and Community Health, 42,* 213–219.

Winneke, G., Brockhaus, A., Ewers, U., Kramer, U., & Neuf, M. (1990). Results from the European multicenter study on lead neurotoxicity in children: Implications for risk assessment. *Neurotoxicology and Teratology, 12,* 553–559.

World Health Organization (WHO), International Programme on Chemical Safety. (1995). *Environmental health criteria 165-inorganic lead.* Geneva: Author.

Woodcock, R., McGrew, K., & Mather, N. (2001). *Woodcock-Johnson Tests of Achievement* (3rd ed.). Itasca, IL: Riverside.

Yeates, K., Ris, M., & Taylor, H. (Eds.). (2000). *Pediatric neuropsychology: Research, theory, and practice.* New York: Guilford Press.

Yuan, W., Holland, S., Cecil, K., Dietrich, K., Wessel, S., Altaye, M., et al. (2006). The impact of early childhood lead exposure on brain organization: A functional magnetic resonance imaging study of language function. *Pediatrics, 118,* 971–977.

CHAPTER FOURTEEN

# Leukemia

Julie K. Ries, PsyD, and Susan A. Scarvalone, MSW, LCSW-C

Childhood leukemia is the most common form of childhood cancer, affecting approximately 3,250 children each year in the United States (Ries et al., 2007). Leukemia is a cancer of the white blood cells, and although it is treatable, and curable in some situations, scientists have not yet found its cause. Due to advances in the treatment for leukemia, the survival rate has improved dramatically since the 1970s. The death rate has fallen nearly 50% (Butler & Haser, 2006), resulting in a current survival rate of approximately 80%. Scientific research also has guided the development of new treatments that are less toxic, therefore decreasing the risk that a child will have cognitive or learning difficulties.

## DESCRIPTION OF THE DISORDER

To understand more about leukemia, it is helpful to review what is known about blood. There are three types of blood cells: red cells, white cells, and platelets, all of which originate in the bone marrow, the spongy material found inside the long bones of the body. These immature cells grow and mature, until they are released into the circulating blood to serve vital, life-sustaining functions.

The red blood cells contain hemoglobin, a protein that collects oxygen from the lungs and carries it to other parts of the body. This is important to prevent anemia (i.e., low red blood cell count). The white cells serve to fight infections in the body. There are three types of white cells: monocytes, lymphocytes, and granulocytes. When leukemia is diagnosed, it is identified by the specific type of white cells affected. Platelets are the cells that assist in forming clots to stop bleeding and to heal bruising.

When the abnormal white cells begin to multiply and are unable to develop into mature white cells, they have no function, yet they continue to grow and take up space within the marrow that would have been occupied by healthy red cells, platelets, and white cells. These leukemia cells also can invade the central nervous system (CNS), the brain, and spinal cord. Even though leukemia is a cancer of the white cells, all blood cells are affected when a child has leukemia. Children become anemic due to a low red blood cell count, are at risk for infection due to a decreased number of healthy white cells, and are prone to bruising and bleeding due to low platelet counts.

## Types of Leukemia

Leukemia can be classified as either acute (i.e., fast growing) or chronic (i.e., slow growing). The majority of childhood leukemias are acute, and the most common form of childhood leukemia is acute lymphoblastic leukemia, also referred to as ALL (Ries et al., 2007). This form of cancer is fast growing and affects the developing lymphocytes. Of the 3,250 children diagnosed with leukemia each year, 75% will have ALL and 20% will have acute monocytic leukemia, also referred to as AMoL (Ries et al., 2007). AMoL is also fast growing and affects the developing monocytes.

The diagnosis of childhood leukemia is most common in children ages 2 to 7 years, with the highest incidence at approximately 3 years of age (Ries et al., 2007). Boys are at slightly higher risk for leukemia than girls, and in the United States, it is seen more often in Whites than in African Americans (Mulhern & Butler, 2004; Ries et al.). The incidence of children diagnosed with leukemia has increased over the past 2 decades (Ries et al.). Gender differences are also noted in long-term survivors' sequelae from the chemotherapy and irradiation, such that irradiation appears to have more harmful cognitive effects for females, whereas males tend to exhibit more learning problems (Brown & Madan-Swain, 1993).

Scientists are studying the genetic and environmental factors that may cause leukemia. They are interested in what happens genetically to cause a normal cell to become a leukemia cell. They are also looking at environmental factors, such as exposure to high doses of radiation or radiation therapy used to treat other types of cancer, or exposure to other chemotherapy agents used for treating prior cancers (Holland & Rowland, 1991).

There is evidence that some genetic diseases increase the risk of developing leukemia, although this is still very rare. These conditions include Down syndrome, neurofibromatosis—type 1, Shwachman syndrome, Bloom syndrome, Fanconi anemia, Kostmann syndrome, and ataxia telangiectasia (Ries et al., 2007). With identical twins, if one develops leukemia before the age of 6 years, there is a 25% chance that the other twin will also develop it within 1 year (Keene, 2002).

## MEDICAL TREATMENT

### Signs and Symptoms

The diagnosis of ALL is usually made after the parents have begun to notice certain signs and symptoms. Children may have one or many of the following symptoms: paleness; more bruises, especially bruises that do not fade; black-and-blue marks for no apparent reason; tiredness; aches in the arms and legs; low stamina; enlarged lymph nodes; and fever. All of these symptoms are seen in far less serious childhood conditions, so the diagnosis of childhood leukemia is often not the initial diagnosis. However, as the symptoms continue to develop, the trained pediatrician will form the diagnosis of leukemia, although it may take several visits. The diagnosis is made by a physical examination and blood work and is confirmed with a bone marrow aspiration and biopsy. Under the microscope, pathologists will see the exact type of leukemia; further tests are then performed for more exact information to guide medical intervention.

### Types of Treatment

The primary medical intervention for ALL is chemotherapy. However, if a child relapses (i.e., if leukemia returns) or is in a high-risk subgroup, a child may receive a combination of chemotherapy and cranial irradiation. Current treatment consists of multiple phases, one of which is CNS therapy. This CNS prophylactic treatment is largely responsible for the marked increase in long-term survival of children with ALL because the CNS houses the leukemic cells; therefore, the prophylactic treatment tackles these cells at their source to reduce the probability of relapse. This phase of therapy general consists of intrathecal chemotherapy (ITC), or the administration of the agent directly into the CNS via cerebrospinal fluid. Cranial or craniospinal irradiation is typically reserved for leukemia that is high risk or for patients who have had a CNS relapse.

### Phases of Treatment

Medical treatment for leukemia can be broken down into four phases, each with a specific purpose: remission induction, CNS preventative therapy or prophylaxis, consolidation, and maintenance (Mulhern & Butler, 2004). The remission induction phase is aimed at rapid elimination of the leukemia cells from the bone marrow and circulatory system. The CNS preventative therapy or prophylaxis involves the use of intrathecal chemotherapy with methotrexate or a combination of methotrexate and other drugs to eradicate leukemia where it is housed in the body. As noted above, certain subgroups (i.e., high risk or relapse) may also receive cranial and/or craniospinal irradiation. Consolidation is used to intensify therapy after remission has occurred. Finally, maintenance therapy involves continued treatment of the less detectable cells for approximately 2.5 to 3 years.

## PSYCHOLOGICAL IMPACT OF ALL

### Initial Diagnosis

When a child is diagnosed with leukemia, it affects the entire family profoundly (Holland & Rowland, 1991). For parents, it means asking how they will be able to care for their child who now has a life-threatening illness. Initial emotional reactions are intense and range from confusion, denial, and fear to anxiety, anger or guilt, and grief or sadness. It is difficult for families to absorb the complicated medical information. They may be unable to accept the serious nature of their child's illness. They may be overwhelmed with guilt over their inability to protect their child from getting leukemia and blame themselves for causing the leukemia or delays in detecting the illness. They also struggle with feelings of helplessness, as they lose control of their child's daily life, and suddenly the medical treatment team is making decisions for their child. Parents may feel very sad and grief stricken, as they realize that their family life will never be the same. In these early days of adjusting to the diagnosis, parents also turn to hope as they begin to absorb the fact that the majority of children with leukemia do conquer their disease (Keene, 2002).

For children, a diagnosis of leukemia means entering a new, unfamiliar world involving painful medical procedures and treatment. They may be aware of how serious their illness is as they see their parents looking frightened and grief stricken. In addition to feeling unwell physically, they have emotional reactions as well. Infants, toddlers, and preschool children may have fears of separation, abandonment, and loneliness during this time. They look to their parents for comfort and safety and now find that their parents are not in control of their environment as they previously were.

School-age children will also feel this disruption, but their primary fears are often more related to physical injury and bodily harm. It is not uncommon for children to view their illness as a punishment for their own thoughts and actions and to feel guilty about this (Leukemia and Lymphoma Society, 2005); this is especially the case because no one yet knows what causes leukemia. In addition, the children are now exposed to the hospital unit where they see that other children who are going through treatment look different because of their medical treatment. All of this is quite unsettling for the school-age child.

Older school-age children and adolescents also respond emotionally to the diagnosis and early days of therapy. They are able to cognitively understand the serious nature of the disease, the specific medical information (when delivered in age-appropriate terms), and how the illness is affecting them, their family, and friends. At this age, they are more worried about illness and the possibility of death, and when this is coupled with the reality of having a life-threatening illness, older children and adolescents can feel vulnerable and frightened for their own future.

The early days following the diagnosis are very intense for both the child and family, but as treatment starts, there is also a new focus on being hopeful about the future. Because most children with leukemia respond so positively in the early stages of their treatment, both the child and family can see that the treatment is working, which helps them to feel positive about the remaining treatment.

Because the early stages of treatment for leukemia are so intensive, the child will be spending much time in the hospital, either as an inpatient or for clinic visits. There will be both anticipated and unanticipated hospital visits, given that children at this stage are also very vulnerable to infections in their immunocompromised state of health.

As a result, school-age children will face disruption in their school attendance and participation. This has far-reaching effects for children with leukemia; in addition to missing important academic lessons, they are also missing opportunities for learning important socialization skills and developing and maintaining friendships. Because school is so central to the lives of children, this disruption is often a source of great concern and worry for both children and parents.

For many children with leukemia, returning to school is not possible until they are in remission and the therapy enters the less intensive maintenance phase. This phase of treatment signals a time when life is usually more predictable. The child is still susceptible to infections, which could mean further time as an inpatient. However, although children are still having frequent clinic visits, they are now stable enough to tolerate school attendance and participation (Steen & Mirro, 2000). Fortunately, many programs are available to assist when children are unable to return to school (Leukemia and Lymphoma Society, 2005). Homebound or hospital-based educational programs exist and are mandated by law to provide educational opportunities for all children who have disabilities.

## SEQUELAE OF THE DISORDER AND TREATMENT

### Acute Sequelae

During the acute phase of treatment, or the period from diagnosis through treatment, children with leukemia may be absent from school due to frequent illness (e.g., nausea, fever, fatigue) because of their compromised immune system, ALL, or side effects from the treatment regimen. A child may be referred for a neuropsychological evaluation during this phase as part of a research protocol to assess the impact of the treatment regimen on the child's functioning. In addition, the school psychologist can potentially serve a valuable role at this time by supporting the child's adjustment to the diagnosis and treatment, as well as facilitating the child's ability to have homework sent home and ensuring that services are maintained through the homebound or hospital-based tutor so that the child is able to keep up with peers.

### Postacute Sequelae

Most children will transition back to school. A neuropsychological evaluation may be done during this phase in order to identify the child's profile of strengths and limitations. The strengths can be used to mitigate some of the limitations (e.g., a strength in auditory memory may be used to facilitate learning for a child who has visual memory difficulties). The child may benefit from an individualized education plan (IEP) in order to address any potential limitations that may be identified during the neuropsychological evaluation. The school psychologist can assist a parent by providing information regarding the procedure to initiate an IEP and may also potentially do some school-based assessment in preparation for the IEP meeting. The school psychologist will serve a critical role in helping the child transition back to school and to adjust to life posttreatment.

## Late Effects

Late effects "are temporally defined as occurring after the successful completion of medical therapy, usually two or more years from the time of diagnosis, and it is generally assumed that late effects are chronic, if not progressive in their course" (Mulhern & Butler, 2004, p. 1). One of the more common late effects is fatigue. It may not be apparent until a year posttreatment, especially following cranial radiation therapy (CRT). For a comprehensive list of potential late effects of each system of the body, see *Late Effects of Treatment for Childhood Cancer* as listed in the Resources section at the end of this chapter.

Children may be referred for a neuropsychological evaluation to determine the impact of their treatment on their current functioning as late effects can occur several years following treatment. As noted above, ALL treatment may negatively impact the developing myelin, resulting in problems with higher order cognitive functioning that may not be apparent until a child reaches a particular developmental level.

# NEUROPSYCHOLOGICAL ASPECTS OF LEUKEMIA

## Overview

Due to advances in medicine, more than 80% of children diagnosed with ALL are cured of the disease (Mulhern & Butler, 2004); however, long-term survivors may face overt and covert neuropsychological sequelae faced by long-term survivors. Some studies have found global effects on some children's cognitive function (Mulhern et al., 1987), whereas other studies have highlighted changes in specific neuropsychological functions (Iuvone et al., 2002; Peckham, Meadows, Bartel, & Marrero, 1988), or both global and specific effects (Campbell et al., 2007; Mulhern & Butler). These discrepancies are due in part to the fact that the older research focused solely on intellectual assessment and academic achievement, which was not sensitive enough to target specific neuropsychological deficits associated with the CNS prophylaxis (intrathecal methotrexate and CRT; Butler & Haser, 2006).

In addition, some of the sequelae may be overt and noticed immediately (i.e., tingling of the fingers, slowed processing, hearing loss), whereas other sequelae may be more subtle and not manifest until a child reaches a developmental level in which the skill must be utilized (i.e., increased executive function demands in middle school and high school). In a sample of long-term survivors of acute lymphocytic leukemia who had received high doses of cranial irradiation (2,400 cGy), Peckham and colleagues (1988) observed deficits on school performance approximately

8 to 10 years after treatment. Research has guided medical advances, so that the dose of cranial irradiation has been decreased from 2,400 cGy to 1,800 cGy, resulting in a decrease in the severity of the neurocognitive impact on long-term survivors (Peckham et al.). Therefore, less deficit might be revealed in more recent studies that include children who received lower doses of irradiation compared to children who received highers dose of irradiation.

Several researchers have examined the neuropathology of the neuropsychological sequelae of the CNS prophylaxis. Cognitive functions including memory, attention, and processing speed are mediated by myelin in the brain. Research by Burger and Boyko (1991) found that the CNS prophylaxis (i.e., cranial irradiation and intrathecal methotrexate) resulted in demyelination and radiation produced necrosis (i.e., cell death) of this white matter. The amount or volume of cerebral white matter was also found to play an important role in attention (Reddick et al., 2006; Mulhern, White, et al., 2004), specifically, cerebral white matter volumes in the prefrontal/frontal lobe and cingulated gyrus. The rate of development of this white matter was found to be an important factor in the neuropsychological sequelae exhibited by childhood cancer survivors (Butler & Haser, 2006). In addition, some studies revealed that some of the deficits in immediate and delayed verbal recall and difficulty shifting set from one task to another may be at least partially due to cerebral calcifications located in the basal ganglia, which has extensive connections to the frontal lobes of the brain (Brouwers & Poplack, 1990; Brown & Madan-Swain, 1993).

## Cognitive/Intellectual Functioning

Although medical advances have improved the treatment of ALL, neurocognitive impairment continues to be a risk for specific interventions. "The risks for neurocognitive impairment, even among those treated without cranial radiation therapy (CRT), remains significant in that approximately 30% of those treated with intrathecal chemotherapy will exhibit cognitive dysfunction" (Mulhern & Butler, 2004, p. 10). Intrathecal chemotherapy is infused into the CNS via the cerebrospinal fluid. Methotrexate is believed to be one of the more neurotoxic intrathecal chemotherapies (Cole & Kamen, 2006; Waber & Mullenix, 2000), in addition to cytarabine and hydrocortisone.

Some studies have noted that children were at higher risk for potential neurocognitive deficits if they were diagnosed at a younger age (Peckham et al., 1988), female, or treated with 2,400 cGy of cranial irradiation, intrathecal and IV methotrexate, and corticosteroids (Eiser, 2004; Mulhern & Butler, 2004). The neurocognitive deficits may not be apparent until after the maintenance therapy (Jansen et al., 2005) and may be temporary, persist for years, or be permanent (Cole & Kamen, 2006).

During the mid- to late 1980s, researchers examined the impact of cranial irradiation on higher cortical and subcortical neuropsychological functions (Copeland et al., 1988). Irradiation appeared to have the greatest impact on perceptual reasoning, arithmetic, visual-motor integration, and reduced processing speed. Some studies have found that CNS prophylaxis (intrathecal chemotherapy) in combination with cranial irradiation is directly related to learning problems found in children with ALL (Précourt et al., 2002; Van Dongen-Melman, De Groot, Van Dongen, Verhulst, & Hählen, 1997). Delayed neurotoxic effects, known as late effects, appear to be due to this combination (Mulhern et al., 1987; Waber et al., 1995) because CRT reportedly increases the ability of the neurotoxic chemotherapy to cross the blood-brain barrier (Griffin, Rasey, & Bleyer, 1977).

## Attention and Executive Functioning

One of the first studies to examine underlying neuropsychological sequelae that were negatively impacted by CNS prophylaxis (intrathecal chemotherapy and a dose of 2,400 cGy of CRT) focused on the role of the nondominant hemisphere and subcortical functions (Rowland et al., 1984). Specifically, deficits included shortened attention span, increased distractibility, poor concentration, and academic underachievement, most notably in arithmetic. Another study (Butler, Hill, Steinherz, Meyers, & Finlay, 1994) examining various combinations of CNS prophylaxis yielded similar results, supporting the hypothesis that cranial irradiation in combination with intrathecal methotrexate was significantly associated with impaired neuropsychological functions of the nondominant hemisphere, including nonverbal intelligence, perceptual localization, nondominant-hand motor skills, visual-motor integration, and problems with regulation of attention.

In a study of 23 children who were long-term survivors of acute lymphocytic leukemia who were given high doses of irradiation (2,400 cGy), 83% (19 out of 23) reportedly had problems with attention or concentration described as "lapses, floats, not listening, or short circuits" (Peckham et al., 1988, p. 129). Even with reductions in the dose of radiation (from 2,400 cGy to 1,800 cGy), researchers continued to see problems with cancer survivors' attention regulation systems (Lockwood, Bell, & Colegrove, 1999). Specifically, children who received cranial irradiation before the age of 54 months demonstrated difficulty executing basic and more complex attention skills, including tracking, focusing, shifting, active mental switching, problem solving, and sustained attention, whereas those children who received cranial irradiation later in childhood (older than 54 months) demonstrated milder problems with sustained attention and mental switching. One study pinpointed underlying attentional deficits that negatively impact the encoding stage of memory processing as a factor contributing to short-term memory impairments (Brouwers & Poplack, 1990).

## Memory and Learning

Memory problems were also reported in the literature. A study of 23 children (Peckham et al., 1988) who were long-term survivors of acute lymphocytic leukemia reported visual memory problems (65%, 15 out of 23) and auditory memory problems (52%, 12 of 23). Another study found that regardless of the combination of CNS prophylaxis, children treated for ALL performed significantly lower than age-corrected norms on a test of visual-spatial memory (Mulhern, Wasserman, Fairclough, & Ochs, 1988). Another study examined the late effects of a combination of intrathecal chemotherapy and CRT compared with intrathecal chemotherapy alone with a sample of 19 females, ages 7 to 11 years. Results of the study revealed a deficit primarily impacting auditory attention and verbal learning in girls who received the combination therapy. This deficit was seen on measures of reading comprehension, auditory working memory, and the later learning trials of the second half of a verbal learning measure (Précourt et al., 2002).

## Visual-Motor, Visual-Perceptual, Visual-Spatial, and Motor Functioning

The right frontal lobe of the brain is involved in visual and spatial reasoning. It has increased myelin and is therefore particularly vulnerable to the effects of CRT (Cole & Kamen, 2006). One study by Hockenberry and colleagues (2007) revealed that children with ALL experienced significant and persistent visual-motor difficulties during their treatment or more than 2 years later. Fine motor and visual-motor processing skills are necessary for higher level cognitive functions including nonverbal intelligence and academic achievement, particularly in tasks of arithmetic and written language. Another study (Regan & Reeb, 1998) examined ALL survivors and found that their visual-motor system was vulnerable to increased demands in design complexity, attention, processing speed, and memory. Deficits were noted both in the input of visual organization of a task as well as the output or fine motor coordination.

Treatment with CRT can reportedly contribute to growth problems in this population and subsequent problems with poor weight gain or obesity (Leung et al., 2000). The biological reason for this variability in weight gain is unknown. One study found that a majority of the sample was physically heavier than same-age peers (17 of 18 subjects; Peckham et al., 1988), most of whom were reported to demonstrate problems with motor coordination.

## Academic Achievement

Peckham and colleagues (1988) touted their work as the first study investigating the educational achievement of long-term survivors of acute lymphocytic leukemia (who had high doses of cranial irradiation) whose pretreatment ability levels were known and whose educational outcomes had been determined. Although more children in this group received reading intervention, their parents and teachers frequently identified learning difficulties in mathematics. Results of this study revealed that 74% (17 out of 23) reported difficulty in learning basic mathematics facts related to problems with short-term memory, memory for processes, and sequencing the order of operations.

In contrast, 40% (9 of the 23 subjects) cited difficulties with reading comprehension. A statistically significant difference between actual and expected reading achievement ($p$=.0025) and math achievement ($p$=.0032) was noted. In addition, 14 of the 23 children reported difficulty telling time on a circular clock. A majority of the children (70%, 16 of 23) reported problems with remembering, sequencing, and following multiple directions. Approximately 65% (15 of 23 subjects) were observed to exhibit poor performance under pressure, forgetting previously learned material, and testing below homework or class work performance. It is important to note that two of the children excelled in reading, and one excelled in mathematics. Some studies have revealed a higher incidence of academic difficulties, particularly reading and math performance, when a child received CRT and was younger at diagnosis (Campbell, et al., 2007; Kumar, Mulhern, Regine, Rivera, & Kun, 1995; Leung et al., 2000). Leung and colleagues estimated that the probability of academic difficulties decreased by approximately 50% if CRT was delayed until the child was 2 years of age instead of occurring soon after diagnosis in infants.

## Psychological, Emotional, and Behavioral Functioning

Some studies have examined the psychological, behavioral, and social adjustment of children following a cancer diagnosis and treatment, yielding variable results. One large sibling-controlled, multisite study of young adult survivors of childhood leukemia (this study examined acute myelogenous leukemia [AML]), Hodgkin's disease, and non-Hodgkin's lymphoma revealed a significantly increased risk (1.6 to 1.7 times more likely) of symptoms of depression and somatic distress, and intensive chemotherapy added to this risk (Zebrack et al., 2002). However, the investigators noted that being a cancer survivor did not compound the risk for depression and distress associated with these demographic characteristics (i.e., female gender and low socioeconomic status). Levin-Newby, Brown, Pawletko, Gold, & Whitt (2000) studied cancer survivors several years posttreatment. They found that although their sample generally experienced normal social development and few internalizing or externalizing behavioral problems, approximately 14 percent of the survivors met criteria for poor adjustment as rated by their parents. This study highlights the need for multiple raters in various contexts in order to fully assess a child's psychological well-being.

Other studies have suggested that many survivors of childhood cancer were at increased risk for maladaptive psychosocial sequelae, including depression (Koocher & O'Malley, 1981) and posttraumatic stress disorder. Peckham and colleagues (1988) reported that slightly more than half of their sample (15 of 23 children) was described as more immature than their peers based on parent and teacher report.

## Case Studies of Leukemia

Two case studies are presented below in order to illustrate examples of potential neuropsychological patterns of performance based on treatment types (chemotherapy only versus chemotherapy and irradiation). It is important to note that these two patients do not represent all children with ALL due to the variability in genetics, family environment, socioeconomic status (SES), gender, culture, and medical disorders; therefore, caution should be taken in making conclusions based on these specific cases. The first case is that of a 10-year-old female who had "standard risk" or more common ALL that was treated with only chemotherapy; the second case is that of a 7.5-year-old male who presented with high-risk ALL due to a relapse and was treated with chemotherapy and irradiation.

### *Case 1: Sarah*

The first case is that of a 10-year-old female named Sarah. She was diagnosed with ALL at 4 years of age. Sarah was described as attaining her developmental milestones on time or earlier than expected. As a toddler, she was noted to have infrequent staring spells of unknown etiology, mild seasonal allergies, and sleeping difficulties. Family history is significant for anxiety and depression, as well as for left-handedness and astigmatism. A combination of side effects of chemotherapy reportedly caused a thrombosis (i.e., blood clot) and a seizure at age 4 years. This was reportedly treated pharmaceutically and has not reoccurred.

At the time of the evaluation, Sarah lived with her biological parents and two younger siblings. She was a fifth-grade student, receiving primarily A's with the exception of some B's in written expression. No academic concerns were noted; however, her mother expressed concern that Sarah had a tendency to exhibit "messy" or "sloppy" printing, but said that her handwriting was "neat." Her parents also expressed some concern regarding Sarah's reported lack of motivation at school and her tendency to put her friends first. She was an athlete involved in soccer, and she played the flute. Sarah underwent a neuropsychological evaluation approximately 6 years after her diagnosis.

### *Case 2: Timothy*

The second case describes Timothy, a 7.5-year-old male diagnosed with B-cell ALL at 3.5 years of age. Timothy lived with his biological parents and was an only child. He was active in Cub Scouts and played several sports. Timothy reportedly had no history of neuropsychological problems, and there was no family history of learning, emotional, or medical problems.

During his kindergarten year, Timothy had a tutor come to his home because of his frequent absences due to his medical appointments and ALL treatment. Upon his return to school, a 504 plan was created to assist Timothy with homework completion. The following accommodations were provided: extra time to complete tasks, chunk work into smaller, more manageable pieces, modify work load as needed, praise attempts to begin and continue work, provision of preferential seating, provision of small group instruction as needed, and allowing him to complete class work at home as needed. In addition, Timothy received one-to-one reading/phonics assistance due to his difficulty in this area; however, he reportedly was not eligible for participation in a remediation group despite some problems with sound discrimination of "b" versus "d" and "q" versus "p", and some reversals of first and last letters of words.

Timothy repeated the first grade because his parents decided to hold him back following significant academic difficulties during his chemotherapy treatment, subsequent frequent trips to the school nurse, and difficulty with homework completion. At the time of the evaluation, he was a first-grade student in mainstream classes and was doing well academically. Timothy's parents observed that he had difficulty remembering what he had learned immediately after it was taught or when asked to demonstrate his newly learned knowledge the next day.

Regarding his medical care for ALL, Timothy underwent an aggressive treatment regimen of chemotherapy; however, CNS recurrence was noted after 14 months. As a result, Timothy received a combination treatment of more chemotherapy and craniospinal irradiation per protocol (total dose to the cranium: 2400 cGy, 150 cGy per day for 3 weeks; total dose to the spine: 1500 cGy, 150 cGy per day for 2 weeks). At the time of the evaluation, he had been in remission for approximately 7 months. The referral was initiated by his oncologist as part of his treatment regimen.

## General Findings

Sarah and Timothy's neuropsychological profiles are presented in Table 14.1. As you can see from the results of their neuropsychological evaluations, their performance is generally consistent with what is described in the literature, given their relative weaknesses in processing speed, working memory, auditory attention, subtle executive function difficulties, intact language, variable memory, and some motor problems. However, their profiles were inconsistent with the literature given their relative strength in perceptual reasoning and intact mathematical skills.

Sarah and Timothy's visual attention abilities were more variable. They both demonstrated a relative strength in target detection (focused attention); however, Timothy's search speed was significantly below that of his same-age peers. Sarah's problems with automaticity were most notable in her relative weakness on academic fluency measures and phonemic fluency. Sarah and Timothy also demonstrated variability in their motor and memory abilities, the latter being possibly negatively influenced by fluctuations in attention. Sarah exhibited average to high average verbal learning, contextual memory, and nonverbal memory, but a weakness was noted in her ability to encode complex visual stimuli via visual-motor input and output and organization. Timothy demonstrated significant variability in both domains. His verbal learning abilities and contextual verbal memory were within the borderline range, whereas

**TABLE 14.1 Neuropsychological Profiles of Two Children With ALL**

| | Sarah (ITC) | Timothy (ITC & CRT) |
|---|---|---|
| Intellectual Functioning | | |
| WISC-IV | | |
| Full Scale IQ | Average | Low average |
| Verbal Comprehension | High average | Low average |
| Perceptual Reasoning | High average | Average |
| Working Memory | Average | Low average |
| Processing Speed | Average | Low average |
| Academic Achievement | | |
| WJ-III | | |
| Letter-Word Identification | Average | Average |
| Passage Comprehension | Average | |
| Reading Fluency | Borderline | |
| Calculation | High average | Average |
| Applied Problems | High average | |
| Math Fluency | Average | |
| Spelling | Average | Average |
| Writing Samples | High average | |
| Writing Fluency | Average | |
| Executive Functioning | | |
| TEA-Ch Sky Search | | |
| Targets | High average | Low average |
| Time | Average | Deficient |
| Attention | Average | Deficient |
| TEA-Ch Score! | Deficient | Borderline |
| TEA-Ch Score DT! | Average | |
| TEA-Ch Creature Counting | | |
| Accuracy | Deficient | Borderline |
| Time | n/a | n/a |
| TEA-Ch Sky Search DT | Average | Deficient |

*Continued*

**TABLE 14.1** *(Continued)*

| | Sarah (ITC) | Timothy (ITC & CRT) |
|---|---|---|
| NEPSY | | |
| Visual Attention | | Low average |
| Verbal Fluency | | Borderline |
| Tower | | Average |
| D-KEFS Trail Making Test | | |
| Visual Scanning | Average | |
| Number Sequencing | Average | |
| Letter Sequencing | Average | |
| Number-Letter Sequencing | Average | |
| D-KEFS Verbal Fluency Test | | |
| Letter Fluency | Low average | |
| Category Fluency | High average | |
| Category Switching | Average | |
| Category Switching Accuracy | Average | |
| D-KEFS Color-Word Interference | | |
| Color Naming | Average | |
| Word Reading | High average | |
| Inhibition | High average | |
| Inhibition/Switching | High average | |
| Language Functioning | | |
| CELF-IV | | |
| Formulated Sentences | High average | |
| Concepts and Following Directions | Average | |
| BNT | Average | |
| NEPSY | | |
| Phonological Processing | | Average |
| Comprehension of Instructions | | Average |
| CTOPP | | |

**TABLE 14.1** *(Continued)*

| | Sarah (ITC) | Timothy (ITC & CRT) |
|---|---|---|
| Rapid Digit Naming | | Low average |
| Rapid Letter Naming | | Average |
| **Learning/Memory** | | |
| CMS Dot Locations | | |
| Learning | | Average |
| Total Score | | Average |
| Long Delay | | Average |
| CMS Stories | | |
| Immediate | High average | Borderline |
| Delayed | High average | Deficient |
| Delayed Recognition | Average | Average |
| CMS Faces | | |
| Immediate | Average | Average |
| Delayed | High average | Low average |
| CVLT-C | | |
| Total Trials 1–5 | Average | Borderline |
| Short-Delay Free Recall | Average | Average |
| Short-Delay Cued Recall | Average | Low average |
| Long-Delay Free Recall | Average | Deficient |
| Long-Delay Cued Recall | Average | Borderline |
| Recognition | High average | Borderline |
| RCFT | | |
| Immediate Recall | Low average | |
| Delayed Recall | Borderline | |
| Recognition | Borderline | |
| **Visual-Spatial and Visual-Motor Functioning** | | |
| VMI-V | | |
| VMI | Low average | Average |
| Visual Perception | Low average | |

*Continued*

**TABLE 14.1** *(Continued)*

| | Sarah (ITC) | Timothy (ITC & CRT) |
|---|---|---|
| Motor Coordination | Low average | |
| NEPSY | | |
| Arrows | | High average |
| Visual-motor Precision | | High average |
| RCFT | | |
| Copy Accuracy | Low average | |
| Copy Time | Low average | |
| **Fine Motor Skills** | | |
| Hand Dynamometer | | |
| Right hand | Deficient | Borderline |
| Left hand | Deficient | Borderline |
| Grooved Pegboard | | |
| Right hand | Average | Low average |
| Left hand | Average | Low average |
| Finger Tapping Test | | |
| Right hand | Low average | Low average |
| Left hand | Borderline | Borderline |

*Note.* Blank cells indicate tasks that were not administered; n/a, not applicable due to the significant number of errors, unable to calculate speed/efficiency; d/c=discontinued; BNT, Boston Naming Test (Kaplan, Goodglass, Weintraub, & Segal, 1983); CELF-IV, Clinical Evaluation of Language Fundamentals—Fourth Edition (Semel, Wigg, & Secord, 2003); CMS, Children's Memory Scale (Cohen, 1997); CRT, Craniospinal irradiation; CTOPP, Comprehensive Test of Phonological Processing (Wagner, Torgesen, & Rashotte, 1999); CVLT-C, California Verbal Learning Test—Children's Version (Delis, Kramer, Kaplan, & Ober, 1994); D-KEFS, Delis-Kaplan Executive Function System (Delis, Kaplan, & Kramer, 2001); Finger Tapping Test (Reitan, 1969); Grooved Pegboard Test (Trites, 1989); ITC, Intrathecal chemotherapy; NEPSY, Developmental Neuropsychological Assessment (Korkman, Kirk, & Kemp, 1997); RCFT, Rey Complex Figure Test (Meyers & Meyers, 1995); Smedley Hand Dynamometer (Smedley, n.d.); TEA-Ch, Test of Everyday Attention for Children (Manly, Robertson, Anderson, & Nimmo-Smith, 1999); VMI-V, Beery-Buktenica Developmental Test of Visual-Motor Integration—Fifth Edition (Beery, Buktenica, & Beery, 2005); WISC-IV, Wechsler Intelligence Scale for Children—Fourth Edition (Wechsler, 2003); and WJ-III, Woodcock-Johnson Tests of Achievement—Third Edition (Woodcock, McGrew, & Mather, 2001).

his visual memory was within the average range. Timothy demonstrated variable benefit from retrieval cues, and both Sarah and Timothy demonstrated relative strengths among their motor skills on a measure of fine motor speed and coordination and weaknesses in grip strength.

Sarah and Timothy were reportedly coping well and adjusting to their life posttreatment. Adaptive skills were also generally age appropriate and no significant emotional or behavioral problems were noted by them, their parents, or teachers. As noted above, intrathecal chemotherapy and cranial irradiation result in diffuse injury to the white matter of the brain that negatively impacts the cognitive functions of this region, including attention, processing speed, visual perception, and motor function.

## INTERVENTIONS

The focus of intervention has shifted from survival to quality of life considerations due to advances in treatment of leukemia that have increased the survival rates and decreased the neuropsychological sequelae of the disorder and its treatment. However, recent studies have examined the negative impact of subtle sequelae on a child's long-term functioning in the academic, occupational, and social arenas (Mulhern & Butler, 2004; Peckham et al., 1988). Mulhern and Butler proposed alterations in environmental demands combined with rehabilitation as most likely to result in maximal therapeutic gains.

### Pharmacological Intervention

Mulhern, Khan, and colleagues (2004) examined the impact of medication to improve a child's attention and learning. Results of the study revealed that, compared to the placebo, children who received methylphenidate showed a significant improvement, at least temporarily, in their attention and social interactions.

### Neuropsychological Intervention and Accommodation

Butler and Copeland (2002) have created a model of cognitive rehabilitation drawing from the literature on traumatic brain injury, special education/educational psychology, and clinical psychology. The cognitive remediation program targets the attention system, particularly sustained, selective, divided, and executive control. This program has shown some success in improving a child's cognitive functioning (Butler & Haser, 2006; Mulhern & Butler, 2004). It also involves teaching a child metacognitive strategies, including self-monitoring, and utilizes cognitive-behavioral therapeutic approaches including problem-solving skills, social skills, relaxation training, and anger management.

## Academic Modification and Intervention

Based on some of the work with brain-injured patients (Baron & Goldberger, 1993), ecological or environmentally based treatment has been the focus of intervention. Some examples are shown in Table 14.2. Mulhern and Butler (2004) cautioned, "one of the greatest dangers in not communicating these new problems to the patient's teachers is that the patient's struggles in the classroom can be falsely attributed to a lack of motivation, attitude problems, daydreaming or emotional adjustment" (p. 10). It is imperative to plan and prepare for a child's future through the Transition portion of an IEP. In particular, goals and specific steps should be outlined to address a child's occupational interests, financial planning, navigating the adult health system, and social and emotional well-being. Mulhern and Butler also noted that "successful completion of school and the acquisition of academic concepts and information are the foundation for adult productivity. Now that cure rates are high, waiting until the patient is known to be a long-term survivor before providing intervention for neurocognitive deficits is no longer defensible" (p. 11). Baron and Goldberger (1993) highlighted some of the potential strategies that can be implemented in order to mitigate or support a child's limitations, as noted in the table below.

Peckham and colleagues (1988) found that few children in their study had attendance problems after the initial period of illness. It was believed that the excessive absences (30 to 60 school days per year) of three of the children in their study were due to social and emotional problems rather than physical illness. It is interesting that Peckham and colleagues also found that children who were older at the time of diagnosis tended to achieve less than expected. It was hypothesized that this subgroup of children were more affected by the academic interruptions due to absences.

Due to the destruction of white matter caused by CRT, Rourke (1987) proposed the need for intensive intervention aimed at increasing sensory-motor integration. The intervention would focus on stimulating the remaining white matter to encourage the growth of grey matter in the brain that relied on white matter for proper development. As a result of this white matter damage, Rourke suggested that a child may need to learn some compensatory strategies, including verbal mediation.

Teachers play a challenging role when a child in their class is diagnosed with leukemia. At that point, the child is vulnerable to infections, and the teacher does needs to be vigilant about the health environment

**TABLE 14.2 Environmental Adaptations to Facilitate Academic Achievement**

| Neuropsychological Weakness | Intervention |
|---|---|
| Slowed processing speed, writing difficulties | Extended time limits for examination |
| Memory retrieval difficulties | Use of true/false or multiple-choice formats for exams rather than essays |
| Auditory difficulties; fine motor problems; organizational difficulties | Recordings of classroom lectures |
| Fine motor or visual-motor problems | Written handouts of lecture materials and preprinted assignments to decrease note-taking demands and reduce copying from a blackboard; permission to compose assignments on the computer rather than handwriting them; removal of time constraints for written work; use of tape recorder to record lectures; use of calculators in an attempt to avoid mechanical errors (e.g., carrying numbers to the wrong column); regular evaluation of needs resulting in support for that student within the classroom |
| Fatigue | Decreased expectations for volume of homework; reduced number of items on exams |
| Attention problems | Preferential seating |

*Note.* Adapted from Baron and Goldberger (1993) and Armstrong and Horn (1995).

of the classroom. The teacher will need to work closely with the parents to help communicate with the other children and their parents about the need for close surveillance to prevent infection. The teacher will need to be sensitive to both protecting the child with cancer while continuing to provide an environment where the child has a normal learning environment.

## Psychological Intervention and Treatment

Returning to school is a challenge for children with leukemia and their families. Some of the challenges are driven by the leukemia and treatment, and these include missing school for medical appointments, unexpected hospital admissions, and susceptibility to infections. Other factors include psychosocial barriers; parents of school-age children may fear that the school will not be able to care for their child. Parents take on much responsibility for managing the medical needs of their children at home, and suddenly they are now sharing this responsibility with the school. They may worry that their child will develop infections from other children or will be teased by other children. Levin-Newby and colleagues (2000) highlighted the role of positive family functioning (cohesiveness) and academic functioning on a child's social and emotional adjustment.

Children also may be fearful of returning to school. They may look different, especially when they have lost hair and their weight has drastically increased or decreased, and they may worry about being accepted by their peers. They have been unable to turn in schoolwork and may worry whether they can keep up with their classmates. They have also missed the opportunity to develop or strengthen friendships and may be concerned that they will be unable to find friends at school. This can be a time of great anxiety (Holland & Rowland, 1991).

Fortunately, there are many approaches that the family, medical team, and school personnel can take to assist in successful reentry to school. One of the most important components for any successful reentry plan is open communication about the child's illness, treatment, side effects, and the capacities for learning and being treated normally within the classroom setting (Leukemia & Lymphoma Society, 2002). Parents need to feel that the school understands their child's needs and is invested in their child's future. The school needs to feel comfortable about the expectations for having a child with leukemia in their care. Additional school reentry programs have been developed that focus on teacher, peer, and parent education and on support (Benner & Marlow, 1991; Charlton, Pearson, & Morris-Jones, 1986; Cleave & Charlton, 1997; Katz, Varni, Rubenstein, Blew, & Hubert, 1992; Larcombe & Charlton, 1996; Pallmeyer et al., 1986; Varni, Katz, Colegrove, & Dolgin, 1993).

The majority of children in the maintenance phase will go on to end their treatment successfully and enter into a phase of long-term survivorship, still needing medical attention and surveillance, but with the expectation that they will no longer need treatment for leukemia. Unfortunately, some children with leukemia will have a relapse of their disease. This is a very difficult time for everyone. The child has been put through so much already, and there is a sense of betrayal (Keene, 2002) that the initial treatment did not work. This means that more treatment, or different treatment such as a bone marrow transplant, is needed. Both the child and family know more this time around and are aware of other children who faced relapse and were not successful in getting well again. The emotional toll on the family can be immense. As treatment continues, once again family life is disrupted, including school participation. This may be a time when home-based schooling is again considered, and there are new challenges for maintaining connections between the child and classmates (Steen & Mirro, 2000).

Siblings of children with leukemia have their own concerns. Depending on their ages, they may not fully comprehend the complexity of their sibling's illness and treatment, but they are fully aware of the impact it has on their family life. The family focus is now understandably on the sick child, and siblings may react with feelings of abandonment, fear, jealousy, and guilt (Keene, 2002). It is important for parents to try to balance the needs of their entire family when their attention is drawn to the sick child.

There is a growing awareness that although we have made great strides in treating childhood leukemia, these children will face long-term side effects from their treatment. This is especially true for school-age children, with implications for their long-term learning needs.

Caregivers and teachers play a critical role in the child's development and recovery from cancer through advocacy and early identification of obstacles to their child's success in the academic environment (Eiser, 2004). Peckham and colleagues (1988) indicated that a small number of children in their study achieved greater than expected levels of academic success, indicating that individualized instruction, tutoring, and parental support may reduce some learning deficits; they recommended early educational intervention.

Zebrack and colleagues (2002) highlighted the need for further research that examines the dynamic interplay between biological and psychosocial pathways by which cancer and its treatment influence future psychosocial functioning. They also emphasized the need for further research to tease out biological factors (i.e., late health effects from chemotherapy or irradiation) from socioeconomic influences (i.e., the potential fallout that arises from missed school, limited career opportunities, poor medical monitoring and access to health care) that may contribute to emotional difficulties following treatment.

## CONCLUSION

There have been great strides in treatment for childhood leukemia. Many more children are now cured of this disease and will become long-term survivors of cancer. Although this is cause for great satisfaction, these children continue to face long-term side effects from their disease and their treatment, which may impact their future growth and development. This is especially true for school-age children as they learn the building blocks for their future educational needs. As more children survive childhood leukemia, it becomes even more important to be knowledgeable about the implications for their long-term educational needs.

## RESOURCES

### Books

Henry, C. S., & Gosselin, K. (2001). *Taking cancer to school.* Plainview, NY: Jayjo Books.

Leukemia and Lymphoma Society. (2002). *The Trish Green back-to-school program for children with cancer* [Handbook]. White Plains, NY: Author.

Steen, G., & Mirro, J. (2000). *Childhood cancer: A handbook from St. Jude's Children's Research Hospital.* Cambridge, MA: Perseus.

Sullivan, N. A. (2004). *Walking with a shadow: Surviving childhood leukemia.* Westport, CT: Praeger Publishers.

### Organizations and Web Sites

American Cancer Society (ACS)

The ACS provides information, publications about cancer and various aspects of living with cancer, cancer camps, support groups, and research and educational programs.

Mailing Address: 1599 Clifton Road Northeast
Atlanta, Georgia 30329-4251
Phone Number: (800) 227-2345
Web Site: www.cancer.org

Candlelighters Childhood Cancer Foundation

Founded in 1970 by parents of children with cancer, Candlelighters offers a toll-free information hotline, publications, local support group chapters, and national advocacy.

Mailing Address: P.O. Box 498
Kensington, Maryland 20895-0498
Phone Number: (800) 366-2223
Web Site: www.candlelighters.org

Children's Oncology Camping Association International

This organization provides over 65 camping experiences in the United States for children who have endured cancer.

Mailing Address: P.O. Box 41433
Des Moines, Iowa 50311
Phone Number: (515) 491-4999
Web Site: coca-intl.org

Late Effects of Treatment for Childhood Cancer

WebMD is an online reference page that allows individuals to search for specific information. If the above information is inserted into the web site's search box, several different links will appear that will allow the reader to discover general late effects, as well as more specific information about how treatment for childhood cancer effects the digestive, reproductive, and muscoloskeletal system.

Web Site: www.webmd.com

Leukemia and Lymphoma Society

The society provides information; publications on all aspects of leukemia, lymphoma and Hodgkins disease; and financial assistance for travel-related costs for treatment.

Mailing Address: 1311 Mamaroneck Avenue
White Plains, New York 10605
Phone Number: (800) 955-4572
Web Site: www.leukemia.org

National Cancer Institute (NCI)

The NCI provides comprehensive information about all aspects of cancer-related topics, including treatment options, clinical trials, and complementary and alternative medicines.

Mailing Address: Cancer Information Service
NCI Public Inquiries Office
Bethesda, Maryland 20892
Phone Number: (800) 422-6237
Web Site: www.nci.nih.gov

National Coalition for Cancer Survivorship

The coalition provides publications on all aspects of survivorship, advocacy and support as well as a search tool to find resources on the Internet.

Mailing Address: 1010 Wayne Avenue, Suite 770
Silver Spring, Maryland 20910
Phone Number: (877) 622-7937
Web Site: www.cansearch.org

Pediatric Oncology Resource Center

The resource center provides a Web site for and by parents, friends, and families of children who have childhood cancer with various groups for support and information.

Web Site: acor.org/ped-onc

Surveillance Epidemiology and End Results (SEER) Program

As part of the National Cancer Institute (NCI), this is the authoritative source of information on cancer incidence and survival in the United States.

Web Site: www.seer.cancer.gov

## REFERENCES


Armstrong, D., & Horn, M. (1995). Educational issues in childhood cancer. *School Psychology Quarterly, 10,* 292–304.

Baron, I.S., & Goldberger, E. (1993). Neuropsychological disturbances of hydrocephalic children with implications for special education and rehabilitation. *Neuropsychological Rehabilitation, 3,* 389–410.

Beery, K.E., Buktenica, N.A., & Beery, N.A. (2005). *Beery-Buktenica Developmental Test of Visual-Motor Integration* (5th ed.). Lutz, FL: Psychological Assessment Resources.

Benner, A.E., & Marlow, A.S. (1991). The effect of a workshop on childhood cancer on student's knowledge, concerns, and desire to interact with a classmate with cancer. *Children's Health Care, 20,* 101–107.

Brouwers, P., & Poplack, D. (1990). Memory and learning sequelae in long-term survivors of acute lymphoblastic leukemia: Association with attention deficits. *American Journal of Pediatric Hematology/Oncology, 12,* 174–181.

Brown, R.T., & Madan-Swain, A. (1993). Cognitive, neuropsychological, and academic sequelae in children with leukemia. *Journal of Learning Disabilities, 26,* 74–90.

Burger, P.C., & Boyko, O.B. (1991). The pathology of central nervous system radiation injury. In P.J. Gutin, S.A. Leibel, & G.E. Sheline (Eds.), *Radiation injury to the nervous system* (pp. 3–15). New York: Raven Press.

Butler, R.T., & Copeland, D.R. (2002). Attentional processes and their remediation in children treated for cancer: A literature review and the development of a therapeutic approach. *Journal of the International Neuropsychological Society, 8,* 113–124.

Butler, R.W., & Haser, J.K. (2006). Neurocognitive effects of treatment for childhood cancer. *Mental Retardation and Developmental Disabilities Research Reviews, 12,* 184–191.

Butler, R.W., Hill, J.M., Steinherz, P.G., Meyers, P.A., & Finlay, J.L. (1994). Neuropsychologic effects of cranial irradiation, intrathecal methotrexate, and systemic methotrexate in childhood cancer. *Journal of Clinical Oncology, 12,* 2621–2629.

Campbell, L.K., Scaduto, M., Sharp, W., Dufton, L., Van Slyke, D., Whitlock, J.A., et al. (2007). A meta-analysis of the neurocognitive sequelae of treatment for childhood acute lymphocytic leukemia. *Pediatric Blood Cancer, 49,* 65–73.

Charlton, A., Pearson, D., & Morris-Jones, P.H. (1986). Children return to school after treatment for solid tumors. *Social Science and Medicine, 22,* 1337–1346.

Cleave, H., & Charlton, A. (1997). Evaluation of a cancer based coping and caring course used in three different settings. *Child Care Health and Development, 23,* 399–413.

Cohen, M.J. (1997). *Children's Memory Scale.* New York: The Psychological Corporation.

Cole, P.D., & Kamen, B.A. (2006). Delayed neurotoxicity associated with therapy for children with acute lymphoblastic leukemia. *Mental Retardation and Developmental Disabilities Research Reviews, 12,* 174–183.

Copeland, D.R., Dowell, R.E., Jr., Fletcher, J.M., Sullivan, M.P., Jaffe, N., Cangir, A., et al. (1988). Neuropsychological test performance of pediatric cancer patients at diagnosis and one year later. *Journal of Pediatric Psychology, 13,* 183–196.

Delis, D., Kaplan, E., & Kramer, J. (2001). *The Delis-Kaplan Executive Function System: Examiner's manual.* San Antonio, TX: The Psychological Corporation.

Delis, D.C., Kramer, J.H., Kaplan, E., & Ober, B.A. (1994). *California Verbal Learning Test—Children's Version.* San Antonio, TX: The Psychological Corporation.

Eiser, C. (2004). Neurocognitive sequelae of childhood cancers and their treatment: A comment on Mulhern and Butler. *Pediatric Rehabilitation, 7,* 15–16.

Griffin, T.W., Rasey, J.S., & Bleyer, W.A. (1977). The effect of photon irradiation on blood-brain-barrier permeability to methotrexate in mice. *Cancer, 40,* 1109–1111.

Hockenberry, M., Krull, K., Moore, K., Gregurich, M.A., Casey, M.E., & Kaemingk, K. (2007). Longitudinal evaluation of fine motor skills in children with leukemia. *American Journal of Pediatric Hematology/Oncology, 29,* 535–539.

Holland, J.C., & Rowland, J.H. (1991). *Handbook of psycho-oncology: Psychological care of the patient with cancer.* New York: Oxford University Press.

Iuvone, L., Mariotti, P., Colosimo, C., Guzzetta, F., Ruggiero, A., & Riccardi, R. (2002). Long-term cognitive outcome, brain computed tomography scan, and magnetic resonance imaging in children cured for acute lymphoblastic leukemia. *Cancer, 95,* 2562–2570.

Jansen, N.C., Kingma, A., Tellegen, P., van Dommelen, R.I., Bouma, A., Veerman, A., et al. (2005). Feasibility of neuropsychological assessment in leukaemia patients shortly after diagnosis: Directions for future prospective research. *Archives of Disease in Childhood, 90,* 301–304.

Kaplan, E., Goodglass, H., Weintraub, S., & Segal, O. (1983). *Boston Naming Test.* Philadelphia: Lea & Febiger.

Katz, E.R., Varni, J.W., Rubenstein, C.L., Blew, A., & Hubert, N. (1992). Teacher, parent, and child evaluative ratings of a school reintegration intervention for children with newly diagnosed cancer. *Children's Health Care, 2,* 69–75.

Keene, N. (2002). *Childhood leukemia: A guide for families, friends and caregivers* (3rd ed.). Sebastopol, CA: O'Reilly & Associates.

Koocher, G., & O'Malley, J. (1981). *The Damocles syndrome.* New York: McGraw Hill.

Korkman, M., Kirk, U., & Kemp, S. (1997). *NEPSY: A Developmental Neuropsychological Assessment.* San Antonio, TX: The Psychological Corporation.

Kumar, P., Mulhern, R.K., Regine, W.F., Rivera, G. K., & Kun, L.E. (1995). A prospective neurocognitive evaluation of children treated with additional chemotherapy and craniospinal irradiation following isolated central nervous system relapse in acute lymphoblastic leukemia. *International Journal of Radiation, Oncology, Biology, Physics, 31,* 561–566.

Larcombe, I.J., & Charlton, A. (1996). Children's return to school after treatment for cancer: Study days for teachers. *Journal of Cancer Education, 11,* 102–105.

Leukemia and Lymphoma Society. (2002). *The Trish Green back-to-school program for children with cancer* [Handbook]. White Plains, NY: Author.

Leukemia and Lymphoma Society. (2005). *Emotional aspects of childhood blood cancers* [Handbook]. White Plains, NY: Author.

Leung, W., Hudson, M., Zhu, Y., Rivera, G.K., Ribeiro, R.C., Sandlund, J.T., et al. (2000). Late effects in survivors of infant leukemia. *Leukemia, 14,* 1185–1190.

Levin-Newby, W., Brown, R.T., Pawletko, T.M., Gold, S.H., & Whitt, J.K. (2000). Social skills and psychological adjustment of child and adolescent cancer survivors. *Psycho-Oncology, 9,* 113–126.

Lockwood, K.A., Bell, T.S., & Colegrove, R.W. (1999). Long-term effects of cranial radiation therapy on attention functioning in survivors of childhood leukemia. *Journal of Pediatric Psychology, 24, 55–66.*

Manly, T., Robertson, T., Anderson, V., & Nimmo-Smith, I. (1999). *Test of Everyday Attention for Children.* Suffolk, England: Thames Valley Test Company.

Meyers, J.E., & Meyers, K.R. (1995). *Rey Complex Figure Test and Recognition Trial professional manual.* Lutz, FL: Psychological Assessment Resource.

Mulhern, R.K., & Butler, R.W. (2004). Neurocognitive sequelae of childhood cancers and their treatment. *Pediatric Rehabilitation, 7,* 1–14.

Mulhern, R.K., Khan, R.B., Kaplan, S., Helton, S., Christensen, R., Bonner, M., et al. (2004). Short-term efficacy of methylphenidate: A randomized, double-blind, placebo-controlled trial among survivors of childhood cancer. *Journal of Clinical Oncology, 22,* 4795–4803.

Mulhern, R.K., Ochs, J., Fairclough, D., Wasserman, A.L., Davis, K.S., & Williams, J.M. (1987). Intellectual and academic achievement status after CNS relapse: A retrospective analysis of 40 children treated for acute lymphoblastic leukemia. *Journal of Clinical Oncology, 5,* 933–940.

Mulhern, R.K., Wasserman, A.L., Fairclough, D., & Ochs, J. (1988). Memory function in disease-free survivors of childhood acute lymphocytic leukemia given CNS prophylaxis with or without 1,800 cGy cranial irradiation. *Journal of Clinical Oncology, 6,* 315–320.

Mulhern, R.K., White, H.A., Glass, J.O., Kun, L.E., Leigh, L., Thompson, S.J., et al. (2004). Attentional functioning and white matter integrity among survivors of malignant brain tumors of childhood. *Journal of the International Neuropsychological Society, 10,* 180–189.

Pallmeyer, T.P., Saylor, C.F., Treiber, F.A., Eason, L.J., Finch, A.J., & Carek, D.J. (1986). Helping school personnel understand the student with cancer: Workshop evaluation. *Child Psychiatry and Human Development, 16,* 206–217.

Peckham, V.C., Meadows, A.T., Bartel, N., & Marrero, O. (1988). Educational late effects in long-term survivors of childhood acute lymphocytic leukemia. *Pediatrics, 81,* 127–133.

Précourt, S., Robaey, P., Lamothe, I., Lassonde, M., Sauerwein, H.C., & Moghrabi, A. (2002). Verbal cognitive functioning and learning in girls treated for acute lymphoblastic leukemia by chemotherapy with or without cranial irradiation. *Developmental Neuropsychology, 21,* 173–195.

Reddick, W.E., Shan, Z.Y., Glass, J.O., Helton, S., Xiong, X., Wu, S., et al. (2006). Smaller white-matter volumes are associated with larger deficits in attention and learning among long-term survivors of acute lymphoblastic leukemia. *Cancer, 106,* 941–949.

Regan, J.M., & Reeb, R.N. (1998). Neuropsychological functioning in survivors of childhood leukemia. *Child Study Journal, 28*(3), 179–199.

Reitan, R. (1969). *Finger Tapping Test.* Tucson: Reitan Neuropsychological Laboratories, University of Arizona.

Ries, L.A., Eisner, M.P., Kosary, C.L., Hankey, B.F., Miller, B. A., Clegg, L., et al. (Eds.). (2007). *SEER Cancer Statistics Review, 1975–2004.* Bethesda, MD: National Cancer Institute. Retrieved October 12, 2007, from http://seer.cancer.gov/csr/1975_2004/

Rourke, B. (1987). Syndrome of nonverbal learning disabilities; The final common pathway for white matter disease/dysfunction? *The Clinical Neuropsychologist, 1,* 209–234.

Rowland, J.H., Glidewell, O.J., Sibley, R.F., Holland, J.C., Tull, R., Berman, A., et al. (1984). Effects of different forms of CNS prophylaxis on neurologic function in childhood leukemia. *Journal of Clinical Oncology, 12,* 1327–1355.

Semel, E., Wigg, E.H., & Secord, W.A. (2003). *Clinical Evaluation of Language Fundamentals* (4th ed.). San Antonio, TX: The Psychological Corporation.

Smedley, F. (n.d.). *Smedley Hand Dynamometer.* Wood Dale, IL: Stoelting.

Trites, R. (1989). *Grooved Pegboard Test.* Lafayette, IN: Lafayette Instruments.

Van Dongen-Melman, J.E.W.M., De Groot, A., Van Dongen, J.J.M., Verhulst, F.C., & Hählen, K. (1997). Cranial irradiation is the major cause of learning problems in children treated for leukemia and lymphoma: A comparative study. *Leukemia, 11,* 1197–1200.

Varni, J.W., Katz, E.R., Colegrove, R., & Dolgin, M. (1993). The impact of social skills training on the adjustment of children with newly diagnosed cancer. *Journal of Pediatric Psychology, 18,* 751–767.

Waber, D.P., & Mullenix, P.J. (2000). Acute lymphoblastic leukemia. In K.O. Yeates, M.D. Ris, & H.G. Taylor (Eds.), *Pediatric neuropsychology: Research, theory, and practice* (pp. 300–319). New York: Guilford Press.

Waber, D.P., Tarbell, N.J., Fairclough, D., Atmore, K., Castro, R., Isquith, P., et al. (1995). Cognitive sequelae of treatment of childhood acute lymphoblastic leukemia: Cranial radiation requires an accomplice. *Journal of Clinical Oncology, 13,* 2490–2496.

Wagner, R.K., Torgesen, J.K., & Rashotte, C.A. (1999). *Examiner's manual: The Comprehensive Test of Phonological Processing.* Austin, TX: PRO-ED.

Wechsler, D. (2003). *Wechsler Intelligence Scale for Children* (4th ed.). San Antonio, TX: The Psychological Corporation.

Woodcock, R.W., McGrew, K.S., & Mather, N. (2001). *Woodcock-Johnson Tests of Achievement* (3rd ed.). Rolling Meadows, IL: Riverside.

Zebrack, B.J., Zeltzer, L.K., Whitton, J., Mertens, A.C., Odom, L., Berkow, R., et al. (2002). Psychological outcomes in long-term survivors of childhood leukemia, Hodgkin's disease, and non-Hodgkin's lymphoma: A report from the Childhood Cancer Survivor Study. *Pediatrics, 110,* 42–52.

CHAPTER FIFTEEN

# Migraine Headache

Laura Slap-Shelton, PsyD

*"I'm opening out like the largest telescope that ever was! Goodbye feet!" (for when she looked down at her feet, they seemed to be almost out of sight, they were getting so far off). "Oh, my poor little feet, I wonder who will put on your shoes and stockings now, dears? I shall be a great deal too far off to trouble myself about you: you must manage the best way you can—but I must be kind to them," thought Alice.*

(*Alice's Adventures in Wonderland*; Lewis Carroll, 1865)

## DESCRIPTION OF THE DISORDER

Migraine headaches have plagued and fascinated human beings from the beginning of time. Descriptions of migraine can be found in ancient Sumerian writings, in the writings of Socrates, and in literature, philosophy, and medical writings throughout history (Bille, 1962). Lewis Carroll, a migraineur (i.e., migraine sufferer), knew about the more exotic effects of migraine disorder and was able to translate them into his classic book, *Alice in Wonderland* (Bille). In fact, one variety of migraine has been named the *Alice in Wonderland syndrome.* [Medical awareness of migraine headache in children can be found as early as the 18th century, and Bille's study represents one of the seminal studies of migraine disorder in children.]

Migraine headaches are characterized by severely painful throbbing headaches that are often debilitating. They are recurrent and frequently, in addition to severe pain, have other symptoms associated with them, such as nausea, abdominal pain, vomiting, light and sound sensitivity (i.e., photophobia and phonophobia, respectively), and auras that often present as unusual visual or perceptual experiences that are harbingers of the headache that is about to arrive (Bille, 1962; Headache Classification Committee of the International Headache Society, 2004).

Migraine headaches can occur as early as infancy but are difficult to recognize before the child is able to communicate information about his or her internal state. Approximately half of all people with migraines have had their first one by the age of 20 years. Many studies have examined prevalence rates of migraine in children, with varying results. Some studies indicate an increase in prevalence at around the age of 7 years, with prevalence rates in the range of 2.5%. Before puberty, more boys than girls have migraines; with the onset of puberty, the numbers shift and more girls than boys have migraines. Prevalence rates at age 17 years are approximately 8% of boys and 23% of girls (Bille, 1962; Curse, 2007; Hoelscher & Lichstein, 1984). There is generally a family history associated with migraine. Some studies have indicated that with each decade the prevalence of childhood migraine has increased; they point to environmental concerns that may be contributing to this increase. Sillanpää and Anttila (1996) wrote of this phenomenon:

> Although no significant association could be shown in the present study, changes in the social environment might explain the significantly increased prevalence. That is an alarming sign of the stressful life and ill-being of children. It may even reflect the ill-being of society. (p. 470)

Kabbouche, Bentti Vockell, LeCates, Powers, and Hershey (2001) note that 10% of U.S. children with migraine will miss 1 day of school out of 10 and that approximately 1% missed 4 days out of 10. They calculated that this was the equivalent of 164,454 missed days of school.

Causes of migraine include genetics, stress, environmental triggers, or certain activities or events that will predictably bring on a migraine. For some people, triggers may be foods such as chocolate or cheese. For other people, intense activity is predictably followed by a migraine once the activity is over (Bille, 1962; Headache Classification Committee of the International Headache Society, 2004; Sillanpää & Anttila, 1996). Aromaa, Sillanpää, Rautava, and Helenius (1998) found that fear and anxiety triggered headache in children with migraine more than they triggered headache in children without migraine. Researchers of childhood migraine have noted a connection between stress at school and migraine. Bener and colleagues (2000) found a correlation between migraines and timing of examinations. In this study, computer use, loud noise, and a hot environment were the most common environmental triggers of migraine.

The underlying mechanism of migraines was previously believed to be dilatation of cranial blood vessels, and this theory continues to be popularly held. According to this theory, the aura was caused by the constriction of cranial blood vessels (Curse, 2007). Currently, however, the phenomenon of vasodilation is understood as a symptom of the migraine rather than its cause. No single gene or genetic pathway has been identified as a cause of migraine, and migraine is understood to be polygenetic (i.e., due to multiple genetic factors) and also caused by environmental factors (Curse; Weiller et al., 1995; Welch, Barkley, Tepley, & Ramadan, 1993).

The current pathophysiological model of migraine proposes that they arise in the brain stem and involve the locus ceruleus (Curse, 2007; Micieli et al., 1995). The locus ceruleus is believed to initiate an event known as cortical spreading depression, in which a wave of depolarization spreads across the neuronal and glial cells of the brain. This is believed to be the event that sets off the aura. This event spreads to the trigeminal nerve afferents, which release a variety of polypeptides, including Substance P, and vasoactive peptides, which lead to the pain and vasodilation or the migraine itself. The blood-brain barrier permeability also is believed to be altered during this course of events (Curse; Weiller et al., 1995; Welch et al., 1993).

The two children presented in this chapter illustrate the course of onset of abdominal migraines at a very young age and a more typical case of migraine in childhood. Because of a variety of behavioral and medical issues, Matthew was seen for a neuropsychological evaluation at 8 years of age when he was in the second grade. He was a White child in a middle-class family and had one older sibling. His parents reported that they were not able to help him regulate his behavior, which was growing increasingly out of control at home, in addition to increasing behavioral issues at school. Matthew's migraines presented before the age of 2 years and were a mystery to his parents and physicians. He would lie on the floor, engaging in repetitive body movements for periods ranging from a few minutes to as long as 5 hours. It was possible to interrupt this activity and gain his attention. Vomiting also occurred. Previous endoscopic testing had been negative. At 2 years of age, a medical evaluation ruled out the presence of a seizure disorder, and imaging studies of his brain were negative. It was suggested that he was engaging in self-stimulatory stereotypic behaviors consistent with a pervasive developmental disorder. His behaviors persisted, and he was reevaluated at age 3 and diagnosed with abdominal migraines. At this point, the presence of headaches accompanying these episodes was becoming clearer. In addition, Matthew's repetitive movements were more clearly seen to be efforts to put pressure on his abdomen. His headaches could be characterized as midfrontal and as lasting up to 2 hours. He began to have headaches without abdominal pain as well. Treatment with Tegretol was initiated and alleviated both the headache and abdominal pain. However, at age 4, in conjunction with an unrelated stressful event, his headaches and abdominal pain returned. At this point, Matthew's headaches were characterized as being in the occipital region and were accompanied by nausea, photophobia, and phonophobia. Adjustment of his medications again alleviated his symptoms.

Matthew was described as a child whose internal pressure for perfection increased his stress. His level of stress was correlated with his episodes of migraine, with episodes occurring during periods of high stress. Also, due to his many painful and unpleasant experiences, he developed a mild phobia of eating, which became associated with pain. His controlling and demanding behaviors were also understood as deriving from a need for internal control in reaction to his many years of uncontrolled and unpredictable pain.

Heather presented as a 12-year-old, sixth-grade student whose parents were concerned about her slow processing and difficulties with language arts in school. She was doing fairly well in school, was generally well adjusted with friends, and involved in extracurricular activities. She was a fraternal twin, and her twin did not have migraines. Her family was White and middle class. She had an older brother in college who had a nonverbal learning disorder. Heather had been diagnosed with migraine headache at 8 years of age and had been taking daily prophylactic medication for migraine since that time. Initially, her headaches were attributed to environmental factors (i.e., poor air quality, mold) in her school, and she was placed in a different school. The resulting separation from her twin led to some anxiety, and counseling was initiated. Toward the end of the school year, her physician diagnosed her with migraine headaches. Heather reported that she has a migraine approximately one to two times per month in the summer. In contrast, during the school year, she reported mild levels of headache almost daily. Heather related that her headaches usually started in one side of her head and were accompanied by vomiting and light and noise sensitivity. Triggers included changes in the weather, pollen, and stress.

For both Matthew and Heather, the diagnosis of migraine was not initially obvious. In one case it almost led to an erroneous diagnosis of a pervasive developmental disorder, and in another it led to an unnecessary placement in a new school and consequent additional stress. The diagnosis of migraine disorder is made by a physician and is based on the history of the headaches. Children have been found to be reliable reporters of the migraine headache experiences (Labbé, Williamson, & Southard, 1985). Further, several studies have found that children's drawings of their headaches can help to differentiate between migraine and tension headaches (Stafstrom, Rostasy, & Minster, 2002) and can be useful in monitoring the course of treatment (Stafstrom, Goldenholz, & Dulli, 2005).

The diagnostic criteria for migraine in children have been revised and refined over the past two decades (Aromaa et al., 1998; Curse, 2007; Headache Classification Committee of the International Headache Society, 1988; Wöber-Bingöl et al., 1996). In a review of the 1988 criteria, Wöber-Bingöl and colleagues noted that children with migraine would be more accurately identified if the minimum length of the migraine were shortened and if severe headache associated with nausea were sufficient for individuals who did not meet other descriptive criteria. Please see Tables 15.1 through 15.3 for the 2004 International Headache Society (IHS) classification system for the diagnostic criteria of migraine without aura (i.e., common migraine), migraine with aura (i.e., classic migraine), and migraine in children.

Some researchers have specified that for the diagnosis of childhood migraine, the quality of the headache and the associated symptoms may be more important than the established diagnostic criteria. They emphasize that, for children, three of the following symptoms should be present for a diagnosis of migraine: abdominal pain, nausea, or vomiting with headache; unilateral headache; pulsating or throbbing pain; complete relief after a brief rest; a visual, sensory, or motor aura; and a family history of migraine headaches (Curse, 2007). As noted in the IHS criteria, children may have headaches lasting from 1 to 72 hours and may more commonly have bilateral headaches. In young children, inferences about phonophobia and photophobia substitute for patient self-report.

**TABLE 15.1 IHS Diagnostic Criteria for Migraine without Aura**

A. At least five attacks meeting criteria B through D

B. Headaches last 4 to 72 hours either treated or untreated

C. Headache has a minimum of two of the following characteristics:

1. Unilateral location
2. Pulsating quality
3. Moderate to severe pain intensity
4. Aggravated by or causes avoidance of routine physical activity such as walking and climbing stairs

D. During the headache, a minimum of one of the following:

1. Nausea or vomiting or both
2. Photophobia and phonophobia

E. Headache not caused by another disorder

*Note.* Modified from the Headache Classification Committee of the International Headache Society (2004).

**TABLE 15.2 IHS Diagnostic Criteria for Migraine with Typical Aura**

A. At least two attacks of headache meeting the criteria for migraine without aura
B. Aura consisting of a minimum of one of the following (but no motor weakness):
    1. Fully reversible positive visual symptoms (i.e., flickering lights, spots, or lines) or negative visual symptoms (i.e., loss of vision)
    2. Fully reversible sensory symptoms including positive experiences (i.e., pins and needles) and/or negative experiences (i.e., numbness)
    3. Fully reversible dysphasic speech disturbance
C. A minimum of two of the following:
    1. Homonymous visual and/or unilateral sensory symptoms
    2. At least one aura symptom develops gradually over 5 or more minutes, and/or different aura symptoms occur in succession over 5 or more minutes
    3. Each symptom lasts from 5 to 60 minutes
D. Headache meeting criteria for migraine without aura begins during the aura or follows the aura within 60 minutes

*Note.* Modified from the Headache Classification Committee of the International Headache Society (2004).

**TABLE 15.3 IHS Features of Migraine in Children**

A. Attacks may be of shorter duration (1 to 72 hours in children versus 4 to 72 hours in adults)
B. Headache is usually bilateral in children with the adult unilateral pattern emerging in late adolescence or early adulthood
C. Photophobia and phonophobia may be inferred by behavior in young children

*Note.* Modified from the Headache Classification Committee of the International Headache Society (2004).

Abdominal migraines are now classified under the rubric of childhood periodic syndromes (Headache Classification Committee of the International Headache Society, 2004). These are syndromes that are generally precursors of migraine. Abdominal migraine is reported at a frequency of approximately 12% of school-age children. The abdominal pain is generally poorly localized or midline, dull, and moderate to severe in intensity. It is associated with two or more of the following criteria: anorexia, nausea, vomiting, and pallor. There are several other types of migraine headache as well (Curse, 2007).

## RELATED MEDICAL ISSUES

In terms of associated medical issues, studies have not found evidence of a connection between migraines and allergies, head injuries, orthostatic circulatory insufficiency, enuresis and encopresis, or tic disorders (Bille, 1962). Convulsive disorders are sometimes seen in individuals with migraine but are not believed to be directly causative. Paroxysmal tachycardia (i.e., a period of rapid heartbeats that begins and ends suddenly), dysmenorrhea (i.e., pain or discomfort experienced just before or during the menstrual period), some types of sleep disorders, sudden abdominal pain, and cyclical vomiting are associated with migraine in children (Bille). Research reported to the XI Congress of the International Headache Society indicated that a connection probably exists between oppositional defiant disorder and migraine headache in children ages 6 to 17 years (Columbus Children's Hospital, 2003).

## RESULTS FROM NEUROPSYCHOLOGICAL EVALUATION

Using the Wechsler Intelligence Scale for Children—Fourth Edition (WISC-IV; Wechsler, 2003), neuropsychological testing for Matthew yielded a Full Scale IQ in the 79th percentile with a mild relative weakness in his processing speed (47th percentile). This was believed to be related to his careful and neat performance on the Coding subtest, which led to slow task completion and a performance in the 16th percentile. His memory testing indicated the presence of weak delayed verbal memory (12th percentile) as well as weakness on a forced-choice verbal recognition measure (5th percentile). Performance on other tasks indicated functioning in the average to high average range. Issues with anxiety and symptoms of attention-deficit/hyperactivity disorder (ADHD) were identified through behavioral ratings.

Heather's neuropsychological testing results also indicated weakness in processing speed with her Processing Speed index score in the 16th percentile, in contrast to her Verbal Comprehension index score in the 79th percentile and her Perceptual Reasoning score in the 90th percentile. Again, weakness on the Coding subtest (9th percentile) appeared to result from her careful work approach. She demonstrated impaired visual memory for faces (2nd percentile) in contrast to average range performance on other memory tasks. Behavioral ratings completed by one of her parents and by her teachers were consistent in identifying mildly elevated levels of anxiety.

Studies of cognitive and emotional functioning in individuals with migraine disorder have yielded findings of some mild neuropsychological and emotional differences (Bille, 1962; Kalaydjian, Zandi, Swartz, Eaton, & Lyketsos, 2007). Longitudinal and cross-sectional studies evaluating individuals suffering from migraine later in life have not found significant cognitive differences or greater prevalence of dementia or other brain disease in these individuals (Gaist et al., 2005; Kalaydjian et al., 2007). However, brain imaging studies are raising possible concerns regarding increased stroke and possible other difficulties later in life (Elkind & Scher, 2005). In a neuropsychological study of adult migraine sufferers (Le Pira et al., 2000), migraine sufferers with and without auras were weaker than the control group on visual-spatial memory tasks; migraine patients without aura showed impaired verbal memory compared to controls. The investigators hypothesized that both areas of memory deficit were secondary to organizational and strategic weaknesses in learning. Calandre, Bembibre, Arnedo, and Becerra (2002) studied adults with migraine using neuropsychological measures and found weaknesses in memory, attention, and visuomotor speed in migraine sufferers. They also found higher levels of anxiety in patients with migraine as compared to those without migraine.

In a longitudinal study of children with migraine (Aromaa et al., 1998), findings indicated a prevalence of left-handedness; lower performance on tests of verbal ability but not on intelligence measures; and less success on school examinations at ages 15 and 17 in students with migraines. Fewer of the students with migraines went on to earn college degrees.

Bille's (1962) study did not provide any evidence to support an earlier popular belief that children with migraine disorders are more intelligent than their peers. Some differences were found in speed of performance, with greater weakness in girls with migraines. However, the same girls were found to be more accurate than their faster nonmigraine peers. Bille's study also found greater weakness in motion perception in girls with migraines than in girls without. D'Andrea, Nertempi, Ferro Milone, Joseph, and Cananzi (1989) found decreased short- and long-term memory function in children diagnosed with migraine without aura.

Bille (1962) found an increase in generalized anxiety and in anxiety around achievement in children with migraine disorders, with a stronger finding in girls with migraines. D'Andrea and colleagues (1989) did not find abnormal personality traits in children with migraine but noted greater inhibition of aggression and higher levels of anxiety in their subjects with migraine. Likewise, Aromaa and colleagues (1998) found evidence of greater levels of anxiety around school performance.

Thus, although further research about cognitive abilities in children with migraine is needed, the two cases described here, which were selected because of the children's history of migraine (although migraine was not the presenting concern at the time of the evaluation), appear to be consistent with the trend of presence of memory weakness and increased levels of anxiety in children with migraine identified in the literature.

## INTERVENTIONS

Childhood migraine is generally treated with medication and therapy. Medications used to treat migraine include analgesics, triptans, calcium blockers, and antiemetics (Caruso, Brown, Exil, & Gascon, 2000; The Cleveland Clinic Foundation, 2005; Kabbouche et al., 2001; Lewis et al., 2002; Sorge et al., 1988; Winner, 2002). Sometimes children are placed on a daily prophylactic medication, and other times they take medication at the first sign of the migraine. If the migraine becomes unmanageable, a rescue medication may be used to bring the episode to an end. If untreated, the child will often require rest in a quiet, dark environment. As is often the case with medication for children, more studies are needed to evaluate the use of medications that are used with adolescents and adults when they are used with children under the age of 12 (Lewis et al.).

Therapeutic interventions for children with migraine disorders include biofeedback, electromyographic (EMG) biofeedback, relaxation training, cognitive therapy, and anxiety management training (Allen & McKeen, 1991; Hoelscher & Lichstein, 1984; Osterhaus, Lange, Linssen, & Passchier, 1997; Werder & Sargent, 1984). Management of contingencies associated with migraine and role modeling have been proposed as other possible methods of support (Hoelscher & Lichstein).

Matthew's evaluation led to recommendations for refinement of some of the treatment strategies already in place. With a greater awareness of the significance of his anxiety concerns, his school guidance counselor and teacher worked with him to establish a behavioral reward system to help him better comply with school rules. It was recommended that homework demands be decreased temporarily while his parents worked with him to decrease perfectionistic behaviors and overall anxiety levels. His parents took him to counseling with a psychologist in the community to address anxiety issues and behavioral management strategies at home.

Treatment modalities that were recommended for Matthew included implementation of biofeedback, use of relaxation strategies, and implementation of a cognitive-behavioral approach to help him better understand his behavior and develop better coping strategies. His parents were encouraged to participate in his therapy to develop new ways to respond to him when he was experiencing pain and new ways to manage his demanding behavior at home. Matthew's parents continued to work closely with his physician to ensure maximum benefit from his medications. His evaluation also included a recommendation that he learn verbal retrieval strategies to improve his ability to recall information, and recommendations were made for allowing extra time for work and test completion, given his weak processing speed. In terms of his ADHD symptoms, recommendations were made for considering treatment with medication, in particular, if the abatement of his anxiety level did not produce a reduction in his inattentive and hyperactive-impulsive symptom profile.

Heather's overall profile indicated that slow processing speed was contributing to difficulties with her work completion. Recommendations were made to accommodate her need for more time to complete assignments and work on tests. Her school was planning to complete academic testing at the beginning of the coming school year, and the results would also be considered in her overall plan. Because of her report of almost constant headache and greater frequency of migraine during the school year, in contrast to relative freedom from headache and much lower frequency during the summer, it was recommended that Heather learn ways to relax and manage her anxiety levels during the school year. As recommended for Matthew, relaxation training, biofeedback, and cognitive-behavioral therapy were identified as possible means for achieving reduced headache and migraine frequency. The use of a headache diary was recommended to help track the frequency and timing of her headaches, the type of headaches (migraine versus tension), and the severity of the headaches. During therapy, she was encouraged to develop an action plan for the implementation of relaxation, exercise, dietary, sleep, and cognitive strategies.

In the school setting, migraine is generally not identified as a major handicap requiring formal accommodations and an Individualized Educational Plan. However, it is important that classroom teachers and relevant school personnel be aware of students who have migraine disorders. As Bille (1962) wrote:

> The teacher should always be spoken to if there is a child with migraine in the class. He should be given information about the manifestations of the disease, and the special problems of these children. The teacher then often has much more understanding of the child, and considers

> him more carefully. At times it is necessary to advise a change of class or to arrange extra help with lessons. (p. 131)

The school nurse also may play an important role and should be aware of the student's treatment plan, in case the child has a migraine during schooltime. The school psychologist or social worker may also play a helpful role in teaching relaxation and anxiety management strategies to children with migraine disorders.

If a child has severe migraines that lead to multiple school absences, arrangements for making up school work, tutoring after school, or home tutoring will need to be made. It is helpful for teachers to recognize that a child with migraine has frequent experiences of severe pain and sometimes has perceptual experiences that are quite different from those of their peers. This awareness can certainly contribute to their understanding of the student. Awareness of the child's migraine can also help with accommodating a student's need to visit the school nurse or implement anxiety reduction strategies in the classroom.

If a child becomes too fearful, or complains of having a headache as a means of avoiding class work or other anxiety-provoking events at school, a phenomenon known as secondary gain, the teacher also has an important role to play. Consultation with or referral to the school's psychologist or social worker and discussion with the child's parents would be appropriate and important steps to take in order to avoid a downward slide by the student. The development of a plan to help the child manage their anxiety in the classroom without resorting to reporting headache will be very helpful. Given the current trends in the U.S. schools under No Child Left Behind for testing to occur more frequently and to have more weight in determining a child's and a child's school's future, awareness of strategies to reduce classroom stress may be particularly helpful to children with migraine.

In conclusion, migraine headache occurs with significant frequency in school-age children and adolescents. Awareness on the part of the teacher and other school personnel, and communication between school staff, parents, and the student can go a long way to help minimize any negative effects of migraine in school-age children.

## RESOURCES

### Books

Cheyette, S. (2002). *Mommy, my head hurts: A doctor's guide to your child's headache.* New York: Newmarket Press.

Diamond, S., & Diamond, A. (2001). *Headache and your child: The complete guide to understanding and treating migraine and other headaches in children and adolescents.* New York: Fireside.

Hockaday, J. M. (1988). *Migraine in childhood: And other non-epileptic paroxysmal disorders.* London: Butterworth-Heinemann.

Winner, P., & Rothner, A. D. (2001). *Headache in children and adolescents.* Hamilton, Ontario, Canada: B. C. Decker.

## Organizations and Web Sites

The American Chronic Pain Association

This organization facilitates peer support and education for individuals with chronic pain.

Web Site: www.theacpa.org

The American Council for Headache Education (ACHE)

The American Headache Society sponsors this Web site, which provides information regarding headache hygiene, treatment, headache diaries, school nurse information forms, and other helpful resources.

Web Site: www.achenet.org

HeadTalk

This Web site provides educational resources for those suffering with migraines.

Web Site: www.headtalk.com

Migraine Awareness Group: A National Understanding for Migraineurs (MAGNUM)

MAGNUM provides information for migraine sufferers and their family and friends, including information about treatment and management.

Mailing Address: 113 South Saint Asaph, Suite 300
Alexandria, Virginia 22314
Phone Number: (703) 739-9384
Web Site: www.migraines.org

National Headache Foundation

This nonprofit organization provides information to headache sufferers and medical professionals.

Phone Number: (888) NHF-5552
Web Site: www.headaches.org

World Headache Alliance

This Web site provides information to better understand headaches, in addition to links to the latest research and community resources.

Web Site: www.w-h-a.org/wha2/index.asp

## REFERENCES


Allen, K. D., & McKeen, L. R. (1991). Home-based multicomponent treatment of pediatric migraine. *Headache, 31,* 467–472.

Aromaa, M., Sillanpää, M. L., Rautava, P., & Helenius, H. (1998). Childhood headache at school entry: A controlled clinical study. *Neurology, 50,* 1729–1736.

Bener, A., Uduman, S. A., Qassimi, E. M. A., Khalaily, G., Sztriha, L., Kilpelainen, H., et al. (2000). Genetic and environmental factors associated with migraine in schoolchildren. *Headache, 40,* 152–157.

Bille, B. S. (1962). Migraine in school children: A study of the incidence and short-term prognosis, and a clinical, psychological and electroencephalographic comparison between children with migraine and matched controls. *Acta Paediatrica, 136*(Suppl.), 1–151.

Calandre, E. P., Bembibre, J., Arnedo, M. L., & Becerra, D. (2002). Cognitive disturbances and regional cerebral blood flow abnormalities in migraine patients: Their relationship with the clinical manifestations of the illness. *Cephalalgia, 22,* 291–302.

Caruso, J. M., Brown, W. D., Exil, G., & Gascon, G. G. (2000). The efficacy of divalproex sodium in the prophylactic treatment of children with migraine. *Headache, 40,* 672–676.

The Cleveland Clinic Foundation. (2005). *Migraines in children and adolescents.* Retrieved August 25, 2007, from http://www.clevelandclinic.org/health/health-info/docs/2500/2555.asp?index=9637

Columbus Children's Hospital. (2003, September 15). *Link between migraines and behavioral disorders in children.* Retrieved August 26, 2007, from http://mentalhealth.about.com/cs/familyresources/a/kidmigraine.htm

Curse, R. P. (2007, August 25). *Pathophysiology, clinical features, and diagnosis of migraine in children.* Retrieved August 25, 2007, from http://uptodate.com

D'Andrea, G., Nertempi, P., Ferro Milone, F., Joseph, R., & Cananzi, A. R. (1989). Personality and memory in childhood migraine. *Cephalalgia, 9,* 25–28.

Elkind, M. S., & Scher, A. I. (2005). Migraine and cognitive function: Some reassuring news. *Neurology, 64,* 590–591.

Gaist, D., Pedersen, L., Madsen, C., Tsiropoulos, I., Bak, S., Sindrup, S., et al. (2005). Long-term effects of migraine on cognitive function: A population-based study of Danish twins. *Neurology, 64,* 600–607.

Headache Classification Committee of the International Headache Society. (1988). Classification and diagnostic criteria for headache disorders, cranial neuralgias and facial pain. *Cephalalgia, 8*(Suppl. 7), 1–96.

Headache Classification Committee of the International Headache Society. (2004). The international classification of headache disorders (2nd ed.). *Cephalalgia, 24*(Suppl. 1), 8–160.

Hoelscher, T. J., & Lichstein, K. L. (1984). Behavioral assessment and treatment of child migraine: Implications for clinical research and practice. *Headache, 24,* 94–103.

Kabbouche, M. A., Bentti Vockell, A.-L., LeCates, S. L., Powers, S. W., & Hershey, A. D. (2001). Tolerability and effectiveness of prochlorperazine for intractable migraine in children [Electronic version]. *Pediatrics, 107,* e62. Retrieved June 28, 2007, from http://www.pediatrics.org

Kalaydjian, A., Zandi, P. P., Swartz, K. L., Eaton, W. W., & Lyketsos, C. (2007). How migraines impact cognitive functions: Findings from the Baltimore ECA. *Neurology, 68,* 1417–1424.

Labbé, E. E., Williamson, D. A., & Southard, D. R. (1985). Reliability and validity of children's reports of migraine headache symptoms. *Journal of Psychopathology and Behavioral Assessment, 7,* 375–383.

Le Pira, F., Zappalà, G., Giuffrida, S., Lo Bartolo, M. L., Reggio, E., Morana, R., et al. (2000). Memory disturbances in migraine with and without aura: A strategy problem? *Cephalalgia, 20,* 475–478.

Lewis, D. W., Kellstein, D., Dahl, G., Burke, B., Frank, L. M., Toor, S., et al. (2002). Children's ibuprofen suspension for the acute treatment of pediatric migraine. *Headache, 42,* 780–786.

Micieli, G., Tassorelli, C., Bosone, D., Cavallini, A., Bellantonio, P., Rossi, F., et al. (1995). Increased cerebral blood flow velocity induced by cold pressor test in migraine: A possible basis for pathogenesis? *Cephalalgia, 15,* 494–498.

Osterhaus, S. O., Lange, A., Linssen, W. H., & Passchier, J. (1997). A behavioral treatment of young migrainous and nonmigrainous headache patients: Prediction of treatment success. *International Journal of Behavioral Medicine, 4,* 378–396.

Sillanpää, M., & Anttila, P. (1996). Increasing prevalence of headache in 7-year-old schoolchildren. *Headache, 36,* 466–470.

Sorge, F., De Simone, R., Marano, E., Nolano, M., Orefice, G., & Carrieri, P. (1988). Flunarizine in prophylaxis of childhood migraine: A double-blind, placebo-controlled, crossover study. *Cephalalgia, 8,* 1–6.

Stafstrom, C. E., Goldenholz, S. R., & Dulli, D. A. (2005). Serial headache drawings by children with migraine: Correlation with clinical headache status. *Journal of Child Neurology, 20,* 809–813.

Stafstrom, C. E., Rostasy, K., & Minster, A. (2002). The usefulness of children's drawings in the diagnosis of headache. *Pediatrics, 109,* 460–472.

Wechsler, D. (2003). *Wechsler Intelligence Scale for Children* (4th ed.). San Antonio, TX: The Psychological Corporation.

Weiller, C., May, A., Limmroth, V., Jüptner, M., Kaube, H., Schayck, R., et al. (1995). Brain stem activation in spontaneous human migraine attacks. *Nature Medicine, 1,* 658–660.

Welch, K. M., Barkley, G. L., Tepley, N., & Ramadan, N. M. (1993). Central neurogenic mechanisms of migraine. *Neurology, 43*(6 Suppl. 3), S21–25.

Werder, D. S., & Sargent, J. D. (1984). A study of childhood headache using biofeedback as a treatment alternative. *Headache, 24,* 122–126.

Winner, P. (2002). Triptans for migraine management in adolescents. *Headache, 42,* 675–679.

Wöber-Bingöl, C., Wöber, C., Wagner-Ennsgraber, C., Karwautz, A., Vesely, C., Zebenhoizer, K., et al. (1996). IHS criteria for migraine and tension-type headache in children and adolescents. *Headache, 36,* 231–238.

CHAPTER SIXTEEN

# Sickle Cell Disease

Kimberly M. Rennie, PhD, and
Julie A. Panepinto, MD, MSPH

## DESCRIPTION OF THE DISORDER

Sickle cell disease is an inherited red blood cell disorder that results in chronic morbidity and increased mortality. The disease affects approximately 70,000 people in the United States (Ashley-Koch, Yang, & Olney, 2000). One in 400 African American infants will be affected with the disease (Lin-Fu, 1972). In nearly all states, sickle cell disease is diagnosed through newborn screening at birth by hemoglobin electrophoresis. It is caused by the substitution of a valine amino acid for the glutamic amino acid at the sixth position of the beta globin hemoglobin chain. This substitution causes the red blood cell to be rigid and sickle shaped, resulting in increased vascular obstruction and tissue ischemia (i.e., the sickle-shaped red blood cells are rigid and inflexible, causing them to become lodged within blood vessels and restrict blood flow, resulting in damage to the tissue). This contributes to the development of many complications and increased morbidity for those who have sickle cell disease.

## RELATED MEDICAL ISSUES

Common manifestations of sickle cell disease include anemia; frequent painful crises; acute and chronic lung problems; infections; central nervous system infarctions (i.e., strokes), both silent and overt; splenic sequestration (i.e., red blood cells get trapped in the spleen causing a precipitous fall in hemoglobin level and the potential for hypovolemic shock); skin ulcers; and chronic end organ damage. Painful crises, termed vaso-occlusive crises, are the most common event that patients with sickle cell disease experience, as illustrated by the patient in Case 1. Cerebral infarction in sickle cell disease is common and includes both overt stroke (i.e., clinical stroke, with focal signs such as weakness, drooping of the face, difficulty talking and/or walking, lasting more than 24 hours) and silent stroke (i.e., a stroke that can be diagnosed with brain imaging but is difficult to detect without imaging as they tend to occur in the prefrontal cortex and do not have the same obvious motor changes as in an overt stroke). Cases 2 and 3 illustrate this complication of sickle cell disease. The following case studies will address the most common morbidities of patients with sickle cell disease that also have an impact on neurocognitive functioning.

## Case 1: Vaso-Occlusive Crises

John is an 11-year-old male who was diagnosed with sickle cell disease at birth after newborn screening was performed. His medical history is complicated by frequent hospitalizations due to vaso-occlusive crises. He was hospitalized 12 times over the last year due to these crises. During these hospitalizations John is managed with intravenous pain medications that often make him tired. When he is finally well enough to go home, he is usually on oral pain medications that can also cause sleepiness. In addition, he has a history of poor school performance and retention (first grade). John was referred for further neuropsychological testing due to this history.

Upon presentation for his neuropsychological evaluation, it was reported that John's early developmental history was uncomplicated. Aside from his sickle cell disease and its associated complications, medical and neurological histories were unremarkable. The main concern presented, at the time of evaluation, was the impact of his sickle cell disease on his school performance. As previously mentioned, he had a history of frequent hospitalizations, with each one lasting from a few days to up to a week in length.

At the time of the evaluation, John did not have an Individual Education Plan (IEP) or 504 plan, and no previous evaluations had ever been conducted. He presented as a relatively friendly and very polite preadolescent. Rapport was easy to establish and maintain, and he was compliant and cooperative with the examiner's requests. Extra prompting and reinforcement was needed when he was faced with difficult items.

Results of the evaluation indicated intact intellectual functioning and below-average to average academic skills. Difficulties with attentional regulation, fluency, verbal memory, and fine motor coordination were noted. Recommendations were made for consultation with a pain psychologist and an IEP under the Other Health Impairment (OHI) category. Specific school recommendations included extra time for completion of class work and other assignments, modified length of assignments, provision of class notes ahead of time, and occupational therapy consultation.

Many children with sickle cell disease who experience recurrent hospitalizations do not typically return to school the first day following discharge from the hospital. Thus, many children may miss up to a week or more of school as a result of one hospitalization. Unfortunately, given the state and district mandates for the provision of homebound instruction, oftentimes children with sickle cell disease do not receive homebound instruction. In fact, retention is not uncommon among children with sickle cell disease due to the number of school days missed. However, this does not seem to be an appropriate solution, as many of these children end up with significant educational problems as they advance through school.

Typically, children with sickle cell disease who do not have a history of sickle cell–related stroke tend to have average intellectual functioning, as was seen in this case. Common deficits include weaknesses in the areas of executive functioning, including attentional regulation. Less common but not atypical are fluency and fine motor coordination problems. Thus, compared to their healthy peers, these children tend to have more difficulty paying attention in school, need more time to process information, and may have difficulty with efficient note taking.

Patients with sickle cell disease have an average pain rate (number of episodes per patient year) of 1 (Platt et al., 1991). There is considerable variability in the pain rate of patients with sickle cell disease, and, as patients get older, vaso-occlusive events happen more frequently (Panepinto, Brousseau, Hillery, & Scott, 2005). A small subset of patients will experience 3 to 10 episodes a year, whereas up to 40% of patients will have no painful episodes (Platt et al.). Adults who experience higher pain rates have an increased rate of mortality (Platt et al.). Supportive care is the most common treatment used during painful crises. Typically, patients who are hospitalized with painful crises are managed with intravenous pain medications, either given as a continuous infusion (i.e., the administration of a fluid into a blood vessel, usually over a prolonged period of time) or by intermittent bolus infusion (i.e., a single dose of drug usually injected into a blood vessel over a short period of time). They also receive intravenous fluids as needed. They are then gradually transitioned to oral pain medications, which they often continue to take at home. These medications commonly cause drowsiness and can make return to school and work difficult, as noted above in John. In addition, the average length of stay for a vaso-occlusive crisis is 4 days (Panepinto et al., 2005). Thus, John spends a substantial number of days per year in the hospital. This prevents him from attending school, and his pain medications contribute to additional constraints due to the common side effect of sleepiness.

## Case 2: Overt Stroke

Tom is a 9-year-old boy who has residual right-sided hemiparesis (i.e., weakness on the right side of his body). At 3.5 years of age, he presented to the emergency department with acute onset of right arm and leg weakness and an inability to walk. He was noted upon presentation to have right-sided hemiparesis and aphasia (i.e., inability to speak). Magnetic resonance imaging (MRI) and magnetic resonance angiography (MRA) of his brain revealed a right-middle cerebral artery stroke with occlusion (i.e., obstruction) of that vessel. Tom was referred to the neuropsychology service for further evaluation of his neurocognitive abilities.

Tom was seen approximately 7 years after his stroke for neuropsychological evaluation. Until the time of his stroke, early development was reportedly unremarkable. Following his stroke, his handedness switched from right to left, and he began to have difficulties with language. At the time of his stroke, he also suffered a seizure. No further seizures or strokes have been reported.

He presented as a very friendly child, albeit somewhat disinhibited, and was easy to engage. Tom was distractible at times and required frequent redirection, to which he responded well. Overall, he appeared to put forth good effort and was generally cooperative.

Results of the current evaluation indicated a significant discrepancy (23 points) between his well-below-average verbal reasoning ability and his average nonverbal reasoning ability. His academic achievement was generally consistent with his overall intellectual functioning, which fell mainly within normal limits. Significant difficulties with attentional regulation, fine motor coordination, and language-based tasks were noted.

Overall, results of Tom's evaluation are generally consistent with what is seen in children with sickle cell disease who have suffered a stroke. That is, these children tend to have significant deficits in attentional regulation, fluency, and fine motor coordination. Unlike this case, however, following an overt stroke, intellectual functioning tends to fall within the impaired range (i.e., below 70). Remarkably, Tom's overall intellectual functioning remains in the average range. It is also important to note that although deficits in intellectual functioning, executive functioning (including attentional regulation), fluency, and fine motor coordination are common among all who have suffered overt stroke, other neurocognitive deficits will vary depending on the location of the stroke. For example, left-sided strokes tend to result in language impairment, whereas right-sided strokes tend to result in nonverbal impairments.

As mentioned previously, intellectual functioning tends to fall within the mentally retarded range after children with sickle cell disease suffer an overt stroke. In Tom's case, this did not happen. Given his family history, it is hypothesized that Tom would likely have fallen in the superior range of intelligence had he not suffered an overt stroke. This suggests that Tom's cognitive reserve helped buffer the full impact of his stroke. Cognitive reserve is a term that is used to refer to the brain's resiliency (i.e., an individual's ability to protect himself/herself from damage or insult to the brain; Stern, 2002). It is theorized that higher cognitive reserve raises the threshold at which one sees the decline in cognitive functioning as a result of injury to the brain (Stern). Higher cognitive reserve is also thought to be associated with premorbid intellectual functioning and familial antecedents.

The common presenting symptoms of an acute overt stroke include hemiparesis, seizures, a change in mental status, and visual or language problems. Overt stroke occurs in up to 10% of children with sickle cell disease and is characterized by physical and neurocognitive impairment (Craft, Schatz, Glauser, Lee, & DeBaun, 1993; Ohene-Frempong et al., 1998). It is a significant cause of death and morbidity in children with sickle cell disease. The mortality rate for children with sickle cell disease who experience stroke is as high as 11% (Ohene-Frempong et al.). The mainstay of therapy for acute stroke in sickle cell disease is red blood cell transfusion therapy. Red blood cell transfusions are used to lower the amount of sickle hemoglobin in the patient's blood from 80% or more to less than 30%. This therapy is then continued long-term on a chronic basis and is effective in lowering the recurrent stroke risk from as high as 70% if no therapy is instituted to 20% with chronic therapy (Armstrong et al., 1996; Ohene-Frempong et al.). To receive this therapy, a patient spends approximately 1 day a month at a health care facility.

Blood transfusion therapy, however, carries inherent risk that contributes to the overall morbidity of patients with sickle cell disease. Iron overload is a known and expected side effect of chronic blood transfusion therapy. Over the course of 1 to 2 years, monthly blood transfusions lead to iron overload and the deposition of iron into the liver, heart, and other vital organs. Without chelation therapy to reduce iron overload, the liver or heart will ultimately fail and the patient will have an untimely death related to organ failure (i.e., cirrhosis of the liver, fibrosis of the heart). In addition, there is a risk of infection with blood transfusions. Although these risks are not great, contracting these illnesses is devastating and may lead to an increased risk of mortality.

In addition to the above-mentioned risks from transfusion, many families report that their children's level of fatigue seems to increase as they get further out from their last transfusion. In fact, some even report that transfusion seems to make their children have attention-deficit/hyperactivity disorder (ADHD). This phenomenon is likely due to changes in hemoglobin (i.e., a protein that transports oxygen in the red blood cells) levels. As children get further out from their last transfusion, their hemoglobin levels decrease, resulting in anemia, which is associated with fatigue. Once they receive their next scheduled transfusion, their hemoglobin levels go up, which gives them a burst of energy, which is likely what parents refer to as ADHD.

## Case 3: Silent Stroke

The sister of John, Sarah is an 11-year-old female with sickle cell disease who presented with complaints of new-onset headaches. Her mother also reported that she was having more difficulty concentrating in school and getting her homework done at home. Due to these symptoms and the positive family medical history of sickle cell disease, Sarah underwent an MRI of the brain. The MRI showed the presence of an infarct (i.e., tissue that has died due to a lack of oxygen resulting from blockage of an artery) in the left occipital and right frontal lobes of the brain. The imaging study confirmed the presence of silent infarction in this child. Sarah was referred to the neuropsychology service for evaluation due to having experienced a silent stroke and increased difficulties with school.

According to parental report, Sarah experienced relatively normal development and was doing well academically until the onset of her headaches. Aside from her sickle cell disease, her medical and neurological histories were unremarkable. She presented as a somewhat shy preadolescent girl and was slow to warm up to the examiner. She put forth good effort and was generally cooperative with examiner's requests. However, she tended to take a longer-than-typical amount of time to respond to questions.

Results of Sarah's evaluation indicated average intellectual functioning with evenly developed verbal and nonverbal reasoning abilities. Deficits with attentional regulation, fine motor coordination, and processing speed were noted. Academic achievement was within normal limits.

Overall, results of her profile are generally consistent with what we see in children who have suffered a silent infarction. These children tend to have new onset of difficulties with attentional regulation, processing, and fine motor coordination. Unfortunately, due to the nature of silent stroke, many of these children may not be identified at the time of the stroke, and months or years may pass before they are identified. Identification is crucial because silent stroke significantly increases the risk of having an overt stroke. Astute teachers and parents play a critical role in bringing these children to the attention of their hematologists. Oftentimes, either teachers or parents will report a change in the child's handwriting or ability to pay attention. Processing speed issues may also help to identify these children. One teacher reported frustration that Sarah would not respond when asked a question. It turned out that given extra time, she was able to respond appropriately.

Finally, children who have suffered a silent stroke tend to have below-average intellectual functioning; however, Sarah's intellectual functioning remained in the average range, leading some to believe that her silent stroke did not have a major impact on her functioning. This clearly was not the case. Moreover, as was the case with her brother John, it is likely that given the family history, Sarah's level of intellectual functioning was probably above average or better.

Silent stroke, defined as the presence of abnormalities in an imaging study of the brain along with a normal neurological exam and no prior history of any physical findings, occurs in up to 22% of children with sickle cell disease (Pegelow et al., 2002). The risk of recurrent silent stroke and overt stroke is higher in these patients. Like overt stroke, silent stroke is characterized by neurocognitive deficits, especially in attention, resulting in poor school achievement and behavioral problems (Armstrong et al., 1996; Brown et al., 2000). Silent stroke is not associated with physical impairment. Unlike for overt stroke, there is no defined standard treatment for these patients, although ongoing clinical trials are examining the effect of chronic red blood cell transfusions on the risk of recurrent silent stroke or overt stroke.

## Case 4: General

Bobby is a 9-year-old male with sickle cell disease who has had minimal complications from sickle cell disease. He averages one hospitalization a year for pain and has not had an overt stroke. He has a history of obstructive sleep apnea from adenoid and tonsillar hypertrophy (i.e., enlargement), which has resulted in notable nighttime hypoxia (i.e., an inadequate supply of oxygen to the brain) during his hospitalizations. He was referred to the neuropsychology service for further evaluation because his grades recently slipped to C's and D's from A's and B's in the past. His mother also reported that he seemed to know things some days but not other days.

As with the other cases described, Bobby experienced relatively normal early development. Aside from his sickle cell disease and associated complications, his medical and neurological histories were unremarkable. He generally warmed easily to the examiner, and rapport was easily established and maintained with him. He was cooperative on tasks that came naturally for him but resisted slightly and needed reassurance and encouragement for items that were more difficult for him. Bobby had a tendency to make comments such as "I'm stupid" or "I'm never gonna get this" when faced with more challenging tasks.

Results indicated overall intellectual functioning in the below-average range, with significantly better developed nonverbal than verbal reasoning abilities (31 point discrepancy). Attentional regulation was within normal limits. His academic achievement scores fell within the impaired to below-average ranges (ranging from 58–83). Mathematics represented an area of relative strength for Bobby, with his performance in this area yielding his highest scores. In the areas of reading and written language, his scores were generally 70 or below. On expressive and receptive language testing, his performance fell within the very impaired range. Similarly, Bobby had significant difficulty on measures of verbal memory. His visual memory skills, however, were within normal limits. Mild fine motor difficulties were noted. He was diagnosed with a language disorder, with appropriate recommendations made.

In this case, it is impossible to know whether Bobby's sickle cell disease contributed to his language disorder. However, it highlights the fact that regardless of the severity of their disease, children with sickle cell-disease are also at risk for typical developmental disorders (e.g., learning disabilities). In general, children with sickle cell disease who do not have major medical complications tend to have normal intellectual functioning. However, a disproportionately higher percentage of these children have deficits with attentional regulation, although this was not seen in this particular case. It is important to note, however, that these children do not have what many individuals think of as typical ADHD. Instead, they have difficulty sustaining their attention to tasks and tend to need a longer-than-typical time to process information and formulate an appropriate response. Unfortunately, oftentimes these deficits with initiation are mistaken for oppositional behavior in these children.

Sickle cell disease is characterized by its unpredictability and variability. Thus far, it has been difficult to predict the disease severity of these patients. Bobby in Case 4 had a relatively mild course with few complications from his sickle cell disease. Despite this, he exhibited significant impairments in his neuropsychological functioning.

Another common occurrence in children with sickle cell disease is an increased number of somatic complaints (i.e., aches and pains). Due to the nature of their disease, children with sickle cell have a much higher incidence of aches and pains than children without a chronic illness. The impact of this pain cannot be emphasized enough. As a result of their pain, these children may miss school, which not only impacts their academic achievement but also their ability to establish and maintain appropriate peer relationships. As a result of their disease, limitations are placed on the social activities in which they may be able to partake. The socioemotional impact of this disease is just as real as the medical and neuropsychological complications. Consequently, these children need not only medical and academic support but social supports as well.

## SUMMARY

Sickle cell disease is a complicated disease, and complications of the disease can range from mild to severe. One of the most devastating complications is the occurrence of stroke. Approximately 10% of individuals with sickle cell disease will suffer an overt stroke, and another 20% will have a silent stroke (Reese & Smith, 1997). The neuropsychological sequelae of either an overt or silent stroke can be quite severe. The average IQ for individuals who have suffered an overt stroke is 70 (Craft et al., 1993). It is quite devastating for parents and other caregivers to see children who were once experiencing normal development and had the potential to graduate from high school and attend a 4-year university now require special education services for the rest of their academic career and possibly never achieve functional independence as an adult. Although patients who have suffered an overt stroke tend to experience the most severe neurocognitive deficits, others are not free from neurocognitive difficulties. Patients who have suffered a silent stroke tend to have below-average IQs and are at increased risk for academic difficulties (Craft et al.). Moreover, the occurrence of a silent stroke places these children at higher risk for overt stroke. Unfortunately, silent stroke may go unrecognized in many patients who do not receive adequate medical care. Also, as seen from the cases presented, although patients who have not suffered a stroke may have intact intellectual functioning, they are not completely free of cognitive and academic problems. Noll and colleagues (2001) found that children with sickle cell disease who had not suffered a stroke had more academic difficulties than matched controls. Moreover, evidence exists that suggests that over time these children experience declines in their intellectual functioning.

The psychosocial impact of sickle cell disease can be as severe as the medical and neuropsychological sequelae and should not be overlooked. Parents and families of children and adolescents who have experienced strokes have to begin planning for continued support of their child beyond the typical high school or college graduation. These children will usually need a much higher level of support as a result of their decline in functioning. Moreover, it is important to note that sickle cell disease takes a toll on the children who have not yet suffered a stroke as well. Although these children look fine and may appear healthy, they are not and in fact are truly suffering from a devastating disease. Oftentimes, their frequent school absences, the restrictions placed on their activities, academic difficulties, chronic pain, small stature, and frequent hospitalizations collectively impact their ability to maintain friendships.

Finally, it should be noted that in the past, the average life span for individuals with sickle cell disease was around 30 to 40 years. As a result of advances in treatment, individuals with sickle cell are now surviving into their 50s. This is a great accomplishment, but it shows how far we still have to go. To date, the only cure for sickle cell disease is bone marrow transplantation. Unfortunately, the bone marrow transplant may not be successful, and a risk of death is associated with bone marrow transplantation. To further complicate matters, the criteria for a bone marrow transplant are quite stringent, and finding a match is very difficult. Thus, only a tiny percentage of children with sickle cell disease actually undergo a bone marrow transplant. If the bone marrow transplantation is successful, as they get older, these children then also have to cope with infertility.

## RESOURCES

### Books

Bloom, M. (1995). *Understanding sickle cell disease.* Jackson: University Press of Mississippi.

Day, S., & Marion, S. B. (1996). *Educator's guide to sickle cell disease.* Memphis, TN: St. Jude Children's Research Hospital.

Earles, A., Lessing, S., & Vichinsky, E. (Eds.). (1993). *Parents' handbook for sickle cell disease: Part II. Six to eighteen years of age.* Berkeley: State of California Department of Health Services.

Lessing, S., & Vichinsky, E. (1998). *Parents' handbook for sickle cell disease: Part I. Birth to six years of age.* Oakland: State of California Department of Health Services.

Sickle Cell Disease Association of America. (1998). *Parent/teacher guide: How parents and teachers can work together to achieve school success for children with sickle cell anemia.* Baltimore: Author.

### Organizations and Web Sites

Children's Hemiplegia and Stroke Association

This is a nonprofit support group for parents and families of children who have had a stroke.

Web Site: www.chasa.org/

Kids Health for Parents

This Web site provides information about a variety of health issues for parents, children, and teachers. The sickle cell link provides general information about the disease and includes links to additional resources.

Web Site: www.kidshealth.org/parent/medical/heart/sickle_cell_anemia.html

National Heart Lung Blood Association

This organization provides information about sickle cell disease and engages in research for sickle cell disease.

Web Site: www.nhlbi.nih.gov/health/dci/Diseases/Sca/SCA_WhatIs.html

Sickle Cell Disease

This Web site provides general information about sickle cell disease, including symptoms and treatment.

Web Site: www.ygyh.org/sickle/whatisit.htm

Sickle Cell Disease Association of America

This organization is dedicated to finding a cure for sickle cell disease. Its Web site provides general information, research updates, and links to additional resources.

Web Site: www.sicklecelldisease.org/

The Sickle Cell Information Center

The mission of this site is to provide sickle cell patients and professionals with education, news, research updates, and worldwide sickle cell resources.

Web Site: www.scinfo.org/

## Electronic Media

Starbright Explorer Series: The Sickle Cell Slime-O-Rama Game

This CD-ROM for children ages 6 to 15 helps explain sickle cell disease to kids through fun games and interesting facts. The Sickle Cell Slime-O-Rama game asks kids questions about the disease, taking care of their health, and pain management. The CD-ROM also has information about blood tests, radiology, and IVs. Released in 2001, it can be obtained from the Starbright Foundation in Los Angeles, California.

## REFERENCES

Armstrong, F. D., Thompson, R. J., Jr., Wang, W., Zimmerman, R., Pegelow, C. H., Miller, S., et al. (1996). Cognitive functioning and brain magnetic resonance imaging in children with sickle cell disease. Neuropsychology Committee of the Cooperative Study of Sickle Cell Disease. *Pediatrics, 97,* 864–870.

Ashley-Koch, A., Yang, Q., & Olney, R. S. (2000). Sickle hemoglobin (HbS) allele and sickle cell disease: A HuGE review. *American Journal of Epidemiology, 151,* 839–845.

Brown, R. T., Davis, P. C., Lambert, R., Hsu, L., Hopkins, K., & Eckman, J. (2000). Neurocognitive functioning and magnetic resonance imaging in children with sickle cell disease. *Journal of Pediatric Psychology, 25,* 503–513.

Craft, S., Schatz, J., Glauser, T. A., Lee, B., & DeBaun, M. R. (1993). Neuropsychologic effects of stroke in children with sickle cell anemia. *Journal of Pediatrics, 123,* 712–717.

Lin-Fu, J. S. (1972). *Sickle cell anemia: A medical review.* Rockville, MD: U.S. Department of Health, Education, and Welfare.

Noll, R. B., Stith, L., Garstein, M. A., Ris, M. D., Grueneich, R., Vannatta, K., et al. (2001). Neuropsychological functioning of youths with sickle cell disease: Comparison with non-chronically ill peers. *Journal of Pediatric Psychology, 26,* 69–78.

Ohene-Frempong, K., Weiner, S. J., Sleeper, L. A., Miller, S. T., Embury, S., Moohr, J. W., et al. (1998). Cerebrovascular accidents in sickle cell disease: Rates and risk factors. *Blood, 91,* 288–294.

Panepinto, J. A., Brousseau, D. C., Hillery, C. A., & Scott, J. P. (2005). Variation in hospitalizations and hospital length of stay in children with vaso-occlusive crises in sickle cell disease. *Pediatric Blood and Cancer, 44,* 182–186.

Pegelow, C. H., Macklin, E. A., Moser, F. G., Wang, W. C., Bello, J. A., Miller, S. T., et al. (2002). Longitudinal changes in brain magnetic resonance imaging findings in children with sickle cell disease. *Blood, 99,* 3014–3018.

Platt, O. S., Thorington, B. D., Brambilla, D. J., Milner, P. F., Rosse, W. F., Vichinsky, E., et al. (1991). Pain in sickle cell disease: Rates and risk factors. *New England Journal of Medicine, 325,* 11–16.

Reese, F. L., & Smith, W. R. (1997). Psychosocial determinants of health care utilization in sickle cell disease patients. *Annals of Behavioral Medicine, 19,* 171–178.

Stern, Y. (2002). What is cognitive reserve? Theory and research application of the reserve concept. *Journal of the International Neuropsychological Society, 8,* 448–460.

CHAPTER SEVENTEEN

# Sleep-Disordered Breathing

Jennifer A. Janusz, PsyD, ABPP-CN, Joette James, PhD, and Ann C. Halbower, MD

Kelly is an 8-year-old White female with a long-standing history of difficulties with attention, impulsivity, and emotional regulation. These have become increasingly disruptive in the home, school, and social settings, with parents and teachers raising concerns regarding the possibility of a learning or attention disorder.

Kelly was born to her biological parents at full term following an uncomplicated pregnancy. Although Kelly was sociable as an infant, she also exhibited some irritability and was at times difficult to soothe. Kelly's developmental motor and language milestones were achieved within normal parameters. In fact, Kelly's mother reported that she "began to run as soon as she could walk." As a toddler, Kelly required an increased level of parental supervision due to her high activity level. She also had trouble sustaining attention and usually moved quickly from one activity to the next. Further, Kelly exhibited frequent, intense temper tantrums, which typically resulted in hitting, kicking, and biting others. These behaviors persisted into Kelly's preschool years. Given her behavioral difficulties, Kelly attended a small private school for kindergarten and first grade. In that setting, with a lower student-to-teacher ratio and a structured, yet flexible teacher, Kelly did relatively well. Although there were ongoing concerns regarding her attention and activity level, she quickly acquired academic concepts. Kelly's family moved, and she subsequently began attending her current school, in which the second grade is a large, "open concept" classroom with approximately 35 students. Although she describes Kelly as a sweet, outgoing child, Kelly's second-grade teacher notes significant inattention and distractibility in the classroom. Kelly also needs frequent reminders to stay on task and has difficulty completing work within expected time frames. Kelly is described as very talkative, and she often blurts out answers and interrupts others, which can be disruptive in the classroom. Similar behaviors are observed at home as well. Although she is a popular child who is generally well liked by classmates, Kelly can be domineering in her relationships with other children and has trouble maintaining personal space, which sometimes results in alienation from peers. In addition, she is prone to emotional outbursts when thwarted or frustrated.

Kelly's medical history is notable for many years of loud snoring that can be heard in her parents' bedroom and that reportedly occurs every night. At times, it seems as if Kelly is struggling to breathe while asleep, and she often makes gasping sounds. Sometimes her chest seems to be moving up and down, although it does not look like air is flowing, and Kelly's parents have had to shake her awake when this occurs. In addition, Kelly's mother reports that it is occasionally difficult to arouse Kelly in the mornings, and the bedcovers are typically disheveled after a night of very restless sleep. During the daytime, Kelly is noted to breathe through her mouth. She has a muffled voice and tends to drool, especially when she is sleeping. She frequently has dark circles under her eyes, which her mother attributes to poor sleep, although she notes that this is worse during allergy season. Several months ago, Kelly was started on a trial of stimulant medication to address her attention and behavioral control issues; however, the medication seemed to have only a minimal effect and was thus discontinued.

## DESCRIPTION OF THE DISORDER

Sleep-disordered breathing (SDB) is a condition characterized by partial or complete upper airway obstruction during sleep due to collapse or narrowing of the pharynx. This can result in fragmentation of sleep due to brief arousals during the night, as well as disruption or cessation of airflow. SDB has been associated with physical, cognitive, behavioral, and emotional complications in both children and adults (Beebe, 2006; Halbower & Mahone, 2006; Schecter & the Section on Pediatric Pulmonology, 2002).

The severity of the airway obstruction in SDB is considered to be on a continuum (Blunden, Lushington, Kennedy, Martin, & Dawson, 2000).

Primary snoring, defined as snoring without changes in oxygenation, is at the mild end of the spectrum. Upper airway resistance syndrome, in the middle of the continuum, is characterized by snoring with increased breathing effort but no blood oxygen abnormalities. Obstructive sleep apnea (OSA) is considered the most severe form of SDB. OSA is characterized by a repeated obstruction or blocking of the airway that can disrupt normal respiratory gas exchange, resulting in changes in oxygenation, including *hypoxia* (i.e., reduction in oxygen levels in blood) and *hypercarbia* (i.e., increase in carbon dioxide levels in blood). Increased breathing effort, snoring, gasping, and frequent awakenings, during which normal breathing is resumed, are typically seen (Beebe, 2005; Halbower & Mahone, 2006; Hansen & Vandenberg, 1997). Episodes of complete airway obstruction are termed *apneas,* whereas partial obstructions are *hypopneas* (Redline et al., 2007). In children, enlarged tonsils and adenoids are commonly associated with upper airway obstruction (American Academy of Pediatrics, 2002), although abnormal neuromuscular tone can also be a major contributing factor (Arens & Marcus, 2004). An overnight polysomnogram (PSG) completed in a sleep laboratory and measuring sleep-wake states, respiration, cardiac activity, blood levels of oxygen and carbon dioxide, and movement is considered the "gold standard" in diagnosing OSA (American Thoracic Society, 1996).

Prevalence rates of OSA in children range from 1% to 3% in the school-age population (Ali, Pitson, & Stradling, 1993; Brunetti et al., 2001; Redline et al., 1999). It is suspected that upper airway resistance syndrome occurs frequently, although exact rates are unknown (Bao & Guilleminault, 2004). Primary snoring is reported to have a prevalence rate of 7% to 12%, with some studies reporting rates as high as 21% (Corbo et al., 2001; Ferreira et al., 2000; Ipsiroglu et al., 2001; Owen, Canter, & Robinson, 1996). Children with OSA tend to have associated respiratory allergies and asthma (Ievers-Landis & Redline, 2007). Obesity is considered a risk factor for SDB; the risk of OSA is 4.6 times greater for overweight children than for children of normal weight, with this risk greater for adolescents than younger children (Ievers-Landis & Redline). However, clearly not all children who exhibit SDB are obese, given that enlarged tonsils and adenoids, the most common cause of SDB, can occur for a variety of reasons. Lower socioeconomic status (SES) has also been related to SDB, but this relationship may be mediated by increased rates of obesity in this population (Chervin, Clarke, et al., 2003). In contrast, high intelligence may be a protective factor against neuropsychological deficits, especially attention problems (Beebe, 2005; Halbower et al., 2006).

The characteristics of OSA differ between adults and children. Enlarged tonsils and adenoids are more likely to be associated with airway obstruction in children than adults. Although many adults are treated with continuous positive airway pressure, which delivers a stream of compressed air through the nose or mouth to prevent collapse of the airway, children are generally treated with adenotonsillectomy (i.e., surgical removal of the tonsils and adenoids). This is successful in approximately 80% of children with OSA (Lipton & Gozal, 2003; Mitchell & Kelly, 2006). Discrete apneic episodes are more common in adults; in contrast, children typically exhibit hypopneas and persistent hypoventilation (i.e., reduced amount of air entering lungs, resulting in inadequate gas exchange; Rosen, D'Andrea, & Haddad, 1992). As a result, children with OSA may demonstrate milder hypoxia than adults (Lewin, Rosen, England, & Dahl, 2002). Children tend to have less fragmented sleep and report less daytime sleepiness compared to adults. However, hyperactivity and irritability are much more commonly reported in children (Kaemingk et al., 2003).

Children may be especially vulnerable to the negative effects of SDB, as childhood is a time of rapid brain development and skill acquisition. The cognitive and behavioral sequelae of SDB can significantly impact a child's ability to participate effectively and successfully not only in learning situations but also in social settings. If untreated, these problems may alter a child's developmental path and prevent him or her from reaching full cognitive potential (Beebe, 2006; Halbower et al., 2006). Therefore, early identification and treatment of children with SDB is essential to ensure optimal academic and social success.

## CASE CONTINUATION

Due to concerns regarding Kelly's attention and behavioral regulation, she was referred for a neuropsychological evaluation. Kelly presented at the evaluation as friendly and age appropriate in her social interaction with the examiner, and she was quite chatty in informal conversation. Kelly's activity level was elevated, with fidgeting and squirming noted. At times, she stood up to complete tasks. Kelly's sustained attention was generally adequate within the highly structured, individualized testing setting; however, occasional distractibility was noted.

### Assessment Results

The results of the neuropsychological evaluation (see Tables 17.1 and 17.2) indicated average overall cognitive ability. Language skills, nonverbal processing skills, verbal and visual memory, processing speed, and fine motor/graphomotor functioning were all within normal limits for age. Mild weaknesses were noted in Kelly's early academic skills. In this context, significant deficits were noted on formal measures of sustained auditory and visual attention, as well as divided attention. In addition, Kelly exhibited notable weaknesses in multiple aspects of executive functioning, including impulse control, emotional regulation, working memory, and independent planning/organization. Given parental concerns regarding Kelly's sleep, her mother completed the Child Sleep Questionnaire (CSQ; Huntley, Campo, Dahl, & Lewin, 2007; see Figure 17.1, reprinted with author permission), which was significant for several symptoms associated with SDB, including snoring that occurs three to four times per week or more and that is heard outside of the bedroom, as well as parental observation of difficulties with breathing during sleep. Kelly's mother also endorsed symptoms of mild daytime sleepiness; she indicated that Kelly has a "slight chance of dozing" while watching television and riding in a car or on a bus and is difficult to arouse approximately two mornings per week.

As a whole, Kelly's neuropsychological profile appeared to be consistent with the diagnosis of Attention-Deficit/Hyperactivity Disorder (ADHD), Combined Subtype. Given Kelly's history of age-appropriate acquisition of preacademic skills, the current mild academic difficulties were attributed to the impact of her attention and executive weaknesses on her availability for learning, as opposed to a specific learning disorder. In addition, based on screening using the CSQ, Kelly appeared to evidence symptoms of SDB, prompting a referral to a local sleep clinic.

## COMPLICATIONS ASSOCIATED WITH SDB

Untreated OSA is associated with significant morbidity, including systemic and pulmonary hypertension, cardiovascular problems, and failure to thrive (Beebe & Gozal, 2002; Chervin et al., 2006; Lewin et al., 2002; Schecter & the Section on Pediatric Pulmonology, 2002). When hospital stays, medication use, and visits to the emergency room are considered, children with OSA utilize health care services 2.6 times more often than children without OSA (Reuveni, Simon, Tal, Elhayany, & Trasiuk, 2002).

Whereas physical symptoms are linked to more severe untreated OSA, cognitive, behavioral, and emotional difficulties are seen in children along the entire spectrum of SDB. In fact, primary snoring itself, even without PSG findings or oxygen desaturations, is associated with neurobehavioral difficulties (O'Brien, Mervis, Holbrook, Bruner, Klaus, et al., 2004; Urschitz et al., 2004). Given the similar consequences observed in children with primary snoring and OSA, these effects will be considered together under the larger rubric of SDB.

**TABLE 17.1 Neuropsychological Evaluation Test Summary**

| Scale | Scaled Score | Standard Score |
|---|---|---|
| Wechsler Abbreviated Scale of Intelligence | | |
| Full Scale IQ | | 95 |
| Verbal IQ | | 93 |
| Performance IQ | | 95 |
| Wide Range Achievement Test—Third Edition | | |
| Reading | | 89 |
| Spelling | | 96 |
| Arithmetic | | 88 |
| California Verbal Learning Test—Children's Version | | |
| List A Total Trials 1–5 | | 96 |
| List A Trial 1 Free Recall | | 115 |
| List A Trial 5 Free Recall | | 108 |
| Learning Slope | | 93 |
| List A Short-Delay Free Recall | | 115 |
| List A Short-Delay Cued Recall | | 100 |
| List A Long-Delay Free Recall | | 93 |
| List A Long-Delay Cued Recall | | 115 |
| Semantic Cluster | | 78 |
| Perseverations | | 115 |
| Intrusions | | 85 |
| Recall Consistency | | 108 |
| Recognition | | 115 |
| Wide Range Assessment of Memory and Learning—Second Edition | | |
| Story Memory | 9 | |
| Story Memory Recall | 9 | |
| Story Recognition | 12 | |
| Children's Memory Scale | | |
| Dot Locations Learning | 10 | |

**TABLE 17.1** (*Continued*)

| Scale | Scaled Score | Standard Score |
|---|---|---|
| Dot Locations Total Score | 10 | |
| Dot Locations Long Delay | 10 | |
| NEPSY—A Developmental Neuropsychological Assessment | | |
| Comprehension of Instructions | 7 | |
| Verbal Fluency—Semantic | | 81 |
| Verbal Fluency—Categorical | | 101 |
| Beery-Buktenica Developmental Test of Visual-Motor Integration—FifthEdition | | |
| VMI | | 102 |
| Tower of London—Drexel | | |
| Total Move Score | | ≤60 |
| Total Correct Score | | 98 |
| Total Rule Violation Score | | ≤60 |
| Total Initiation Time | | 106 |
| Total Execution Time | | 82 |
| Total Problem-Solving Time | | 78 |
| Rey-Osterrieth Complex Figure Test | | |
| Copy Organization | | 80 |
| Delay Organization | | 81 |
| Test of Everyday Attention for Children | | |
| Sky Search Correct Targets | 9 | |
| Sky Search Time per Target | 2 | |
| Sky Search Attention Score | 1 | |
| Score! | 5 | |
| Creature Count Total Correct | 4 | |
| Walk/Don't Walk | 3 | |
| Sky Search DT | 1 | |

*Continued*

**TABLE 17.1** (*Continued*)

| Scale | Scaled Score | Standard Score |
|---|---|---|
| | Grooved Pegboard | |
| Right (dominant) hand | | 109 |
| Left hand | | 100 |

*Note.* The Beery-Buktenica Developmental Test of Visual-Motor Integration—Fifth Edition (VMI-V; Beery, Buktenica, & Beery, 2004); California Verbal Learning Test—Children's Version (CVLT-C; Delis, Kramer, Kaplan, & Ober, 1994); Children's Memory Scale (CMS; Cohen, 1997); NEPSY: A Developmental Neuropsychological Assessment (Korkman, Kirk, & Kemp, 1997); Rey-Osterrieth Complex Figure (ROCF; Bernstein & Waber, 1996); The Test of Everyday Attention for Children (TEA-Ch; Manly, Robertson, Anderson, & Nimmo-Smith, 1999); Tower of London—Drexel University (TOL; Culbertson & Zilmer, 2000); The Wechsler Abbreviated Scale of Intelligence (WASI; Wechsler, 1999); Wide Range Achievement Test—Third Edition (WRAT-3; Wilkinson, 1995); (Wide Range Assessment of Memory and Learning—Second Edition (WRAML-2; Sheslow & Adams, 2003).

The most commonly reported problems among children with SDB are symptoms associated with ADHD, including elevated rates of hyperactivity and impulsivity. Reports of attentional problems have been less consistent, suggesting that among school-age children, behavioral dysregulation may be more common than inattention (Beebe, 2006; Halbower & Mahone, 2006; Mitchell & Kelly, 2006). ADHD is associated with deficits in executive functions (Barkley, 1997), and problems in this neurocognitive domain are commonly reported in children with SDB as well. Studies have demonstrated problems in mental flexibility (Archbold, Giordani, Ruzicka, & Chervin, 2004; Friedman et al., 2003), verbal fluency (Beebe et al., 2004), and planning (Gottlieb et al., 2004; O'Brien, Mervis, Holbrook, Bruner, Smith, et al., 2004) on office-based tests. Reports from parent and teacher questionnaires, which may provide a better understanding of the child's executive skills in "real world" environments, are consistent with these findings. Parents and teachers of children with SDB report problems with aspects of behavioral regulation and metacognitive skills, such as initiation, working memory, planning, organization, and self-monitoring (Beebe et al., 2004).

Studies have yielded mixed findings regarding the effects of SDB on intellectual ability. As a group, children with SDB score in the average range on IQ tests. Although two studies of older school-age children with severe sleep apnea showed IQ deficits compared to matched normal controls (Halbower et al., 2006; Rhodes et al., 1995), deficits in IQ have usually been found in preschool through first-grade children

**TABLE 17.2 Questionnaire Data**

| Scale | Parent T Score | Teacher T Score |
|---|---|---|
| Behavior Rating Inventory of Executive Function | | |
| Inhibit | 65 | 74 |
| Shift | 68 | 43 |
| Emotional Control | 70 | 78 |
| Behavior Regulation Index | 70 | 63 |
| Initiate | 55 | 91 |
| Working Memory | 75 | 86 |
| Plan/Organize | 69 | 66 |
| Organization of Materials | 59 | 82 |
| Monitor | 65 | 76 |
| Metacognitive Index | 69 | 83 |
| Global Executive Composite | 71 | 79 |
| ADHD-IV Rating Scale (Home, School Versions) | | |
| Attention Problems | 82 | 75 |
| Hyperactivity | 73 | 70 |
| Achenbach Scales (Child Behavior Checklist, Teacher's Report Form) | | |
| Anxious/Depressed | 51 | 59 |
| Withdrawn/Depressed | 53 | 50 |
| Somatic Complaints | 61 | 50 |
| Social Problems | 58 | 64 |
| Thought Problems | 51 | 50 |
| Attention Problems | 70 | 72 |
| Rule-Breaking Behavior | 54 | 58 |
| Aggressive Behavior | 51 | 67 |
| Internalizing Problems | 57 | 54 |
| Externalizing Problems | 51 | 66 |
| Total Problems | 57 | 64 |
| Affective Problems | 55 | 52 |
| Anxiety Problems | 50 | 56 |

*Continued*

**TABLE 17.2** (*Continued*)

| Scale | Parent T Score | Teacher T Score |
|---|---|---|
| Somatic Problems | 57 | 50 |
| Attention-Deficit /Hyperactivity Problems | 75 | 77 |
| Oppositional Defiant Problems | 51 | 69 |
| Conduct Problems | 56 | 61 |

*Note.* ADHD Rating Scale—IV (DuPaul, Power, Anastopoulos, & Reid, 1998); Behavior Rating Inventory of Executive Function (BRIEF; Gioia, Isquith, Guy, & Kenworthy, 2000); Child Behavior Checklist for Ages 6–18 (CBCL; Achenbach, 2001a); Teacher's Report Form for Ages 6–18 (TRF; Achenbach, 2001b).

(Gottlieb et al., 2004; Montgomery-Downs, Crabtree, & Gozal, 2005; O'Brien, Mervis, Holbrook, Bruner, Klaus, et al., 2004; O'Brien, Mervis, Holbrook, Bruner, Smith, et al., 2004). This suggests that age may be a moderating factor in intellectual functioning, with younger children at greater risk (Beebe, 2005). Findings in the areas of visual perception and memory also have been inconsistent. Although language skills appear to be relatively unaffected by SDB, several studies have found deficits in comprehension of oral instructions and early phonological skills (Beebe, 2006). Referring a child for a comprehensive neuropsychological evaluation could assist the school psychologist in identifying areas of deficit that may require intervention and/or accommodation.

As may be expected given high rates of hyperactivity and impulsivity, SDB has been associated with a range of externalizing behaviors including conduct problems, bullying, aggression, and oppositional behavior (Chervin et al., 2002; Chervin, Dillon, Archbold, & Ruzicka, 2003; Rosen et al., 2004; Urschitz et al., 2003). Although chronic mood problems are not typically seen in children with SDB, emotional dysregulation and instability are common (Beebe et al., 2004). Given these factors, it is not surprising that children with SDB tend to have difficulty relating to peers (Lewin et al., 2002; Rosen et al.). The neurocognitive deficits and behavioral problems experienced by children with SDB affect their overall quality of life (QOL), with standardized QOL ratings below those of children with asthma or juvenile rheumatoid arthritis (Mitchell & Kelly, 2006).

Significant school problems are associated with SDB (Gozal, 1998), with some studies suggesting that children with SDB are at two times the risk of academic problems compared to children without SDB (Urschitz et al., 2003). Although children with SDB tend to have lower academic grades, deficits are not found on office-based testing of academic skills. This suggests that poor school performance may be related to other factors, such as behavior problems, hyperactivity, inattention, or weak executive functioning skills, rather than resulting from a skill-based deficit (Beebe, 2006). This is important for school personnel to consider, as traditional academic testing may not adequately capture the factors contributing to a child's academic and classroom performance.

Although still inconclusive, much research has explored the mechanisms responsible for the cognitive, behavioral, and emotional sequelae associated with SDB. Intermittent hypoxia has been proposed as a contributing factor, as this has been related to neurocognitive deficits in adults with OSA and in children with a variety of other disorders presenting with hypoxia. However, hypoxia is likely not the sole cause of difficulties, as children tend to have relatively mild and brief hypoxic episodes. Furthermore, as discussed earlier, children with primary snoring without hypoxia also exhibit similar cognitive and behavioral problems. Sleep disruption and fragmentation have been put forth as contributing factors as well. Certainly, parents of children with SDB consistently report that their children experience daytime sleepiness (Gottlieb et al., 2003; Urschitz et al., 2004), and children have demonstrated increased sleep propensity on objective measures, such as the Multiple Sleep Latency Test (MSLT; Carskadon et al., 1986). However, children rarely reach levels on the MSLT that would be considered pathological in adults (Gozal, Wang, & Pope, 2001). It has also been proposed that both intermittent hypoxia and sleep disruptions may interfere with the restorative processes that occur during sleep (Beebe, 2006; Blunden & Beebe, 2006).

Several brain regions have been considered to be susceptible to SDB, including subcortical gray matter, white matter, the hippocampus, and the prefrontal cortex (PFC; Beebe, 2006; Halbower et al., 2006). The PFC is of particular interest, given its role in attention and executive functioning skills. Furthermore, the PFC is one of the only brain regions that appears to "functionally disconnect from other brain regions during sleep, allowing it to recalibrate" (Kennedy et al., 2004, p. 336), suggesting it may be particularly vulnerable to disruptions during sleep. Finally, compared to other brain regions, the PFC continues to develop through childhood and adolescence, which may make it more prone to adverse effects (Beebe & Gozal, 2002).

## COMORBID DISORDERS AND DIAGNOSTIC CONSIDERATIONS

As discussed earlier, higher rates of inattention, hyperactivity, and conduct problems are reported among children with SDB. Although rates of internalizing disorders are not elevated, problems with emotional regulation are apparent. However, the percentage of children with SDB who meet *Diagnostic and Statistical Manual of Mental Disorders—Fourth Edition* (*DSM-IV*; American Psychiatric Association, 1994) criteria for many behavioral or emotional disorders has not been clearly established.

Not surprisingly, the rate of ADHD in children with SDB has been reported to be higher than the general population, with one study reporting that 28% of their sample met *DSM-IV* criteria (Chervin et al., 2006). Despite the considerable overlap in symptoms of ADHD and SDB, the *DSM-IV* does not include SDB or OSA as a possible differential diagnosis (Hansen & Vandenberg, 1997). SDB is an important consideration when evaluating a child with ADHD-like symptoms, as a portion of children diagnosed with ADHD also have SDB. Among children with severe ADHD, the prevalence of OSA has been reported at 5%. That rate rises to 26% among children with mild ADHD (O'Brien et al., 2003). Misdiagnosis of SDB symptoms as ADHD can result in inappropriate treatment, as children may be unnecessarily treated with medications for ADHD (Huang et al., 2007). It has been recommended that screening of a child's sleep be completed in cases of ADHD or other behavioral and emotional disorders that are not responding as expected to standard treatment interventions (Hansen & Vandenberg). Appropriate intervention is especially important for SDB, as some symptoms seem to improve following treatment. Therefore, delaying treatment can have significant negative implications for a child's future development.

As concerns regarding attention and behavioral regulation are typically first noticed when a child enters school, school psychologists are in the unique position of having early opportunities to help identify symptoms associated with SDB. Although we are certainly not implying that psychologists should diagnose sleep disorders, obtaining information about sleep can help a psychologist determine whether a referral to a pediatrician or sleep specialist for more comprehensive evaluation should be made. Questions regarding the presence and frequency of snoring, gasping during sleep, or "heavy" breathing can be integrated into a typical interview with parents (from the Pediatric Sleep Questionnaire in Chervin, Ruzicka, Archbold, & Dillon, 2005). Reviews of the literature indicate that chronic snoring may be one of the best predictors of cognitive and behavioral problems (Beebe, 2006). Therefore, parental report of significant snoring can be considered a "red flag" that requires further evaluation by a physician.

Standardized questionnaires, such as the CSQ (Huntley et al., 2007; see Figure 17.1), can also be helpful. The CSQ was developed by Daniel Lewin, PhD, DABSM, at Children's National Medical Center in Washington, D.C. It is a 41-item questionnaire that can be given to a caretaker to complete; it screens for common pediatric sleep disorders in children from the ages of 2 through 18. Caretakers are asked to respond to questions assessing sleep habits (e.g., usual bedtime, sleep onset latency, number of awakenings and time awake after sleep onset), general questions regarding symptoms of sleep disorders (e.g., bedtime resistance, snoring, sleepwalking, etc.), and an 8-item modified Epworth Sleepiness Scale (Johns, 1991). Although more comprehensive than available established pediatric sleep questionnaires such as the Pediatric Sleep Questionnaire (Chervin, Hedger, Dillon, & Pituch, 2000) or the Children's Sleep Habits Questionnaire (Owens, Spirito, & McGuinn, 2000), the CSQ has not yet been normed.

## TREATMENT AND LONG-TERM EFFECTS

Many of the cognitive and behavioral problems associated with SDB appear to diminish following adenotonsillectomy. Following surgery, children demonstrate improvements in cognition, including attention (Ali, Pitson, & Stradling, 1996; Avior et al., 2004; Montgomery-Downs et al., 2005), memory (Chervin et al., 2006; Friedman et al., 2003), and executive functions (Beebe, 2006; Friedman et al.). Postsurgical improvements in grades have been reported as long as 1 year after treatment (Gozal, 1998). Behavioral improvements after surgery are also seen, with fewer reports of aggression, inattention, and hyperactivity (Beebe, 2006; Chervin, Dillon, et al., 2003; Chervin et al., 2006). Similar positive effects have been seen in quality of life (Constantin et al., 2007; Tran, Nguyen, Weedon, & Goldstein, 2005).

In children diagnosed with comorbid SDB and ADHD, adenotonsillectomy has been found to be more effective in reducing symptoms of inattention and hyperactivity than treatment with methylphenidate (Huang et al., 2007). Furthermore, in one study, 50% of children with SDB diagnosed with ADHD no longer met criteria for ADHD after surgery (Chervin et al., 2006). This again emphasizes the importance of appropriate diagnosis, and resulting intervention, when considering ADHD symptoms.

Few studies have investigated the longer-term risk associated with both treated and untreated SBD. Snoring at a young age appears to be predictive of hyperactivity and poor school performance in elementary and middle school (Chervin et al., 2005; Gozal & Pope, 2001). This is even seen in children whose snoring had spontaneously resolved (Beebe, 2006) or in children who underwent adenotonsillectomy (Gozal & Pope). These findings are important to consider, as they not only highlight chronic snoring as an important risk factor for later problems but also suggest that residual deficits may still be apparent up to 10 years after snoring resolves. As such, some children may require ongoing school-based interventions even after medical treatment has been completed.

## CASE CONTINUATION

Given the possibility of SDB potentially causing or exacerbating Kelly's symptoms of ADHD, she was referred to the sleep clinic at a local children's hospital; there she was evaluated by a multidisciplinary team of sleep specialists, including ear, nose and throat physicians, pulmonologists, psychologists, and psychiatrists. The evaluation determined that Kelly had enlarged adenoids and tonsils. An overnight PSG in a sleep laboratory was performed to determine whether there was any evidence of sleep-disordered breathing. In addition to diagnosis, information gained through PSG, such as oxygen levels and heart rate, aids in predicting whether children may be at risk for complications during surgery (Brown et al., 2003). On the PSG, it was noted that Kelly's oxygen saturations often fell below 75%, suggesting that her sleep apnea was severe enough to pose a significant risk for postoperative complications and that she would need close observation.

With the diagnosis of OSA, it was recommended that Kelly undergo adenotonsillectomy. The surgery was successful, and immediate benefits were noted in terms of a significant reduction in Kelly's snoring, improved continuity of sleep, and the disappearance of symptoms of daytime sleepiness (e.g., difficulties with morning arousal). In addition, over the course of several months, Kelly's parents and teachers observed improvements in her sustained attention, her activity level, and the stability of her mood. She seemed more engaged both academically and socially. Nonetheless, Kelly's ADHD symptoms and associated executive dysfunction continued to have an adverse impact on her learning. As such, it was felt that she would benefit from individualized special education supports and accommodations. Specifically, a well-organized educational program that would provide direct, positive reinforcement for task completion and appropriate behavior was recommended. An individualized education plan (IEP) was created for Kelly under the Other Health Impairment (OHI) category.

## INTERVENTIONS

### General Considerations

Appropriate diagnosis is the first important step in intervention. Given the reported positive effects of surgical treatment in SDB, determining whether ADHD-like symptoms are related to SDB can be critical.

However, as discussed earlier and as illustrated in the case example of Kelly, children can continue to demonstrate problems even after treatment and may require ongoing school-based interventions. Nevertheless, many children improve so much symptomatically that they can be treated with significantly less stimulant medication or come off medical therapy entirely (Chervin et al., 2006).

In a review of the literature, no studies regarding behavioral or cognitive interventions specific to children with SDB were identified. As such, interventions will need to target the cognitive and behavioral profile of the individual child, and interventions that have proven effective for inattention, behavioral dysregulation, and executive functioning deficits in other populations will likely be appropriate for children with SDB.

Throughout the school years, close communication between school personnel and parents is essential to identify areas of need, determine success of interventions, and monitor overall progress. It will be especially important for parents and teachers to discuss any treatment implementation, such as medication or surgery, with school personnel, so that changes in functioning can be monitored. Children with SDB may need frequent review and modification of IEP or Section 504 plans should symptoms change over time.

## Interventions for Preschool-Age Children

As noted earlier, younger children may be at increased risk for cognitive difficulties. As differences seem to be seen in overall cognitive ability among younger children, appropriate academic stimulation, in the form of structured preschool, may be worthwhile. Participation in preschool will allow teachers to monitor a child's progress and refer for psychological assessment, should concerns arise.

In children with ADHD, behavioral dysregulation is a common complaint and is typically the greatest area of need for intervention; the same may be expected for young children with SDB. Classroom strategies that target poor inhibitory control involve (a) identifying antecedents to disruptive behavior and (b) implementing reinforcement systems. In the use of reinforcement systems, it is important to provide immediate feedback about behavior, as well as to change reinforcers frequently. Children may do better in highly structured classrooms with clear rules and expectations and may benefit from visual presentation of rules (Mahone & Slomine, 2007). Preschool children with inhibitory control difficulties may also benefit from frequent breaks, particularly those that involve motor activity, such as handing out pencils to classmates or bringing work to the teacher for review. Such breaks need only be of short duration (1–2 minutes) and can serve as a reward for work completed.

## Interventions for School-Age Children

Once children enter elementary school, the cognitive and/or behavioral effects of SDB may interfere with academic development and may warrant an IEP or Section 504 plan. Similar to children with ADHD, school-age children with SDB would likely benefit from accommodations within the classroom to address symptoms of inattention and behavioral dysregulation. Children with inhibitory control difficulties will continue to need a high level of structure at the outset to promote more appropriately controlled behavior, and the use of a reinforcement system can help promote compliance with rules. Varying the instructional medium and pace will help keep a child engaged and available for learning, and balancing time between tasks that require sustained attention and those that are more active and hands-on in nature is likely to be beneficial. Developmentally, children may be ready to learn simple strategies to promote behavioral control, such as counting to 10 before responding verbally or physically. Teachers can promote better inhibitory control by asking students to verbalize their approach to the task, including articulating goals related to accuracy and time. This may be particularly helpful for children who tend to rush through their work and can assist the child in developing a more organized and strategic approach (Isquith & Gioia, 2002).

Given parent- and teacher-reported deficits in executive functions, interventions for these problems will become more important as the child with SDB progresses through elementary school, with increasing demands for sitting in one's seat, attending to teacher lectures, and completing work independently. Interventions in elementary school should focus on teaching rudimentary strategies of planning and organization that can continue and be elaborated on in middle and high school. It is helpful to teach children how to identify the goal of an assignment and break it down into manageable steps. The process of planning one's approach to tasks should be discussed at all opportunities, both at school and at home. Children also can be taught active listening strategies that compensate for working memory difficulties, such as asking questions and restating or paraphrasing information (Gioia & Isquith, 2001; Mahone & Slomine, 2007).

## Interventions for Adolescents

Behavioral dysregulation can continue into adolescence and can manifest in behavioral problems related to "acting before thinking," or academic difficulties related to rushing through and not checking work. In school, it will be important to reinforce careful completion of work, with strategies taught for proofreading and checking mistakes. Behavior contracts may continue to be helpful in managing inappropriate behavior; however, it is also important to start teaching strategies to help the adolescent "stop and think" before acting. Psychologists can be helpful in this regard.

Executive strategies that started in elementary school can be built on during the high school years. Teenage students would benefit from learning to develop timelines for completing larger projects, and the resource *Executive Skills in Children and Adolescents* (Dawson & Guare, 2004) contains many helpful worksheets that can be used to plan homework and study time. Given the busy schedule of many of today's high school students, a written log of activities, including study time, assignments, due dates, and extracurricular activities, can be essential. As adolescents may have difficulty monitoring their own success at using such systems, it may be helpful for an adult, either a parent or a teacher, to assist the teen in determining the effectiveness of the system and, if problems are identified, brainstorming potential alternatives (Mahone & Slomine, 2007). Coaching can be a useful strategy, especially for adolescents. Coaches help to identify specific goals and work with students to develop ways to help them achieve those goals. The coach also monitors progress and provides rewards for goal attainment. Given the collaborative nature of the relationship, coaching is most successful with children who are willing participants (Palumbo & Diehl, 2007).

Depending on the severity of symptoms and their effect on school functioning, children with SDB may continue to qualify for services in college or other post–high school academic settings. It may be helpful for school psychologists to continue to document problems in school to assist in qualification for services. School counselors can assist students in choosing colleges or programs that may best fit their learning needs.

## Social Skills Training

As discussed earlier in the chapter, children with SDB tend to have poor peer relationships. Although not specifically elucidated within the literature, based on findings for children with ADHD, it may be surmised that these problems result from (a) behavioral impulsivity resulting in inappropriate behaviors in the social setting and/or (b) poor executive functioning skills interfering with social problem solving. Social skills training programs focus on ways to improve peer interactions through teaching and modeling techniques to help resolve conflicts and decrease aggression. Although the authors are unaware of any social skills training groups that have been run specifically for children with SDB, if the child has ADHD-like symptoms, he or she may benefit from a social skills group for children with ADHD (Palumbo & Diehl, 2007).

## CONCLUSION

Children with SDB are at risk for academic difficulties, as well as social and behavioral problems, which can continue even after treatment. Considerable overlap exists between symptoms of SDB and other disorders, specifically ADHD, and these neurobehavioral problems may interfere with a child's academic development. School psychologists are in the important position of being able to identify early symptoms that may be related to SDB, resulting in appropriate treatment and potentially limiting long-term consequences.

## RESOURCES

### Books

Ferber, R. (2006). *Solve your child's sleep problems: New, revised, and expanded edition.* New York: Fireside.

This is the updated and expanded version of the book often considered a classic text on pediatric sleep disorders (focusing on infants, toddlers, and preschoolers), including information regarding bedtime routines, night terrors, sleepwalking, and SDB. It includes an extensive bibliography of children's books on bedtime, sleep, and dreaming.

Mindell, J. A., & Owens, J. A. (2003). *A clinical guide to pediatric sleep.* Philadelphia: Lippincott, Williams, & Wilkins.

Intended for primary care practitioners but useful for all clinicians, this is a practical guide for information regarding common pediatric sleep disorders and their treatment. Includes symptom checklists for specific disorders, as well as chapters on sleep and medication and on sleep problems in special populations.

Owens, J., & Mindell, J. (2005). *Take charge of your child's sleep: The all-in-one resource for solving sleep problems in kids and teens.* New York: Marlowe & Company.

This book offers practical advice for parents on improving sleep in school-age children, including information on the relationship between SDB and attention/behavior disorders.

### Organizations and Web Sites

American Academy of Pediatrics (AAP)

The AAP Web site is a good source of information for a broad range of children and adolescent health issues.

Web Site: www.aap.org

American Sleep Apnea Association

This Web site provides information regarding how to have your child evaluated for sleep apnea, as well as more general information about sleep apnea.

Web Site: www.sleepapnea.org/resources/pubs/child.html

*Revised 06/2006*

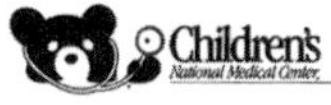

**Child Sleep Questionnaire (ages 2-18)**

Child's Name: ________________________Today's date: ____/____/____

Child's gender: □ male □ female Child's age:____ Child's date of birth: ____/____/____

Your Name: ______________________ Your gender: □ male □ female

Your relationship to the child: □ biological parent □ step parent □ grandparent □ adoptive parent □ foster parent □ other (specify): ______________________

**1.** Has your child ever been diagnosed with a sleep disorder? □ No □ Yes (if yes please specify): □ narcolepsy □ obstructive sleep apnea □ restless leg syndrome Other:______________

**2.** Does your child have any medical problems □ No □ Yes. If yes, please specify:__________

**2a.** Does your child take any medications □ No □ Yes. If yes, please specify:__________

**2b.** Does your child have symptoms of reflux (heart burn, frequent spit-ups after meals) □ No □ Yes

**For questions think about your child's sleep during the last 3 months:**

**Weekday Schedule**

**3.** What time does your child **go to bed on weeknights** (school nights)? ________ pm/am

**4.** What time does your child **wake up on weekdays** (school mornings)? ________ pm/am

**5.** On average, how many hours does your child sleep on **weeknights** (school nights)? _____ hours

**6.** On how many **weekdays** (school mornings) does your child: **Please circle one number**

| | |
|---|---|
| a. Wake up on her/his own? | 0 1 2 3 4 5 |
| b. Use an alarm to wake up? | 0 1 2 3 4 5 |
| c. Is awakened by a parent, sibling or other caretaker? | 0 1 2 3 4 5 |
| d. Need to be awakened several times before getting out of bed? | 0 1 2 3 4 5 |

**7.** On **weekdays** (school days), how much does your child's bedtime and wake up time change from day to day? Please check **one**: □ Less than 15min. □ 15 to 30min. □ 30 to 60min. □ More than 60min.

**Weekend/Vacation Schedule**

**8.** What time does your child **go to bed on weekends**? ________ pm/am

**9.** What time does your child **wake up on weekends**? ________ pm/am

**10.** On average, how many hours does your child sleep on **weekends**? _____ hours

**11.** If your child sets her/his own schedule, which would s/he prefer (think about sleep habits during summers and weekends) Please check **one**: □ Go to bed early and wake up early □ Go to bed late and wake up late □ No preference

**12.** Has your child ever taken over-the-counter or prescription medications at bed time to help her/him calm down and/or fall asleep? □ No □ Yes

**12a.** If yes, please list the medications and dose: ______________________

**13.** Which of the following items does your child have in her/his bedroom? Please check **all** that apply:□ TV □ DVD/VCR □ Computer □ Internet access □ Video game system □ telephone/cell phone

**Instructions:** Below is a list of questions about various sleep problems. For each question please think about the **last three weeks** and answer all items even if some do not apply to your child.

| | Never | Not during the past month | Less than once a week | Once or twice a week | 3 or 4 times a Week | 5 or more times a week |
|---|---|---|---|---|---|---|
| **14.** Does your child drink caffeinated beverages (for example: colas, Mountain Dew, energy drinks, Sunkist, iced tea, chocolate milk) or eat foods that contain caffeine (for example, chocolate)? | ☐ | ☐ | ☐ | ☐ | ☐ | ☐ |
| **15.** Does your child have difficulty waking up in the morning on **weekdays/school days**? | ☐ | ☐ | ☐ | ☐ | ☐ | ☐ |
| **16.** Does your child nap? | ☐ | ☐ | ☐ | ☐ | ☐ | ☐ |
| **16a.** If so, how long is a typical nap? ________hrs. ________ min. | | | | | | |
| **17.** Does your child resist going to bed? | ☐ | ☐ | ☐ | ☐ | ☐ | ☐ |
| **18.** Is there a regular bedtime routine in your home? | ☐ | ☐ | ☐ | ☐ | ☐ | ☐ |
| **19.** After bedtime, does your child call you back to the bedroom more than 2 times? | ☐ | ☐ | ☐ | ☐ | ☐ | ☐ |
| **20.** Is bedtime and the hour leading up to it a stressful time for your child? | ☐ | ☐ | ☐ | ☐ | ☐ | ☐ |
| **21.** Does your child have difficulty falling asleep at night? | ☐ | ☐ | ☐ | ☐ | ☐ | ☐ |
| **21a.** How much time does it **usually** take her/him to fall asleep after going to bed? __________ hrs. __________ min. | | | | | | |
| **21b.** What is the **longest** time it has taken your child to fall asleep after being put to bed? _________ hrs. _________ min. | | | | | | |
| **22.** Does your child wake up in the middle of the night and take 10 or more minutes to fall back to sleep? | ☐ | ☐ | ☐ | ☐ | ☐ | ☐ |
| **22a.** How much time does it **usually** take her/him to fall back to sleep after waking in the night? _______ hrs. _______ min. | | | | | | |
| **22b.** What is the **longest** time it has taken your child to fall back to sleep after waking in the night? _____ hrs. ____ min. | | | | | | |
| **23.** Does your child grind her/his teeth while sleeping? | ☐ | ☐ | ☐ | ☐ | ☐ | ☐ |

**2**

| | Never | Not during the past month | Less than once a week | Once or twice a week | 3 or 4 times a Week | 5 or more times a week |
|---|---|---|---|---|---|---|
| **24.** Does your child sleep in a caretaker's bed? | □ | □ | □ | □ | □ | □ |
| **25.** Does your child share a bedroom with another family member? | □ | □ | □ | □ | □ | □ |
| **26.** Does your child have difficulty waking up in the morning on **weekends**? | □ | □ | □ | □ | □ | □ |
| **27.** Does your child wake up screaming, agitated or confused? | □ | □ | □ | □ | □ | □ |
| **27a.** If yes, does s/he calm down after being comforted? Please check **one**: □ No □ Yes Please provide any additional details: ______________________ | | | | | | |
| **27b.** If yes, does s/he remember waking up the next morning? Please check **one**: □ No □ Yes | | | | | | |
| **28.** Does your child sleep walk? | □ | □ | □ | □ | □ | □ |
| **28a.** If yes, while sleepwalking has your child ever: Please check **all** that apply: □ been at risk of injury □ been injured □ attempted to leave the bedroom □ attempted to leave the home | | | | | | |
| **29.** Does your child have repetitive movements during sleep? Please check **all** that apply: □ leg jerks □ head banging □ lip smacking □ other (please specify):__________________ | | | | | | |
| **29a.** If your child has repetitive movements, how often do they occur during sleep? | □ | □ | □ | □ | □ | □ |
| **30.** Does your child report having nightmares or frightening dreams? | □ | □ | □ | □ | □ | □ |
| **31.** Does your child report that s/he could not move when s/he tried to get up in the morning? | □ | □ | □ | □ | □ | □ |
| **32.** Does your child fall asleep suddenly at unexpected times? | □ | □ | □ | □ | □ | □ |
| **33.** Does your child report having very real dreams like there is a person or animal in her/his room? | □ | □ | □ | □ | □ | □ |
| **34.** Does your child have uncomfortable feelings in the legs or arms (occurring at bed time or when sitting for a long period of time) that are relieved by movement or rubbing? | □ | □ | □ | □ | □ | □ |
| **35.** Does your child snore? | □ | □ | □ | □ | □ | □ |
| **35a.** Snoring can be heard from: Check **one**: □ only in her/his bedroom □ one room away □ two or more rooms away on the same floor □ throughout the entire house | | | | | | |

| | Never | Not during the past month | Less than once a week | Once or twice a week | 3 or 4 times a Week | 5 or more times a week |
|---|---|---|---|---|---|---|
| **36.** While your child is sleeping, does your child: Please check **all** that apply: □ struggle to breath □ gasp □ hold her/his breath □ stop breathing for short periods of time | | | | | | |
| **36a.** If yes, how often do these breathing problems occur? | □ | □ | □ | □ | □ | □ |
| **37.** How often is your child a restless sleeper? | □ | □ | □ | □ | □ | □ |
| **38.** How often does your child wet her/his bed at night? | □ | □ | □ | □ | □ | □ |
| **38a.** If your child wets the bed has he/she ever been completely dry for more than one week? □ No □ Yes | | | | | | |
| **39.** How often do you observe your child while s/he sleeps? | □ | □ | □ | □ | □ | □ |

**40.** Please read each situation below carefully. After reading each situation, please rate your child's chances of dozing on a typical day.

Please check only **one** box in each row

| **Situation** | **Would never doze** | **Slight chance of dozing** | **Moderate chance of dozing** | **High chance of dozing** |
|---|---|---|---|---|
| **a.** In school (while in a classroom) | □ | □ | □ | □ |
| **b.** Watching TV | □ | □ | □ | □ |
| **c.** Sitting quietly in public (in church, at a movie or lecture) | □ | □ | □ | □ |
| **d.** Riding in a car or on a bus | □ | □ | □ | □ |
| **e.** Lying down to rest in the afternoon | □ | □ | □ | □ |
| **f.** While sitting and talking to someone | □ | □ | □ | □ |
| **g.** While playing alone quietly or reading | □ | □ | □ | □ |
| **h.** While playing with friends | □ | □ | □ | □ |

**41.** How concerned are you about your child's sleep? Please place an X between the asterisks.

*______________________________________________________________*

Not concerned at all                                                                 Extremely concerned

**4**

**Child Sleep Questionnaire (CSQ)**

**Description**

Sleep variables, were derived from a 41-item pediatric sleep questionnaire that is used as a clinical screen for common sleep problems in children ages 2 - 18. Caretakers respond to questions that assess sleep habits (usual bedtime, sleep onset latency, number of awakenings and time awake after sleep onset), general questions regarding symptoms of sleep disorders (bedtime resistance, snoring, sleep walking, etc.) and an 8-item modified Epworth Sleepiness Scale (ESS) (scores range from 0 – 24) that assesses daytime sleep propensity. When answering questions caretakers are asked to report on the frequency of relevant events associated with of sleep habits, sleep schedules and the presence of common sleep disorder symptoms occurring in the past month using a 5-point Likert-type scale (anchors for scale include; 1 = never, 2 = less than once a week, 3 = 1 or two times a week, 4 = 3 or 4 times a week, and 5 = 5 or more times a week). While participants are not formally diagnosed with sleep disorders, clinically significant criteria were used to characterize the following sleep problems: behavioral sleep disorders (BSD), insomnia, excessive daytime somnolence (EDS), sleep disordered breathing (SDB), insufficient sleep, parasomnias, nightmares, and enuresis (see scoring algorithm below).

**Scoring Algorithm**

The CSQ categorizes several categories of common childhood sleep problems using the criteria below:

1.) Behavioral Sleep Disorders (BSD)
- Bedtime resistance with a frequency ≥ 3-4x a week
- Call back during the night with a frequency ≥ 3-4x a week

2.) Enuresis
- Bed wetting with a frequency ≥ 1-2x a week for children ≥ 4 years of age

3.) Excessive Daytime Somnolence (EDS)
- ESS score > 10*
- Nap frequency with a frequency ≥ 3-4x a week for children ≥ 7 years of age
- Difficulty waking up in the morning ≥ 3-4x a week for children ≤ 11 years of age

4.) Insomnia
- Difficulty initiating sleep with a frequency ≥ 3-4x a week
- SOL ≥ 30 minutes
- Sleep maintenance problems with a frequency ≥ 3-4x a week
- WASO ≥ 20 minutes

5.) Insufficient Sleep
- Total estimated sleep time < 7 hours for children ≥ 12 years of age **or** < 8 hours for children ≤ 11 years of age.

6.) Nightmares
- Nightmares with a frequency ≥ 3-4x a week

7.) Parasomnias
- Night terrors with a frequency ≥ 1-2x a week
- Sleep walking with a frequency ≥ 1-2x a week

8.) Sleep Disordered Breathing (SDB)
- Snoring with a frequency ≥ 3-4x a week **and** snoring is heard outside of the bedroom
- Snoring with a frequency ≥ 3-4x a week **and** any of the following behaviors observed by care taker: child struggles to breath, holds her breath, stops breathing or gasps for breath

*Note: earlier versions of the CSQ may have used a 7-item ESS so scores would range from 0-21 and an ESS > 8 would be clinically significant.

**Questions concerning the use of the CSQ may be referred to:**

**Daniel S. Lewin, Ph.D., D.ABSM**
**Children's National Medical Center**
**111 Michigan Avenue, N.W.**
**Washington, DC 20010-2970**
**Email: dlewin@cnmc.org**

FIGURE 17.1 Child Sleep Questionnaire.

National Heart, Lung and Blood Institute (NHLBI) Star Sleeper Web Site

This is a Web site designed to promote healthy sleep habits through online games for children and information for parents, teachers and pediatricians. It includes lesson plans and activities that can be incorporated by teachers into their curricula (e.g., keeping a sleep diary).

Web Site: www.nhlbi.nih.gov/health/public/sleep/starslp/index.htm

National Sleep Foundation

The NSF provides extensive information for parents and professionals about sleep through the life span, from infancy to adulthood, including a searchable topic-based database and tips on healthy sleep habits.

Web Site: www.sleepfoundation.org

Sleep Net

This is an online sleep resource with numerous links.

Web Site: www.sleepnet.com

Talk About Sleep

This is an online resource with a wealth of information about sleep and sleep disorders from infancy through adulthood.

Web Site: www.talkaboutsleep.com

## REFERENCES


Achenbach, T. M. (2001a). *Child Behavior Checklist for Ages 6–18*. Burlington: University of Vermont Department of Psychiatry.

Achenbach, T. M. (2001b). *Teacher's Report Form for Ages 6–18*. Burlington: University of Vermont Department of Psychiatry.

Ali, N. J., Pitson, D. J., & Stradling, J. R. (1993). Snoring, sleep disturbance, and behaviour in 4–5 year olds. *Archives of Diseases of Childhood, 68,* 360–366.

Ali, N. J., Pitson, D. J., & Stradling, J. R. (1996). Sleep disordered breathing: Effects of adenotonsillectomy on behaviour and psychological functioning. *European Journal of Pediatrics, 155,* 56–62.

American Academy of Pediatrics, Section on Pediatric Pulmonology, Subcommittee on Obstructive Sleep Apnea Syndrome. (2002). Clinical practice guidelines: Diagnosis and management of childhood obstructive sleep apnea. *Pediatrics, 109,* 704–712.

American Psychiatric Association. (1994). *Diagnostic and statistical manual of mental disorders* (4th ed.). Washington, DC: Author.

American Thoracic Society. (1996). Standards and indications for cardiopulmonary sleep studies in children. *American Journal of Respiratory and Critical Care Medicine, 153,* 866–878.

Archbold, K. H., Giordani, B., Ruzicka, D. L., & Chervin, R. D. (2004). Cognitive executive dysfunction in children with mild sleep-disordered breathing. *Biological Research for Nursing, 5,* 168–176.

Arens, R., & Marcus, C. L. (2004). Pathophysiology of upper airway obstruction: A developmental perspective. *Sleep, 27,* 997–1019.

Avior, G., Fishman, G., Leor, A., Sivan, Y., Kaysar, N., & Derowe, A. (2004). The effect of tonsillectomy and adenoidectomy on inattention and impulsivity as measured by the Test of Variables of Attention (TOVA) in children with obstructive sleep apnea syndrome. *Otolaryngology, Head, and Neck Surgery, 131,* 367–371.

Bao, G., & Guilleminault, C. (2004). Upper airway resistance syndrome: One decade later. *Current Opinions in Pulmonary Medicine, 10,* 461–467.

Barkley, R. A. (1997). Behavioral inhibition, sustained attention, and executive functions: Constructing a unifying theory of ADHD. *Psychological Bulletin, 121,* 65–94.

Beebe, D. W. (2005). Neurobehavioral effects of obstructive sleep apnea: An overview and heuristic model. *Current Opinions in Pulmonary Medicine, 11,* 494–500.

Beebe, D. W. (2006). Neurobehavioral morbidity associated with disordered breathing during sleep in children: A comprehensive review. *Sleep, 29,* 1115–1134.

Beebe, D. W., & Gozal, D. (2002). Obstructive sleep apnea and the prefrontal cortex: Towards a comprehensive model linking nocturnal upper airway obstruction to daytime cognitive and behavioral deficits. *Journal of Sleep Research, 11,* 1–16.

Beebe, D. W., Wells, C. T., Jeffries, J., Chini, B., Kalra, M., & Amin, R. (2004). Neuropsychological effects of pediatric obstructive sleep apnea. *Journal of the International Neuropsychological Society, 10,* 962–975.

Beery, K. E., Buktenica, N. A., & Beery, N. A. (2004). *The Beery-Buktenica Developmental Test of Visual-Motor Integration* (5th ed.). Minneapolis, MN: NCS Pearson.

Bernstein, J. H., & Waber, D. P. (1996). *Developmental scoring system for the Rey-Osterrieth Complex Figure: Professional manual.* Odessa, FL: Psychological Assessment Resources.

Blunden, S., Lushington, K., Kennedy, D., Martin, J., & Dawson, D. (2000). Behavior and neurocognitive performance in children aged 5–10 years who snore compared to controls. *Journal of Clinical and Experimental Psychology, 22,* 554–568.

Blunden, S. L., & Beebe, D. W. (2006). The contribution of intermittent hypoxemia, sleep debt, and sleep disruption to daytime performance deficits in children: Consideration of respiratory and non-respiratory sleep disorders. *Sleep Medicine Reviews, 10,* 109–118.

Brown, K. A., Morin, I., Hickey, C., Manoukian, J. J., Nixon, G. M., & Brouillette, R. T. (2003). Urgent adenotonsillectomy: An analysis of risk factors associated with postoperative respiratory morbidity. *Anesthesiology, 99,* 586–595.

Brunetti, L., Rana, M. L., Lospalluti, A., Pietrafesa, R., Francavilla, M., Fanelli, M., et al. (2001). Prevalence of obstructive sleep apnea syndrome in a cohort of 1,207 children of southern Italy. *Chest, 120,* 1930–1935.

Carskadon, M. A., Dement, W. C., Mitler, M. M., Roth, T., Westbrook, P. R., & Keenan, S. (1986). Guidelines for the Multiple Sleep Latency Test (MSLT): A standard measure of sleepiness. *Sleep, 9,* 519–524.

Chervin, R. D., Archbold, K. H., Dillon, J. E., Panahi, P., Pituch, K., Dahl, R. E., et al. (2002). Inattention, hyperactivity, and symptoms of sleep-disordered breathing. *Pediatrics, 109,* 449–456.

Chervin, R. D., Clarke, D. F., Huffman, J. L., Szymanski, E., Ruzicka, D. L., Miller, V., et al. (2003). School performance, race, and other correlates of sleep-disordered breathing in children. *Sleep Medicine, 4,* 21–27.

Chervin, R. D., Dillon, J. E., Archbold, K. H., & Ruzicka, D. L. (2003). Conduct problems and symptoms of sleep disorders in children. *Journal of the American Academy of Child and Adolescent Psychiatry, 42,* 201–208.

Chervin, R. D., Hedger, K. M., Dillon, J. E., & Pituch, K. J. (2000). Pediatric sleep questionnaire (PSQ): Validity and reliability of scales for sleep-disordered breathing, snoring, sleepiness, and behavioral problems. *Sleep Medicine, 1,* 21–32.

Chervin, R. D., Ruzicka, D. L., Archbold, K. D., & Dillon, J. E. (2005). Snoring predicts hyperactivity four years later. *Sleep, 28,* 885–890.

Chervin, R. D., Ruzicka, D. L., Giordani, B. J., Weatherly, R. A., Dillon, J. E., Hodges, E. K., et al. (2006). Sleep-disordered breathing, behavior, and cognition in children before and after adenotonsillectomy. *Pediatrics, 117,* e769–e778.

Cohen, M. J. (1997). *Children's Memory Scale.* New York: The Psychological Corporation.

Constantin, E., Kermack, A., Nixon, G. M., Tidmarsh, L., Ducharme, F. M., & Brouillette, R. T. (2007). Adenotonsillectomy improves sleep, breathing, and quality of life but not behavior. *Journal of Pediatrics, 150,* 540–546.

Corbo, G. M., Forastiere, F., Agabiti, N., Pistelli, R., Dell'Orco, V., Perucci, C. A., et al. (2001). Snoring in 9- to 15-year old children: Risk factors and clinical relevance. *Pediatrics, 108,* 1149–1154.

Culbertson, W. C., & Zilmer, E. A. (2000). *Tower of London—Drexel University.* Chicago: Multi-Health Systems.

Dawson, P., & Guare, R. (2004). *Executive skills in children and adolescents: A practical guide to assessment and intervention.* New York: Guilford Press.

Delis, D., Kramer, J. H., Kaplan, E., & Ober, B. A. (1994). *California Verbal Learning Test—Children's Version.* San Antonio, TX: The Psychological Corporation.

DuPaul, G. J., Power, T. J., Anastopoulos, A. D., & Reid, R. (1998). *ADHD Rating Scale—IV.* New York: Guilford Press.

Ferreira, A. M., Clemente, V., Gozal, D., Gomes, A., Pissarra, C., Cesar, H., et al. (2000). Snoring in Portuguese primary school children. *Pediatrics, 106,* E64.

Friedman, B. C., Hendeles-Amitai, A., Kozminsky, E., Leiberman, A., Friger, M., Tarasiuk, A., et al. (2003). Adenotonsillectomy improves neurocognitive function in children with obstructive sleep apnea syndrome. *Sleep, 26,* 999–1005.

Gioia, G. A., & Isquith, P. K. (2001). New perspectives on educating children with ADHD: Contributions of the executive functions. *Journal of Health Care Law and Policy, 5,* 124–163.

Gioia, G. A., Isquith, P. K., Guy, S. C., & Kenworthy, L. (2000). *Behavior Rating Inventory of Executive Function.* Odessa, FL: Psychological Assessment Resources.

Gottlieb, D. J., Chase, C., Vezina, R. M., Heeren, T. C., Corwin, M. J., Auerbach, S. H., et al. (2004). Sleep-disordered breathing symptoms are associated with poorer cognitive function in 5-year-old children. *Journal of Pediatrics, 145,* 458–464.

Gottlieb, D. J., Vezina, R. M., Chase, C., Lesko, S. M., Heeren, T. C., Weese-Mayer, D. E., et al. (2003). Symptoms of sleep-disordered breathing in 5-year-old children are associated with sleepiness and problem behaviors. *Pediatrics, 112,* 870–877.

Gozal, D. (1998). Sleep-disordered breathing and school performance in children. *Pediatrics, 102,* 616–620.

Gozal, D., & Pope, D. W. (2001). Snoring during early childhood and academic performance at ages thirteen and fourteen years. *Pediatrics, 107,* 1394–1399.

Gozal, D., Wang, M., & Pope, D. W. (2001). Objective sleepiness measures in pediatric obstructive sleep apnea. *Pediatrics, 108,* 693–697.

Halbower, A. C., Degaonkar, M., Barker, P. B., Earley, C. J., Marcus, C. L., Smith, P. L., et al. (2006). Childhood obstructive sleep apnea associates with neuropsychological deficits and neuronal brain injury. *PLoS Medicine, 3,* e301.

Halbower, A. C., & Mahone, E. M. (2006). Neuropsychological morbidity linked to childhood sleep-disordered breathing. *Sleep Medicine Reviews, 10,* 97–107.

Hansen, D. E., & Vandenberg, B. (1997). Neuropsychological features and differential diagnosis of sleep apnea syndrome in children. *Journal of Clinical Child Psychology, 26,* 304–310.

Huang, Y. S., Guilleminualt, C., Li, H. Y., Yang, C. M., Wu, Y. Y., & Chen, N. H. (2007). Attention-deficit/hyperactivity disorder with obstructive sleep apnea: A treatment outcome study. *Sleep Medicine, 8,* 18–30.

Huntley, E. D., Campo, J. V., Dahl, R. E., & Lewin, D. S. (2007). Sleep characteristics of youth with functional abdominal pain and a healthy comparison group. *Journal of Pediatric Psychology, 32,* 938–949..

Ievers-Landis, C. E., & Redline, S. (2007). Pediatric sleep apnea: Implications of the epidemic of childhood overweight. *American Journal of Respiratory and Critical Care Medicine, 175,* 436–441.

Ipsiroglu, O. S., Fatemi, A., Werner, I., Tiefenthaler, M., Urschitz, M. S., & Schwarz, B. (2001). Häufigkeit von Schlafstörungen bei Schulkindern zwischen 11 und 15 Jahren [Prevalence of sleep disorders in schoolchildren between 11 and 15 years of age]. *Wiener Klinische Wochenschrift, 113,* 235–244.

Isquith, P. K. & Gioia, G. A. (2002). *The Behavior Rating Inventory of Executive Function—Software program* [Scoring and interpretive software]. Lutz, FL: Psychological Assessment Resources.

Johns, M. W. (1991). A new method for measuring daytime sleepiness: The Epworth Sleepiness Scale. *Sleep, 14,* 540–545.

Kaemingk, K. L., Pasvogel, A. E., Goodwin, J. L., Mulvaney, S. A., Martinez, F., Enright, P. L., et al. (2003). Learning in children and sleep disordered breathing: Findings of the Tucson Children's Assessment of Sleep Apnea Study (TuCASA) prospective cohort. *Journal of the International Neuropsychological Society, 9,* 1016–1026.

Kennedy, J. D., Blunden, S., Hirte, C., Parsons, D. W., Martin, A. J., Crowe, E., et al. (2004). Reduced neurocognition in children who snore. *Pediatric Pulmonology, 37,* 330–337.

Korkman, M., Kirk, U., & Kemp, S. (1997). *NEPSY: A Developmental Neuropsychological Assessment.* San Antonio, TX: The Psychological Corporation.

Lewin, D. S., Rosen, R. C., England, S. J., & Dahl, R. E. (2002). Preliminary evidence of behavioral and cognitive sequelae of obstructive sleep apnea in children. *Sleep Medicine, 3,* 5–13.

Lipton, A. J., & Gozal, D. (2003). Treatment of obstructive sleep apnea in children: Do we really know how? *Sleep Medicine Review, 7,* 61–80.

Mahone, E. M., & Slomine, B. S. (2007). Managing dysexecutive disorders. In S. J. Hunter & J. Donders (Eds.), *Pediatric neuropsychological intervention* (pp. 287–313). New York: Cambridge University Press.

Manly, T., Robertson, I. H., Anderson, V., & Nimmo-Smith, I. (1999). *The Test of Everyday Attention for Children.* Bury St. Edmunds, England: Thames Valley Test Company.

Mitchell, R. B., & Kelly, J. (2006). Behavior, neurocognition, and quality-of-life in children with sleep-disordered breathing. *International Journal of Pediatric Otorhinolaryngology, 70,* 395–406.

Montgomery-Downs, H. E., Crabtree, V. M., & Gozal, D. (2005). Cognition, sleep, and respiration in at-risk children treated for obstructive sleep apnoea. *European Respiratory Journal, 25,* 336–342.

O'Brien, L. M., Holbrook, C. R., Mervis, C. B., Klaus, C. B., Bruner, C. J., Raffield, J. L., et al. (2003). Sleep and neurobehavioral characteristics of 5- to 7-year-old children with parentally reported symptoms of attention-deficit/hyperactivity disorder. *Pediatrics, 111,* 554–563.

O'Brien, L. M., Mervis, C. B., Holbrook, C. R., Bruner, J. L., Klaus, C. J., Rutherford, J., et al. (2004). Neurobehavioral implications of habitual snoring in children. *Pediatrics, 114,* 44–49.

O'Brien, L. M., Mervis, C. B., Holbrook, C. R., Bruner, J. L., Smith, N. H., McNally, N., et al. (2004). Neurobehavioral correlates of sleep-disordered breathing in children. *Journal of Sleep Research, 13,* 165–172.

Owen, G. O., Canter, R. J., & Robinson, A. (1996). Snoring, apnoea, and ENT symptoms in the paediatric community. *Clinical Otolaryngology, 21,* 130–134.

Owens, J. A., Spirito, A., & McGuinn, M. (2000). The children's sleep habits questionnaire (CSHQ): Psychometric properties of a survey instrument for school-aged children. *Sleep, 23,* 1043–1051.

Palumbo, D. R., & Diehl, J. (2007). Managing attentional disorders. In S. J. Hunter & J. Donders (Eds.), *Pediatric neuropsychological intervention* (pp. 253–286). New York: Cambridge University Press.

Redline, S., Budhiraja, R., Kapur, V., Marcus, C. L., Mateika, J. H., Mehra, R., et al. (2007). The scoring of respiratory events in sleep: Reliability and validity. *Journal of Clinical Sleep Medicine, 3,* 169–200.

Redline, S., Tishler, P. V., Schluchter, M., Aylor, J., Clark, K., & Graham, G. (1999). Risk factors for sleep-disordered breathing in children: Associations with obesity, race, and respiratory problems. *American Journal of Respiratory and Critical Care Medicine, 159,* 1527–1532.

Reuveni, H., Simon, T., Tal, A., Elhayany, A., & Trasiuk, A. (2002). Health care service utilization in children with obstructive sleep apnea syndrome. *Pediatrics, 110,* 68–72.

Rhodes, S. K., Shimoda, K. C., Waid, L. R., O'Neil, P. M., Oexmann, M. J., Collop, N. A., et al. (1995). Neurocognitive deficits in morbidly obese children with obstructive sleep apnea. *Journal of Pediatrics, 127,* 741–744.

Rosen, C. L., D'Andrea, L., & Haddad, G. G. (1992). Adult criteria for obstructive sleep apnea do not identify children with serious obstruction. *American Review of Respiratory Disease, 146,* 1231–1234.

Rosen, C. L., Storfer-Isser, A., Taylor, G. H., Kirchner, L., Emancipator, J. L., & Redline, S. (2004). Increased behavioral morbidity in school-aged children with sleep-disordered breathing. *Pediatrics, 114,* 1640–1648.

Schecter, M. S., & the Section on Pediatric Pulmonology, Subcommittee on Obstructive Sleep Apnea Syndrome. (2002). Technical report: Diagnosis and management of childhood obstructive sleep apnea syndrome. *Pediatrics, 109,* 1–20.

Sheslow, D., & Adams, W. (2003). *Wide Range Assessment of Memory and Learning* (2nd ed.). Wilmington, DE: Wide Range.

Tran, K. D., Nguyen, C. D., Weedon, J., & Goldstein, N. A. (2005). Child behavior and quality of life in pediatric obstructive sleep apnea. *Archives of Otolaryngology, Head, and Neck Surgery, 131,* 52–57.

Urschitz, M. S., Eitner, S., Guenther, A., Eggebrecht, E., Wolff, J., Urschitz-Duprat, P., et al. (2004). Habitual snoring, intermittent hypoxia, and impaired behavior in primary school children. *Pediatrics, 114,* 1041–1048.

Urschitz, M. S., Guenther, A., Eggebrecht, E., Wolff, J., Urschitz-Duprat, P. M., Schlaud, M., et al. (2003). Snoring, intermittent hypoxia, and academic performance in primary school children. *American Journal of Respiratory and Critical Care Medicine, 168,* 464–468.

Wechsler, D. (1999). *The Wechsler Abbreviated Scale of Intelligence.* San Antonio, TX: The Psychological Corporation.

Wilkinson, G. S. (1995). *Wide Range Achievement Test* (3rd ed.). Wilmington, DE: Wide Range.

# CHAPTER EIGHTEEN

# Solid Organ Transplantation

Crista E. Wetherington, PhD, and Peter J. Duquette, PhD

Pediatric organ transplantation has become a successful medical intervention for many children in recent years. Improvements in the sophistication of technology and an increased understanding of the procedure have resulted in better rates of survival following transplant. As these medical successes have become more evident, concerns about psychosocial, cognitive, and neuropsychological functioning have emerged. When a particular organ is compromised, its inability to perform its usual functions effectively may lead to cognitive dysfunction through direct or indirect pathways. Anticipation and early detection of potential problems are necessary in managing and minimizing the damage they may cause. This chapter will address disorders, medical issues, and neuropsychological research relating to transplantation of the heart, lungs, liver, and kidneys in the pediatric population. A case study of a child who received a liver transplant will also be presented. Relevant interventions and resources will be provided as well.

## HEART TRANSPLANTATION

### Description of the Disorder

Pediatric heart transplantation was not commonly used as an intervention for children with congenital heart defects and other cardiac problems until somewhat recently. Medical advances in the last 20 years have resulted in increased numbers of children receiving heart transplants, with up to 70% (Chinnock, 2006) surviving 5 years posttransplant. Consistent with other medical conditions and their treatments, decreased mortality rates are often accompanied by increases in morbidity as children cope with the effects of chronic cardiac problems and transplantation.

Primary reasons for heart transplant in the pediatric population include structural errors in heart formation, cardiac tumors, infections, and toxins (Chinnock, 2006). Specifically, cardiomyopathy (i.e., a structural or functional disease of the heart muscle, especially overdevelopment of the heart and obstructive damage to the heart), congenital heart disease, heart failure after cardiac surgery, and cardiac neoplasms (i.e., tissue growth/tumor) tend to require transplantation. These problems result in the heart's inability to pump blood effectively to maintain the health of the heart and other organs. At Texas Children's Hospital between November 1984 and October 2005, 53% of transplant patients had a diagnosis of cardiomyopathy, 39% had a congenital heart defect, and 8% were being retransplanted (Morales et al., 2007).

### *Incidence*

Approximately 2,000 heart transplants were performed in individuals of all ages in the United States in 2006 (United Network for Organ Sharing, 2007). Between 2003 and 2005, approximately 700 pediatric heart transplants occurred in the United States (Scientific Registry of Transplant Recipients, 2006). Roughly 300 to 350 children worldwide receive heart transplants each year (Chinnock, 2006), with approximately 360 transplants occurring in 2005 (Boucek et al., 2005).

When examining the age of heart transplant recipients, there are a very large number of transplants in the first year of life relative to those completed during childhood and adolescence. Another peak, although not as significant, occurs in the early teenage years (Boucek et al., 2005). A younger age at transplant has been associated with better rates of long-term survival, with many infant heart recipients alive at follow-up as teenagers (Boucek et al.).

It is generally believed that survival rates have improved tremendously since heart transplants were first begun, but with mixed findings about improvements over the last 10 to 12 years (Morales et al., 2007). Morales and colleagues found that rates of survival increased significantly in the first year posttransplant relative to pre-1995 data, but no consistent improvements in survival were found beyond the first year. Rates of early mortality have declined since the inception of heart and lung transplantation in children, with these improvements in survival rates showing diminished increase over time (Boucek et al., 2005).

*Underlying Genetic or Medical Etiology*

Reasons for pediatric heart transplantation vary by age, with infants, children, and adolescents requiring heart transplants for different reasons. In infants, the most frequent indication for heart transplant is congenital heart malformation, comprising 66% of cases, with cardiomyopathy indicated in approximately 30% of infant heart transplants (Milanesi et al., 2007). After the age of 1 year, these proportions change, with cardiomyopathy becoming a more common indication for heart transplant, whereas congenital heart defect is less common (Milanesi et al.).

Dilated cardiomyopathy (DCM), a leading indication of cardiac transplant, appears to be more common in boys than girls, in blacks than whites, and in infants under the age of 1 year. At 1 and 5 years into the follow-up of a cohort of 1,426 children with DCM in the early 1990s, 31% were deceased or had been transplanted at 1 year, and 46% were deceased or had been transplanted by 5 years (Towbin et al., 2006).

## Cognitive and Neuropsychological Functioning

With increasing rates of survival posttransplant in recent years, more attention has been placed on quality of life issues. Consistent with this shift, a focus on cognitive and neuropsychological effects related to organ failure, treatment for organ disease, and transplant is warranted. Obtaining a clear picture of the functioning of children posttransplant is complicated. Although the adult literature tends to focus on pretransplant functioning, much pediatric literature addresses the posttransplant functioning of children who received transplants as infants. Little research has examined both the pre- and posttransplant functioning of children who received heart transplants. Some authors suggest that improvements in functioning are often observed after a child suffering from end-stage organ failure receives a transplant (Qvist, Jalanko, & Holmberg, 2003).

Literature on the functioning of adult end-stage cardiac patients suggests disproportionate levels of impairment in several areas of neuropsychological functioning, such as verbal learning and memory as well as manual, psychomotor, and mental speed (Putzke et al., 1997). The potential hypoxia (i.e., a deficiency of oxygen reaching the tissues of the body; Chinnock, 2006) and cyanosis (i.e., a bluish or purplish discoloration due to deficient oxygenation of the blood; Stewart, Kennard, Waller, & Fixler, 1994) that may accompany heart defects reduce the flow of oxygen to the brain. Limited cardiac output may also cause arrhythmias that limit the flow of blood to the brain. These issues would be expected to result in the manifestation of cognitive and developmental deficits in children and adolescents experiencing heart disease and its related treatments (Todaro, Fennell, Sears, Rodrigue, & Roche, 2000).

In their review of literature on cognitive functioning after organ transplantation, Stewart and colleagues (1994) suggested that factors related to the course of disease (e.g., growth deficits, hypoxia, and circulation of cerebrotoxins) had the potential to increase children's vulnerability to cognitive deficits. Other factors contributing to susceptibility to deficits include psychosocial functioning related to the illness, disruptions to early brain development, the course of the disease, and the effects of treatment. These factors all have the potential to impact a child's ability to learn, benefit from instruction, develop new skills, and maintain existing skills. Consistent with the idea of improved mortality but higher rates of morbidity, some evidence suggests that heart transplant in infancy impacts cognitive functioning in toddlers, children, and adolescents (Babikian et al., 2003; Freier et al., 2004; Krishnamurthy, Jones, Nichols, Naramor, & Freier, 2006).

The impact of heart transplant on cognition is not completely clear, particularly when examining the effects of transplantation across different developmental stages. Findings suggest mild delays based on developmental and motor testing in the preschool years, with other age groups in the average range (Freier et al., 2004). Some research suggests below-average IQ scores in childhood when heart transplant occurs during infancy, with transplantation occurring during middle childhood (at 7- and 8-years-old) resulting in average mean IQ scores (Babikian et al., 2003). In contrast, some delays have been noted beyond early and middle childhood. Adolescents who received heart transplants as infants demonstrated low average IQ and average academic achievement, with the level of intellectual ability mediating behavioral functioning (Krishnamurthy et al., 2006).

Research on neurodevelopmental outcomes after heart surgeries in infancy and toddlerhood seems to yield similar outcomes to those obtained after heart transplant. Five-year-olds were found to have cognitive, visual-motor, and memory abilities in the average range (Forbess, Visconti, Bellinger, Howe, & Jonas, 2002; Forbess, Visconti, Bellinger, & Jonas, 2001; Forbess, Visconti, Hancock-Friesen, et al., 2002), but with Full Scale and Performance IQ scores that were significantly lower than those obtained by the normative sample (Forbess et al., 2001).

## LUNG TRANSPLANTATION

### Description of the Disorder

Pediatric lung transplantation occurs when a child receives one or two lungs from an organ donor (Children's Hospital Boston, 2007). Although most donors are deceased, some children receive lungs from living donors. Indications for transplantation include cystic fibrosis (CF; a topic covered in more detail in another chapter in this book) and end-stage pulmonary disease, as well as pulmonary hypertension (i.e., high blood pressure in the arteries that supply the lungs; American Heart Association, 2007), pulmonary vein stenosis (i.e., a condition that obstructs the flow of oxygen-rich blood from the lungs back to the heart; Children's Hospital Boston), and pulmonary fibrosis (i.e., scarring or thickening of tissues deep in the lung; Medline Plus, 2005).

Despite advances in pediatric lung transplantation in recent years, the life expectancy for children posttransplant remains limited, with the potential for multiple complications. Findings have suggested a median survival rate of just under 6 years for a cohort of pediatric lung recipients in the midwest from the late 1980s through early 2000s (Myers, de la Morene, Sweet, et al., 2005, cited in Jerkic, Aurora, & Elliot, 2007), with outcomes comparable between adults and children in the cohort.

### *Incidence*

Since the first pediatric lung transplantation in 1986 (Faro et al., 2007), over 1,300 lung and heart-lung transplants have been reported (Wells & Faro, 2006). An estimated 950 lung transplants took place between 1986 and 2004, with an additional 447 heart-lung transplants conducted during that time period (Faro et al.). The number of pediatric lung transplants remained relatively stable during the late 1990s and early 2000s (Boucek et al., 2005).

Improvements in early survival are evident, but rates of long-term survival have not demonstrated significant improvements over time. Less than 50% of recipients survive at 5 years posttransplant (Huddleston, 2006) or over the long term (Boucek et al., 2005). According to abstracts compiled by Jerkic and colleagues (2007), complications in pediatric lung transplantation include infections, kidney disease, gastroesophageal reflux, and Epstein-Barr viremia. Bronchiolitis obliterans (i.e., a pathological process producing obstruction of the bronchiles due to inflammation and fibrosis), infections, and malignancy have been associated with late mortality (Huddleston). Rates of survival are lower for children with CF and infected lungs than for children with other diagnoses (Boucek et al.). Although findings show good functional status posttransplant, about 50% of recipients require rehospitalization in the first 5 years after transplant (Boucek et al.).

### *Underlying Genetic or Medical Etiology*

Pediatric lung transplantation has unique characteristics that distinguish it from transplantation in adults. Although some similarities have been found between adult and pediatric lung transplantation, differences are evident in specific etiologies and indications, complications, pharmacokinetics, and monitoring (Wells & Faro, 2006). Due to the different indications for transplantation in recipients of different ages, generalizability of findings from the adult literature to children remains limited.

Indications for pediatric lung transplantation include end-stage or progressive lung disease and pulmonary vascular disease (Faro et al., 2007). In infants, congenital heart disease is the most common indication due to its deleterious effects on pulmonary functioning, accounting for half of lung transplant procedures (Boucek et al., 2005). Specific to infants, an indication for transplantation is an abnormality in how surfactant (e.g., a surface active agent, specifically one that prevents the lung from filling with water by capillary action) is metabolized, impacting respiration (Huddleston, 2006).

CF, followed by pulmonary vascular disease, is the most common reason for lung transplantation in children (Boucek et al., 2005) and is a much more common indication for transplantation in children than adults (Wells & Faro, 2006). Survival rates, however, are comparable between the two age groups. For children and adolescents, CF is the most common diagnosis, followed by primary pulmonary hypertension and congenital heart disease. Of all adolescents receiving lung transplants, 72% have CF (Boucek et al.).

Findings regarding the long-term outcomes after lung transplant in children have produced mixed findings. Despite a lack of differences in survival rates between adults and children, some literature indicates better outcomes for children. In one pediatric cohort, however, children required more significant medical intervention posttransplant and were more likely to experience immunosuppressive effects (Alvarez et al., 2005). Other research has suggested that lung transplantation may extend length of life for adults with CF but not for children (Liou, Adler, & Huang, 2005). Due to differences in methodology and measurement, the actual discrepancies between children and adults are unclear (Jerkic et al., 2007).

## Cognitive and Neuropsychological Functioning

Some research has examined outcomes after combined heart and lung transplantation. Research has not, however, adequately addressed specific neuropsychological outcomes after pediatric lung transplantation alone. Adults with end-stage pulmonary disease demonstrate memory impairment (Crews et al., 2003; Ruchinskas et al., 2000), elevations on the scales of the Minnesota Multiphasic Personality Inventory-2 (MMPI-2; Butcher, Graham, Williams, & Kaemmer, 1992; Crews et al.), and deficits in attentional set shifting (Ruchinskas et al.). Due to differences in etiologies between pediatric and adult populations, the generalizability of research with adult populations is limited. Factors such as amount of school missed and family psychosocial stressors resulting from lengthy hospitalization would be expected to impact academic functioning and socioemotional outcomes in children.

Evidence exists that heart or heart-lung transplantation in childhood is followed by a normal, stable course of cognitive and academic development (Wray & Radley-Smith, 2006) but with scores that are lower than those of comparison groups (Wray, Pot-Mees, Zeitlin, Radley-Smith, & Yacoub, 1994; Wray & Radley-Smith, 2005). In contrast to a lack of significant problems in cognitive development, approximately one-third of patients who had received heart or heart-lung transplantation were found to have behavior problems (Wray & Radley-Smith, 2006). Evidence suggested that congenital heart disease was associated with lower cognitive and behavioral problems than cardiomyopathy. Other research, however, suggests significant cognitive delay, increased rates of special education placement, and academic and behavioral concerns in a small group of children who received heart, lung, or heart-lung transplantation (Brosig, Hintermeyer, Zlotocha, Behrens, & Mao, 2006). Cognitive problems posttransplant were not related to specific medical factors but were significantly correlated with socioeconomic status (SES) and parental marital status. Children with cognitive problems tended to be of lower SES and have unmarried parents; academic problems were also related to SES.

Some research has examined neuropsychological outcomes posttransplant in adult lung recipients; literature has not, however, extensively addressed such outcomes in children and adolescents. Despite limited data on the impact of lung transplantation on the cognitive and neuropsychological functioning of children, other factors associated with lung transplantation would be expected to impact typical development. Psychosocial functioning, school absences, anxiety about organ rejection, and other family stressors may impact a child's ability to learn effectively and do well in school.

## LIVER TRANSPLANTATION

### Description of the Disorder

Over the past 40 years, liver transplantation has become the standard of care for treatment of a child with failing liver function (Tiao, Alonso, & Ryckman, 2006). Children with liver dysfunction are at risk for a variety of medical, neurocognitive, and academic complications due to the liver's failure to use bile effectively to eliminate toxins from the blood or to process, digest, and absorb medications, fat, and vitamins A, D, E, and K (Arya & Balistreri, 2002). Children requiring liver transplantation pose a number of logistical problems for surgeons (e.g., scarcity of age-matched donors; congenital absence of bile duct in pediatric transplant recipients). As a result, several surgical procedures, including reduced-size, living donor, and split-liver transplantations, have been developed specifically for pediatric patients. These innovations have allowed children with end-stage liver disease to survive longer into adolescence and adulthood than previously expected. Current estimates of 5-year liver graft survival rates (80%–90%) suggest continued improvements in the overall health of pediatric liver transplant recipients (Goss et al., 1998; Tiao et al., 2006). A consistent shortage of appropriate donors represents the largest contributor to patient mortality (Tiao et al.). Concerns also have been raised regarding the impact on cognitive and neurological functioning resulting from (a) prolonged hospitalization following surgery and (b) chronic immunosuppression, used to eliminate or reduce the likelihood of host rejection of a liver transplant (Adams et al., 1987; Grimm et al., 1996).

### *Incidence*

The incidence of liver disease is significantly lower in children than in adult patients, but the potential impact on health-related quality of life, family stress, and health care expenses is much greater (Arya & Balistreri, 2002). Current estimates of incidence among infants suggest that liver disease affects approximately 1 in 2,500 live births (Balistreri, 1998). Although the actual prevalence of pediatric liver disease is not known, researchers have estimated that 15,000 to 20,000 children are hospitalized for liver disease each year (Arya & Balistreri).

Based on Organ Procurement and Transplantation Network (OPTN) data as of April 2007, approximately 17,000 individuals nationwide are currently awaiting liver transplantation (OPTN, 2007). Potential pediatric liver transplant recipients ($n$ = 724) represent only a small portion of these potential recipients. Approximately three-fourths of children awaiting liver transplant are White, and approximately 60% are male (OPTN). In 2006, approximately 6,650 liver transplants were conducted nationwide, with pediatric liver transplant recipients from birth to 17 years comprising 9% ($n$ = 576) of this figure (OPTN).

### *Underlying Genetic or Medical Etiology*

The underlying causes of liver dysfunction in children are numerous. Biliary atresia represents the most common etiology of liver disease and is the leading indication for liver transplantation, accounting for nearly half of all pediatric cases (Arya & Balistreri, 2002; Goss et al., 1998). This condition involves the obstruction of the bile ducts, which prevents bile from properly passing into the intestines from the liver. Epidemiological surveys among American children suggest that biliary atresia is more common among African American than White children, in addition to being more common among girls than boys (Balistreri et al., 1996; Bates, Bucuvalas, Alonso, & Ryckman, 1998; Yoon, Bresee, Olney, James, & Khoury, 1997).

Several other disease entities specific to liver disease make up the remainder of potential underlying causes. Children with viral hepatitis, hereditary disorders (e.g., Alpha-1-antitrypsin deficiency, Wilson disease), and genetic disorders (e.g., Alagille syndrome, hemochromatosis, tyrosinemia) also represent a portion of those who require liver transplantation (Balistreri et al., 1996). Acute liver failure resulting from an adverse reaction to a virus or medication also may necessitate liver transplantation.

## Cognitive and Neuropsychological Functioning

As the number of liver transplantations that occur in school-age children continues to increase, research examining cognitive outcomes in these children generally suggests both global and specific deficits. In general, deficits in visual-spatial functioning, motor control, receptive language, and intelligence have been cited as potential neurocognitive outcomes of pediatric liver transplantation (Krull, Fuchs, Yurk, Boone, & Alonso, 2003; Stewart et al., 1991; Wayman, Cox, & Esquivel, 1997). In addition, deficits in specific aspects of memory (e.g., list learning) have been determined to be a risk in these children (Krull et al.; Stewart et al.). However, longitudinal studies of school-age children or adolescents who underwent liver transplantation during infancy or early childhood have not been conducted to date. Therefore, making long-term conclusions regarding the progression of neurocognitive status in this population can be problematic.

Researchers have been able to identify a number of pre- and post-transplant factors that may predispose children undergoing liver transplantation to cognitive impairment. Earlier onset of liver disease in children has been associated with both cognitive and motor deficits (Stewart et al., 1988). Increased levels of cerebrotoxic substances (e.g., elevated blood ammonia, elevated bilirubin levels) prior to transplantation have been correlated with deficits in overall cognitive functioning, particularly in adults (Amodio et al., 1998; Krull et al., 2003). Prolonged exposure to immunosuppressive medications (e.g., cyclosporine) or corticosteroids (e.g., prednisone) to prevent host rejection of the transplant may also have late effects on overall cognitive performance (Adams et al., 1987; Keenan et al., 1996). Furthermore, prolonged hospitalization following pediatric liver transplant has been identified as a risk factor for lower intellectual, language, academic, and visual-motor functioning in this population (Krull et al.).

## KIDNEY TRANSPLANTATION

### Description of the Disorder

Kidney transplantation has become the treatment of choice for children with kidney failure, also referred to as end-stage renal disease (ESRD). Advances in pharmacological and transplant therapies over the past three decades have decreased the morbidity and mortality rates of children and adolescents undergoing kidney transplantation. The kidneys serve the main functions of regulating body composition (e.g., volume, concentration, and acidity of fluids) and excreting metabolic end products such as urea (Briggs, Kriz, & Schnermann, 2005). Generalized dysfunction in the kidneys, often referred to as chronic kidney disease (CKD), has been defined as the progressive loss of kidney function below approximately 75% of normal as measured by the glomerular filtration rate (GFR). Dysfunction includes those individuals with mild, moderate, or severe reductions in GFR as well as those with ESRD requiring dialysis or transplantation (Schieppati, Pisoni, & Remuzzi, 2005). Over the years, surgeons have become proficient in utilizing both living donor and cadaveric transplantation procedures for children and adolescents with ESRD. According to OPTN data (2007), these advances have increased the overall kidney graft survival rates (1 year, 93%–95%; 5 years, 68%–85%) and patient survival rates (1 year, 97%–99%; 5 years, 94%–96%) for pediatric kidney transplantation patients. Despite these improvements in medical care and increased rates of patient survival, the literature continues to identify neurocognitive concerns in children who progress to ESRD with dialysis or transplant dependence (Gipson, Wetherington, Duquette, & Hooper, 2004).

#### *Incidence*

The incidence of kidney failure is much lower in children than in adults, but the long-term effects on family functioning, medical costs, and quality of life are likely larger (Gipson et al., 2004). Estimates obtained from the United States Renal Data System (USRDS, 2005) indicate that approximately 1,200 new cases of ESRD are diagnosed each year in the

United States for individuals from birth to 19 years of age. Nationwide, ESRD affects nearly 15 per one million children in the general population nationwide, based on the most recent data compilation from 2003. This number represents only a small portion of the nearly 100,000 total new cases of ESRD diagnosed each year (USRDS). The total prevalence of ESRD in the United States was estimated to be over 440,000, with individuals from birth to 19 years of age representing less than 2% ($n$ = 6684) of this figure (USRDS).

According to data obtained from OPTN (2007), over 75,000 patients nationwide are awaiting a kidney transplant. Pediatric patients comprise only 1% ($n$ = 775) of this number (OPTN). In 2006, over 17,000 kidney transplants were conducted nationwide, with pediatric kidney transplant recipients from birth to 17 years comprising only 5% ($n$ = 894) of this figure (OPTN). Approximately 42% of children awaiting a kidney transplant are White, and nearly 60% are male (OPTN). Approximately 37% of all kidney transplants were reportedly from living donors, with the remainder being from cadveric donors.

Researchers using OPTN data have examined the relative influence of various transplant factors on long-term graft survival. Gjertson and Cecka (2001) have posited that pediatric kidney transplant recipients who were in their teenage years, were of African American descent, and received transplants before 1994 were at increased risk for poorer outcomes with regards to long-term graft survival. These researchers also indicated that nearly half of all pediatric kidney transplant recipients would likely need a second graft before the age of 25 years (Gjertson & Cecka). Living donor recipients tended to fare better than cadaveric donor recipients with regards to long-term graft survival (Gjertson & Cecka).

### *Underlying Genetic or Medical Etiology*

The specific etiologies of kidney dysfunction are inherently different in children and adults. For adults, and increasingly for adolescents who are overweight or obese, diabetes and hypertension are the two most common causes of CKD and ESRD (National Kidney Foundation [NKF], 2007). For children, the three most common causes of kidney dysfunction and failure according to the NKF (2007) are (a) disruptions in the urinary tract that prevent the normal flow of urine (e.g., obstructive uropathy/dysplasia), (b) damaged filtration processes in the kidney (e.g., focal segmental glomerularsclerosis [FSGS]), and (c) genetic/acquired disorders or syndromes with renal involvement (e.g., polycystic kidney disease, hemolytic uremic syndrome).

Gipson, Duquette, Icard, and Hooper (2007) have identified a number of additional inherited disorders that affect both the central nervous system (CNS) and kidney function. Children with Galloway Mowatt syndrome or Joubert syndrome typically present with concurrent structural CNS abnormalities and congenital kidney dysfunction. Congenital kidney dysfunction with intact CNS structure is found in children with cystinosis or Lowe syndrome. In addition, children with systemic lupus erythematosus are reported to have difficulties with seizures and/or stroke following the onset of the disorder late in childhood, despite otherwise normal CNS development during infancy and early childhood (Gipson et al.).

## Cognitive and Neuropsychological Functioning

To date, there have unfortunately been no large-scale prospective studies conducted to examine the neurocognitive functions of pediatric kidney transplant recipients. In this sense, accurate predictions of the prevalence, incidence, and magnitude of developmental delays or neurocognitive deficits are problematic for this population. However, the extant literature has examined aspects of neuroimaging, electrophysiological, and neurocognitive findings in a number of cross-sectional studies with children who have previously undergone a kidney transplant.

Neuroimaging findings have supported the possible presence of cerebral atrophy, white matter lesions, and/or silent infarcts in the vast majority of pediatric kidney transplant recipients (Qvist et al., 2002; Valanne, Qvist, Jalanko, Holmberg, & Pihko, 2004). Cerebral structural abnormalities have been associated with transplantation at a later age, longer time spent on dialysis, and enrollment in special education services (Qvist et al.; Valanne et al.). These researchers also reported abnormalities on electrophysiological measures in more than one-third of patients in their sample (Qvist et al.), and previous research has suggested the possibility of delayed myelination or synaptogenesis with earlier onset of CKD pathology (Hurkx et al., 1995).

Several studies have examined the neurocognitive status of small samples of children either at posttransplant or comparing across renal replacement therapy modalities. Lawry, Brouhard, and Cunningham (1994) compared transplanted children ($n$ = 13) with dialysis-dependent children ($n$ = 11). They found a higher mean intelligence in the transplant group, although both groups fell largely within the average range. Conversely, Brouhard and colleagues (2000) found no differences in the intellectual functioning of their transplant versus dialysis-dependent groups. Mendley and Zelko (1999) have also found that attention improved following pediatric kidney transplantation in a study with a small sample size. Similarly, preliminary evidence suggests that memory, attention, motor skills, and speed of mental processing may all improve following kidney transplantation in children (Brouhard et al., 2000; Fennell, Fennell, Carter, Mings, & Klausner, 1990; Lawry et al., 1994; Qvist et al., 2002), although the frequency of residual deficits in the pediatric kidney transplant population has been documented to be greater than in the general population (Gipson et al., 2004).

## RESULTS FROM NEUROPSYCHOLOGICAL EVALUATION

The following case study summarizes neuropsychological evaluations of a 12-year-old boy before and after receiving a liver transplant.

### Background and Demographic Information

Alfonso, a 12-year-old male, was referred for neuropsychological evaluations by the hepatology department to assess his cognitive and behavioral functioning before and after liver transplant. Baseline testing was conducted 2 months prior to Alfonso's liver transplant, and posttransplant testing was conducted 6 months after his successful liver transplant. Alfonso underwent liver transplantation following liver failure secondary to hepatitis A virus. Referral questions prior to transplant focused mainly on concerns about Alfonso's functioning at school. Specifically, he was struggling to maintain attention and focus, behaving impulsively at times, exhibiting poor fine motor coordination, and performing below expectation in the areas of written language and reading. Furthermore, he reportedly began to exhibit social withdrawal, irritability, poor self-esteem, and reduced tolerance for frustration. Parent report also indicated concern that Alfonso may have developed symptoms of depression prior to transplant.

The following information was gained via interview with Alfonso's parents and grandmother and a review of available medical records. Alfonso was the product of an uncomplicated pregnancy and was born at full term weighing 7 pounds. No neonatal complications were reported, and Alfonso reached all early developmental milestones within age-appropriate time frames. Other than his liver disease, he was described as a generally healthy child. Parent report indicated that Alfonso seemed to regress in some cognitive skills prior to the liver transplant. Alfonso participated in individual psychotherapy with a pediatric psychologist to address adjustment to his liver transplant and possible mood symptoms.

Alfonso resided with his biological parents and two brothers (ages 13 and 10 years). Both of Alfonso's brothers were said to be developing typically and in several areas were functioning at a higher level than Alfonso was. As a result, his parents believed that Alfonso's self-esteem was declining, and he was becoming increasingly withdrawn. Prior to transplant, Alfonso was often irritable, made self-deprecating statements (e.g., "I'm stupid"), had poor tolerance for frustration, and preferred to be by himself. His irritability was most notable when he was tired. Alfonso's parents agreed that he appeared to be growing increasingly depressed and socially isolated. Even when other children were present to play with his siblings, Alfonso frequently went off by himself. He was not typically invited to play dates or birthday parties by classmates, did not talk to friends on the phone, and did not usually have friends over to play. Ratings of Alfonso's social-behavioral functioning revealed clinically significant concerns by both his parents in the areas of hyperactivity and aggression. One parent also rated attention problems and somatization highly; the other parent's ratings indicated that Alfonso's depression and social withdrawal were in the clinically significant range as well. On ratings of executive functioning, both parents reported difficulties with inhibition, shifting, and working memory that were clinically significant. One parent also rated Alfonso's level of emotional control in the clinically significant range.

Alfonso underwent liver transplantation in December of his sixth-grade school year at 12 years 3 months of age. He was served in all regular education courses prior to transplant. According to his parents, Alfonso struggled across all academic areas, though his performance was quite variable over time. This caused significant problems with his teachers, who interpreted poor performance as a lack of effort and motivation rather than as a true educational deficiency.

Alfonso also seemed to have some difficulty adjusting to middle school. He was increasingly required to attend lunchtime in-school detention due to oppositional behavior or failure to complete work. The tasks required during detention were largely written, which is an area of great difficulty for Alfonso. As a result, he tended not to finish the assignments, leading to more detention. According to his parents, his most recent grades were all passing, though they noted that his grades are modified compared to his classmates. With the increased difficulty at school during sixth grade, Alfonso began to exhibit avoidant behavior (e.g., saying he is ill).

Several of his teachers provided written notes in preparation for the neuropsychological evaluation. Reports consistently indicated that attentional focus was an area of weakness. Teacher reports also noted the variability in performance across days, the presence of occasional oppositional behavior, and failure to complete assignments. It also was notable that Alfonso's teachers all cited frequent absences as a contributing factor to his academic difficulties.

## Behavioral Observations

Alfonso was accompanied to both appointments by his parents. Although he lives in a bilingual household, both Alfonso and his mother stated that English was his primary language, and therefore the evaluations were conducted entirely in English. No significant differences were observed in Alfonso's behavioral presentation between the pre- and posttransplant evaluations. Overall, Alfonso presented as a socially engaging boy who appeared eager to perform well. He put forth good effort on all measures, though his behavior was variable in terms of attention span and focus. During testing, he was quite fidgety, made frequent noises, and was very restless in his chair. Alfonso responded impulsively at times but often self-corrected his impulsive errors. He displayed right-hand dominance for graphomotor (paper and pencil) tasks and had good pencil control. Due to Alfonso's good effort, the results of these evaluations are believed to provide valid estimates of his functioning at the time of each assessment.

## Test Results

Data from the tests administered to Alfonso at pre- and posttransplant testing are displayed in Table 18.1. Results from both evaluations revealed patterns of specific neurocognitive strengths and weaknesses, which is generally consistent with the patterns for many children with suboptimal filtration of toxins in the body and immunosuppression for a large organ transplant.

Results from the initial evaluation indicated that Alfonso demonstrated a significant relative weakness across language-mediated tasks, which affects receptive, expressive, and written language skills. Fine motor skills also were determined to be an area of relative weakness, along with attention span and focus. In the area of academics, weaknesses were apparent for written language and basic reading skills. Adaptive functioning was rated as well below age expectations. It was determined that he met diagnostic criteria for attention-deficit/hyperactivity disorder (ADHD).

Results from the posttransplant evaluation were quite consistent with previous findings. Academically, significant relative weaknesses continued to be evident for receptive language and written language skills. Furthermore, Alfonso demonstrated borderline skills in terms of reading comprehension and single-word spelling. It was concluded that Alfonso's

**TABLE 18.1 Neuropsychological Testing Standard Scores of Patient Before and After Liver Transplant**

| Scale | Pretransplant | Posttransplant |
|---|---|---|
| | WISC-IV | |
| Full Scale IQ | 85 | 89 |
| Verbal Comprehension index | 86 | 86 |
| Perceptual Reasoning index | 88 | 96 |
| Working Memory index | 86 | 90 |
| Processing Speed index | 81 | 80 |
| | WRAT-4 | |
| Reading Composite | 80 | 79 |
| Sentence Comprehension | 79 | 77 |
| Word Reading | 85 | 84 |
| Spelling | 77 | 73 |
| Math Computation | 89 | 87 |
| | TOWL-3 | |
| Spontaneous Writing | 75 | 71 |
| | VMI-V | |
| VMI Total score | 92 | 96 |
| | PPT | |
| Dominant (right) hand | 75 | 77 |
| Nondominant (left) hand | 80 | 78 |
| Simultaneous/both hands | 81 | 82 |
| | GDS | |
| Total Correct | 75 | 73 |
| Total Commissions | 78 | 65 |
| Total Response Latencies | 95 | 97 |
| | D-KEFS | |
| Tower: Total Achievement | 95 | 100 |
| Letter Fluency | 85 | 90 |
| Category Fluency | 90 | 90 |

**TABLE 18.1** *(Continued)*

| Scale | Pretransplant | Posttransplant |
|---|---|---|
| TOMAL | | |
| Visual Selective Reminding | 110 | 115 |
| Visual Selective Reminding (Delay) | 105 | 120 |
| Word Selective Reminding | 100 | 105 |
| Word Selective Reminding (Delay) | 110 | 115 |
| CMS | | |
| Stories Immediate Recall | 100 | 105 |
| Stories Delayed Recall | 95 | 105 |
| CELF-4 | | |
| Concepts and Directions | 75 | 65 |
| Formulated Sentences | 75 | 70 |
| ABAS-II | | |
| General Adaptive Composite | 59 | 48 |
| Social Skills | 70 | 61 |
| Conceptual Skills | 66 | 53 |
| Practical Skills | 49 | 48 |

*Note.* ABAS-II, Adaptive Behavior Assessment System—Second Edition (Harrison & Oakland, 2003); CELF-4, Clinical Evaluation of Language Fundamentals—Fourth Edition (Semel, Wigg, & Secord, 2003); CMS, Children's Memory Scale (Cohen, 1997); D-KEFS, Delis-Kaplan Executive Function System (Delis, Kaplan, & Kramer, 2001); GDS, Gordon Diagnostic System (Gordon, 1983); PPT, Purdue Pegboard Test (Tiffin, 1968); TOMAL, Test of Memory and Learning (Reynolds & Bigler, 1994); TOWL-3, Test of Written Language—Third Edition (Hammill & Larsen, 1996); VMI-V, Beery-Buktenica Developmental Test of Visual-Motor Integration (Beery, Buktenica, & Beery, 2004); WISC-IV, Wechsler Intelligence Scale for Children—Fourth Edition (Wechsler, 2003); and WRAT-4, Wide Range Achievement Test—Fourth Edition (Wilkinson & Robertson, 2006).

language-based difficulties were likely to impact his ability to function in all classes, in particular as he advances through the grades and as greater emphasis is placed on note taking in lecture-type classes. Although math skills were somewhat better developed than other academic skills, to the extent that application of mathematical concepts depends on comprehension of verbal instructions, he was determined to be at risk for experiencing difficulties in this area as well. As such, resource assistance in all areas was recommended as detailed below.

Alfonso demonstrated well-developed problem-solving skills on both verbal and nonverbal tasks. Likewise, both verbal and nonverbal memory skills appeared intact. Visual-motor integration (e.g., visual perception and paper-and-pencil control) fell consistently at age expectation, though fine motor speed emerged as an area of relative weakness. This deficit could potentially impact Alfonso's written language skills even further in the classroom environment. His mother's ratings of his adaptive skills were once again generally lower than expected based on his current estimated level of intellectual functioning, with overall adaptive functioning falling within the impaired range. Because this finding was consistent across evaluations, it suggested that behavioral or emotional factors may be interfering with his ability to participate in self-care activities to the degree that he is capable of.

Alfonso's mother rated her son as experiencing an increased number of depressive symptoms affecting self-esteem, social functioning, and likely behavioral functioning. Further, reports from current teachers consistently noted decreased attention span and poor focus. Although emotional factors also may be playing a role in Alfonso's difficulties with sustained attention, his difficulties appear pervasive enough to suggest that a medication trial should be considered to help alleviate difficulties with inattention and impulsivity.

## Case-Specific Interventions

Several recommendations specific to this particular case were provided to Alfonso and his parents, including the following:

1. In an effort to address his ADHD-like symptoms, Alfonso's parents were encouraged to consult with his pediatrician or medical team to discuss the possibility of a medication trial to improve his attention and impulsivity. Instructional and behavioral modifications also were provided to target Alfonso's regulation of his attention and disruptive behavior at home and school.
2. To address depressive symptoms reported by his mother, it was recommended that Alfonso participate in individual psychotherapy to intervene with his self-esteem, social/behavioral functioning, adaptability, and overall adjustment to his medical status and treatment. A combination of cognitive-behavioral techniques, supportive counseling, and family-focused problem solving was recommended for use with Alfonso.

3. It also was recommended that his parents advocate for special education services for their son under the Other Health Impairment (OHI) classification, as Alfonso's educational difficulties were likely related, at least in part, to his medical history. Continued placement in the regular classroom environment with resource room services across all academic areas also was recommended to help Alfonso gain essential academic skills and learn from other students. His parents were advised to request an individualized education plan (IEP) meeting at Alfonso's school to document the need for special education services. In particular, it was recommended that Alfonso participate in speech/language therapy and occupational therapy in order to address significant relative weaknesses in receptive/expressive language and fine motor skills, respectively. In addition, it was strongly recommended that a behavioral plan be put into place to address problem areas. In particular, in-school detention requiring a written language product was determined not to be the most appropriate punishment for negative behavior. Instead, completion of math computations, reading assignments with true/false quizzes, or projects were recommended for consideration. Offering Alfonso options that do not tap his greatest areas of weakness would more likely lead to his successful completion of the punishment and return to normal activities.
4. It was strongly recommended that Alfonso attend school regularly to the fullest extent possible to foster more consistent acquisition of information. Daily attendance also will allow him the opportunity to engage in social experiences, complete homework regularly, and increase his motivation to learn. In addition, regular attendance will make it less likely that he will fall behind, get frustrated, or miss essential information.
5. Given Alfonso's weakness in the area of adaptive skills, it also was strongly recommended that he be encouraged to participate in self-care activities to the best of his ability whenever possible. His parents were encouraged to support his efforts to engage in such activities, particularly as his medical care is involved, to avoid undesired consequences.

## General Recommendations

To determine the most appropriate interventions for a child, it is best to examine his or her profile of neuropsychological functioning and consider his or her individual needs. Several ideas are listed below for recommendations and interventions that may prove useful for pediatric transplant recipients in general.

Due to the potential for changes in neuropsychological functioning over the course of treatment and/or transplant, closely observing a child's functioning over time could provide useful information. Consider implementing a standard protocol of pre- and posttransplant testing to determine if any intra-individual differences are apparent after transplant. Curriculum-based assessments might be a useful tool for tracking a student's academic progress at frequent intervals.

Some evidence suggests that children may have comprised neuropsychological functioning posttransplant. Because transplants are often scheduled in advance, it is possible to prepare for these transitions. Strategies include gathering information about the child's pretransplant functioning and following him or her posttransplant, and establishing a plan prior to transplant for monitoring the student's progress. Due to the significant amount of school missed for transplantation and complications, it might be beneficial to have a plan in place as the child leaves for transplantation regarding how he/she will be followed and by whom. When medically necessary, consider homebound services to help the child maintain schoolwork while at home recovering from transplant. Reintegrate the child back into school once medically appropriate, even if only for partial days; if needed, make the transition back to school gradually. For example, after transplant, children may be reluctant to return to school because they have missed a significant amount of work, are not sure how other children will respond, and are concerned that they may become sick while at school. A gradual transition back to school may ease these concerns and make the process smoother. Such a transition might include having the child start by joining other students for lunch, then for lunch and a class, then for half days, and finally for a full school day.

Although many children may not show adverse neuropsychological effects posttransplant, research has demonstrated that children who face significant psychosocial stressors prior to transplant are at greater risk for negative outcomes posttransplant. Therefore, psychologists and mental health professionals should screen for potential psychosocial stressors and mood disorders. The presence of such difficulties could negatively impact a family's level of organization and stress, making it more difficult to follow through with schoolwork and medical compliance. Areas to screen for include psychosocial stressors and mood disorders. Psychosocial stressors include medical expenses, missed work for parents, insurance coverage, and ability to pay bills. In addition, the routines of other children in the family may be disrupted due to the patient's medical needs. Siblings may receive less attention from parents than usual. Parents often feel the pressure of trying to meet all their children's needs adequately, which may create stress in the family. In addition, after a transplant, families face rigorous, complex, and challenging medical and treatment regimens. These psychosocial stressors often make following through with necessary regimens quite challenging. Premorbid mood and anxiety disorders, or emergent adjustment disorders, may surface after transplantation. Children and their families awaiting and undergoing transplantation face worries about the procedure, the risk for possible reject or infection, and sometimes the need for retransplantation. Frequent anxious thoughts are likely to impair a child's ability to concentrate and complete schoolwork as needed. Children may benefit from therapeutic interventions by child life specialists, licensed psychologists, or special education counselors that target coping.

Children who receive transplants tend to miss significant amounts of school due to their illness, transplant, hospitalization, and follow-up doctor's visits. In considering the negative impact that extended absences have on school functioning, as well as neuropsychological deficits that may emerge due to the illness or transplant, a child may require additional supports in the school environment to have instructional needs met. Consider enrollment in Section 504 of regular education or in special education.

For children who demonstrate language difficulties, assessments and interventions that target this specific area may be helpful. Consider speech and language assessment and intervention for language problems. Give one-step directions, avoiding complex multistep instructions and unnecessary language. Similarly, some children may benefit from interventions that target motor problems. Consider occupational therapy assessment and intervention for motor deficits. Practice coordinating motor movements with visual information through completion of wooden or plastic puzzles with a picture as a guide, model airplanes, and fossil models.

For children who present with attentional weaknesses following transplant, interventions that would work for children with ADHD may be effective. In coordination with their physician, families should consider a stimulant medication trial when ADHD symptoms are present. At home, maintain one location to study and keep school books. Make use of a table or desk, and gather materials (e.g., paper, pencil) in advance. Schedule quiet time in the evening for homework. Teacher monitoring of attention in the classroom may be very beneficial. Specifically, teachers can redirect behavior quietly and positively. They should establish eye contact before giving directions. Special cues as a reminder to focus attention should be developed. Minimize visual and auditory distractions by preferential seating. Teachers or an assigned peer can check the assignment book to be sure homework has been recorded.

Behavioral and emotional issues related to health concerns may arise for children who are anticipating or who have undergone transplant. Individual psychotherapy, especially provided by a pediatric psychologist or child life specialist, is strongly recommended. Therapy should address issues related to mood, fear of needles, frustrations regarding medical setbacks, relaxation techniques, adjustment to new diagnosis, pain management, and the transition back to school. Peer support groups with children with other complicated medical needs and social skills training also may be helpful. Lastly, educating other children at school about the student's medical condition may be warranted.

In addition to interventions that may be effective in the school setting, parents may benefit from education about strategies to implement in the home environment to address areas of concern. Parents may wish to consider pursuing private services for speech and language therapy and occupational therapy to maximize the intensity of the intervention. Collaboration is very strongly encouraged between the school, family, and the medical treatment team.

## SUMMARY

Research, although still somewhat limited, has produced variable findings on the impact of organ transplantation in the pediatric population. Some evidence exists that heart transplantation in infancy may result in decreased overall cognitive scores in childhood and adolescence, which might be related to the effects of cyanotic episodes and arrhythmias prior to transplantation. Literature on renal transplant, however, suggests improved functioning posttransplant, likely related to improved functioning of the kidneys and their increased ability to filter toxins that may have been contributing to cognitive deficits prior to transplantation. Despite the different medical diagnoses and etiologies underlying pediatric organ transplantation, children undergoing organ transplantation may share several potential psychosocial problems. For example, extended absences from school, fear about medical procedures, uncertainty about the future, and concerns about the effectiveness of the transplantation may affect transplant recipients. Considering the potential problems that may emerge and proactively implementing prevention and intervention strategies may potentially minimize or ameliorate some of these negative effects. For other concerns, such as cognitive functioning, screening and assessment will be important to determine an individual child's needs.

## RESOURCES

Children's Organ Transplant Association (COTA)

COTA is an association that assists patients who need life-saving organ, bone marrow, cord blood, or stem cell transplants. This Web site describes the support COTA offers, which includes helping families who are raising funds for transplantation. Also listed are links to patient information, transplant centers, organ procurement centers, and charitable organizations.

Mailing Address: 2501 COTA Drive
Bloomington, Indiana 47403
Phone Number: (800) 366-2682
Web Site: www.cota.org

International Society for Heart and Lung Transplantation
This Web site lists links that provide information and education on heart and lung transplantation and organ donation.

Web Site: www.ishlt.org/links/organDonation.asp

National Kidney Foundation
The National Kidney Foundation Web site offers information about kidney disease, comorbid conditions, treatments, and transplantation.

Web Site: www.kidney.org

Texas Children's Hospital
This section of the Texas Children's Hospital Web site provides links to lung transplantation resource Web sites.

Web Site: www.texaschildrenshospital.org/carecenters/Lung_Transplant/Resources.aspx

United Network for Organ Sharing (UNOS)
UNOS facilitates organ sharing between transplant centers and organ procurement organizations. Their Web site describes their mission, helps promote organ donation, and provides data on the rates of transplantation and number of individuals awaiting transplant.

Web Site: www.unos.org

## REFERENCES

Adams, D. H., Ponsford, S., Gunson, B., Boon, A., Honigsberger, L., Williams, A., et al. (1987). Neurological complications following liver transplantation. *Lancet, 1,* 949–951.

Alvarez, A., Algar, F. J., Santos, F., Lama, R., Baamonde, C., Cerezo, F., et al. (2005). Pediatric lung transplantation. *Transplantation Proceedings, 37,* 1519–1522.

American Heart Association. (2007). *Pulmonary hypertension.* Retrieved April 10, 2007, from http://www.americanheart.org/presenter.jhtml?identifier=11076

Amodio, P., Marchetti, P., Del Piccolo, F., Campo, G., Rizzo, C., Iemmolo, R. M., et al. (1998). Visual attention in cirrhotic patients: A study on covert visual attention orienting. *Hepatology, 27,* 1517–1523.

Arya, G., & Balistreri, W. F. (2002). Pediatric liver disease in the United States: Epidemiology and impact. *Journal of Gastroenterology and Hepatology, 17,* 521–525.

Babikian, T., Freier, M. C., Burley Aaen, T. R., Pivonka, J., Gardner, J. M., Baum, M., et al. (2003). Long-term neuropsychological sequelae of infant cardiac transplant recipients: Trends and predictors of outcome [Abstract]. *Journal of Heart and Lung Transplantation, 22,* S144–S145.

Balistreri, W. F. (1998). Transplantation for childhood liver disease: An overview. *Liver Transplantation and Surgery, 4,* S18–S23.

Balistreri, W. F., Grand, R., Suchy, F. J., Ryckman, F. C., Perlmutter, D. H., & Sokol, R. J. (1996). Biliary atresia: Summary of a symposium. *Hepatology, 23,* 1682–1697.

Bates, M. D., Bucuvalas, J. C., Alonso, M. H., & Ryckman, F. C. (1998). Biliary atresia: Pathogenesis and treatment. *Seminars in Hepatology, 18,* 281–294.

Beery, K. E., Buktenica, N. A., & Beery, N. A. (2004). *Beery-Buktenica Developmental Test of Visual-Motor Integration* (5th ed.). Bloomington, MN: Pearson Assessments.

Boucek, M. M., Edwards, L. B., Keck, B. M., Trulock, E. P., Taylor, D. O., & Hertz, M. (2005). Registry of the International Society for Heart and Lung Transplantation: Eighth Official Pediatric Report—2005. *Journal of Heart and Lung Transplantation, 24,* 968–982.

Briggs, J. P., Kriz, W., & Schnermann, J. B. (2005). Overview of kidney function and structure. In A. Greenberg (Ed.), *Primer on kidney diseases* (4th ed., pp. 2–19). Philadelphia: Elsevier Saunders.

Brosig, C., Hintermeyer, H., Zlotocha, J., Behrens, D., & Mao, J. (2006). An exploratory study of the cognitive, academic, and behavioral functioning of pediatric cardiothoracic transplant recipients. *Progress in Transplantation, 16,* 38–45.

Brouhard, B. H., Donaldson, L. A., Lawry, K. W., McGowan, K. R., Drotar, D., Davis, I., et al. (2000). Cognitive functioning in children on dialysis and post-transplantation. *Pediatric Transplant, 4,* 261–267.

Butcher, J. N., Graham, J. R., Williams, C. L., & Kaemmer, B. (1992). Minnesota Multiphasic Personality Inventory—Adolescent. Minneapolis: University of Minnesota Press.

Children's Hospital Boston. (2007). *About lung transplants.* Retrieved April 4, 2007, from http://www.childrenshospital.org/clinicalservices/Site2022/mainpage S2022P4.html

Chinnock, R. E. (2006). *Heart transplantation.* Retrieved March 6, 2007, from http://www.emedicine.com/ped/topic2797.htm

Cohen, M. (1997). *Children's Memory Scale.* San Antonio, TX: The Psychological Corporation.

Crews, W. D., Jr., Jefferson, A. L., Broshek, D. K., Rhodes, R. D., Williamson, J., & Brazil, A. M. (2003). Neuropsychological dysfunction in patients with end-stage pulmonary disease: Lung transplant evaluation. *Archives of Clinical Neuropsychology, 18,* 353–362.

Delis, D. C., Kaplan, E., & Kramer, J. H. (2001). *Delis-Kaplan Executive Function System.* San Antonio, TX: The Psychological Corporation.

Faro, A., Mallory, G. B., Visner, G. A., Elidemir, O., Mogayzel, P. J., Jr., Danziger-Isakov, L., et al. (2007). American Society of Transplantation executive summary on pediatric lung transplantation. *American Journal of Transplantation, 7,* 285–292.

Fennell, R., Fennell, E., Carter, R., Mings, E., & Klausner, A. (1990). Association between renal function and cognition in childhood chronic renal failure. *Pediatric Nephrology, 4,* 16–20.

Forbess, J. M., Visconti, K. J., Bellinger, D. C., Howe, R. J., & Jonas, R. A. (2002). Neurodevelopmental outcomes after biventricular repair of congenital heart defects. *Journal of Thoracic and Cardiovascular Surgery, 123,* 631–639.

Forbess, J. M., Visconti, K. J., Bellinger, D. C., & Jonas, R. A. (2001). Neurodevelopmental outcomes in children after the Fontan Operation. *Circulation, 104,* 127–132.

Forbess, J. M., Visconti, K. J., Hancock-Friesen, C., Howe, R. C., Bellinger, D. C., & Jonas, R. A. (2002). Neurodevelopmental outcome after congenital heart surgery: Results from an institutional registry. *Circulation, 106,* 95–102.

Freier, M. C., Babikian, T., Pivonka, J., Burley Aaen, T., Gardner, J. M., Baum, M., et al. (2004). A longitudinal perspective on neurodevelopmental outcome after infant cardiac transplantation. *Journal of Heart and Lung Transplantation, 23,* 857–864.

Gipson, D. S., Duquette, P. J., Icard, P. F., & Hooper, S. R. (2007). The central nervous system in childhood chronic kidney disease. *Pediatric Nephrology.* Pre-print retrieved April 15, 2007, from http://springerlink.metapress.com/content/n327770813j66t83/?p=f41c945445794e9d8fd2165cb22650ce&pi=12

Gipson, D. S., Wetherington, C. E., Duquette, P. J., & Hooper, S. R. (2004). The nervous system and chronic kidney disease in children. *Pediatric Nephrology, 19,* 832–839.

Gjertson, D. W., & Cecka, J. M. (2001). Determinants of long-term survival of pediatric kidney grafts reported to the United Network for Organ Sharing kidney transplant registry. *Pediatric Transplantation, 5,* 5–15.

Gordon, M. (1983). *The Gordon Diagnostic System.* DeWitt, NY: Gordon Systems.

Goss, J. A., Shackleton, C. R., McDiarmid, S. V., Maggard, M., Swenson, K., Seu, P., et al. (1998). Long-term results of pediatric liver transplantation: An analysis of 569 transplants. *Annals of Surgery, 228,* 411–420.

Grimm, M., Yeganehfar, W., Laufer, G., Madl, C., Kramer, L., Eisenhuber, E., et al. (1996). Cyclosporine may affect improvement of cognitive brain function after successful cardiac transplantation. *Circulation, 94,* 1339–1345.

Hammill, D. D., & Larsen, S. C. (1996). *Test of Written Language* (3rd ed.). Austin, TX: Pro-Ed.

Harrison, P. L., & Oakland, T. (2003). *Adaptive Behavior Assessment System* (2nd ed.). San Antonio, TX: The Psychological Corporation.

Huddleston, C. B. (2006). Pediatric lung transplantation. *Seminars in Pediatric Surgery, 15,* 199–207.

Hurkx, W., Hulstijn, D., Pasman, J., Rotteveel, J., Visco, Y., & Schroder, C. (1995). Evoked potentials in children with chronic renal failure, treated conservatively or by continuous ambulatory peritoneal dialysis. *Pediatric Nephrology, 9,* 325–328.

Jerkic, P., Aurora, P., & Elliot, M. J. (2007). Pediatric lung transplantation: Literature review 2005. *Pediatric Transplantation, 11,* 14–20.

Keenan, P. A., Jacobson, M. W., Soleymani, R. M., Mayes, M. D., Stress, M. E., & Yaldoo, D. T. (1996). The effect on memory of chronic prednisone treatment in patients with systemic disease. *Neurology, 47,* 1396–1402.

Krishnamurthy, V., Jones, J. P., Nichols, J. G., Naramor, T., & Freier, M. C. (2006). Cognitive and emotional development in infant heart transplant recipients. *Journal of Heart and Lung Transplantation, 25*(Suppl. 1), 51.

Krull, K., Fuchs, C., Yurk, H., Boone, P., & Alonso, E. (2003). Neurocognitive outcome in pediatric liver transplant recipients. *Pediatric Transplantation, 7,* 111–118.

Lawry, K. W., Brouhard, B. H., & Cunningham, R. J. (1994). Cognitive functioning and school performance in children with renal failure. *Pediatric Nephrology, 8,* 326–329.

Liou, T. G., Adler, F. R., & Huang, D. (2005). Use of lung transplantation survival models to refine patient selection in cystic fibrosis. *American Journal of Respiratory and Critical Care Medicine, 173,* 246–247.

Medline Plus. (2005). *Idiopathic pulmonary fibrosis.* Retrieved April 10, 2007, from http://www.nlm.nih.gov/medlineplus/ency/article/000069.htm

Mendley, S. R., & Zelko, F. A. (1999). Improvement in specific aspects of neurocognitive performance in children after renal transplantation. *Kidney International, 56,* 318–323.

Milanesi, O., Cerutti, A., Biffanti, R., Salvadori, S., Gambino, A., & Stellin, G. (2007). Heart transplantation in pediatric age. *Journal of Cardiovascular Medicine, 8,* 67–71.

Morales, D. L. S., Dreyer, W. J., Denfield, S. W., Heinle, J. S., McKenzie, E. D., Graves, D. E., et al. (2007). Over two decades of pediatric heart transplantation: How has survival changed? *Journal of Thoracic and Cardiovascular Surgery, 133,* 632–639.

National Kidney Foundation. (2007). *High blood pressure and chronic kidney disease in children: A guide for parents.* Retrieved April 15, 2007, from http://www.kidney.org/atoz/atozItem.cfm?id=164

Organ Procurement and Transplantation Network. (2007). *The 2006 OPTN/SRTR Annual Report: Transplant Data 1996–2005.* Retrieved April 15, 2007, from http://www.optn.org/AR2006/default.htm

Putzke, J. D., Williams, M. A., Millsaps, C. L., Azrin, R. L., LaMarche, J. A., Bourge, R. C., et al. (1997). Heart transplant candidates: A neuropsychological descriptive database. *Journal of Clinical Psychology in Medical Settings, 4,* 343–355.

Qvist, E., Jalanko, H., & Holmberg, C. (2003). Psychosocial adaptation after solid organ transplantation in children. *Pediatric Clinics of North America, 50,* 1505–1519.

Qvist, E., Pihko, H., Fagerudd, P., Valanne, L., Lamminranta, S., Karikoski, J., et al. (2002). Neurodevelopmental outcome in high-risk patients after renal transplantation in early childhood. *Pediatric Transplant, 6,* 53–62.

Reynolds, C. R., & Bigler, E. D. (1994). *Test of Memory and Learning.* Austin, TX: Pro-ED.

Ruchinskas, R. A., Broshek, D. K., Crews, W. D., Jr., Barth, J. T., Francis, J. P., & Robbins, M. K. (2000). A neuropsychological normative database for lung transplant candidates. *Journal of Clinical Psychology in Medical Settings, 7,* 107–112.

Schieppati, A., Pisoni, R., & Remuzzi, G. (2005). Pathophysiology and management of chronic kidney disease. In A. Greenberg (Ed.), *Primer on kidney diseases* (4th ed., pp. 444–454). Philadelphia: Elsevier Saunders.

Scientific Registry of Transplant Recipients. (2006). *The U.S. Organ Procurement and Transplantation Network and the Scientific Registry of Transplant Recipients.* Retrieved March 6, 2007, from http://www.ustransplant.org/csr/current/nats.aspx

Semel, E., Wigg, E. H., & Secord, W. A. (2003). *Clinical Evaluation of Language Fundamentals* (4th ed.). San Antonio, TX: The Psychological Corporation.

Stewart, S., Hiltebeitel, C., Nici, J., Waller, D., Uauy, R., & Andrews, W. (1991). Neuropsychological outcome of pediatric liver transplantation. *Pediatrics, 87,* 367–376.

Stewart, S., Kennard, B. D., Waller, D. A., & Fixler, D. (1994). Cognitive function in children who receive organ transplantation. *Health Psychology, 13,* 3–13.

Stewart, S., Uauy, R., Kennard, B., Waller, D., Benser, M., & Andrews, W. (1988). Mental development and growth in children with chronic liver disease of early and late onset. *Pediatrics, 82,* 167–172.

Tiao, G. M., Alonso, M. H., & Ryckman, F. C. (2006). Pediatric liver transplantation. *Seminars in Pediatric Surgery, 15,* 218–227.

Tiffin, J. (1968). *Purdue Pegboard examiner's manual.* Rosemont, IL: London House.

Todaro, J. F., Fennell, E. B., Sears, S. F., Rodrigue, J. R., & Roche, A. K. (2000). Review: Cognitive and psychological outcomes in pediatric heart transplantation. *Journal of Pediatric Psychology, 25,* 567–576.

Towbin, J. A., Lowe, A. M., Colan, S. D., Sleeper, L. A., Orav, E. J., Clunie, S., et al. (2006). Incidence, causes, and outcomes of dilated cardiomyopathy in children. *Journal of the American Medical Association, 296,* 1867–1876.

United Network for Organ Sharing. (2007). *Transplant living organ facts.* Retrieved March 6, 2007, from http://www.transplantliving.org/beforethetransplant/organfacts/heart.aspx

United States Renal Data System. (2005). *USRDS 2005 annual data report: Atlas of end-stage renal disease in the United States.* Bethesda, MD: National Institutes of Health, National Institutes of Diabetes and Digestive and Kidney Diseases.

Valanne, L., Qvist, E., Jalanko, H., Holmberg, C., & Pihko, H. (2004). Neuroradiologic findings in children with renal transplantation under 5 years of age. *Pediatric Transplantation, 8,* 44–51.

Wayman, K., Cox, K., & Esquivel, C. (1997). Neurodevelopmental outcome of young children with extrahepatic biliary atresia 1 year after liver transplantation. *Journal of Pediatrics, 131,* 894–898.

Wechsler, D. (2003). *Wechsler Intelligence Scale for Children* (4th ed.). San Antonio, TX: Harcourt Assessment.

Wells, A., & Faro, A. (2006). Special considerations in pediatric lung transplantation. *Seminars in Respiratory and Critical Care Medicine, 27,* 552–560.

Wilkinson, G. S., & Robertson, G. J. (2006). *Wide Range Achievement Test* (4th ed.). Lutz, FL: Psychological Assessment Resources.

Wray, J., Pot-Mees, C., Zeitlin, H., Radley-Smith, R., & Yacoub, M. (1994). Cognitive function and behavioural status in paediatric heart and heart-lung transplant recipients: The Harefield experience. *British Medical Journal, 309,* 837–841.

Wray, J., & Radley-Smith, R. (2005). Beyond the first year after pediatric heart or heart-lung transplantation: Changes in cognitive function and behaviour. *Pediatric Transplantation, 9,* 170–177.

Wray, J., & Radley-Smith, R. (2006). Longitudinal assessment of psychological functioning in children after heart or heart-lung transplantation. *Journal of Heart and Lung Transplantation, 25,* 345–352.

Yoon, P. W., Bresee, J. S., Olney, R. S., James, L. M., & Khoury, M. J. (1997). Epidemiology of biliary atresia: A population-based study. *Pediatrics, 99,* 376–382.

CHAPTER NINETEEN

# Spina Bifida

Denise Phalon Cascio, MS, and Julie K. Ries, PsyD

## DESCRIPTION OF THE DISORDER

Spina bifida is defined as a congenital neural tube defect that occurs between the first 3 (Copp, Fleming, & Greene, 1998) and 6 weeks of gestation, during a process called *neurulation,* during which the brain and spinal cord are formed (Mitchell et al., 2004). In spina bifida, the neural tube, which eventually forms the spine, fails to fuse (typically at the caudal portion of the spine), resulting in a protruding spinal cord (Mitchell et al.; Wills, 1993). There are three classifications of spina bifida: (1) occulta, in which the neural tube closure fails, but spinal cord tissue is not involved and no neurological deficit is present; (2) meningocele, in which the spinal cord meninges herniate through the spinal column defect, but spinal cord neural tissue is not involved and few neurological consequences are present; and (3) myelomeningocele, in which incompletely formed meninges and malformed spinal cord protrude from the spinal cord resulting in many sensory, motor, and neurological consequences (Kaplan, Spivak, & Bendo, 2005). In myelomeningocele, a balloon-like sac containing the spinal cord lies outside the body and must be surgically closed within 48 hours of birth (Mitchell et al.; Wills). Typically, the sac protrudes from the lower part of the body, close to the tailbone; however, it can occur at any level of the spine, and the level of the lesion dictates the level of motor problems and function loss that the individual will experience (Wills). Specifically, the higher up the spine that the lesion occurs, the greater the likelihood of more loss of function and potential neurological issues (e.g., hydrocephalus) and neuropsychological sequelae (e.g., attention problems).

Although it is the second most common birth defect, the cause of spina bifida remains largely unknown. Studies have implicated folic acid deficiencies, and there is some indication that heredity, maternal diabetes, and environmental toxins (such as anticonvulsant drugs) may also play a role (Mitchell et al., 2004; Williams, Rasmussen, Flores, Kirby, & Edmonds, 2005; Wills, 1993). Spina bifida occurs in about 3,000 U.S. births per year, with a higher prevalence observed in women of Hispanic ethnicity and the lowest occurrence observed among Asian and African American ethnicities (Williams et al.). Research has shown that preconception intake of folic acid can reduce the risk of spina bifida by 50% to 70% (Williams et al.).

Children with spina bifida represent a diverse and varied group of individuals who display a wide range of behaviors and experience variable levels of functioning. It should not be assumed that every child with spina bifida will fit the clinical picture described in this chapter; rather, this chapter is intended to provide the reader with comprehensive information about the complications and presentations that occur most frequently within the spina bifida myelomeningocele (SBM) population as a direct result of the physical condition and related medical complications and from secondary conditions that result directly or indirectly from spina bifida and the related medical issues.

## RELATED MEDICAL ISSUES

Although there is no cure for spina bifida, it can be medically managed such that about 78% of people born with the disorder survive to at least age 17 (Mitchell et al., 2004). Because it is a complex disorder with physiological and psychological components, individuals born with spina bifida myelomeningocele often face a lifetime of medical, psychological, and neuropsychological complications either as a direct result of this condition or as a secondary condition related to the effects of spina bifida. These complications include lower limb weakness or paralysis, sensory loss, lack of bladder and/or bowel control, orthopedic problems such as scoliosis, latex allergies, seizures, skin sores, obesity, precocious puberty, muscle contractures, chronic urinary tract infections, hydrocephalus, and spinal cord tethering and Chiari malformation, which are described below (Baron, Fennell, & Voeller, 1995; Mitchell et al.; Simeonsson,

2002). All of these secondary conditions require medical attention, including prevention and remediation, as they greatly impact the individual's participation in and enjoyment of life.

Chiari malformation refers to a condition in which a portion of the brain stem descends into the cervical spine, causing pain, apnea (i.e., episodes of breathing cessation while sleeping), swallowing difficulties, headache, paresis (i.e., motor weakness), and balance problems. This malformation occurs in approximately 75% of individuals with spina bifida (Mitchell et al., 2004). Along with the problems mentioned above, Chiari malformations can also contribute to eye movement disorders and motor difficulties experienced by children with spina bifida and often are the main cause of the obstruction that leads to hydrocephalus (Wills, 1993), which is an increase or blockage of the cerebrospinal fluid (CSF) that normally cushions the brain.

Spinal cord tethering occurs because the spinal cord in patients with spina bifida is attached to the surrounding structures, preventing it from ascending normally so the spinal cord is low-lying or tethered. With growth, the spinal cord can become stretched, and blood flow to the cord can be inhibited. A tethered cord can cause symptoms such as back and leg pain, changes in leg strength, progressive muscle contractures, deformities of the legs, scoliosis, and bowel and bladder dysfunctions. About 20% to 50% of spina bifida patients require surgery to untether the spinal cord. Untethering operations are undertaken primarily to prevent further deterioration, rather than to improve what has already occurred (Spina Bifida Association of America, 2007).

Catheterization for bladder dysfunction or sensory loss is common and can lead to frequent urinary tract infections (Baron et al., 1995). Struggles with incontinence and catheterization can lead to embarrassment and social isolation for children with spina bifida as they get older (Verhoef et al., 2005). Furthermore, confinement to a wheelchair and lack of mobility can lead to obesity in children with spina bifida. As a secondary condition, obesity warrants attention, particularly because it can be prevented and also because it can further limit or impair the child who already has difficulties with mobility. Research has indicated that close to 50% of children with spina bifida had a larger percentage of body fat compared to age-matched controls (Mita, Akataki, & Itoch, 1993). Because of immobility, these children also may be at higher risk for pressure sores, which can become infected and can create a serious medical problem if severe and left untreated.

Scoliosis and muscle contractures occur in about 90% of children with spina bifida as a result of wheelchair confinement (Simeonsson, 2002). Muscle contractures can be very painful and often require surgery to correct or release them (Baron et al., 1995). Scoliosis and other spine curvatures can become so severe that they cause respiratory difficulties for the individual with spina bifida (Baron et al.). Children with spina bifida are also at risk for accidental self-injurious behavior, often as a result of diminished pain sensitivity in extremities and limbs (Simeonsson).

About 60% of children with spina bifida demonstrate an allergy to latex (Simeonsson, 2002). Symptoms of latex allergy include skin rash, hives, eye tearing and irritation, wheezing, and itching. More severe reactions can include rapid heart beat, tremors, chest pain, difficulty breathing, hypotension (i.e., low blood pressure), anaphylactic shock, temporary loss of consciousness, or potentially death. Given the frequency of medical exams and procedures during which latex gloves may be worn, and the presence of latex in many common materials, it is important to consider this allergy when working with individuals with this disorder. Table 19.1 shows a list of many common foods and items that contain latex and may trigger latex-associated allergies.

Seventy percent of children who receive the diagnosis of spina bifida actually have the lesion categorized as myelomeningocele. Of these, approximately 90% experience hydrocephalus; as a result, this chapter will focus on myelomeningocele (hereafter MM) with hydrocephalus (hereafter HC), as this is the population readers are most likely to interact with. Given the high percentage of individuals with spina bifida who also develop HC, and because HC is the most commonly implicated

**TABLE 19.1 Products that Contain Latex**

| Foods That Contain Protein found in Latex | Common Items that Contain Latex |
|---|---|
| Banana | Balloons |
| Avocado | Rubber bands |
| Chestnut | Other elastic (e.g.) on clothing |
| Kiwi | Some adhesive tapes and bandages |
| Pear | Rubber balls |
| Mango | Pacifiers |
| Potato | Beach Toys |
| Celery | Art supplies |
| Fig | Glue and paste |

*Note.* This is not an exhaustive list; any item that is light brown in color and can be stretched may contain latex. Please see the Resources section for a website containing more latex items.

condition in neuropsychological findings with this population, please refer to the chapter on hydrocephalus in this volume, as it will only be mentioned briefly in this chapter as it relates to MM. HC is defined as "an imbalance in the production and absorption of cerebrospinal fluid [that] . . . enlarges the ventricular system, exerting pressure upward, downward, and outward on surrounding brain structures" (Baron et al., 1995, p. 221).

HC is typically treated with shunt placement, which allows the CSF to leave the brain, restoring normal pressure inside the skull. The most common shunt for reducing HC is a ventriculoperitoneal (VP) shunt, which drains CSF from the brain into the peritoneal (abdominal) cavity where it can be reabsorbed by the body and excreted (Baron et al., 1995). Eighty-five percent of children with MM/HC are shunt-dependent; they cannot function without a properly working shunt (Wills, 1993).

Although shunt placement has been vital in extending and improving the lives of those with HC, this procedure is not without problems. Each time a shunt is replaced or revised, a brain lesion is an unavoidable side effect. This lesion is usually in the right parietal region (Wills, 1993), which is the portion of the brain largely responsible for visual-spatial and sensory motor functioning (Walsh & Darby, 1999). In addition, shunts can lead to infections and/or hemorrhages, and furthermore malfunctions and obstructions are common. When shunt failures occur, they can have significant consequences for the child with HC (Baron et al., 1995). Table 19.2 lists common signs that a child might exhibit if experiencing a shunt failure. Shunts often need to be revised due to failure or to accommodate changes as the child grows physically (Baron et al.), and unfortunately some research suggests that IQ scores decline as the number of shunt revisions in a child's life increases (Wills). All of the complications related to shunt placement and revision can have their own impact on the child's health and functioning, including cognitive functioning, in addition to the effects of MM/HC themselves.

**TABLE 19.2 Symptoms of Shunt Failure**

| Physical Symptoms | Behavioral Symptoms |
|---|---|
| Headache | Confusion |
| Vomiting | Stupor |
| Balance or coordination problems | Irritability |
| Seizure | Fatigue |
| Vision problems | Personality change |

## NEUROPSYCHOLOGICAL SEQUELAE OF SPINA BIFIDA

Although most children who have spina bifida without HC tend to obtain average or above-average scores on neuropsychological tests (Iddon, Morgan, Loveday, Sahakian, and Pickard, 2004), the 90% of children with MM who also have HC often present with a complex neuropsychological profile. Typical neuropsychological problems seen in children who have been shunted for HC include lower IQ scores, social immaturity, academic difficulties in varied areas, as well as difficulties with memory, motor abilities, nonverbal abilities, and executive functions (Baron et al., 1995). Neuropsychological research findings related to MM/HC discussed in this chapter will be described in the following 10 categories of ability or function: overall cognitive ability, adaptive functioning, academic skills, executive functioning, language functioning, memory abilities, fine motor, visual-motor, visual-perceptual skills, and emotional and behavioral functioning.

### Overall Cognitive Ability

On formal intelligence testing, children with MM/HC tend in general to have "normal" or average intelligence, even if they have significant motor impairment (Manning-Courtney, 1999). In addition, children with MM/HC typically demonstrate higher verbal than nonverbal scores. In particular, research with this population has shown lower processing speed (PSI) and perceptual organizational (POI) scores on the Wechsler Intelligence Scale for Children—Third Edition (WISC-III; Wechsler, 1991) than on verbal components of the same test (Baron et al., 1995; Calhoun & Mayes, 2005).

### Adaptive Functioning

Adaptive skills are daily living or self-help skills required for self-sufficiency and independence. Children with spina bifida often have more skill requirements due to their disorder, including catheterization (e.g., draining of the bladder with the use of a device), transfers (i.e., moving from the wheelchair to the bed), exercises (e.g., pushing themselves up off of the wheelchair on a regular basis to prevent skin breakdown on the buttocks), use of leg braces, and medication regimens. The level of the lesion on the spine may directly affect the degree of motor impairment, potentially limiting a child's ability to perform some tasks (Manning-Courtney, 1999). A higher lesion may negatively impact a child's ability to walk and issues involving toileting, dressing, and bathing. Children with MM/HC can learn to assist to the best of their ability in performing these skills or the task can be adapted for them (e.g., use of special adaptive utensils to allow a child with fine motor problems to eat more independently).

## Academic Skills

Seven out of 10 children with spina bifida may exhibit developmental delays or learning problems that warrant special education (Shelov, 2005). In a controlled study of mathematical ability, a group of children with spina bifida solved fewer problems than children without this disorder. The spina bifida group was also less accurate in their calculations and required longer response time (Barnes et al., 2006). Another study by Barnes, Dennis, and Hetherington (2004) found that young adults with MM/HC exhibited deficient reading comprehension skills and writing fluency that may have potential consequences for educational attainment and functional independence. Research has also found that children with MM/HC demonstrate many of the features of the syndrome of nonverbal learning disabilities (NLD). Yeates, Loss, Colvin, and Enrile (2003) found that about half of the children with MM displayed a pattern of strengths and limitations consistent with NLD syndrome; however, the authors encourage caution in making generalizations regarding the use of this model in understanding children with MM/HC.

## Executive Functioning and Attention

Even children with MM/HC with average or above-average IQ scores present with difficulties in memory, learning, and executive functions such as planning, shifting, flexibility, and sustained attention (Iddon et al., 2004). Some research has shown that children with HC experience particular impairment on complex activities that may require more than one cognitive process (e.g., self-monitoring), as well as an inability to develop and use strategies to improve performance on difficult tasks (Iddon et al.). Furthermore, children with MM/HC often have attention difficulties that may be consistent with criteria for Attention-Deficit/Hyperactivity Disorder (ADHD), Predominantly Inattentive Type (Baron et al., 1995). The incidence of ADHD in children with MM/HC is about 30% to 40%, a number that greatly exceeds the population incidence rate of 5% to 17%. It has been noted that diagnoses of ADHD given to children with MM/HC likely reflect problems with inattention more than hyperactivity (Burmeister et al., 2005; Davidovitch et al., 1999).

## Language Functioning

Although children with spina bifida and HC typically demonstrate higher verbal than nonverbal skills on intelligence testing, language functioning can still be impacted. Children with spina bifida and HC have been observed to have difficulties in both receptive and expressive language, including vocabulary, verbal fluency, sentence repetition, and complex grammar (Baron et al., 1995). There also is evidence that these children struggle with word finding and may use over-learned phrases to compensate for lack of fluency, resulting in what might sound like "empty chatter" (Baron et al.).

## Memory Abilities

Memory difficulties have been observed in this population but are not as well studied as other neuropsychological aspects. Current literature suggests that children with MM/HC have memory difficulties, but these problems may in fact be related to problems with attention (Baron et al., 1995). A study by Scott and colleagues (1998) concluded that children who had been treated with a shunt to relieve HC performed more poorly on memory tasks than children who did not suffer from HC. In addition, problems with encoding and retrieval on nonverbal and verbal tasks were observed in children with HC, regardless of etiology (spina bifida or another cause).

## Fine Motor, Visual-Motor, and Visual-Perceptual Skills

Fine and gross motor dysfunction and poor eye-hand coordination are typical in children with MM/HC, all of which may manifest in poor handwriting, poor coordination, low dexterity, problems with design or letter copying, and slower writing or copying speed (Baron et al., 1995). Deficits in perceptual and motor timing were noted in children with MM/HC on duration-perception tasks and rhythmic tapping tasks in a study by Dennis and colleagues (2004). These deficits appeared to correlate with volume reductions in the cerebellum (Dennis et al., 2004). Furthermore, it has been noted that children with MM/HC demonstrate perceptual motor problems that particularly affect graphomotor skills, such as performance on tasks measuring the ability to copy designs. These children also tend to do more poorly on timed tasks, in particular those that involve motor skills (Baron et al.).

## Emotional and Behavioral Functioning

A recent study showed that children with MM/HC, compared to typically developing children, were rated by their parents or caregivers as being less adaptable; having increased difficulty initiating social interactions with strangers; displaying greater withdrawal; being more distractible and less attentive and persistent; and possessing a less predictable rhythm in terms of sleeping, waking, and eating. This implies that the temperaments of children with MM/HC may place them at risk for misunderstanding social cues and will likely impact learning, as well as participation in home and community activities (Vachha & Adams, 2005).

As rated by their caregivers, children with MM/HC displayed more symptomatic behaviors than a control group; specifically, the group with MM/HC scored higher on measures of ADHD, oppositional disorders, phobias, and obsessions (Ammerman, 2003). Ammerman also found that mothers of children with MM/HC reported more symptoms of depression in their children; however, this did not correlate with the child's own perception of depressive symptoms. In addition, studies have shown that children with MM/HC are more socially immature, more passive, more dependent on adults, less scholastically independent, less physically active, and more likely to have attention and concentration difficulties than their non-MM/HC counterparts (Holmbeck et al., 2003). In a study of social problem solving, children with congenital disorders, including spina bifida, came up with fewer solutions to hypothetical problems than did a group of children with acquired brain injuries, suggesting subtle differences in neuropsychological deficits that lead to social difficulties (Warschausky, Argento, Hurvitz, & Berg, 2003).

Psychosocial issues are salient for these children as well, including problems with self-image, self-esteem, anxiety, and depression (Baron et al., 1995). The most stressful developmental period for children with MM/HC and their families may be adolescence, when issues regarding independence and vocational goals emerge. The self-perceptions of children with MM/HC have been evaluated in controlled studies; Antle (2004) found that self-worth among this population was related to friendships and perceived social support from parents. Unfortunately, it was also noted that a sense of global self-worth in this population tends to decline with age, likely due to increased awareness and internalization of negative perceptions by others who view them as disabled (Antle).

## NEUROPSYCHOLOGICAL CASE FORMULATION

### Relevant History and Reason for Referral

The neuropsychological case presented is that of Jason, a 7-year-old, right-handed White male. A comprehensive evaluation was requested to assess neuropsychological factors, clarify areas of strength and weakness, and assist in educational/therapeutic program planning in light of a history of spina bifida myelomeningocele with shunted HC and related medical complications.

Jason was reportedly delivered full-term and underwent surgery to close the neural tube and to place a shunt shortly after his birth. He remained in the hospital for 4 weeks. Jason's achievement of motor and language developmental milestones was delayed. He was able to crawl at 6 months but currently ambulates via a wheelchair. He began using single words around his second birthday. With regard to toileting issues, he continues to require assistance with catheterization, although he expresses a desire to do this himself.

With regard to his medical history, Jason has experienced mild ear infections and repeated urinary tract infections. At 18 months of age, he had a hernia surgically repaired. At 3 years of age, he fractured his kneecap when he attempted to stand. Jason has undergone several shunt revisions, the last of which occurred when he was 6 years old. Just prior to this last surgery, Jason had a fever of 103 degrees for several weeks, which resolved after the shunt revision and was likely related to shunt failure. At the time of the evaluation, he was scheduled to have surgery to address a Chiari malformation. Jason receives Bactrim on a daily basis to prevent recurrent urinary tract infections. There are no significant concerns with regard to his vision or hearing. He has an allergy to latex.

Jason is enrolled in his second year of kindergarten under a homeschool program. He is repeating kindergarten due to missing school because of multiple surgeries over the past year. Prior to homeschooling, Jason was enrolled in a small private school. He reportedly made friends easily and enjoyed school; however, his mother withdrew him due to her concerns about the school environment and its ability to meet his needs. Academically, Jason finds numbers easy, but he reportedly often demonstrates poor motivation and effort. He also demonstrates day-to-day changes in memory abilities. Tests administered and Jason's scores are presented in Tables 19.3 and 19.4.

## Behavioral Observations

At the time of the evaluation, Jason was a few weeks away from neurosurgery to reduce compression from a Chiari malformation, and the results of the evaluation likely reflect his abilities and behaviors, given his dynamic neurological condition.

Jason was evaluated over the course of two sessions approximately a week apart. Both sessions were in the morning. Jason presented as a very outgoing and friendly child who was very eager to meet the examiner. He

**TABLE 19.3 Neuropsychological Testing Data**

| | Scaled Score | Standard Score |
|---|---|---|
| **Intellectual Functioning** | | |
| DAS Verbal Ability | | 83 |
| Spatial Reasoning | | 68 |
| Nonverbal Reasoning | | 86 |
| Global Composite | | 77 |
| **Academic Skills** | | |
| DAS Basic Number Skills | | 76 |
| Spelling | | 68 |
| Word Reading | | 85 |
| BBCS-R School Readiness Composite | 8 | |
| **Language Functioning** | | |
| CELF-2 Concepts & Following Directions | 6 | |
| **Visual-motor Skills** | | |
| VMI-V VMI | | 80 |
| Visual Perception | | 100 |
| Motor Coordination | | 70 |

*Note.* BBCS-R, Bracken Basic Concept Scales – Revised (Bracken, 1998); CELF-2, Clinical Evaluation of Language Fundamentals Preschool – Second Edition (Wiig, Secord, & Semel, 2004); DAS, Differential Ability Scales (Elliott, 1990); VMI, Beery-Buktenica Developmental Test of Visual-Motor Integration – Fifth Edition (Beery, Buktenica, & Beery, 2004).

was seated in a wheelchair and was appropriately dressed and groomed. He appeared very excited and eager to go with the examiner to the evaluation room. Rapport was easily established but not easily maintained. Once engaged in the evaluation tasks, Jason often complained or asked for a break. His interest in testing waned very quickly, and he became very difficult to encourage. He rarely responded to redirection or encouragement in an attempt to bring him back to tasks. Jason would continually wheel himself out of the examination room and explore the hallways, entering other staff's offices in curious exploration. He would also switch the lights in the exam room on and off and was unresponsive

**TABLE 19.4 T Scores from Parent and Teacher Ratings of Adaptive, Behavioral, and Emotional Functioning**

| Scale | Parent | Teacher |
|---|---|---|
| ABAS-II | | |
| Conceptual | 89 | 98 |
| Social | 96 | 108 |
| Practical | 72 | 91 |
| Global Ability Composite | 81 | 94 |
| BASC | | |
| Externalizing Problems | 50 | 47 |
| Internalizing Problems | 58 | 73 |
| Behavioral Symptoms Index | 49 | 49 |
| Adaptive Skills | 51 | 55 |
| BRIEF[a] | | |
| Inhibit | 39 | 66 |
| Shift | 41 | 64 |
| Emotional Control | 48 | 60 |
| Initiate | 63 | 63 |
| Working Memory | 37 | 80 |
| Plan/Organize | 52 | |
| Organization of Materials | 50 | |
| Monitor | 36 | 65 |

*Note.* ABAS-II, Adaptive Behavior Assessment System – Second Edition (Harrison & Oakland, 2003); BASC, Behavior Assessment Scale for Children (Reynolds & Kamphaus, 1998); BRIEF, Behavior Rating Inventory of Executive Functioning (Gioia, Isquith, Guy, & Kenworthy, 2000). [a]Blank cells indicate scores that were not able to be calculated due to numerous missing responses on the questionnaire.

to redirection from the examiner. When he became frustrated with the examiner's attempts to keep him in the room and resume tasks, Jason put his head down, became red in the face, wheeled himself into the corner of the room, and said "No! I don't want to!" Jason also frequently wheeled his wheelchair into the table in frustration or sometimes in an attempt to be silly.

Throughout the evaluation, Jason's affect and mood were relatively labile, ranging from very excitable to extremely frustrated. Jason had difficulty with sustained attention and constantly had to be encouraged to look at stimuli. Attempts at redirection had to be made repeatedly, and he was frequently distracted by auditory and visual stimuli. He responded well to frequent change of tasks, which seemed to lead to greater ability to attend. When he was engaged in a task, the behavioral momentum seemed to provide him with some encouragement and motivation to continue the task. However, any lapse of continuity between tasks resulted in work refusal and distraction. As the evaluation continued, he had greater difficulty attending to tasks, and requests for attention became more frequent and less effective. He responded well to praise and attention from the second examiner and medical resident who were in the room and would complete tasks to gain this attention.

In general, Jason demonstrated variable motivation. On tasks he clearly enjoyed, including a task involving blocks, he worked hard; however, on other tasks he perceived as more arduous or boring, he became very obstinate and refused to do the task, several times backing away from the table or rolling his wheelchair to another part of the room. He demonstrated impulsivity on many tasks requiring nonverbal responses or pointing to the correct answer; therefore, many times throughout the evaluation he was encouraged by the examiner to look at all of the choices prior to making his answer known. His overall activity level was higher than expected for his age.

His comprehension of most instructions appeared to be within expectations, and directions did not typically need to be repeated. He did not demonstrate any significant articulation errors or dysfluencies. He engaged in much spontaneous conversation, often in an attempt to get out of completing certain tasks. His conversation was appropriate, although off topic at times. His conversations revolved around pretend play at times, and the examiner was able to use pretend play about "Power Rangers" to motivate and engage him in the testing. Jason was able to respond appropriately to the examiner when asked questions about himself. However, on more complex tasks, he occasionally had to be asked to repeat or expand on his answers in order to clarify and adequately score his response. Jason was not typically aware of it when he was making errors but occasionally benefited from feedback. He was right-hand dominant for writing and drawing and demonstrated an emerging tripod pencil grip. When completing sensorimotor tasks, he demonstrated proximal overflow (i.e., reduced ability to isolate muscles); for example, he often stuck out his tongue while attempting to write or draw.

Overall, Jason exhibited extremely variable rates of attention/concentration, cooperation, task perseverance, and motivation. And, as mentioned above, he was in a state of physical discomfort given the complications from his Chiari condition. Therefore, the test results discussed in this case presentation may reflect his medical condition and should be considered a lower bound estimate of Jason's neuropsychological functioning.

## Neuropsychological Findings

Jason's overall cognitive ability fell within the borderline range (6th percentile). His performance on the various tasks was relatively stable, and he obtained low average scores on tasks measuring verbal and nonverbal skills. He performed in the mildly impaired range on tasks measuring spatial abilities (4th percentile). This pattern of performance indicates that Jason's cognitive abilities are relatively unitary across verbal and nonverbal domains with a relative weakness in spatial abilities.

On a measure of adaptive functioning, it appears that Jason's overall abilities, as perceived by his mother on the parent rating, were within the low average range. Jason's mother reported relative strengths in communication and social abilities. Relative weaknesses were noted in self-care and community use, which are not surprising given his medical condition, which requires an increased self-care regimen and limits his mobility greatly. When his mother completed the rating from the perspective of his homeschool teacher, she perceived Jason's abilities to be within the average range with relative strengths in communication and social abilities as well as a relative weakness in self-direction. With this in mind, he is demonstrating adaptive skills consistent with what might be expected given his level of cognitive ability.

An evaluation of Jason's early academic skills was also completed. He performed within the borderline range on tasks measuring basic number skills (5th percentile), within the mildly impaired range on tasks measuring spelling (2nd percentile), and within the low average range on tasks measuring word reading (16th percentile). Jason performed within the average range on tasks measuring school readiness skills (25th percentile). He was noted to have nystagmus, a lateral "shaking" of the eyes, which can impact vision and reading.

On measures of emerging executive functioning, Jason's behaviors and effort compromised the validity of the task. He obtained scores within the borderline range on a task of simple visual attention; however, he refused to complete the task, rendering his score invalid. Jason's mother responded to a questionnaire detailing her perceptions of his executive functioning ability. She did not report any significant difficulties with behavioral regulation, metacognition, or general executive skills. However, she indicated concerns with Jason's ability to initiate activity. In addition, a teacher rating of Jason's executive functioning ability found that he exhibits difficulties in the areas of working memory, emotional control, and behavior regulation. The significant difference between these two reports indicates that Jason may have more difficulty in the more demanding school environment as opposed to home living. Given that his parent is his caregiver and current teacher, caution should be taken in this interpretation, as it does not reflect the breadth of collateral information of his behavior in multiple environments, nor does it demonstrate his breadth of experience.

With regard to language functioning, Jason performed within the borderline range on a receptive language task that required him to follow simple and complex verbal directions. Based on a parent questionnaire, Jason is demonstrating age-appropriate pragmatic language skills.

Because of significant difficulty with sustained attention and motivation, the tasks presented to assess Jason's memory abilities were not valid. On these tasks, his performance could not be scored as he was unable to complete the task within the valid time parameters due to his behavior of leaving the room and not focusing on the stimuli.

On tasks that measured Jason's fine motor, visual-motor, and visual-perceptual skills, he demonstrated an emerging tripod pencil grip appropriate for his age. His ability to copy increasingly complex single figures fell within the low average range. His visual perception abilities fell within the average range, and his motor coordination performance was within the borderline range, suggesting that his motor skills were a relative weakness and may limit his ability to complete visual-spatial tasks that require fine motor involvement. His ability to create patterns out of colored blocks to match a picture fell within the mildly impaired range.

Jason's emotional and behavioral functioning were also evaluated. His mother completed a parent questionnaire detailing her perceptions of Jason's functioning in this domain, where she indicated significant concerns with somatization (i.e., stress expressed in physical discomfort). However, this result is typically seen in children with chronic medical conditions. Jason's mother also indicated some concerns with hyperactivity and attention problems. When the teacher's version of the same questionnaire was completed, similar concerns with somatization, attention, and hyperactivity were noted. In addition, significant anxiety was observed in Jason in the school environment. As previously mentioned, these findings are limited as a result of the single rating of his behaviors due to his homeschool status.

## Conclusions

An area of vulnerability noted in the evaluation was in Jason's ability to sustain attention. His poor overall vigilance and sustained attention clearly impeded his successful performance on several of the tasks presented to him and resulted in the lack of additional evaluation of his memory skills. Jason became less attentive after several minutes of testing and had to be constantly redirected to the tasks presented to him. This clearly impacted his ability to perform tasks that require at least average attentional skills, including receptive language measures.

Differences were noted in his mother's perception of Jason's emotional and executive functioning between the home and school environment. From her responses, it appears that Jason exhibits more anxiety, less self-direction, poorer emotional control, and more difficulties with shifting, inhibiting, and monitoring his behavior while engaged in school tasks or new learning than in the normal home environment. It appears that structured yet flexible instructions and tasks provide an environment in which he is better able to maintain attention. Also, children with spina bifida have problems with initiation (an executive function) that can appear as poor motivation. As a result, increased support, prompting, and a behavioral reinforcement system are required to improve his performance. Although he suffers from other medical issues that likely impact his diagnostic profile, a diagnosis of ADHD cannot be ruled out.

Many children with shunted HC show a pattern of performance in which verbal skills are better developed than spatial skills due to a combination of factors including stretching of the white matter tracts that line ventricles and typical shunt placement in the right parietal lobe, which is thought to be associated with spatial skills. Jason's profile is consistent with this finding. These issues put him at increased risk for mathematics difficulties, particularly as the curriculum becomes more visual and abstract, requiring increased spatial abilities.

Research has shown that language skills in children with spina bifida typically reflect good fluency and social reciprocity with less-developed complex, higher order language. Jason's profile is consistent with this given his less-developed comprehension skills. In addition, it appears that Jason's language abilities and long-term memory are relatively stable and can serve as strengths during times of medical instability.

## INTERVENTIONS

A disability can be described as a "gap between a person's capability and the demands of the environment" (Simeonsson, 2002, p. 199). With this in mind, it is clear that the interaction between a person and his or her environment, including family, school, and community, can all exacerbate and/or mediate a disability (Wills, 1993). It is crucial to provide early and effective interventions for children with MM/HC because of the myriad of medical, neuropsychological, emotional, and social complications that impact children with this disorder. The school setting is an important location for intervention as many of the complications experienced by MM/HC children directly affect skills that they need to learn and be productive in school. What follows is a review of specific interventions to address each of the areas discussed in this chapter.

Specific recommendations for remediation and prevention of secondary conditions include parent and family education and support with regard to the individual's participation in home living, physical modifications at school and home to facilitate accessibility for the individual with spina bifida, training for parents and caregivers about positioning to reduce scoliosis and skin sores, and accessible school and community resources for exercise and involvement as well as education about nutrition and fitness to prevent and treat obesity (Simeonsson, 2002). Furthermore, Table 19.5 shows specific interventions that are likely to be most appropriate at particular education levels and developmental periods, according to the difficulties that are most salient during each time period.

## RESOURCES

### Books

Lutkenhoff, M. (Ed.). (1999). *Children with spina bifida: A parent's guide.* Bethesda, MD: Woodbine House.

Lutkenhoff, M., & Oppenheimer, S. G. (Eds.). (1997). *Spinabilities: A young person's guide to spina bifida.* Bethesda, MD: Woodbine House.

Rowley-Kelly, F. L. (1992). *Teaching the student with spina bifida.* Baltimore: Paul H. Brookes.

Sandler, A. (1997). *Living with spina bifida: A guide for families and professionals.* Chapel Hill: University of North Carolina Press.

### Organizations and Web Sites

Association for Spina Bifida and Hydrocephalus

This organization provides information, research findings, and contact information for local associations.

Web Site: www.asbah.org/

Children and Adults With Spina Bifida and Hydrocephalus

This organization's Web site is replete with information about spina bifida and its related medical issues.

Web Site: www.waisman.wisc.edu/~rowley/sb-kids

**TABLE 19.5 General Interventions Based on Developmental Stage**

| Specific Concerns | Related Interventions |
|---|---|
| Preschool | |
| Safety | Supervision and implementation of environmental modifications |
| Mobility | Provision of physical therapy, use of orthopeditic devices (leg braces, wheelchair, crutches) |
| Attention | Implementation of environmental modifications |
| Medical issues | Referral to the medical provider |
| Elementary school | |
| Academic functioning | Involvement of the school team through an IEP |
| Social skills | Social involvement through school and community |
| Medical issues | Referral to the medical provider |
| Middle school | |
| Academic functioning | Involvement of the school team through an IEP |
| Social skills | Social involvement through school and community |
| Executive functioning | Implementation of environmental modifications |
| Continence issues | Referral to the medical provider |
| Obesity | Referral to the medical provider, sharing of information with the caregiver, referral to a nutritionist |
| Medical issues | Referral to the medical provider |
| High school | |
| Social isolation | Social involvement through school and community |
| Obesity | Referral to the medical provider, sharing of information with the caregiver, referral to a nutritionist |
| Continence issues | Referral to the medical provider |
| Independence/Transition to Adulthood | Involvement by the medical team & school team through an IEP |
| Mobility | Provision of physical therapy |
| Self Care | Provision of occupational therapy, promoting caregiver's encouragement of independence |
| Dating | Social involvement |

National Information Center for Children and Youth With Disabilities (NICHCY)

The NICHCY specializes in educational program information and other issues important to families and children with disabilities.

| | |
|---|---|
| Mailing Address: | P.O. Box 1492<br>Washington, D.C. 20013-1492 |
| Phone Number: | (800) 695-0285 |
| Web Site: | http://www.nichcy.org |

SB-Teens

The following Web site is a mailing list for adolescents with spina bifida and their families. It allows teenagers with spina bifida to communicate with each other for support and fun.

Web Site: www._sb_teens.homestead.com/

Spina Bifida Association of America

This association offers numerous resources for parents and care providers, advocates for individuals with spina bifida, and conducts conferences for parents and professionals. The Web site also includes a fact sheet that lists information related to latex allergies.

| | |
|---|---|
| Mailing Address: | 4590 MacArthur Boulevard NW, Suite 250<br>Washington, D.C. 20007-4226 |
| Phone Number: | (800) 621-3141 |
| Web Site: | www.sbaa.org |

## REFERENCES


Ammerman, R. T. (2003, August). *Psychopathology in children and adolescents with spina bifida*. Paper presented at the meeting of the American Psychological Association, Washington, DC.

Antle, B. J. (2004). Factors associated with self-worth in young people with physical disabilities. *Health and Social Work, 29,* 167–175.

Barnes, M., Dennis, M., & Hetherington, R. (2004). Reading and writing skills in young adults with spina bifida and hydrocephalus. *Journal of the International Neuropsychological Society, 10,* 655–663.

Barnes, M. A., Wilkinson, M., Khemani, E., Boudesquie, A., Dennis, M., & Fletcher, J. M. (2006). Arithmetic processing in children with spina bifida: Calculation accuracy, strategy use, and fact retrieval fluency. *Journal of Learning Disabilities, 39,* 174–187.

Baron, I. S., Fennell, E. B., & Voeller, K.K.S. (1995). Hydrocephalus and myelomeningocele. In I. S. Baron, E. B. Fennel, & K.K.S. Voeller (Eds.), *Pediatric neuropsychology in the medical setting* (pp. 221–240). New York: Oxford University Press.

Beery, K. E., Buktenica, N. A., & Beery, N. A. (2004). *Beery-Buktenica Developmental Test of Visual-Motor Integration* (5th ed.). Bloomington, MN: Pearson Assessments.

Bracken, B. A. (1998). *Bracken Basic Concept Scales examiner's manual* (rev. ed.). San Antonio, TX: The Psychological Corporation.

Burmeister, R., Hannay, H. J., Copeland, K., Fletcher, J. M., Boudousquie, A., & Dennis, M. (2005). Attention problems and executive functions in children with spina bifida and hydrocephalus. *Child Neuropsychology, 11,* 265–283.

Calhoun, S. L., & Mayes, S. D. (2005). Processing speed in children with clinical disorders. *Psychology in the Schools, 42,* 333–343.

Copp, A. J., Fleming, A., & Greene, N. D. E. (1998). Embryonic mechanisms underlying the prevention of neural tube defects. *Mental Retardation and Developmental Disabilities Research Reviews, 4,* 264–268.

Davidovitch, M., Manning-Courtney, P., Hartmann, L. A., Watson, J., Lutkenhoff, M., & Oppenheimer, S. (1999). The prevalence of attentional problems and the effect of methylphenidate in children with myelomeningocele. *Pediatric Rehabilitation, 3,* 29–35.

Dennis, M., Edelstein, K., Hetherington, R., Copeland, K., Frederick, J., Blaser, S. E., et al. (2004). Neurobiology of perceptual and motor timing in children with spina bifida in relation to cerebellar volume. *Brain, 127,* 1292–1301.

Elliott, C. D. (1990). *Differential Ability Scales: Administration and scoring manual.* San Antonio, TX: The Psychological Corporation.

Gioia, G. A., Isquith, P. K., Guy, S. C., and Kenworthy, L. (2000). *Behavior Rating Inventory of Executive Function.* Odessa, FL: Psychological Assessment Resources.

Harrison, P. L., & Oakland, T. (2003). *Adaptive Behavior Assessment System* (2nd ed.). San Antonio, TX: The Psychological Corporation.

Holmbeck, G. N., Westhoven, V. C., Phillips, W. S., Bowers, R., Gruse, C., Nikolopoulos, T., et al. (2003). A multimethod, multi-informant, and multidimensional perspective on psychosocial adjustment in preadolescents with spina bifida. *Journal of Consulting and Clinical Psychology, 71,* 782–796.

Iddon, J. L., Morgan, D. R., Loveday, C., Sahakian, B. J., & Pickard, J. D. (2004). Neuropsychological profile of young adults with spina bifida with or without hydrocephalus. *Journal of Neurology, Neurosurgery, and Psychiatry, 75,* 1112–1118.

Kaplan, K. M., Spivak, J. M., & Bendo, J. A. (2005). Embryology of the spine and associated congenital abnormalities. *The Spine Journal, 5,* 564–576.

Manning-Courtney, P. (1999). Your child's development. In M. Lutkenhoff (Ed.), *Children with spina bifida: A parent's guide* (pp. 183–201). Bethesda, MD: Woodbine House.

Mita, K., Akataki, K., & Itoch, K. (1993). Assessment of obesity in children with spina bifida. *Developmental Medicine and Child Neurology, 35,* 305–311.

Mitchell, L. E., Adzick, N. S., Melchionne, J., Pasquariello, P. S., Sutton, L. N., & Whitehead, A. S. (2004). Spina bifida. *Lancet, 364,* 1885–1895.

Reynolds, C. R., & Kamphaus R. W. (1998). *Behavior Assessment System for Children.* Circle Pines, MN: American Guidance Service.

Scott, M. A., Fletcher, J. M., Brookshire, B. L., Davidson, K. C., Landry, S. H., Bohan, T. C., et al. (1998). Memory functions in children with early hydrocephalus. *Neuropsychology, 12,* 578–589.

Shelov, S. (Ed.). (2005). *Your baby's first year.* New York: Bantam Books.

Simeonsson, R. J. (2002). Secondary conditions in children with disabilities: Spina bifida as a case example. *Mental Retardation and Developmental Disabilities Research Reviews, 8,* 198–205.

Spina Bifida Association of America. (2007). *Tethering spinal cord.* Retrieved August 8, 2007, from http://www.sbaa.org/site/c.liKWL7PLLrF/b.2700295/k.6B9E/Tethering_Spinal_Cord.htm

Vachha, B., & Adams, R. (2005). Myelomeningocele, temperament patterns, and parental perceptions. *Pediatrics, 115,* 58–63.

Verhoef, M., Lurvink, M., Barf, H. A., Post, M. M., van Asbeck, F. A., Goosekens, R. M., et al. (2005). High prevalence of incontinence among young adults with spina bifida: Description, prediction, and problem perception. *Spinal Cord, 43,* 331–340.

Walsh, K., & Darby, D. (1999). *Neuropsychology: A clinical approach.* New York: Churchill Livingstone.

Warschausky, S., Argento, A. G., Hurvitz, E., & Berg, M. (2003). Neuropsychological status and social problem solving in children with congenital or acquired brain dysfunction. *Rehabilitation Psychology, 48,* 250–254.

Wechsler, D. (1991). *Wechsler Intelligence Scale for Children* (3rd ed.). New York: Psychological Corporation.

Wiig, E. H., Secord, W. A., & Semel, E. (2004). *Clinical Evaluation of Language Fundamentals Preschool* (2nd ed.). San Antonio, TX: Harcourt Assessment.

Williams, L. J., Rasmussen, S. A., Flores, A., Kirby, R., & Edmonds, L. D. (2005). Decline in the prevalence of spina bifida and anencephaly by race/ethnicity: 1995–2002. *Pediatrics, 116,* 580–586.

Wills, K. E. (1993). Neuropsychological functioning in children with spina bifida and/or hydrocephalus. *Journal of Clinical Child Psychology, 22,* 247–265.

Yeates, K. O., Loss, N., Colvin, A. N., & Enrile, B. G. (2003). Do children with myelomeningocele and hydrocephalus display nonverbal learning disabilities? An empirical approach to classification. *Journal of the International Neuropsychological Society, 9,* 653–662.

CHAPTER TWENTY

# Stroke

Cynthia A. Smith, PhD

Sara had been experiencing a headache that would not go away. She was excited about her upcoming lacrosse match and had also been studying for finals. She decided that the headache was due to excitement and too much studying. Suddenly, she experienced a sharp stabbing pain that brought nausea and blindness. She groped for the bathroom to vomit. The room turned sideways, and the world went black. When Sara opened her eyes, she was lying in a dark room with a tube in her throat, surrounded by monitors. There were people in her room, and Sara recognized her mother. She could not focus her eyes, speak out loud, or understand what was being said. She slipped back into the darkness. Sara had experienced an aneurysm in her left frontal lobe.

## DESCRIPTION OF THE DISORDER

The human brain relies on a complex network of arteries and veins for oxygen and nutrients. The arteries deliver oxygenated blood, glucose, and other nutrients to the brain; the veins carry deoxygenated blood back to the heart, removing carbon dioxide, lactic acid, and other metabolic products. Ischemia and hemorrhage are two primary disruptions to this blood flow. An arterial ischemic stroke (AIS) results from a blockage of the inflow of arterial blood. A hemorrhagic stroke occurs when a blood vessel in the brain breaks or ruptures (deVeber, 1999). Cerebrovascular disorders are one of the 10 major causes of death in children under the age of 18. It is estimated that half of these children will experience lasting cognitive or motor disabilities (Jordan, 2006; see also Lynch, Hirtz, deVeber, & Nelson, 2002; Sofronas et al., 2006).

## Ischemic Stroke

In children, ischemic stroke is more common than hemorrhagic stroke. AIS around the time of birth is recognized in 1 in 4,000 full-term infants. During childhood, AIS ranges from 2 to 13 per 100,000 children. The incidence of hemorrhagic stroke in children is estimated at 1.5 to 5.1 per 100,000 children per year (deVeber, 1999).

The child's brain is very vulnerable to compromises in its blood supply as there is no oxygen reserve in the brain and very little energy reserve (deVeber, 1999). Rapid loss of neuronal functioning occurs with interruption of the oxygen supply. With adequate oxygen supply, glucose supply (i.e., energy) can sustain the brain tissue for up to 90 minutes. Although a very young brain (fetal and infant) can experience some recovery (plasticity) of cognitive functioning, the immature brain has greater vulnerability than the adult brain, as it is still developing. The risk factor for ischemic strokes for adults is typically arteriosclerosis. For children, the greatest risk factors are infections or inflammatory disorders such as cardiac disease (up to 50%), coagulation disorders (14%), dehydration (11%), infection (6%), vasculitis (7%), cancer (4%), metabolic disorders (3%) and other miscellaneous disorders (15%). In approximately one-third of cases, there is no identifiable risk factor (deVeber).

Cardiac disorders or heart diseases are the most common cause of ischemic stroke in children. The risk of stroke in children with congenital heart disease is related to the abnormality, diagnostic and surgical procedures, and associated genetic or acquired factors that predispose children to thrombosis (i.e., the formation of a clot within the blood vessel). Cardiac disorders can lead to the development of heart clots that may travel to the brain or can lead to blood vessel blockage in oxygen-deprived patients with anemia (deVeber, 1999; Jordan, 2006; Lynch et al., 2002).

Hematological (i.e., blood) disorders are the second most common cause of stroke in children. These hematological disorders include sickle cell disease (refer to the chapter on sickle cell disease in this volume) and coagulation disorders. Coagulation disorders can result in clotting or hemorrhaging. The risk of stroke is increased in children who have multiple genetic factors. Recurrence of stroke in both of these groups is common (deVeber, 1999; Jordan, 2006; Lynch et al., 2002).

Infectious disorders also are considered to be a common risk factor for stroke in children. Meningitis and encephalitis are two of the most familiar infectious disorders. Varicella infection (i.e., chicken pox) has also been linked to stroke in children. Between 1 in 6,500 to 15,000 children with chicken pox can experience a stroke. In addition, vascular disorders are related to strokes in children. One study indicted that 23% of children with vascular disorders may experience stroke. Vascular disorders include Moyamoya disease (i.e., chronic noninflammatory occlusive of intracranial vasculopathy of an unknown cause) and arterial dissection (typically secondary to trauma). Finally, numerous rare disorders can result in pediatric ischemic stroke (deVeber, 1999; Jordan, 2006; Lynch et al., 2002), as shown in Table 20.1.

The diagnosis of an AIS can be delayed in children because the clinical manifestations can be accounted for by many other etiologies. Typically, a nonresolving neurological deficit (i.e., body weakness on one side of the body, slurred speech, change in cognitive abilities) will first signal an injury. However, such an injury could be accounted for by focal encephalitis, migraine, or focal seizures. Focal seizures at the onset of stroke are relatively frequent in children in comparison to adults. Children also experience transitory ischemic attacks (TIAs) that result in transitory (i.e., temporary) neurological deficits (deVeber, 1999).

## Hemorrhagic Stroke

A hemorrhagic stroke occurs when the child's blood vessels break, weaken, or are injured. This injury results in bleeding into the brain and can cause swelling or blood clotting. Not only is there injury to the site in the brain where the blood clots and pools, but also the brain regions that typically receive the oxygen and nutrients by the blood are deprived and further damage is incurred. Hemorrhagic strokes have four primary causes: malformed blood vessels, poor blood clotting, weakened blood vessels, and trauma (deVeber, 1999; Lynch et al., 2002), as detailed in Table 20.2.

The body has three types of blood vessels to carry blood through the body, specifically, arteries, veins, and capillaries. The largest blood vessels are the arteries, which are thick and strong in order to direct the pressured blood coming from the heart. Typically, the major arteries break off into smaller arteries to enter the veins, which are generally weaker blood vessels the blood flow pressure is less. The capillaries are the weakest blood vessels by necessity. There are three major types of hemorrhages: intracerebral/intraparenchymal hemorrhage (i.e., stroke occurring within the brain), subarachnoid hemorrhage (i.e., stroke occurring between the pial lining and the arachnoid lining of the brain), and trauma hemorrhages (deVeber, 1999; Lynch et al., 2002).

**TABLE 20.1 Disorders Causing Ischemic Stroke**

| Intravascular | Vascular | Embolic |
|---|---|---|
| Sickle cell disease | Meningitis | Congenital heart disease |
| Leukemia | Systemic lupus erythematosus | Acquired heart disease |
| Prothrombotic medications | Rheumatoid arthritis | Rheumatic heart disease |
| Pregnancy and postpartum | Dermatomyositis | Bacterial endocarditis |
| Lupus anticoagulant | Inflammatory bowel disease | Arrhythmia |
| Congenital prothrombotic states | Drug abuse | Amniotic fluid/placenta embolism |
| Metabolic disorders | Early atherosclerosis | Fat/air embolism |
| | Diabetes | Foreign body embolism |
| | Vasculopathies | Cardiac catheterization |
| | Vasospastic disorders (vasospasm, migraines) | |
| | Brain herniation and arterial compression | |
| | Posttraumatic arterial dissection | |
| | Intraoral trauma | |
| | Carotid ligation | |
| | Arteriography | |

Intracerebral hemorrhages occur when the arteries or veins within the brain rupture and bleed into the brain tissue, resulting in a hematoma. The neuronal structures within that brain tissue are disrupted, causing focal damage. Cerebral edema (i.e., swelling) is caused by the presence of blood products and damage to the blood-brain barrier. This edema results in possible severe initial neurological deficits. A large hematoma and the secondary edema can become similar to a mass lesion and result in increased intracranial pressure and focal brain herniation syndromes. In some cases, neurosurgical evacuation or removal of a skull flap is required to reduce pressure. In infants, secondary obstructive hydrocephalus may

**TABLE 20.2 Disorders Causing Hemorrhagic Stroke**

| Vascular Disorders | |
|---|---|
| Congenital anomalies | Arteriovenous malformation, venous angioma, cavernous malformation, hereditary hemorrhagic talangiectasia, intracranial aneurysm |
| Vasculopathies | Sickle Cell disease, Moyamoya disease |
| Vasculitis | Drug abuse, hemolytic-uremic syndrome |
| Trauma | Child abuse, angioplasty, penetrating intracranial trauma |
| Other | Systemic hypertension |
| **Intravascular Disorders** | |
| Hematologic events | Immune thrombocytopenic purpura, Thrombotic thrombocytopenic purpura |
| Hemophilic states | Congenital serum C2 deficiency, Liver dysfunction with coagulation defect vitamin K deficiency, factor deficiencies |

occur and require shunt placement. These children may initially present with severe headaches, focal neurological signs, rapid decreases in consciousness, and seizures. Smaller hemorrhages may exhibit more subtle neurological symptoms. If the brain stem and/or posterior fossa region is involved, ataxia, coma, and other cranial nerve symptoms can occur (deVeber, 1999).

Subarachnoid hemorrhages occur within the multiple linings of the brain and include the circle of Willis (i.e., a circle of arteries that create redundancies in cerebral blood circulation). The space between the pial and arachnoid lining of the brain is typically filled with cerebrospinal fluid (CSF) that is absorbed into the subarachnoid space from the superior sagittal sinus. Children with a subarachnoid hemorrhage typically present with a severe headache, meningeal signs (i.e., neck stiffness), and elevated intracranial pressure. A low-grade fever and leukocytosis (i.e., an abnormally large number of white blood cells) also can be present (deVeber, 1999).

Head trauma is the most common cause for intracranial head injury. Intracerebral hemorrhage caused by trauma can involve one or multiple hemorrhages. In the case of a diffuse shear injury, multiple small hemorrhagic foci throughout the white matter can be found with multiple traumatic subarachnoid hemorrhages. Shaken baby syndrome can be an example of intracranial head injury (deVeber, 1999).

## BRIEF REVIEW OF VASCULAR ANATOMY AND CLINICAL FEATURES

The three major arteries of the cerebral cortex are the anterior cerebral artery (ACA), middle cerebral artery (MCA), and posterior cerebral artery (PCA). These arteries are joined by the anterior communicating artery (AComm) and posterior communicating artery (PComm).

The ACA goes forward to travel in the interhemispheric fissure (i.e., the split between the two hemispheres of the brain) and then travels back to the corpus callosum (i.e., a bundle of white matter fiber that assists the two hemispheres in communicating and working conjointly). The ACA supports the anterior cortex from the frontal to the anterior parietal lobes, including the medial sensorimotor cortex. Clinical features of strokes to the ACA include poor grasp reflex and frontal lobe behavioral abnormalities, which may include impaired judgment, flat affect, apraxia (i.e., inability to make purposeful voluntary movements despite normal muscle function), abulia (i.e., lack of volition), and incontinence. Infarctions (i.e., strokes) to the left ACA can result in right leg weakness and sensory loss and aphasia (i.e., language difficulties). Larger infarctions can result in right hemiplegia (i.e., paralysis affecting one side of the body). Infarctions to the right ACA can result in left leg weakness and sensory loss and left hemineglect (i.e., poor awareness of the left side). Larger infarctions can result in left hemiplegia (Blumenfeld, 2002).

The MCA is divided into the superior division, inferior division, and deep territory. The superior division supports the frontal region superior to the sylvian fissure. Infarctions in this region can result in contralateral (i.e., side opposite to the lesion) face and arm weakness with occasional sensory loss. Infarctions to the left hemisphere can cause an expressive aphasia, and infarctions to the right hemisphere can cause a hemineglect. The inferior division supports the parietal and some of the temporal region. Infarctions to this region in the left hemisphere can result in a receptive aphasia and a right visual field deficit. Some sensory loss may occur in the right face and arm. Right-sided weakness may be present at the onset of symptoms. Infarctions to the right hemisphere in this region can result in profound left hemineglect, left visual field impairments, and somatosensory deficits. Mild left hemiparesis may also be present. The left MCA deep territory supports the basal ganglia. Infarctions may result in contralateral hemiparesis as well as aphasia and neglect (Blumenfeld, 2002).

The PCA supports the thalamus, occipital cortex, and the corpus callosum. Infarctions in this region can result in contralateral field cuts, reading disorders, aphasia, sensory losses, and contralateral hemiparesis (i.e., weakness on one side of the body; Blumenfeld, 2002).

## CASE CONTINUATION

Sara's head hurt, and her throat was sore. She tried to lift her right arm, but it would not respond. She wanted to call out to someone, but the words would not come. Sara's father appeared at the side of her bed. He sat down and tried to reassure her. She could pick out words but not fully comprehend what he was saying. However, his presence was calming to her. Sara had experienced an intracerebral hemorrhagic stroke secondary to an aneurysm in the left middle superior cerebral artery. She had made it to the bathroom and experienced a generalized tonic-clonic seizure.

Her parents called for emergency services, and Sara was brought to the emergency department (ED) at a major hospital. Upon arrival at the ED, she received antiepileptic medication to prevent further seizures and a Computerized Tomography (CT) scan of her brain for diagnostic purposes. The aneurysm was diagnosed, and a successful neurosurgical resection followed. Because of increased intracranial pressure, the bone flap that was removed during surgery was not replaced in order to allow healing. She would now be required to wear a helmet until the flap was replaced.

Sara's beautiful hair was shorn, and her face was swollen. She could move her right leg but not her toes. She was unable to move her arm. Although she generally understood what others were saying, she could not speak. She was able to answer simple yes/no questions by blinking. The nurses and doctors were very kind to her. They always spoke directly to her and would orient her to her location and dates. Sara was starting to understand what happened to her and worried about her recovery.

After 2 weeks in intensive care, Sara was transferred to an acute rehabilitation hospital. By this time, she had regained some movement in her right hand and leg but could not walk. She was confined to a wheelchair. Despite being right-handed, she was unable to use her right hand for any activity. She now was able to understand what was being said to her and use a "thumbs up-thumbs down" reliably for communication. Sara soon realized that she could still read and, to her great relief, started to use a communication board to spell out her needs. At the rehabilitation hospital, she received speech, occupational, and physical therapy. Although previously very athletic, she now found that she fatigued quickly following any sustained activity. She required assistance to learn how to walk once more. However, the most frightening aspect of recovery was the loss of her speech. She was able to have thoughts in her head, but when she tried to speak, her speech was stilted, disorganized, and painstakingly slow. Despite her fear and frustration, Sara persevered in her therapies and made great gains.

During her tenure at the rehabilitation hospital, Sara made significant gains. She was able to walk for short distances with a quad cane and regained some fine motor mobility in her right hand. She commenced utilizing her right arm to stabilize objects and began to use her left hand and arm with more fluidity. Sara also began to speak. Her voice remained rather flat, halting, and monotone, and she offered little spontaneous speech. She exhibited no difficulty with mono- and disyllabic words but needed to give forethought to polysyllabic words. Her rate of processing appeared slightly slower than expected. Just prior to leaving the rehabilitation hospital, Sara received a neuropsychological evaluation. The following are the results of her evaluation 2 months following the aneurysm.

## RESULTS OF NEUROPSYCHOLOGICAL EVALUATION

The neuropsychological evaluation took place over a series of sessions toward the end of Sara's stay in the acute rehabilitation hospital. Sara presented as a friendly and cooperative young lady who developed a good rapport with the examiner. She was dressed in comfortable clothing. Sara was required to wear a helmet as her skull flap had not been replaced. Although she had regained many of her cognitive and motor abilities from the initial stroke, she fatigued quickly; testing was discontinued whenever fatigue was exhibited. Typically, Sara was able to maintain good alertness for approximately 1 hour. Sara's mood and range of affect were appropriate to the situation. She did not appear anxious or depressed. Her speech continued to be slightly flat and stilted, but she readily engaged in conversation with the examiner. During formal testing and conversation, Sara demonstrated word retrieval difficulties, and frequently "talked around" specific words.

Sara exhibited excellent problem-solving skills and perseverance in difficult tasks. Prior to the aneurysm, Sara was right-handed. At the time of the evaluation, she was unable to use the right hand for small motor tasks such as writing or using utensils. She used her left hand for writing and drawing and demonstrated good dexterity. Sara actively used her right arm to steady or hold objects. Overall, Sara exhibited good rates of attention and concentration, cooperation, task perseverance, and motivation. Therefore, the following test results (specific test scores displayed in Table 20.3) are an accurate reflection of Sara's daily level of cognitive functioning.

## Cognitive Functioning

Within the intelligence testing, Sara demonstrated significant variability in subtests ranging from the impaired to high average range. Because of this variability, the "average" overall descriptor is not an adequate reflection of her true cognitive capabilities. In children with average intellectual abilities, a 35-point discrepancy between the Verbal Comprehension and Processing Speed indexes occurred in only 1.1% of the standardization sample (Wechsler, 2003). It is likely that her premorbid intellectual abilities fell in the average to high average range given her strong performance on more factual measures such as Vocabulary and Comprehension. Sara struggled with the Similarities subtest, as she frequently experienced word retrieval problems with specific words and subsequently attempted to describe the missing word. On the Vocabulary and Comprehension measures, she used the word for which she was providing a definition in her response. However, she was able to eventually convey her knowledge regarding these words and concepts.

On the subtests of the Perceptual Reasoning Index, Sara had difficulty with manipulating the blocks of Block Design. The test was administered with no time bonus to account for some of her difficulty. She experienced no difficulty on the two subtests that were not motorically involved. On the two Processing Speed indexes that required the use of a pencil, she was once again hampered by her fine motor limitations. However, it was also apparent on these two measures that her speed of processing had been reduced as well.

## Academic Achievement

On measures of academic achievement, Sara's overall academic ability fell in the average range, which was somewhat below expectations given that she was in gifted and talented classes prior to her stroke. In particular, Sara experienced difficulty with fluency measures that require speed and automatic processing. Her performance on a mathematics measure fell in the borderline range. Sara experienced significant difficulty with rote multiplication. She appeared to have adequate knowledge of mathematical concepts but struggled with calculations. Sara also experienced difficulty on a reading fluency measure, suggesting that she will require extended time for reading assignments.

**TABLE 20.3 Neuropsychological Testing Data**

| | Scaled Score | Standard Score |
|---|---|---|
| Wechsler Intelligence Scale for Children—Fourth Edition | | |
| Full Scale IQ | | 94 |
| Verbal Comprehension index | | 110 |
| Perceptual Reasoning index | | 108 |
| Working Memory index | | 77 |
| Processing Speed index | | 75 |
| Woodcock-Johnson Tests of Achievement—Third Edition | | |
| Academic Skills | | 104 |
| Letter-Word Identification | | 109 |
| Reading Fluency | | 87 |
| Passage Comprehension | | 118 |
| Calculations | | 93 |
| Math Fluency | | 75 |
| Applied Problems | | 93 |
| Spelling | | 107 |
| Children's Memory Scale | | |
| Dot Locations | | |
| Learning | 10 | |
| Total Score | 12 | |
| Long Delay | 12 | |
| Stories | | |
| Immediate | 14 | |
| Delayed | 13 | |
| Delayed Recognition | 15 | |
| Faces | | |
| Immediate | 11 | |
| Delayed | 11 | |
| Word Pairs | | |
| Learning | 9 | |
| Total Score | 10 | |
| Long Delay | 11 | |
| Delayed Recognition | 11 | |
| Numbers | 4 | |
| Sequences | 7 | |

**TABLE 20.3** *(Continued)*

| | Scaled Score | Standard Score |
|---|---|---|
| **Delis-Kaplan Executive Function System** | | |
| Trail Making Test | | |
| Visual Scanning | 9 | |
| Number Scanning | 11 | |
| Letter Sequencing | 7 | |
| Number-Letter Sequencing | 7 | |
| Motor Speed | 4 | |
| Verbal Fluency Test | | |
| Letter Fluency | 7 | |
| Category Fluency | 12 | |
| Tower Total Achievement | 13 | |
| **Boston Naming Test** | | |
| Confrontation Naming | | 104 |
| **Peabody Picture Vocabulary Test—Third Edition** | | |
| Receptive Vocabulary | | 115 |
| **Clinical Evaluation of Language Fundamentals—Fourth Edition** | | |
| Receptive Language | | 102 |
| Expressive Language | | 108 |
| **Beery-Buktenica Developmental Test of Visual-Motor Integration—Fifth Edition** | | |
| VMI | | 72 |
| **Wide Range Assessment of Memory and Learning** | | |
| Finger Window | 13 | |

*Note.* Beery-Buktenica Developmental Test of Visual-Motor Integration—Fifth Edition (VMI-V; Beery, Buktenica, & Beery, 2005); Boston Naming Test (BNT; Kaplan, Goodglass, & Weintraub, 1983); Children's Memory Scale (CMS; Cohen, 1997); Clinical Evaluation of Language Fundamentals—Fourth Edition (CELF-4; Semel, Wigg, & Secord, 2003); The Delis-Kaplan Executive Function System (D-KEFS; Delis, Kaplan, & Kramer, 2001); Peabody Picture Vocabulary Test—Third Edition (PPVT-3; Dunn, Dunn, & Dunn, 1997); Wechsler Intelligence Scale for Children—Fourth Edition (WISC-IV; Wechsler, 2003); Wide Range Assessment of Memory and Learning (WRAML; Sheslow & Adams, 1990); Woodcock-Johnson Tests of Achievement—Third Edition (WJ-III; Woodcock, McGrew, & Mather, 2001).

### Neuropsychological Functioning

On measures of neuropsychological abilities, Sara exhibited selective deficits in verbal working memory, fine motor speed, phonemic fluency, and visuomotor integration. Her performance on all other measures of higher cognitive functioning (receptive and expressive language, immediate and delayed visual and verbal memory, visual working memory, and complex problem solving) all fell within normal limits.

Sara exhibited difficulty with some measures of executive system functioning. She exhibited a restricted verbal working memory (i.e., ability to hold information in memory and subsequently manipulate it by contrasting, comparing, and sequencing) and poorer-than-expected phonemic fluency. On all other measures of executive system functioning (complex problem solving, cognitive set shifting, and semantic fluency), her performance fell within normal limits. Her poor working memory and retrieval abilities probably contributed to her mathematical difficulties.

Sara also exhibited difficulty with fine motor speed and visuomotor integration. Her poor performance on these measures likely reflected her difficulty in attempting to use her nondominant left hand in fine motor tasks.

Sara's difficulty with executive system functioning (working memory and fluency) was consistent with her known left hemisphere arteriovenous malformation (AVM) that was the cause of her stroke. Her fine motor difficulties are consistent given her right hemiparesis. As Sara was in the beginning of her recovery, she was expected to continue to make spontaneous physical and cognitive gains. The greater parts of these gains were expected to be made in the first year of recovery. During this year of recovery, Sara would benefit from changes in her typically rigorous academic program, and appropriate recommendations were suggested.

## RECOMMENDATIONS BASED ON THE NEUROPSYCHOLOGICAL EVALUATION

In considering appropriate recommendations for children like Sara, it is important to consider four converging factors: premorbid cognitive and physical status, current developmental stage, coping capacity, and current cognitive and physical status. Sara is a teenager who was a gifted student and athlete prior to the stroke. She had good family support and continued to demonstrate good coping skills.

Cognitive and physical fatigue is common in patients with similar brain injuries. Not only is the brain still recovering from the injury, but the child often has to exert more energy to accomplish activities. For the first semester, it was recommended that Sara receive a reduced class load. Also, it was recommended that her enrollment in her Spanish class be postponed due to her fluency and expressive language problems. For classroom discussions, it was recommended that the instructor let Sara know in advance what questions she may be asked. This will assist her in finding and saying the words correctly and allow her to formulate and rehearse her response without undue pressure. Sara often knows the answer, but her inability to express the answer limits her class participation. Working memory deficits also impact word and information retrieval. Teenagers with these difficulties frequently experience the "tip of the tongue" phenomenon or may produce the wrong details within the correct concept. Sara may need additional time to retrieve details when answering a question. Cues may be necessary to help her focus on the correct bit of information or specific word. It is often helpful to avoid open-ended questions and to rely more on recognition testing, which does not require retrieval.

With regard to her right hemiparesis, an assessment from the school occupational therapist for accommodations and recommendations was strongly encouraged. Sara would require accommodations in her art class, and, because it would be difficult for Sara to complete lengthy writing assignments, it was recommended that these assignments be reduced in number and volume. She should receive a one-handed keyboard or instruction on how to type using only one hand on a regular keyboard to complete her assignments. Access to a laptop computer to type assignments would be beneficial. The laptop computer would also be useful to help her keep assignments organized. In addition, Sara's ability to take notes and listen to lectures simultaneously will be impacted because of the fine motor and working memory demands. It was suggested that lecture outlines be provided to her prior to the lecture and/or that she be given access to another student's notes. Sara could benefit from having two sets of textbooks (one set for home and one set for school) to assist her in her homework organization and to decrease the weight of what she needs to carry to and from school.

Sara had difficulty with speed of processing, which would result in processing and performing schoolwork at a slower pace. She would require extended time on classroom and standardized tests. This slow rate of processing could impact her ability to comprehend reading material as well. It was recommended that, if poor comprehension occurs, she read along with textbooks on tape to increase her comprehension and retention.

Many teenagers with sudden brain injuries will go through a period of grief and anger at the loss of cognitive and motor skills. Sara previously excelled in athletics and academic endeavors. Many of these pursuits may not come as easily to Sara after her stroke, and she may become frustrated. Sara should be followed closely for symptoms of anxiety or depression. It is possible that she will benefit from individual psychotherapy. It is also common for teenagers to refuse any technological aid or assistance from others. They are striving to be independent, and it is important for them to appear "normal." Sara may need to be reminded that these various aids and adjustments allow her to be as independent as possible and ultimately to appear as normal as possible. For example, struggling to complete a written assignment with her left hand will be difficult and frustrating. Provision of extra time will allow her to demonstrate what she really knows and to continue to function at her high level. Finally, it is very important for Sara's peers, teachers, and family members to remember that she is a very capable and bright young lady. Her expressive language struggles and right hemiparesis may make it tempting to underestimate her cognitive abilities.

It is helpful for the individualized education program (IEP) team to know the neuroanatomical location of the stroke in order to make effective and appropriate recommendations. The following is a list of common recommendations for children with cognitive damage following a stroke, beyond those already listed for Sara.

## Visual Field Cuts

1. The child should be placed near the front of the classroom on the side where vision was affected. Children with strokes in the right hemisphere of the brain should be placed on the left side of the classroom facing the chalkboard. Children with left-sided strokes should be placed on the right side of the classroom facing the chalkboard.
2. The child's "center placement" for work should align with the unaffected visual field's shoulder. Therefore, classroom assignments and tests for children with right-sided stroke should be aligned with the right shoulder; materials for children with left-sided stroke should be aligned with the left shoulder.
3. When addressing or working next to the child, caregivers should ensure that they are within the field of vision. For children with right-sided stroke, the caregiver should be on the right. For children with left-sided stroke, the caregiver should be on the left. As children mature, they should be proactive in asking others to move into their field of vision.
4. When reading or doing workbook activities, it is useful to mark the edge of the page in the affected field of vision with a ribbon.

## Language Difficulties

Children who have had a left-sided stroke can have a range of receptive and expressive language difficulties. It is important to take the time to ensure that the child fully comprehends information that is important and to give plenty of time for expression of thoughts and ideas. Children who have had a right-sided stroke may have difficulty with speech organization and prosody (i.e., the melody of the voice). If a speech or language disorder is suspected, it is important to have a speech/language evaluation with a speech therapist who has experience with children with neurological deficits.

1. For difficulties with language comprehension, adults should keep several general "rules" in mind while interacting with the child. Eye contact needs to be ensured. A prompt to look at the speaker before directions are presented will be helpful. Keep instructions and directions short, simple, and concrete. Limit requests to single commands and convey as much meaning as possible using a few words, pairing instructions with demonstrations. Break complex tasks down into smaller components or steps. Repeat instructions, and ask the child to repeat what he or she understands. Permit recognition (rather than free recall) of correct responses, and limit the number of possible choices. Incorporate visual and auditory teaching strategies to assist children in learning more effectively. Teachers may consider increasing use of overheads or a chalkboard and drawing attention to the picture cues in textbooks.
2. The child's ability to learn new information will be optimized when the information is presented in both a visual and verbal format. Presenting auditory information in conjunction with pictures, images, patterns, or diagrams will be useful. The child's learning potential can also be increased when information is presented musically or rhythmically.
3. It is important for the child to be given a liberal amount of time to respond. Frequently there is a delay as the child formulates and than executes the cognitive and motor actions of speech. In the classroom, the child should be given alternative methods to demonstrate knowledge instead of an oral presentation or response.

## Nonverbal Difficulties

Children who have had a right-sided stroke may experience difficulty with visuospatial information. This type of information can include chalkboard drawings, maps, diagrams, signs, location directions, facial expressions, and nonverbal gestures. This type of deficit is often not as prominent as language disorders but can be debilitating socially and academically.

1. In helping the child compensate for his or her nonverbal deficits, it is important to praise or emphasize verbal strengths. Whenever possible, information should be conveyed in a verbal format. Instructional procedures should help the child associate verbal labels and descriptions with concrete objects, actions, and experiences. Instructors should model verbal mediation and self-direction (talking out loud) to aid the child in self-monitoring and directing.
2. The child may have difficulty with language that describes space and spatial relationships (i.e., directions in two and three dimensions, shapes, etc.) and may require accurate and flexible interpretations of this vocabulary in varied contexts.
3. To increase nonverbal comprehension of social interaction, the child may require instruction in attending to and interpreting facial expressions, gestures, tone of voice, proximity and distance, status and roles of others, grooming and use of dress, and peer participation. This can be obtained through role-play, by analyzing video tape of real life interaction, or through movie interaction. When the child has mastered some of these interactional skills, a small peer counseling group may serve as a useful forum for him or her to practice and to receive feedback regarding these skills.
4. To increase handwriting skills, encourage the child to write about subjects that are interesting and meaningful. Occupational therapy for improving eye-hand coordination may be necessary.
5. For mathematics problems, provide graph paper to decrease spatial difficulties. In addition, encourage the child to verbalize any internal dialogue regarding the mathematics problem and assist the child in breaking mathematical processes into sequential steps that are mastered one at a time before progressing to the next step.
6. Information that is copied from the chalkboard should be limited, and the teacher should review the written information to ensure accuracy. This is particularly important for homework assignments.

## Emotional and Behavioral Issues

With any acute brain injury, children can experience increased feelings of anxiety, sadness, confusion, frustration, anger, and fear. Children and their families will go through a grieving period for any physical or cognitive losses. Increased impulsivity and emotional sensitivity can also be observed. It is important to monitor these children closely to ensure that these feelings are supported and expressed appropriately and do not become of clinical concern through additional interruptions of the child's quality of life. It is also essential for the family to have an ongoing support system for grieving, information, and respite. These symptoms not only result from the physical and cognitive changes but also are caused by changes in the brain's neurochemistry. Symptoms of concern include lengthy episodes of apathy and sadness, social withdrawal, irritability, sleeplessness, fatigue, self-deprecation, and suicidal ideation. If these symptoms are observed by school personnel, the family should be informed, and the child should receive psychotherapy and perhaps a referral to investigate the possible benefits of psychotropic medication.

## RECOVERY AND NEUROPLASTICITY

Recovery of cognitive and motor skills following a stroke results from multiple factors. Initial spontaneous recovery is first observed with reduction of intracerebral pressure and stabilization of the autonomic system. Over a 1- to 2-year period of time, the brain can reorganize by recruiting other parts of the brain to take the function of the injured part of the brain (this is called neuroplasticity). The brain can continue to organize past that period of time, albeit at a lesser rate. Approximately 60% to 85% of children experience lasting functional deficits and neurological abnormalities poststroke (Sofronas et al., 2006). The brain's ability to reorganize depends on the overall health and development of the child and the volume of the infarction. The Canadian Pediatric Ischemic Stroke Registry is the largest sample of children with stroke (Lynch et al., 2002) and indicated that children whose infarction volume was greater than 10% of the intracranial volume have a worse outcome than children whose infarction was less than 10%. This finding is similar to adult stroke outcome research.

A common misconception regarding neuroplasticity is that the younger the brain, the greater the capacity for plasticity. Although the pediatric brain is in general more plastic than an adult brain, the pediatric brain appears to have critical periods in which the capacity for reorganization fluctuates. Pre- or perinatal strokes can affect the ability to acquire language. It has been suggested that, if an injury occurs prior to or within the critical period for acquiring language, the brain has a greater capacity for reorganization than following this critical period.

Some evidence exists that the visuospatial system is less flexible than the language system. Some studies have found that strokes in the left hemisphere disrupt language, whereas strokes in the right hemisphere disrupt visuospatial skills and attention (Max, 2004). A study contrasting right and left hemisphere stroke deficits found no lateralizing deficits on neuropsychological assessment suggesting brain reorganization. However, the children who experienced a stroke exhibited mild diffuse cognitive deficits when compared to same-age peers (Max).

The final consideration for recovery of cognitive and motor functioning following stroke resides in the child's and family's ability to take advantage of rehabilitation opportunities, maintain good health, and demonstrate good coping skills. A strong body of literature indicates that children who have experienced head trauma with intact families tend to have a better outcome (Wade et al., 2006).

There is evidence that children who receive educational and cognitive rehabilitation poststroke experience a higher level of functioning than those children who did not receive such rehabilitation. Rehabilitation programs target a specific cognitive deficit, such as memory or attention, and teach different strategies for the child to use, thereby increasing cognitive abilities (King, White, McKinstry, Noetzel, & DeBaun, 2007). There are also specific rehabilitation programs addressing motor abilities. One such program is termed *constraint-induced movement therapy*. In a hemiparetic child, the limb with greater function is constrained, forcing the child to use the paretic limb for tasks. The child undergoes intensive training of the affected limb with exercises and also performs "real life" tasks. This therapy has been shown to make a substantial improvement in the affected limb (Taub et al., 2007).

## CASE COMPLETION

Sara was finally ready to leave the hospital. She had worked hard to learn how to walk and speak again. She was doing surprisingly well at using her left hand for handwriting. She felt sad that she was unable to join her lacrosse team, but her teammates had visited her and encouraged her to come to all of their games. Sara was anxious about returning to school. Her speech remained slow and halting, and her gait was slow with a slight right-sided bearing. Her beautiful long hair was now a short, stylish bob. She would need to wear a scarf for a while to cover the site of the replaced skull flap. Her head stitches itched, and she longed to have them removed. Although many of her friends had visited her at the hospital, she was concerned about how she would be perceived by others at school, and whether she could keep up with her classmates. She wondered if she would have a date for the prom and how she could take the college boards.

Three years later, Sara continued to write with her left hand and preferred to type. Her right hand had better motor control, and she was able to eat with her right hand and use it for different activities. Her flow of speech was now fairly normal. When she fatigued, she still had word-finding problems. She worked out on a regular basis at the local gym. Her limp was only evident when she was tired. She was a sophomore at a local college and was interested in working in the medical field. She had a boyfriend and was looking forward to homecoming week.

## SUMMARY

Although pediatric stroke is relatively rare, the stroke's effect on a child and the family is potentially devastating. Academic and rehabilitative intervention are complex and must be specifically designed for each individual based on the type and location of the stroke, the child's and the family's ability to cope with the effects of the stroke and subsequent recovery, the developmental stage of the child, and the resources available to the child and family. Consistent with other acute neurological disorders, stroke intervention and rehabilitation requires a team effort with good communication between the team members (neurologist, pediatrician, pediatric physiatrist, psychologist, rehabilitation therapists, educators, family, classmates, and the child). Although the school's focus in developing an IEP is not for rehabilitation purposes, the IEP must be flexible as the child will experience changes in the first year of recovery. It is highly probable that some deficits will resolve and that new problems will present, requiring quick adjustment to the IEP and response from the educational professionals.

As the child is reintegrated into the school and classroom, the school psychologist may wish to consider age-appropriate interventions for the child's peers. Frequently, the child may appear or act differently, to the consternation of their peers. Sensitive education about strokes or the resulting cognitive and motor deficits may answer questions for the peers and result in an easier transition for the child returning to the classroom. Finally, it is critical that these children and their families be treated with respect and kindness. Recovery from the psychological trauma of the stroke and adaptation to the resulting changes require time and care.

## RESOURCES

American Stroke Association

A division of the American Heart Association, the ASA provides information for families and health care providers about the different aspects of stroke.

Mailing Address: 7272 Greenville Avenue
Dallas, Texas 75231-4596
Phone Number: (888) 478-7653
Web Site: www.strokeassociation.org

Brain Aneurysm Foundation

This group attempts to raise public awareness regarding the early detection and treatment of brain aneurysms through support networks and educational resources.

Mailing Address: 612 East Broadway
South Boston, Massachusetts 02127
Phone Number: (888) 272-4602
Web Site: www.bafound.org

Children's Hemiplegia and Stroke Association (CHASA)

This nonprofit group provides support and information to families of infants, children, and young adults who have experienced a stroke.

Mailing Address: 4101 West Green Oaks
Suite 305, #149
Arlington, Texas 76016
Web Site: www.chasa.org

Hemi-Kids

This group provides online support for children with hemiplegia or hemiplegic cerebral palsy.

Web Site: www.hemikids.org/

National Institute of Neurological Disorders and Stroke (NINDS)

NINDS conducts and supports research on brain and nervous system disorders. The first Web site listed below provides information about the recognition and treatment of stroke in children. The second Web site is a general stroke information page.

Web Sites: www.ninds.nih.gov/news_and_events/proceedings/stroke_proceedings/childneurology.htm
www.ninds.nih.gov/disorders/stroke/stroke.htm

National Stroke Association

This organization's Web site is replete with information about stroke prevention, risk factors, and recovery.

| | |
|---|---|
| Mailing Address: | 9707 East Easter Lane, Suite B<br>Centennial, Colorado 80112-3747 |
| Phone Number: | (800) 787-6537 |
| Web Site: | www.stroke.org |

Pediatric Stroke Center

The Pediatric Stroke Center is a basic Web site to inform families about stroke.

Web Site: www.strokecenter.org/peds/

Pediatric Stroke Network

This group is a nonprofit family support organization. The Web site provides information regarding childhood stroke, effects, rehabilitation techniques, and support information.

Web Site: www.pediatricstrokenetwork.com

## REFERENCES

Beery, K.E., Buktenica, N.A., & Beery, N.A. (2005). *Beery-Buktenica Developmental Test of Visual-Motor Integration* (5th ed.). Lutz, FL: Psychological Assessment Resources.

Blumenfeld, H. (2002). *Neuroanatomy through clinical cases.* Sunderland, MA: Sinauer Associates.

Cohen, M.J. (1997). *Children's Memory Scale.* New York: The Psychological Corporation.

Delis, D., Kaplan, E., & Kramer, J. (2001). *The Delis-Kaplan Executive Function System: Examiner's Manual.* San Antonio, TX: The Psychological Corporation.

deVeber, G. (1999). Cerebrovascular disease in children. In K.F. Swaiman & S. Ashwal (Eds.), *Pediatric neurology: Principles and practice* (pp. 1099–1124). St. Louis, MO: Mosby.

Dunn, L.M., Dunn, L.M., & Dunn, D.M. (1997). *Peabody Picture Vocabulary Test* (3rd ed.). Circle Pines, MN: American Guidance Service.

Jordan, L.C. (2006). Stroke in childhood. *The Neurologist, 12,* 94–102.

Kaplan, E., Goodglass, H., & Weintraub, S. (1983). *Boston Naming Test.* Philadelphia: Lea & Febiger.

King, A.A., White, D.A., McKinstry, R.C., Noetzel, M., & DeBaun, M.R. (2007). A pilot randomized education rehabilitation trial is feasible in sickle cell and strokes. *Neurology, 68,* 2008–2011.

Lynch, J.K., Hirtz, D.G., deVeber, G., & Nelson, K.B. (2002). Report of the National Institute of Neurological Disorders and Stroke workshop on perinatal and childhood stroke. *Pediatrics, 109,* 116–123.

Max, J.D. (2004). Effect of side of lesion on neuropsychological performance in childhood stroke. *Journal of International Neuropsychological Society, 10,* 698–708.

Semel, E., Wigg, E.H., & Secord, W.A. (2003). *Clinical Evaluation of Language Fundamentals* (4th ed.). San Antonio, TX: The Psychological Corporation.

Sheslow, D., & Adams, W. (1990). *Wide Range Assessment of Memory and Learning*. Wilmington, DE: Wide Range.

Sofronas, M., Ichord, R.N., Fullerton, H.J., Lynch, J.K., Massicotte, M.P., Wilan, A.R., et al. (2006). Pediatric stroke initiatives and preliminary studies: What is known and what is needed? *Pediatric Neurology, 34,* 439–445.

Taub, E., Griffin, A., Nick, J., Gammons, K., Uswatte, G., & Law, C.R. (2007). Pediatric CI therapy for stroke-induced hemiparesis in young children. *Developmental Rehabilitation, 10,* 3–18.

Wade, S.L., Taylor, G.H., Yeates, K.O., Drotar, D., Stancin, T., Minich, M., et al. (2006). Long-term parental and family adaptation following pediatric brain injury. *Journal of Pediatric Psychology, 31,* 1072–1083.

Wechsler, D. (2003). *Wechsler Intelligence Scale for Children* (4th ed.). San Antonio, TX: The Psychological Corporation.

Woodcock, R.W., McGrew, K.S., & Mather, N. (2001). *Woodcock-Johnson Tests of Achievement* (3rd ed.). Rolling Meadows, IL: Riverside.

CHAPTER TWENTY ONE

# Traumatic Brain Injury

Dixie J. Woolston, PhD, and
Peter L. Stavinoha, PhD

## DESCRIPTION OF THE DISORDER

### Incidence and Prevalence

Traumatic brain injury (TBI) is the number one cause of death in children and accounts for a significant proportion of childhood disabilities (Kuhtz-Buschbeck, Stolze, Golge, & Ritz, 2003). Each year, more than 1 million children sustain a TBI, and over 30,000 of those children become permanently disabled (Hooper et al., 2004). Approximately 1 in 30 children will have sustained a TBI by the age of 21 (Chiu Wong et al., 2006). The annual incidence is estimated to be 180 per 100,000 in children younger than 15 years (Ylvisaker & Feeney, 2007). The highest risk for childhood TBI occurs between birth and 4 years of age, and between 15 and 19 years of age (Centers for Disease Control and Prevention [CDC], 2007). These numbers may underestimate the incidence and prevalence of TBI, as some children may not be documented and/or diagnosed (i.e., they are simply discharged from an urgent care clinic setting) or may never be seen by any medical providers following an injury (Hooper et al.).

### Etiology and Underlying Causes

TBIs occur when the brain is penetrated by an object (i.e., a gunshot wound), when a trauma causes rapid acceleration or deceleration of the brain (i.e., whiplash, when babies are shaken), or when objects strike the head (i.e., falls, physical assault). Competitive contact sports (i.e., football, boxing, wrestling, ice hockey, soccer) and even snow sports carry a risk of acute TBI (Hooper et al., 2004). According to the CDC (2007), the leading causes of TBI are falls (28%); motor vehicle-traffic collisions (20%); being struck by/against objects, including colliding with a stationary or moving object (19%); and assaults (11%).

Young school-age children are most likely to sustain a TBI due to falls, bicycle accidents, and other types of transportation-associated injuries (Keenan & Bratton, 2006). Specifically, young school-age children are likely to be injured in motor vehicle collisions as a result of low utilization of appropriate booster seats and safety restraints. This age group also is likely to sustain a pedestrian injury because young children may dart out into traffic and cross the street unsafely (Hameed, Popkin, Cohn, & Johnson, 2004; Nadler, Courcoulas, Gardner, & Ford, 2001). Similar to younger children, adolescents are at increased risk for a TBI due to motor vehicle accidents. However, older children's risk of head injury because of pedestrian-related incidents is decreased, whereas risk of head injury via sporting injuries increases dramatically (Agran, Winn, Anderson, Trent, & Walton-Haynes, 2001; Keenan & Bratton). Due to the multiple etiologies and variable ways in which the brain is damaged, there are many types and combinations of TBI. Open head injuries occur when the skull has been fractured or split open, or when the brain has been pierced by an object. Closed head injuries occur when the brain is bruised or bumped inside of the skull, and the injury occurs because the brain is rapidly changing speed and direction. See Table 21.1 for a brief definition of common types of brain injuries.

## FACTORS AFFECTING NEUROPSYCHOLOGICAL OUTCOME

### Injury-Related Factors

#### *Injury Severity*

One of the main factors affecting neuropsychological outcome following TBI is injury severity. The most common means of determining injury severity is through the use of the Glasgow Coma Scale (GCS; Teasdale & Jennett, 1974). Essentially, the scale measures an individual's level of

**TABLE 21.1 Common Types of Brain Injuries**

| | |
|---|---|
| Diffuse ischemic injury | Occurs when the gray matter in the brain, which consists of neurons, is injured. |
| Contusion | Bruising of the brain due to trauma or blood leaks. |
| Coup-contrecoup injury | This initial impact of the brain against the skull is called the coup injury. The force of the initial impact is sometimes strong enough to cause the brain to bounce back and hit the opposite side of the skull, resulting in an injury on the opposite side from where the head hit an object. This injury on the opposite side is called the contrecoup injury. |
| Hematoma | Occurs when blood leaks onto the surface of the brain. |
| Concussion | A blow to the head that may result in unconsciousness and microscopic shearing of nerve fibers that are usually undetected by neuroimaging techniques (such as a CT or MRI brain scan). |
| Anoxia/hypoxia | These words relate to oxygen supply to the brain. A period of anoxia indicates brain cells were receiving no oxygen (like being submerged in water). Hypoxia indicates brain cells had a reduced, insufficient oxygen supply (this could happen during a fire). Both anoxia and hypoxia result in brain cell death due to the lack of oxygen. |
| Focal injury | The brain damage done by the injury is relatively confined to the site(s) of impact or contusion. |
| Diffuse injury | This is indicative of global brain dysfunction and is generally the result of diffuse ischemic injury, diffuse axonal injury, and/or severe brain swelling. |

*Note.* The information in this figure was created by Dixie J. Woolston and Peter L. Stavinoha for an internal brochure for the Brain and Nerve Injury Center at Children's Medical Center Dallas, 2005.

consciousness on a scale from 3 to 15 by assessing eye movements (rated from "does not open eyes" to "opens eyes spontaneously"), motor functioning (rated from "makes no movements" to "follows commands"), and verbal output (rated from "makes no sounds" to "converses normally"). A score of 3 on the GCS indicates death or deep coma, and a score of 15 indicates a fully awake and conscious individual. A mild TBI is usually defined as a GCS score of 13 to 15 with no abnormal findings on neuroimaging. A moderate TBI is a GCS score of 9 to 12; children with a GCS score of less than 8 are considered to have sustained a severe TBI (Bishop, 2006; Chung et al., 2006; Keenan & Bratton, 2006). Although the GCS is commonly used to assess brain injury severity, the GCS has been criticized for inaccurately predicting cognitive outcomes in the pediatric population. Thus, time to first motor response and number of visible lesions on neuroimaging are being explored as improved predictors of neurocognitive outcome (Bishop; Taylor, 2004).

Another instrument that is commonly used to predict outcome following a head injury is the Rancho Los Amigos Levels of Cognitive Function Scale (LCFS; Hagen, Malkmus, & Durham, 1979). The revised version of the scale ranks the individual's levels of cognitive functioning on a numerical scale from I to X, with I indicating "No Response: Total Assistance" when the individual is presented with visual, auditory, tactile, proprioceptive, vestibular, or painful stimuli. A score of X indicates that the individual can handle multiple tasks simultaneously, initiate and carry out familiar and unfamiliar tasks, think independently about the consequences of decisions or actions, and recognize the needs and feelings of others and respond appropriately. Although the individual can independently perform the tasks listed above (as well as others listed in the scale criteria), he or she may still require additional time, periodic breaks, and other accommodations and modifications. Thus, a score of X indicates the individual has "Purposeful, Appropriate: Modified Independent" levels of cognition.

Notwithstanding the problems with defining injury severity and predicting outcome, in general, milder TBIs (or higher scores on the GCS) are associated with better neuropsychological outcomes and postinjury functioning (Chung et al., 2006; Taylor et al., 2002; Yeates et al., 2002). A long-term study examining the neuropsychological function in a group of patients 25 years after they sustained minor head injuries as children and adolescents found that injury severity was significantly related to neuropsychological functioning, indicating that even mild pediatric head injury may increase the chances of developing neurocognitive impairments later in life (Hessen, Nestvold, & Sundet, 2006).

Even though mild TBIs (including concussions and terms like subtle, minor, or minimal brain injury) are thought to have better outcomes and fewer long-term effects than moderate or severe head injuries, research indicates these children still experience physical, cognitive, and behavioral symptoms (Cook, Schweer, Shebesta, Hartjes, & Falcone, 2006). For instance, children may report physical complaints such as headaches, dizziness, nausea, vomiting, hypersensitivity to light or noise, blurry vision, fatigue, and sleep problems. Cognitively, children with mild brain injuries may experience decreased concentration, memory dysfunction, and trouble with multitasking, organizing information, or engaging in complex thought processes. Behaviorally, following a mild brain injury, children may have increased irritability, lack of emotional control, anxiety, depression, or posttraumatic stress disorder. These symptoms usually remit within the first 3 months following injury but may persist beyond 6 months postinjury (Gordon, 2006; Hessen et al., 2006; Keenan & Bratton, 2006; Khoshyomn & Tranmer, 2004). Thus, school reeentry immediately after a concussion or mild brain injury can be problematic in the acute stages of recovery. In fact, research indicates that children with mild injuries manifested more school-related behavioral problems and learning difficulties 4 months after injury compared to 1 month after injury, suggesting that the recovery process and school reentry following a TBI requires ongoing, long-term follow-up (Hooper et al., 2004).

### *Secondary Brain Injuries*

Research has shown other injury-related factors to be important in predicting neuropsychological outcome. Hessen and colleagues ( 2006), in their study looking at individuals 25 years after sustaining a "minor" TBI during childhood or adolescence, found that the most important predictors of neuropsychological outcome were length of posttraumatic amnesia at injury, electroencephalography (EEG) pathology, and loss of consciousness at injury. In addition, secondary brain injury often occurs following the initial TBI. For instance, after being injured, the brain releases toxic metabolites, which then cause adjacent brain areas to swell. This edema of the brain can cause further neurological deterioration and possible herniation (Bishop, 2006). Neurosurgical intervention may be required to release the pressure on the brain and reduce the risk of herniation, which unfortunately increases the risk of further complications, leading to a poorer outcome (Khoshyomn & Tranmer, 2004).

Secondary brain injury also may occur if the child experiences posttraumatic seizures following the initial TBI, as seizures increase intracranial pressure and metabolic demands on the brain (Formisano et al., 2007). Research indicates that 10% to 20% of children with severe TBI develop recurrent, spontaneous, chronic seizures, known as posttraumatic epilepsy. Unfortunately, medical management may not reduce seizure activity altogether, and children who develop posttraumatic epilepsy have worse functional outcomes (Statler, 2006). Other mechanisms of secondary brain injury include cerebral blood flow dysregulation, excitotoxicity (i.e., brain cell death), apoptosis (i.e., DNA disruption that leads to cell death), necrosis (i.e., cellular swelling and breaking that leads to cell death), and inflammation (Bishop, 2006).

Another important injury-related predictor of outcome is intracranial hypertension. Increased risk for death is seen in pediatric patients with intracranial pressures persistently greater than 20 mmHG (Jankowitz & Adelson, 2006). If the patient survives, long-term neurological impairment may occur due to the extensive exposure of the injured and healthy brain areas to hypoperfusion (i.e., lack of oxygen or reduced delivery of oxygen to brain areas).

### *Injury Location*

Another factor affecting neuropsychological outcome is which part of the brain has been injured, as different brain areas have different neurocognitive functions. Although an exhaustive description of brain locations and functions is beyond the scope of this chapter, a few general principles are presented in Table 21.2.

The human brain is about the size of two fists put together and rests in the skull cushioned by cerebrospinal fluid (CSF). When the brain is injured due to rapid acceleration/deceleration (like in a car crash), the most vulnerable sites of injury are the inferior frontal and temporal areas, as the brain may impact the bony skull in these regions and can be sheared (i.e., torn) and/or bruised during this type of injury (Khoshyomn & Tranmer, 2004). Further, volumetric analyses showed that, following moderate to severe TBI, children had significantly reduced whole brain and prefrontal and temporal volumes compared to uninjured children, and that larger volumetric measures of preserved tissue predicted better recovery (Wilde et al., 2005). Therefore, common neuropsychological sequelae reported after a brain injury are often related to the cognitive functions/systems located in the frontotemporal regions (Yeates et al., 2004). Frequent cognitive symptoms following this type of injury include memory impairment, reduced social competence, difficulty solvng problems, decreased attention/concentration, trouble organizing, impaired mental flexibility, slowed processing speed, and lack of impulse and/or emotional control (Brenner et al., 2007; Hawley, Ward, Magnay, & Long, 2002; Hooper et al., 2004; Yeates et al.).

**TABLE 21.2 Abilities and Functions Related to Brain Areas**

| | |
|---|---|
| Hemispheric dominance | The brain is conceptually divided into dominant and nondominant sides, or hemispheres. If speech and language are located on the left side of the brain, then the left side is considered the dominant hemisphere. The nondominant hemisphere is thought to have primarily nonlanguage functions, such as spatial awareness and visual reasoning. Most children and adults are left-hemisphere dominant. Thus, if the dominant side is injured, language skills may be affected. |
| Frontal lobes | This area of the brain is involved with higher order cognitive functions like problem solving, attention, prioritizing, planning, expressive language, and motor skills. The frontal lobes also help regulate emotion and personality features. |
| Parietal lobes | This area is associated with visual/spatial skills, sensation (touch), awareness of body position in relation to physical environment, and other nonverbal reasoning skills. |
| Temporal lobes | The primary functions of the temporal lobes include memory, language comprehension, and auditory processing. |
| Occipital lobes | The primary functions of the occipital lobes are vision and interpretation of visual information. |
| Cerebellum | The cerebellum is known principally for controlling coordination and balance of movement. However, it also has extensive connections to all areas of the brain. Damage to the cerebellum can have a significant impact on cognitive functions, such as working memory, mental rotation, and speech fluency. |
| Brain stem | The brain stem is responsible for basic, vital life functions such as heart rate, breathing, temperature, blood pressure, and alertness |

*Note.* The information in this figure was created by Dixie J. Woolston and Peter L. Stavinoha for an internal brochure for the Brain and Nerve Injury Center at Children's Medical Center Dallas, 2005.

## Other Variables Affecting Outcome

### *Premorbid Functioning*

Premorbid functioning, or level of functioning prior to the injury, has been another factor thought to mediate outcome following a TBI. Many studies have shown that recovery of abilities, academic success, and overall levels of functioning are better in individuals who had high preinjury academic ability and levels of functioning (Catroppa & Anderson, 2007; Ewing-Cobbs et al., 2004). Premorbid learning and behavior problems increase the risk of a poor outcome following a TBI (Taylor, 2004; Wechsler, Kim, Gallagher, DiScala, & Stineman, 2005).

### *Age at Time of Injury*

Age may be another factor affecting outcome. Young children may be more likely to sustain a head injury due to a thinner skull, larger space within the skull for the brain to move freely, weaker neck muscles, and a larger head-to-body ratio (Cook et al., 2006). In addition, because children have less myelin (i.e., protective cover for the brain's axons, or communication fibers), they may be more likely to sustain a severe diffuse axonal injury. Despite the theory that the developing brain has greater potential for recovery and more plasticity compared to the adult brain, research indicates that brain injuries at an earlier age may, in fact, be more detrimental, as the development of neural networks that support higher cognitive functioning may be permanently disrupted (Chiu Wong et al., 2006; Ewing-Cobbs et al., 2004). Therefore, cognitive and behavioral deficits related to an early childhood injury may emerge as development and maturation unfold, leading to latent effects of a TBI sustained in early childhood.

### *Recently Acquired Academic Skills*

Competencies that were just emerging prior to the injury and the acquisition of new skills after the injury may be especially vulnerable to disruption from TBI (Brenner et al., 2007). Ewing-Cobbs and colleagues (2004) performed a prospective longitudinal study looking at academic achievement from baseline to 5 years after a TBI. They found that younger children had a deceleration in their academic learning curve, lending support to the hypothesis that early brain injuries disrupt the acquisition of some abilities. Slomine and colleagues (2002) found that younger children displayed greater deficits on measures of executive functioning than older children, even when controlling for attention-deficit/hyperactivity disorder (ADHD) and brain injury variables. Pediatric TBI can lead to persistent neuropsychological and behavioral impairments and adjustment issues in the arenas of intellectual, academic, social, personality, and adaptive functioning (Hawley et al., 2002; Schwartz et al., 2003). Children with TBIs may be at more risk for developmentally related impairments throughout their life span, suggesting the need for long-term management and interventions (Brenner et al.).

### *Additional Injuries*

It is common for children suffering a TBI to have multiple other physical injuries as well, such as broken bones, abdominal injuries, bruised kidneys, and internal organ dysfunction, among others. The presence of severe organ injuries in addition to a brain injury increases the risk of poor outcome. Cardiopulmonary resuscitation (CPR) at the time of injury also is associated with worse outcomes (Bishop, 2006).

## Related Biopsychosocial Issues

### *ADHD*

A common sequela of TBI is the development of symptoms of ADHD or the worsening of preexisting ADHD symptoms (Max et al., 2004). Max and colleagues demonstrated that almost one-third of the children with a severe TBI developed ADHD, and other researchers have found that 16% to 19% of children sustaining a moderate-to-severe TBI met full ADHD diagnostic criteria (Bloom et al., 2001; Max et al., 2005). Thus, the presence of ADHD may exacerbate or contribute to the behavioral and cognitive impairments of a child with a TBI and may further impede successful school reentry and other rehabilitation efforts.

### *Development of Psychiatric Disorders*

Emotionally, children who have sustained TBIs may be more vulnerable to developing psychiatric disorders such as depression and anxiety (Bloom et al., 2001; Hooper et al., 2004; Luis & Mittenberg, 2002). Kirkwood and colleagues (2000) found increased rates of depression in children following a TBI. Other commonly reported emotional problems include temper outbursts, staring spells, and symptoms of posttraumatic stress disorder. Reported rates of new-onset psychiatric illness in children approximately 1 year after injury varied from 20% (Hooper et al.) to 60% (Bloom et al.). Further, these research studies indicated that some psychological sequelae (particularly ADHD and anxiety disorders) following a TBI tended to be persistent and refractory to treatment.

### *Persistent Behavior Problems*

Many studies have shown that children who sustain severe TBI are more likely to develop behavior problems. Further, these behavioral issues are likely to be persistent and difficult to modify (Bloom et al., 2001; Schwartz et al., 2003). Other risk factors for developing postinjury behavioral problems include social disadvantages and preinjury behavioral concerns. Schwartz and colleagues also found an association between increased behavioral symptoms and greater postinjury family distress and burdens. It is interesting that the above study did not find strong correlations between neuropsychological testing and behavioral problems, indicating a need for the development of more specific assessment instruments and procedures to examine behavioral correlates and outcomes over time following a TBI.

### *Social Outcomes*

Children with TBI often have poor social outcomes, with severely injured children demonstrating decreased social competency (Yeates et al., 2004). This may result from the vulnerability of frontotemporal regions to injury (discussed above), as these areas have been implicated in the "social circuit" of the brain. Poor social outcomes may further be related to executive functioning deficits and decreased pragmatic and discourse language skills (Dennis, Guger, Roncadin, Barnes, & Schachar, 2001). In addition, the family environment may moderate social outcome following TBI (Yeates et al., 2004), though social deficits evident 1 year after injury tended to persist.

### *Headaches*

Neurologically, headaches are a persistent complaint following a TBI, with moderate to severe headaches reported even 10 months after injury (Hooper et al., 2004). Guidelines for mild TBIs and management of headaches include sleep and nutrition recommendations, namely encouraging eight glasses of fluids per day and use of acetaminophen as opposed to ibuprofen for pain. Ibuprofen is not recommended due to the potential for rebound headaches and withdrawal (Cook et al., 2006).

### *Sleep Issues*

Another neurological problem that has been the focus of recent studies has been disturbed sleep and nocturnal effects following a TBI. Many caregivers report increased problems with fatigue, trouble sleeping, daytime sleepiness, increased nightmares, talking or walking in sleep, and bed-wetting problems in their children, especially following a severe TBI (Beebe et al., 2007). Although sleep-related clinical guidelines have been developed for adults following brain injuries, procedures have not yet been developed for the pediatric population.

### *Decreased Mobility/Balance*

Many children experience mobility issues following a TBI such as decreased balance, poor coordination, and a reduction in abilities to walk or run (Gagnon, Swaine, Friedman, & Forget, 2004; Hawley et al., 2002). Children who have sustained a TBI often have trouble with gait, which may be characterized by asymmetry in step lengths and increased foot rotation. Decreased balance and gait disturbance often place children at risk for falling, which increases their risk of sustaining an additional TBI. Thus, these types of deficits should be taken into consideration when transitioning back to school, particularly in determining the appropriateness of participating in physical activities (Gagnon et al.). Some trauma centers offer postural stability testing, which can determine whether the individual is ready to return to sports. Sometimes a more comprehensive evaluation at a rehabilitation or sports medicine clinic may be indicated, which can help optimize recovery in athletes (Cook et al., 2006). In addition, the child may need to receive physical therapy, occupational therapy, or adapted physical education via the school.

### *School Transition Following the Injury*

Findings from recent research (Ewing-Cobbs et al., 2004; Hooper et al., 2004) indicate the need for school personnel to be involved in the student's transition back to school, beginning in the early phases of recovery from a brain injury. This research also suggests the need for school personnel to monitor the child's progress long-term, as Hooper and colleagues found an increase in behavioral issues evident at school and the emergence of new learning difficulties occurring 4 months after injury. Thus, it is critical to develop procedures and programs to assist and monitor a child's transition back to the school setting following even a mild TBI.

## Case Study

As mechanisms and outcomes of TBIs are extremely variable, a definitive neuropsychological profile of pediatric brain injury does not exist. The following case was selected as it represents many of the issues that patients, families, and school/medical personnel face when facilitating an individual's recovery from TBI.

## Background and Demographic Information

Chris is a 13-year-old left-handed White male referred for neuropsychological evaluation to assess his current cognitive functioning 6 months after sustaining a TBI. Prior to his injury, Chris was an above-average student, and his parents reported no significant preexisting behavioral or emotional symptoms.

Chris was participating in motorcross with full protective gear (including a helmet) when he lost control of the motorcycle and flipped over the handlebars, landing face-first on the ground. His initial GCS score was 3. He was rapidly intubated at the scene and flown to a pediatric trauma center. Initial brain imaging showed multifocal and diffuse axonal injury (DAI), with many areas of cortical contusion (i.e., brain bleeding and swelling). After a month of inpatient hospitalization, Chris was transferred to a pediatric rehabilitation center. Brain imaging 2 weeks after discharge showed generalized volume loss and gliosis (i.e., a proliferation of cells that accumulate in areas of the brain where damage has occurred) involving the left basal ganglia, orbital surface of the left frontal lobe, and the left temporal lobe.

After completing 8 weeks of rehabilitation, his family transferred him to a specialty day treatment center for an additional 8 weeks of intense cognitive, physical, occupational, speech, and educational rehabilitation. Following that, Chris attended daily intensive physical, occupational, and speech therapies on an outpatient basis.

Physical symptoms at the time of evaluation included hemiparesis (i.e., weakness) of his right arm and leg and a significant right visual field cut (i.e., unable to see things on the right). He was easily fatigued and slept at least 11 hours a night in addition to daily 1- to 2-hour naps. Chris's father also reported that he had an increased sensitivity to noise and decreased pain tolerance. Cognitively, his parents reported increased distractibility, decreased processing speed, word-finding trouble, and memory deficits. Regarding emotions, they indicated that Chris was more impulsive, impatient, and overly friendly than he was before. For example, during a rehabilitation session, Chris ran up to an unfamiliar nurse and exclaimed, "I want to touch your head" and proceeded to rub the nurse's head. His physical therapist reported that Chris had a "short fuse," acted out frequently during sessions, and had a tendency to talk about inappropriate subjects (e.g., commenting about sexual attributes of the women who worked at the facility).

Essentially, Chris sustained extensive DAI with left cerebral hemorrhaging (i.e., bleeding). DAI occurs when axons shear and tear because of rapid acceleration or deceleration of the brain. Axons are long, thin nerve fibers that connect different parts of the brain. These axonal tracks are critical to brain communication, and DAI can result in global brain dysfunction due to the broad nature of the damage. In Chris's case, the shearing and tearing was significantly worse on the left side of the brain, which explains his right extremity weakness and right visual field cut.

At the time of the neuropsychological evaluation, Chris had not returned to school. However, he was on homebound status, and a teacher came to his home 5 days a week for 2 hours a day. The teacher reported concerns regarding Chris's decreased stamina, poor attention, temper outbursts, and reduced social skills, indicating that these issues would impede his ability to be successful in the school environment.

## Behavioral Observations

Chris appeared somewhat small for his age and was appropriately groomed. Hearing and vision were adequate for testing purposes. Even though the examiner made sure to place visual stimuli in his field of view, Chris continued to neglect some stimuli on the right side of the page and did not use his right arm during the testing session. Chris was left-handed, and his pencil grip was awkward. His gait was extremely unsteady, and he tended to swing his right leg. He required cues to maintain conversation with the examiner and needed frequent repetition. Chris became overwhelmed with complex instructions, and the examiner frequently had to repeat or clarify standardized directions. His skills at initiating and maintaining conversation were below expectations for his age. He made some inappropriate comments during testing such as, "The chicks on the fourth floor are cool and they have nice knockers!" He was frequently distracted but usually responded appropriately to redirection. He needed additional prompting when he was tired. Overall, he was cooperative and put forth adequate effort, and these results are thought to be representative of his cognitive and emotional functioning at the time of the evaluation.

## Test Results

For a review of specific test scores, please refer to Tables 21.3 and 21.4. In brief, Chris's performance was impaired in nearly all neurocognitive domains assessed (memory, attention, processing speed, and executive functioning), except for aspects of language. Chris's intellectual functioning was in the low average to average range, which most likely represented a decline from suspected premorbid above-average functioning. His academic aptitude was low average to average, suggesting that Chris benefited from his intensive outpatient therapies, educational experiences, and efforts from his parents to promote cognitive rehabilitation since his injury. However, Chris evidenced a severe deficit in processing speed and significant fluctuations in attention. His performance tended to suffer under time pressure, which was noted particularly in his academic abilities, as his performance dropped from average to moderately impaired when under time constraints. These deficits in attention, processing speed, memory, and executive functioning are consistent with an individual who suffered a moderate-to-severe TBI. In terms of emotional functioning, as measured by parent questionnaires and clinical interview, Chris's parents did not report any significant problems except for attention difficulties and impulsive behavior.

## RECOMMENDATIONS AND INTERVENTIONS

### Case-Specific Interventions

One of the most devastating consequences of TBI is that some problems and symptoms persist and may never entirely remit, even under the best of conditions. Thus, most interventions will not be a panacea; instead, they are targeted to manage and/or improve residual issues from the injury. With regard to Chris, at the outset, he will benefit from a full individual evaluation (FIE) and will need to be evaluated for special education services as an individual who suffered a TBI. Some suggestions to consider when designing a plan for Chris's transition back to home and school are listed below.

#### *Impulsivity and Inhibition*

Chris continued to behave very impulsively and appeared to lack social "brakes" or inhibition. It is important to understand that this is a common sequela of a brain injury, especially the type of frontal lobe damage that Chris sustained. However, it is crucial that Chris be redirected and/or have consequences for inappropriate behavior, and his parents were advised that they would have to be very consistent in how they handle Chris when he makes inappropriate comments or acts out impulsively. For instance, if Chris uses an inappropriate word, it will be important to correct him each time he does it and to establish a consequence for the behavior. It will also be important to provide Chris with positive reinforcement and rewards for improved behavior. The *Love and Logic* books,

**TABLE 21.3 Neuropsychological Testing Data**

| Scale | Scaled Score | T Score | Standard Score |
|---|---|---|---|
| Wechsler Intelligence Scale for Children—Fourth Edition | | | |
| Full Scale IQ | | | 75 |
| General Ability index | | | 87 |
| Verbal Comprehension index | | | 87 |
| Perceptual Reasoning index | | | 88 |
| Working Memory index | | | 91 |
| Processing Speed index | | | 50 |
| Woodcock-Johnson Tests of Achievement—Third Edition | | | |
| Letter-Word Identification | | | 88 |
| Reading Fluency | | | 72 |
| Understanding Directions | | | 83 |
| Calculations | | | 94 |
| Math Fluency | | | 67 |
| Spelling | | | 108 |
| Writing Fluency | | | 66 |
| Passage Comprehension | | | 85 |
| Applied Problems | | | 86 |
| California Verbal Learning Test—Children's Version | | | |
| List A Total Trials 1–5 | | 23 | |
| List A Trial 1 Free Recall | | 35 | |
| List A Trial 5 Free Recall | | 20 | |
| List B Free Recall | | 45 | |
| List A Short-Delay Free Recall | | 20 | |
| List A Short-Delay Cued Recall | | 25 | |
| List A Long-Delay Free Recall | | 25 | |
| List A Long-Delay Cued Recall | | 30 | |
| Recognition | | 45 | |

*Continued*

**TABLE 21.3** *(Continued)*

| Scale | Scaled Score | T Score | Standard Score |
|---|---|---|---|
| | Children's Memory Scale | | |
| Stories Immediate | 4 | | |
| Stories Delayed | 5 | | |
| Stories Delayed Recognition | 8 | | |
| Family Pictures Immediate | 1 | | |
| Family Pictures Delayed | 1 | | |
| Dot Locations Learning | 9 | | |
| Dot Locations Total Score | 8 | | |
| Dot Locations Long Delay | 8 | | |
| | Delis-Kaplan Executive Function System | | |
| Verbal Fluency Test | | | |
| Letter Fluency | 9 | | |
| Category Fluency | 6 | | |
| Total Switching Accuracy | 8 | | |
| Color-Word Interference Test | | | |
| Color Naming | 1 | | |
| Word Reading | 1 | | |
| Inhibition | 1 | | |
| Inhibition/Switching | 1 | | |
| | Trail Making Test | | |
| Form A | | <13 | |
| Form B | | <13 | |

*Note.* California Verbal Learning Test—Children's Version (CVLT-C; Delis, Kramer, Kaplan, & Ober, 1994); Children's Memory Scale (CMS; Cohen, 1997); Delis-Kaplan Executive Function System (D-KEFS; Delis, Kaplan, & Kramer, 2001); Trail Making Test (Reitan, 1971); Wechsler Intelligence Scale for Children—Fourth Edition (WISC-IV; Wechsler, 2003); Woodcock-Johnson Tests of Achievement—Third Edition (WJ-III; Woodcock, McGrew, & Mather, 2001).

**TABLE 21.4 T Scores From Parent and Teacher Ratings of Behavioral and Emotional Functioning**

| Scale | Parent | Teacher |
|---|---|---|
| Behavior Assessment System for Children—Second Edition | | |
| Externalizing Problems | 49 | 55 |
| Hyperactivity | 64 | 66 |
| Aggression | 42 | 48 |
| Conduct Problems | 41 | 49 |
| Internalizing Problems | 37 | 48 |
| Anxiety | 38 | 46 |
| Depression | 39 | 53 |
| Somatization | 41 | 47 |
| Behavioral Symptoms Index | 54 | 59 |
| Atypicality | 55 | 65 |
| Withdrawal | 45 | 47 |
| Attention Problems | 41 | 64 |
| School Problems | | 61 |
| Learning Problems | | 57 |
| Adaptive Skills | 42 | 41 |
| Adaptability | 55 | 39 |
| Social Skills | 45 | 42 |
| Leadership | 41 | 44 |
| Activities of Daily Living | 36 | |
| Functional Communication | 41 | 44 |
| Study Skills | | 41 |
| Behavior Rating Inventory of Executive Function | | |
| Behavioral Regulation Index | 61 | 77 |
| Inhibit | 78 | 78 |
| Shift | 59 | 77 |
| Emotional Control | 40 | 66 |
| Metacognition Index | 61 | 69 |

*Continued*

**TABLE 21.4** *(Continued)*

| Scale | Parent | Teacher |
|---|---|---|
| Initiate | 56 | 66 |
| Working Memory | 71 | 71 |
| Plan/Organize | 53 | 66 |
| Organization of Materials | 57 | 64 |
| Monitor | 63 | 69 |
| General Executive Composite | 62 | 73 |

*Note.* Behavior Assessment System for Children—Second Edition (BASC-2; Reynolds & Kamphaus, 2004); Behavior Rating Inventory of Executive Function (BRIEF; Gioia, Isquith, Guy, & Kenworthy, 2000).

workshops, and/or online material (http://www.loveandlogic.com) may be helpful in generating ideas for optimizing Chris's behavior.

Chris is also evidencing impulsivity and trouble with inhibition and social judgment due to his head injury. As a result, it is recommended that the school have a behavioral intervention plan (BIP) in place for Chris. Although these behaviors are a result of his injury and are not Chris's fault, the school should have consequences for his inappropriate behavior. This will help him become more functional socially, as a behavior plan will help manage his problem behaviors by minimizing and containing disruptions and potentially extinguishing some behaviors. The school should reward Chris's progress and encourage/reinforce positive behaviors. Developing a behavior intervention plan for Chris will require a functional behavior assessment (FBA), which should be completed as soon as possible to identify specific problematic behaviors and develop strategies for managing those behaviors.

### *Organization*

As Chris has a difficult time with planning and organization, his family is encouraged to create a very structured environment. For instance, they should designate a specific place for Chris's personal items and train him to always put things back in their proper place. His parents may want to use a basket or bin system with clearly marked labels/pictures of what goes where. Making his schedule very routine (i.e., keeping it the same as much as possible) will also be beneficial. Chris will benefit from learning to write down important information and developing the skill of utilizing an agenda/day planner. These suggestions will help him develop compensatory strategies for his poor organizational skills.

### *Academic Issues*

It is recommended that Chris not be timed when taking tests and that his teachers allow him extra time to complete his homework and projects. His teachers may need to reduce the number of items when testing Chris (i.e., completing only the odd- or even-numbered items), as it will take him much longer to complete problems and questions than his classmates. Possible strategies to assist Chris include reading the test problems to him and allowing him to provide oral answers rather than written responses. Chris should be provided a place free of distraction when taking tests.

The school should modify or reduce his assignment load, for example, by giving Chris 5 math problems instead of 20, identifying how long it takes him to complete those problems, and then adjusting accordingly. Similarly reading, writing, and other assignments should be reduced. Chris's teachers should coordinate their efforts so that he has no more than 60 minutes of homework daily. Also, his teachers should avoid sending home unfinished schoolwork in addition to homework. It is most important that his teachers help Chris avoid frustration by assigning him homework graded to his capabilities.

### *Language Functioning*

Chris evidenced mild word-finding problems in the evaluation. Therefore, the school should perform a speech and language evaluation to determine whether Chris would benefit from speech therapy at school. If school speech therapy services are provided, the school therapist should coordinate with his outpatient speech therapist to ensure Chris's goals are consistent between the two settings.

### *Gross Motor Functioning*

Chris's gait is extremely unsteady, and he may be at risk for falling. The school's physical therapist should evaluate Chris and his safety in the school environment and make recommendations, accommodations, and/or modifications to help prevent Chris from falling and sustaining any further injuries. Coordination is encouraged between his school physical therapist and private therapist.

### *Fine Motor Functioning*

The school should assess whether occupational therapy would be indicated for Chris. If therapy is provided, coordination between Chris's school occupational therapist and private therapist is encouraged.

### *Memory*

Chris has trouble remembering things and will need to learn compensatory strategies to overcome his memory problems. To compensate for memory deficits, Chris's family and teachers are encouraged to play games that require him to remember things. Some examples of appropriate games include memory/concentration games, Clue™, and/or Cranium educational games (http://www.cranium.com) like Zigity™. Chris may need to have open-book tests or an extra study hour to review materials before taking exams, especially in subjects like science that require knowledge of memorized material. He may need to be provided with copies of the teacher's lecture notes or presentation slides to allow for extra review of the material covered in the class.

### *Attention and Multitasking*

Chris evidenced deficits in attention and multitasking. His parents and teachers should help him perform tasks one at a time, break projects down into small steps, and find ways to self-structure by creating prioritized lists, timelines, and reminder cards and by using an agenda or daily planner. Using a ruler or other device to "frame" his attention on part of a worksheet or problem may also be beneficial. Chris may need to be paired with an attentive, organized peer when working on group assignments to increase his efficiency. In addition, when others are communicating with him, they may need to use brief statements and ask Chris to repeat back what he has heard/understood.

### *Social and Emotional Functioning*

Chris is in the process of adjusting to new weaknesses as the result of his brain injury. As a result, he may find his return to school incredibly frustrating, as some tasks that he was easily able to perform before his head injury may now be difficult for him. Emotionally, this can be an extremely rocky time. Chris's teachers and parents should monitor his emotional adjustment. He may be at risk for depression and/or anxiety due to his TBI, as his deficits may become more apparent to him in the classroom setting than in his home or rehabilitation settings. It may be helpful to designate a "safe area" in the class or school for Chris to go if he becomes overwhelmed or frustrated.

### *Instructional Setting*

Chris should be placed in a class with a low teacher/student ratio whenever possible. This may be achieved through activities such as placing him in small groups and/or pairing him with an attentive peer. As Chris has a visual field cut, he should sit in the front row of the class to the far right. This will minimize the impact of his visual impairment.

## General Recommendations

The recommendations listed above were specific to Chris's case. As he experienced a devastating severe head injury, he required multifaceted interventions to help with the complex cognitive, physical, and socio-emotional sequelae from his TBI. Chris's case was unique in that he was able to participate in many levels of rehabilitative services after discharge from the hospital to facilitate his recovery. However, many children do not have the advantages that Chris had, and the following are some general recommendations for any child that experiences a TBI.

### *Information Dissemination*

One extensive study (Hawley et al., 2002) in the United Kingdom found that fewer than two-thirds of the parents of children with moderate to severe TBIs received information about the difficulties their child might experience after the brain injury. Parents commonly requested information on long-term effects, symptoms to monitor, and additional resources and services to facilitate recovery from a TBI. Team conferences while the child is hospitalized may minimize confusion and decrease inconsistencies in information from various medical providers. Families and patients should be provided with information about expected symptoms, probable recovery timeline, and coping with common problems following a brain injury. Education to families has been shown to minimize postinjury stress and optimize treatment outcomes of emerging symptoms postinjury (Cook et al., 2006).

### *Clinical Follow-Up*

Unfortunately, outcome studies reveal that the majority of children experiencing a TBI do not receive adequate follow-up. Follow-up can include neuroimaging of the brain; physical, occupational, and speech therapies;

neuropsychological consultations; and psychotherapy services (Hawley et al., 2002). When parents were surveyed about their needs when coping with a child who has sustained a TBI, most parents reported they did not understand the postdischarge care requirements necessary for their child and were confused about follow-up (Aitken, Mele, & Barrett, 2004). The parent survey performed by Aitken and colleagues suggested that telephone follow-ups, continued discharge planning, and exit interviews may provide solutions to these identified needs. It is recommended that children receive initial evaluations from physical, speech, and occupational therapists following a head injury to ensure implementation of appropriate rehabilitation services.

### *School Reentry*

Studies suggest that many schools are never notified when a child has sustained a mild TBI, even though children with TBIs demonstrate new problems with learning and exhibit behavioral and emotional symptoms at school following an injury (Ewing-Cobbs et al., 2004; Hawley et al., 2002; Hooper et al., 2004; Luis & Mittenberg, 2002). Hawley and colleagues found that only 20% of their large British survey sample received special accommodations from the school, and these usually consisted of restricted physical activity and/or excused physical education classes. In addition, their study found that even when special education needs were identified, special education services were actually provided to less than two-thirds of the sample. Further, the invisibility of brain injuries, as opposed to physical acknowledgment of a broken leg or arm, may contribute to the lack of identified need and provisions for special education services. Thus, more communication among medical personnel, key school faculty, and families of children with TBIs is recommended to ensure that adequate school services are provided. Finally, as brain injuries often have long-term effects, sometimes a gap in the information chain occurs from teacher to teacher when the child changes classrooms (Hawley et al.). Thus, it is important for school personnel to be fully informed about the nature of TBI, and schools need to develop processes and procedures to ensure information is passed on with the student (Ylvisaker et al., 2005).

### *Family Burden and Stress*

Many studies show that siblings of the injured child suffer increased emotional distress and may in some cases develop posttraumatic stress syndrome (Hawley et al., 2002). Parents may experience hardship due to time, financial, emotional, and other burdens following their child's injury (Aitken et al., 2004). It is recommended that child life specialists work with siblings of the brain-injured child to educate them and reduce emotional distress following the trauma. In addition, parents may need to participate in peer support groups and be referred to social services for help in coping with financial/insurance problems and emotional distress.

### *Activity Restriction*

Activity restriction may be necessary for all levels of TBI, even if the child experiences only a mild concussion. Animal and human studies have shown that repeated minor trauma leads to brain atrophy (i.e., deterioration/decline) and decreased neuropsychological performance (Swaine & Friedman, 2001). In addition, second impact syndrome has occurred in some athletes who obtained a second head injury before symptoms from a previous injury had resolved, which can result in death (Cook et al., 2006). No formal guidelines for children exist, but children with mild concussions with no loss of consciousness are recommended to refrain from physical activity for 1 week, and children with any loss of consciousness with symptoms of concussion (i.e., headache, nausea, vomiting, drowsiness) are recommended to be restricted for 4 weeks (Swaine & Friedman). Physicians may recommend that children with moderate to severe injuries be on physical activity restriction for 6 months or more. Lee's (2006) paper provides a comprehensive list of practical recommendations for the management of concussions in adolescents. Again, it is important to emphasize that every concussion and brain injury is different, and guidance on specific activity restrictions will need to come from the physicians working directly with the child.

### *Cognitive Services*

The frequent unmet need reported by parents of brain-injured children was for cognitive services (Slomine et al., 2006). Subtle cognitive deficits may not be detected by the child's physician, and many traditional psychoeducational measures are not sensitive to cognitive sequelae associated with TBI. Thus, it is recommended that the child's primary caregiver or school personnel request referrals for neuropsychological consultation and evaluation following a head injury.

### *Cognitive Rehabilitation*

Ylvisaker and colleagues (2001) provide a list of context-sensitive approaches to cognitive rehabilitation for children with head injuries. These included specific lists of sensitive, supportive behavioral interventions (i.e., functional behavioral analyses, lifestyle changes, controlling antecedents, interventions provided in natural settings), instructional strategies (i.e., appropriate pacing, task analysis procedures, errorless learning, teaching to mastery, ongoing assessment, flexibility in curricular modification), and biopsychosocial interventions for commonly experienced problems following a TBI. Clearly, there is a need for integrating interventions across domains of cognition, executive functions, communication abilities, self-regulation, social skills, and academic performance. In addition, increasing context sensitivity and working with children with head injuries in natural settings is strongly advised (Ylvisaker et al., 2005).

## SUMMARY

It is obvious that recovery from a pediatric TBI can be a complex, lengthy process. Cooperation and treatment integration from multiple systems and disciplines (i.e., health care providers, school personnel, families, rehabilitation therapists) is necessary in order to implement the comprehensive postinjury care that is recommended to facilitate an optimal outcome.

## RESOURCES

### Books

Crimmins, C. (2000). *Where is the mango princess?* New York: Vintage Books.

Gronwall, D., Wrightson, P., & Waddel, P. (1998). *Head injury: The facts* (2nd ed.). New York: Oxford University Press.

Schoenbrodt, L. (Ed). (2001). *Children with traumatic brain injury: A parent's guide (The special needs collection)*. Bethesda, MD: Woodbine House.

Senelick, R. C., & Dougherty, K. (2001). *Living with brain injury: A guide for families* (2nd ed.). Albuquerque, NM: HealthSouth Press.

Sturm, C. D., Forget, T. R., Jr., & Sturm, J. L. (1998). *Head injury: Information and answers to commonly asked questions: A family's guide to coping*. St. Louis, MO: Quality Medical Publishing.

### Organizations and Web Sites

Brain Injury Association of America

This is a national organization serving and representing individuals, families, and professionals who are touched by a TBI. This group provides information, education, and support to assist the 5.3 million Americans currently living with TBI and their families.

Mailing Address: 1608 Spring Hill Road, Suite 110
Vienna, Virginia 22182
Phone Number: (800) 444-6443
Web Site: www.biausa.org

Brain Injury Society

This group is committed to empowering persons living with conditions caused by a brain injury. The organization works with clients, families, and caregivers to identify strategies and techniques to maximize the newfound potentials for a stronger recovery.

Phone Number: (718) 645-4401
Web Site: www.bisociety.org

Centre for Neuro Skills

This is a comprehensive Web site with the latest information specifically for individuals with a TBI.

Web Site: www.neuroskills.com

Head Injury Hotline

This is a nonprofit clearinghouse founded and operated by head injury survivors where visitors can get information, join a discussion group, build advocacy skills, and learn self-care skills. The site integrates resources from diverse organizations including support groups, rehabilitation, and research sites, as well as lay and professional journals and more.

Phone Number: (206) 621-8558
Web Site: www.headinjury.com

National Institute of Neurological Disorders and Stroke (NINDS)

This link provides the National Institutes of Health scientific fact sheet on TBI.

Web Site: www.ninds.nih.gov/disorders/tbi/tbi.htm

Protection and Advocacy for Persons With Traumatic Brain Injury (TBI)

This program provides assistance in accessing and/or obtaining appropriate rehabilitation therapies, assistive technology, durable medical equipment, case management, and in-home supports for individuals who have experienced a TBI and have resulting disabilities.

Web Site: www.advocacyinc.org

Traumatic Brain Injury Survival Guide

This is an online book written in practical, easy-to-understand language for survivors and families coping with a TBI.

Web Site: www.tbiguide.com

## REFERENCES

Agran, P. F., Winn, D., Anderson, C., Trent, R., & Walton-Haynes, L. (2001). Rates of pediatric and adolescent injuries by year of age [Abstract]. *Pediatrics, 108,* 752–753.

Aitken, M. E., Mele, N., & Barrett, K. W. (2004). Recovery of injured children: Parent perspectives on family needs. *Archives of Physical Medicine and Rehabilitation, 85,* 567–573.

Beebe, D. W., Krivitzky, L., Wells, C. T., Wade, S. L., Taylor, H. G., & Yeates, K. O. (2007). Brief report: Parental report of sleep behaviors following moderate or severe pediatric traumatic brain injury. *Journal of Pediatric Psychology, 32,* 845–850.

Bishop, N. B. (2006). Traumatic brain injury: A primer for primary care physicians. *Current Problems in Pediatric and Adolescent Health Care, 36,* 318–331.

Bloom, D. R., Levin, H. S., Ewing-Cobbs, L., Saunders, A. E., Song, J., Fletcher, J. M., et al. (2001). Lifetime and novel psychiatric disorders after pediatric traumatic brain injury. *Journal of the American Academy of Child and Adolescent Psychiatry, 40,* 572–579.

Brenner, L. A., Dise-Lewis, J. E., Bartles, S. K., O'Brien, S. E., Godleski, M., & Selinger, M. (2007). The long-term impact and rehabilitation of pediatric traumatic brain injury: A 50-year follow-up case study. *Journal of Head Trauma Rehabilitation, 22,* 56–64.

Catroppa, C., & Anderson, V. (2007). Recovery in memory function, and its relationship to academic success, at 24 months following pediatric TBI. *Child Neuropsychology, 13,* 240–261.

Centers for Disease Control and Prevention (CDC). (2007). *What is traumatic brain injury.* Retrieved August 24, 2007, from http://www.cdc.gov/ncipc/tbi/TBI.htm

Chiu Wong, S. B., Chapman, S. B., Cook, L. G., Anand, R., Gamino, J. F., & Devous, M. D., Sr. (2006). A SPECT study of language and brain reorganization three years after pediatric brain injury. *Progress in Brain Research, 157,* 173–185.

Chung, C. Y., Chen, C. L., Cheng, P. T., See, L. C., Tang, S. F., & Wong, A. M. (2006). Critical score of Glasgow Coma Scale for pediatric traumatic brain injury. *Pediatric Neurology, 34,* 379–387.

Cohen, M. (1997). *Children's Memory Scale.* San Antonio, TX: The Psychological Corporation.

Cook, R. S., Schweer, L., Shebesta, K. F., Hartjes, K., & Falcone, R. A., Jr. (2006). Mild traumatic brain injury in children: Just another bump on the head? *Journal of Trauma Nursing, 13,* 58–65.

Delis, D. C., Kaplan, E., & Kramer, J. H. (2001). *Delis-Kaplan Executive Function System.* San Antonio, TX: The Psychological Corporation.

Delis, D. C., Kramer, J. H., Kaplan, E., & Ober, B. A. (1994). *California Verbal Learning Test—Children's Version.* San Antonio, TX: The Psychological Corporation.

Dennis, M., Guger, S., Roncadin, C., Barnes, M., & Schachar, R. (2001). Attentional-inhibitory control and social-behavioral regulation after childhood closed head injury: Do biological, developmental, and recovery variables predict outcome? *Journal of the International Neuropsychological Society, 7,* 683–692.

Ewing-Cobbs, L., Barnes, M., Fletcher, J. M., Levin, H. S., Swank, P. R., & Song, J. (2004). Modeling of longitudinal academic achievement scores after pediatric traumatic brain injury. *Developmental Neuropsychology, 25,* 107–133.

Formisano, R., Barba, C., Buzzi, M. G., Newcomb-Fernandez, J., Menniti-Ippolito, F., Zafonte, R., et al. (2007). The impact of prophylactic treatment on post-traumatic epilepsy after severe traumatic brain injury. *Brain Injury, 21,* 499–504.

Gagnon, I., Swaine, B., Friedman, D., & Forget, R. (2004). Children show decreased dynamic balance after mild traumatic brain injury. *Archives of Physical Medicine and Rehabilitation, 85,* 444–452.

Gioia, G. A., Isquith, P. K., Guy, S. C., & Kenworthy, L. (2000). *Behavior Rating Inventory of Executive Function.* Odessa, FL: Psychological Assessment Resources.

Gordon, K. E. (2006). Pediatric minor traumatic brain injury. *Seminars in Pediatric Neurology, 13,* 243–255.

Hagen, C., Malkmus, D., & Durham, P. (1979). Levels of cognitive functioning. In Professional Staff Association of Rancho Los Amigos Hospital (Ed.), *Rehabilitation of the head injured adult.* Downey, CA: Rancho Los Amigos Hospital.

Hameed, S. M., Popkin, C. A., Cohn, S. M., & Johnson, E. W. (2004). The epidemic of pediatric traffic injuries in South Florida: A review of the problem and initial results of a prospective surveillance strategy. *American Journal of Public Health, 94,* 554–556.

Hawley, C. A., Ward, A. B., Magnay, A. R., & Long, J. (2002). Children's brain injury: A postal follow-up of 525 children from one health region in the UK. *Brain Injury, 16,* 969–985.

Hessen, E., Nestvold, K., & Sundet, K. (2006). Neuropsychological function in a group of patients 25 years after sustaining minor head injuries as children and adolescents. *Scandinavian Journal of Psychology, 47,* 245–251.

Hooper, S. R., Alexander, J., Moore, D., Sasser, H. C., Laurent, S., King, J., et al. (2004). Caregiver reports of common symptoms in children following a traumatic brain injury. *NeuroRehabilitation, 19,* 175–189.

Jankowitz, B. T., & Adelson, P. D. (2006). Pediatric traumatic brain injury: Past, present and future. *Developmental Neuroscience, 28,* 264–275.

Keenan, H. T., & Bratton, S. L. (2006). Epidemiology and outcomes of pediatric traumatic brain injury. *Developmental Neuroscience, 28,* 256–263.

Khoshyomn, S., & Tranmer, B. I. (2004). Diagnosis and management of pediatric closed head injury. *Seminars in Pediatric Surgery, 13,* 80–86.

Kirkwood, M., Janusz, J., Yeates, K. O., Taylor, H. G., Wade, S. L., Stancin, T, et al. (2000). Prevalence and correlates of depressive symptoms following traumatic brain injuries in children. *Child Neuropsychology, 6,* 195–208.

Kuhtz-Buschbeck, J. P., Stolze, H., Golge, M., & Ritz, A. (2003). Analyses of gait, reaching, and grasping in children after traumatic brain injury. *Archives of Physical Medicine and Rehabilitation, 84,* 424–430.

Lee, M. A. (2006). Adolescent concussions-management recommendations: A practical approach. *Connecticut Medicine, 70,* 377–380.

Luis, C. A., & Mittenberg, W. (2002). Mood and anxiety disorders following pediatric traumatic brain injury: A prospective study. *Journal of Clinical and Experimental Neuropsychology, 24,* 270–279.

Max, J. E., Lansing, A. E., Koele, S. L., Castillo, C. S., Bokura, H., Schachar, R., et al. (2004). Attention deficit hyperactivity disorder in children and adolescents following traumatic brain injury. *Developmental Neuropsychology, 25,* 159–177.

Max, J. E., Schachar, R. J., Levin, H. S., Ewing-Cobbs, L., Chapman, S. B., Dennis, M., et al. (2005). Predictors of attention-deficit/hyperactivity disorder within 6 months after pediatric traumatic brain injury. *Journal of the American Academy of Child and Adolescent Psychiatry, 44,* 1032–1040.

Nadler, E. P., Courcoulas, A. P., Gardner, M. J., & Ford, H. R. (2001). Driveway injuries in children: Risk factors, morbidity, and mortality. *Pediatrics, 108,* 326–328.

Reitan, R. M. (1971). Trail Making Test results for normal and brain-damaged children. *Perceptual and Motor Skills, 33,* 575–581.

Reynolds, C. R., & Kamphaus, R. W. (2004). *Behavior Assessment System for Children* (2nd ed.). Circle Pines, MN: AGS Publishing.

Schwartz, L., Taylor, H. G., Drotar, D., Yeates, K. O., Wade, S. L., & Stancin, T. (2003). Long-term behavior problems following pediatric traumatic brain injury: Prevalence, predictors, and correlates. *Journal of Pediatric Psychology, 28,* 251–263.

Slomine, B. S., Gerring, J. P., Grados, M. A., Vasa, R., Brady, K. D., Christensen, J. R., et al. (2002). Performance on measures of executive function following pediatric traumatic brain injury. *Brain Injury, 16,* 759–772.

Slomine, B. S., McCarthy, M. L., Ding, R., MacKenzie, E. J., Jaffe, K. M., Aitken, M. E., et al. (2006). Health care utilization and needs after pediatric traumatic brain injury. *Pediatrics, 117,* e663–e674.

Statler, K. D. (2006). Pediatric posttraumatic seizures: Epidemiology, putative mechanisms of epileptogenesis and promising investigational progress. *Developmental Neuroscience, 28,* 354–363.

Swaine, B. R., & Friedman, D. S. (2001). Activity restrictions as part of the discharge management for children with a traumatic head injury. *Journal of Head Trauma Rehabilitation, 16,* 292–301.

Taylor, H. G. (2004). Research on outcomes of pediatric traumatic brain injury: Current advances and future directions. *Developmental Neuropsychology, 25,* 199–225.

Taylor, H. G., Yeates, K. O., Wade, S. L., Drotar, D., Stancin, T., & Minich, N. (2002). A prospective study of short- and long-term outcomes after traumatic brain injury in children: Behavior and achievement. *Neuropsychology, 16,* 15–27.

Teasdale, G., & Jennett, B. (1974). Assessment of coma and impaired consciousness: A practical scale. *Lancet, 2,* 81–84.

Wechsler, B., Kim, H., Gallagher, P. R., DiScala, C., & Stineman, M. G. (2005). Functional status after childhood traumatic brain injury. *Journal of Trauma, 58,* 940–949.

Wechsler, D. (2003). *Wechsler Intelligence Scale for Children* (4th ed.). San Antonio, TX: The Psychological Corporation.

Wilde, E. A., Hunter, J. V., Newsome, M. R., Scheibel, R. S., Bigler, E. D., Johnson, J. L., et al. (2005). Frontal and temporal morphometric findings on MRI in children after moderate to severe traumatic brain injury. *Journal of Neurotrauma, 22,* 333–344.

Woodcock, R. W., McGrew, K. S., & Mather, N. (2001). *Woodcock-Johnson Tests of Achievement* (3rd ed.). Rolling Meadows, IL: Riverside.

Yeates, K. O., Swift, E., Taylor, H. G., Wade, S. L., Drotar, D., Stancin, T., et al. (2004). Short- and long-term social outcomes following pediatric traumatic brain injury. *Journal of the International Neuropsychological Society, 10,* 412–426.

Yeates, K. O., Taylor, H. G., Wade, S. L., Drotar, D., Stancin, T., & Minich, N. (2002). A prospective study of short- and long-term neuropsychological outcomes after traumatic brain injury in children. *Neuropsychology, 16,* 514–523.

Ylvisaker, M., Adelson, P. D., Braga, L. W., Burnett, S. M., Glang, A., Feeney, T., et al. (2005). Rehabilitation and ongoing support after pediatric TBI: Twenty years of progress. *Journal of Head Trauma and Rehabilitation, 20,* 95–109.

Ylvisaker, M., & Feeney, T. (2007). Pediatric brain injury: Social, behavioral, and communication disability. *Physical Medicine and Rehabilitation Clinics of North America, 18,* 133–144.

Ylvisaker, M., Todis, B., Glang, A., Urbanczyk, B., Franklin, C., DePompei, R., et al. (2001). Educating students with TBI: Themes and recommendations. *Journal of Head Trauma and Rehabilitation, 16,* 76–93.

# Index